Register Now for Online Access to Your Book!

SPRINGER PUBLISHING
CONNECT™

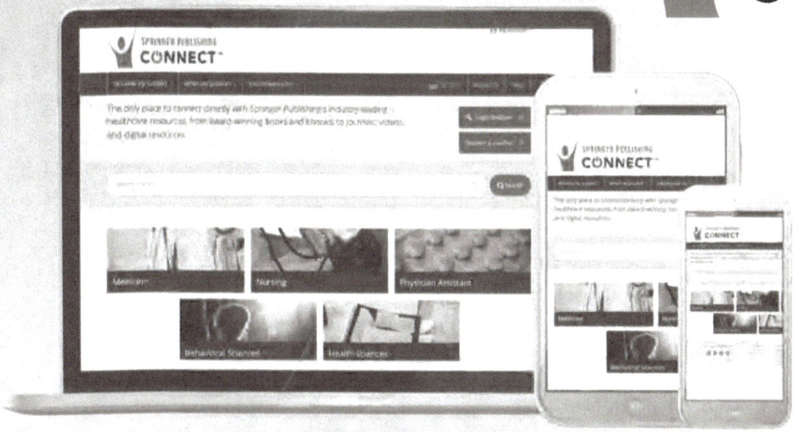

Your print purchase of *Public Health Emergencies: Case Studies, Competencies, and Essential Services of Public Health* **includes online access to the contents of your book**—increasing accessibility, portability, and searchability!

Access today at:
http://connect.springerpub.com/content/book/978-0-8261-4903-9
or scan the QR code at the right with your smartphone. Log in or register, then click "Redeem a voucher" and use the code below.

B6FBA41C

Scan here for quick access.

Having trouble redeeming a voucher code?
Go to https://connect.springerpub.com/redeeming-voucher-code

If you are experiencing problems accessing the digital component of this product, please contact our customer service department at cs@springerpub.com

The online access with your print purchase is available at the publisher's discretion and may be removed at any time without notice.

Publisher's Note: New and used products purchased from third-party sellers are not guaranteed for quality, authenticity, or access to any included digital components.

SPRINGER PUBLISHING
View all our products at springerpub.com

PUBLIC HEALTH EMERGENCIES

Tanya Telfair LeBlanc, PhD, MS (formerly Tanya Telfair Sharpe) is senior health scientist with the Centers for Disease Control and Prevention (CDC). Her career began there as a disease detective, an Epidemic Intelligence Service (EIS 2000) officer working with core and behavioral surveillance systems. Dr. LeBlanc was deployed in one of the anthrax outbreak investigations post–September 11, 2001, and received a number of awards for service during national emergencies. For 8.5 years, she served as senior health scientist/deputy director with the Office of Health Equity in CDC's National Center for HIV/AIDS, Viral Hepatitis, STDs, and TB Prevention, where she co-led an agency-wide initiative to address social determinants of health in disease prevention. She also served as a science team lead in national public health emergency preparedness, leading efforts to advance the science and evidence-based practice of public health emergency preparedness. She conceptualized and was a co-guest editor of three supplements to the *American Journal of Public Health* on topics including the evolution of public health emergency management, medical countermeasures, and community preparedness. She developed and taught a college course—HSEM Medical Management in Mass Emergencies—at Clayton State University. In 2020, she was deployed for 5 months on the State, Tribal, Local and Territorial COVID-19 Task Force as deputy and associate director for science.

Dr. LeBlanc is the author of numerous public health publications, including *Behind the Eight Ball: Sex for Crack Cocaine Exchange and Poor Black Women* (as Sharpe, for Taylor & Francis, 2005), a monograph used in college courses, described as a seminal work in the field. She is an associate editor with the *American Journal of Public Health* and writes children's books under the name T. T. Telfair. Currently, she serves as senior health scientist/epidemiologist for the National Center for Environmental Health, working to reduce lead exposure among children and advance environmental justice. Dr. LeBlanc earned degrees in anthropology and communications at Florida State University and sociology from Georgia State University, where she received a National Research Service Award from the National Institutes of Health. Other experiences include traditional and online university teaching and world travel.

Dr. LeBlanc co-edited this book in her personal capacity. The views expressed are her own and do not represent the views of the Centers for Disease Control and Prevention, the Department of Health and Human Services, or the U.S. government.

Robert J. Kim-Farley, MD, MPH is a professor-in-residence at the University of California, Los Angeles (UCLA) Fielding School of Public Health. He previously served in senior positions in the LA County Department of Public Health (LAC DPH), the Centers for Disease Control and Prevention (CDC), and the World Health Organization (WHO). Dr. Kim-Farley has extensive experience with public health emergencies. He developed, in collaboration with others, the LAC DPH Smallpox Preparedness, Response, and Recovery Plan, setting priorities in communication, coordination, and planning of bioterrorism response activities. He coordinated the development of a Phase 1 Smallpox Vaccination Plan for LA County, facilitated enhancements of the 24/7 reporting system and the health alert network system, and coordinated the development of the Strategic National Stockpile Plan for LA County. As director of communicable disease control and prevention, he coordinated LAC DPH's public health disease control efforts for emerging infectious diseases (e.g., pandemic influenza, Zika, Ebola, and West Nile virus diseases) with the Emergency Medical Services (EMS) Agency and outside hospitals and agencies, as well as integrated bioterrorism preparedness program activities across public health units. At UCLA, he developed and taught a course on Preparing for a Smallpox or Other Bioterrorist Event and lectured in the course on Terrorism, Counter-terrorism and Weapons of Mass Destruction. As associate editor of the *American Journal of Public Health* he has served as the responsible associate editor for three special Preparedness Supplements and written editorials on "Public Health Disasters," "Medical Countermeasures," and "Community Preparedness." Dr. Kim-Farley received special recognition by the regional director, South-East Asia Regional Office, WHO, for extraordinary dedication and valuable support during the emergency response and rehabilitation stages consequent to the earthquake in the State of Gujarat, India. He also received a Department of State Speaker and Specialist grant for lecturing and consulting on avian influenza and pandemic influenza in Ukraine. Dr. Kim-Farley holds degrees in electronic engineering, public health, and medicine from the University of California and is the author of numerous articles and publications in the field of public health.

Dr. Kim-Farley co-edited this book and wrote the chapters authored by him in his personal capacity. The views expressed are his own and do not represent the views of the University of California, Los Angeles.

PUBLIC HEALTH EMERGENCIES

Case Studies, Competencies, and Essential Services of Public Health

Editors

Tanya Telfair LeBlanc, PhD, MS

Robert J. Kim-Farley, MD, MPH

SPRINGER PUBLISHING

Springer Publishing Company, LLC
11 West 42nd Street, New York, NY 10036
www.springerpub.com
connect.springerpub.com/

Acquisitions Editor: David D'Addona
Compositor: Exeter Premedia Services Private Ltd.

ISBN: 978-0-8261-4902-2
ebook ISBN: 978-0-8261-4903-9
DOI: 10.1891/9780826149039

SUPPLEMENTS:
Instructor materials:

SPRINGER PUBLISHING CONNECT™

A robust set of instructor resources designed to supplement this text is located at **http://connect.springerpub.com/content/book/978-0-8261-4903-9.** Qualifying instructors may request access by emailing **textbook@springerpub.com.**

Instructor's Manual: 978-0-8261-4901-4
Instructor's PowerPoint Slides: 978-0-8261-4904-9
Instructor's Test Bank: 978-0-8261-4907-3 (Also available on Respondus®.)

21 22 23 24 / 5 4 3 2 1

Library of Congress Control Number: 2021948856

Printed in the United States of America.

Dedicated to the courageous public health professionals, healthcare personnel, and frontline workers who have tirelessly and sacrificially worked to combat the pandemic of COVID-19 at local, state, national, and international levels to save lives, alleviate suffering, and prevent disability.

Dedicated with love to my daughter . . . Lois J. Sharpe, Summa Cum Laude and Phi Beta Kappa graduate of Agnes Scott College and currently a third-year medical student at the Morehouse School of Medicine. You are truly my inspiration!
—Tanya Telfair LeBlanc, PhD, MS

Dedicated to my wife, Han Ju, for her always kind support and encouragement for my coediting of this book amid the pandemic of COVID-19. What a bounty!
—Robert Kim-Farley, MD, MPH

CONTENTS

CONTRIBUTORS

Howard D. Backer, MD, MPH, Chief Medical Officer, California Medical Assistance Team Program, California Emergency Medical Services Authority, Piedmont, California

Sharon Balter, MD, Director, Division of Communicable Disease Control and Prevention, Acute Communicable Disease Control Program, Department of Public Health, County of Los Angeles, Los Angeles, California

June E. Bancroft, MPH, CIC, Senior Epidemiology and Laboratory Capacity Epidemiologist, Acute and Communicable Disease Prevention, Oregon Public Health Division, Portland, Oregon

Nancy T. Blake, PhD, RN, CCRN-K, NHDP-BC, NEA-BC, FAAN, Chief Nursing Officer, Harbor-UCLA Medical Center, Carson, California; Assistant Adjunct Professor, UCLA School of Nursing, Los Angeles, California

Alexander H. Chang, MD Candidate, Lewis Katz School of Medicine, Temple University, Philadelphia, Pennsylvania

Allison P. Chen, Research Associate, Department of Biology, Johns Hopkins University, Baltimore, Maryland

Zhirui Chen, MSW, PhD Student, School of Social Work, University of Texas at Arlington, Arlington, Texas

Esther D. Chernak, MD, MPH, Associate Clinical Professor, Drexel University Dornsife School of Public Health and Drexel University College of Medicine, Philadelphia, Pennsylvania

Zhen Cong, PhD, Associate Professor, School of Social Work, University of Texas at Arlington, Arlington, Texas

Lauren T. Dunning, JD, MPH, Director, Center for the Future of Aging, Milken Institute, Santa Monica, California

***Denise M. Gaughan, ScD,** Epidemiologist, National Center for Environmental Health, Centers for Disease Control and Prevention, Atlanta, Georgia

---

* Authors serving in their personal capacity and not representing the Centers for Disease Control and Prevention, the Department of Health and Human Services, or the U.S. government.

Catherine J. Goodhue, MN, CPNP, Pediatric Nurse Practitioner, Division of Pediatric Surgery/Trauma Program, Children's Hospital Los Angeles, Los Angeles, California

Aaron Hagedorn, PhD, Assistant Dean for Research and Faculty Affairs, School of Social Work, University of Texas at Arlington, Arlington, Texas

James G. Hodge, Jr., JD, LLM, Peter Kiewit Foundation Professor of Law; Director, Center for Public Health Law and Policy; Director, Western Region Office–Network for Public Health Law, Sandra Day O'Connor College of Law, Arizona State University, Phoenix, Arizona

Mark D. Hoover, PhD, Guest Researcher, Respiratory Health Division, National Institute for Occupational Safety and Health, Morgantown, West Virginia

Edbert B. Hsu, MD, MPH, Associate Professor, Department of Emergency Medicine, Johns Hopkins University, Baltimore, Maryland

Maryam Karimi, MPA, PhD, Assistant Professor, Department of Environmental Health Science, School of Public Health, The University of Alabama at Birmingham, Birmingham, Alabama

Moon Kim, MD, MPH, Medical Epidemiologist, Acute Communicable Disease Control Program, Department of Public Health, County of Los Angeles, Los Angeles, California

Robert J. Kim-Farley, MD, MPH, Professor-in-Residence, Departments of Epidemiology and Community Health Sciences, Fielding School of Public Health, University of California, Los Angeles

Christopher A. Kirby, District Fire Management Officer, Forest Service, U.S. Department of Agriculture, Tijeras, New Mexico

***Tanya Telfair LeBlanc, PhD, MS,** Senior Health Scientist, Centers for Disease Control and Prevention, Atlanta, Georgia

Stephen S. Leonard, PhD, Research Biologist, Health Effects Laboratory Division, National Institute for Occupational Safety and Health, Morgantown, West Virginia

Robert M. Levin, MD, Health Officer, Ventura County Public Health, Ventura, California

Ann Levy, MS, Senior Environmental Program Manager, Water Quality Division, Portland Water Bureau, Portland, Oregon

Glen P. Mays, PhD, MPH, Professor and Chair, Department of Health Systems, Management and Policy, Colorado School of Public Health, University of Colorado, Aurora, Colorado

Rouzbeh Nazari, PhD, Associate Professor, Department of Civil, Construction, and Environmental Engineering, School of Engineering, The University of Alabama at Birmingham, Birmingham, Alabama

***John Person, MPH,** Epidemiologist, Waterborne Disease Prevention Branch, Division of Foodborne, Waterborne, and Environmental Disease, Centers for Disease Control and Prevention, Atlanta, Georgia

Jennifer L. Piatt, JD, Research Scholar, Center for Public Health Law and Policy; Senior Attorney, Western Region Office—Network for Public Health Law, Sandra Day O'Connor College of Law, Arizona State University, Phoenix, Arizona

Taylor S. Pinsent, MPH, Senior Communicable Disease Epidemiologist, Multnomah County Public Health, Portland, Oregon

***David S. Rickless, MS,** GIS Analyst, Geospatial Research, Analysis, and Services Program, Centers for Disease Control and Prevention/Agency for Toxic Substances and Disease Registry, Atlanta, Georgia

Samain Sabrin, MS, Graduate Research Assistant, Department of Civil, Construction, and Environmental Engineering, School of Engineering, The University of Alabama at Birmingham, Birmingham, Alabama

***J. Danielle Sharpe, PhD, MS,** Geospatial Epidemiologist, Coordinator of the Centers for Disease Control and Prevention Social Vulnerability Index, Geospatial Research, Analysis, and Services Program, Centers for Disease Control and Prevention/Agency for Toxic Substances and Disease Registry, Atlanta, Georgia

Kimberley Shoaf, DrPH, Professor, Division of Public Health, University of Utah, Salt Lake City, Utah

Dawn Terashita, MD, MPH, Associate Director, Acute Communicable Disease Control Program, Department of Public Health, County of Los Angeles, Los Angeles, California

***Jonathan S. Yoder, MPH,** Lead, Water, Sanitation, and Hygiene (WASH) Team, COVID-19 Response, Centers for Disease Control and Prevention, Atlanta, Georgia

PREFACE

THE ROAD TO *PUBLIC HEALTH EMERGENCIES: CASE STUDIES, COMPETENCIES, AND ESSENTIAL SERVICES OF PUBLIC HEALTH*

The road to the development of this textbook was long and arduous. In the late 1990s, as a National Institutes of Health–National Research Service Award recipient at Georgia State University, I had the opportunity to conduct a social epidemiology and ethnography study of inner-city Black women who were addicted to crack cocaine to ascertain three outcomes: exposure to HIV, contracting sexually transmitted diseases, and unplanned pregnancies in the context of crack cocaine use. This was a life-altering research experience from which I gained critical knowledge regarding the dynamic social and economic structures that shape people's lives, and ultimately influence health outcomes and access to care. The findings of this research were published in 2005 in a monograph titled *Behind the Eight Ball: Sex for Crack Cocaine Exchange and Poor Black Women* (Taylor & Francis). The work made a lasting impression and helped me understand that vulnerable populations are everywhere in the country, hidden in plain sight and largely overlooked by the mainstream of society.

As an epidemic intelligence service officer with the Centers for Disease Control and Prevention, I was part of a large team deployed to investigate a fatal case of anthrax exposure in 2001 in New York City. At the time, the suspected cause was contaminated mail. However, in contrast to other cases of inhalation anthrax that occurred in Washington, DC, which were linked to contaminated mail, no connections to contaminated mail could be established for the unfortunate hospital worker who succumbed to the disease. The team also investigated side effects of medicines provided to thousands of postal workers for postexposure prophylaxis, out of precaution and concern for the welfare of those employees. From that point, I understood the importance of public health emergency preparedness activities for the safety and well-being of our nation's people. I also gained insight on the sheer vastness and complexity of the task. There were no easy answers to public health problems, and during that particular emergency on the heels of the 9/11 attacks on the World Trade Center and Pentagon, I observed how the new direction for responses, based on deliberate terrorist threats, took shape.

In another opportunity to serve the public's health, I visited the Rosebud Sioux Indian Reservation in South Dakota. Here, I was exposed to the remoteness of the area, and the dearth of basic necessities that I enjoyed, grocery stores and pharmacies, for example. The amazing and gracious tribal leadership explained the realities of being a sovereign nation within a sovereign nation and how during emergency situations, sometimes no state or local responders were available to serve the reservation, due to unclear chains of command and responsibilities. That information stayed with me.

In subsequent years serving as a science team lead in public health preparedness in a major public health agency, I began to understand the disconnect between policy and practice and the challenges in determining which practices were effective. I worked collaboratively with my team to investigate evidence-based preparedness protocols in communities that could be shared broadly as best practices. In addition, I sought to understand the impact of emergencies on routine medical screenings among high-risk populations (e.g., interruption of HIV testing during Hurricane Sandy), to probe the ecological fear factor and decline in emergency department visits associated with an Ebola fatality in Texas, to explore patterns of hospital medical surges after hurricanes using syndromic surveillance data, to evaluate laboratory capacity for response to outbreaks, and to investigate what it takes to build resilience in communities. I had the opportunity to conceptualize and serve as lead coeditor of three supplements to the *American Journal of Public Health* on the evolution of public health management, medical countermeasures, and community preparedness. Over the years, I have mentored countless junior and young public health scientists, in various internship, fellowship, and other programs.

Thus, the work in this textbook is undergirded by my passions in public health: (a) inclusive national preparedness, (b) addressing social determinants of health and advancing health equity, and (c) education and mentoring of new public health scientists.

When Springer editor Mr. David D'Addona contacted me about considering a textbook project on public health emergency preparedness, in our initial conversation we came to a meeting of the minds for pursuing a practical approach to the content. Having the experience of teaching in brick-and-mortar, as well as online, university settings for more than a decade, I firmly understood the missing element in most college-level textbooks. Many of the books available today present information on public health activities but lack specifics on how to apply the skills in the real world. In our long conversation, I concluded that the textbook should answer the question, "What do students in schools of public health need to know to occupy specific roles in preparedness careers?" Using the Essential Public Health Services and the master's degree of Public Health Competencies as road maps for identification of required skills, we developed a strategy to gather case studies from experts in the field and link specific response activities to skills and competencies at multiple career levels. In addition, sitting in a coffee shop, we outlined three major book sections: foundational, case studies, and additional information. As time went on and we began to flesh out the potential book content, I understood that this project would need the support of more than one editor. I invited my colleague, Dr. Robert Kim-Farley, to co-edit with me, as I was impressed with his experiences in university teaching and in public health emergency response work at the state, national, and international levels. Moreover, we had worked collegially together on producing three supplements to the *American Journal of Public Health* on preparedness where he was the responsible associate editor, as well as our both serving as associate editors with the journal.

The product presented herein is the result of 4 years of research, collaboration, and dedication. In this first edition, we hope that students in schools of public health and other universities will be able to understand preparedness in the context of public health, will be able to see themselves in the case studies, will comprehend the concepts presented as representative of real-world activities, and will be able to chart a clearer course ahead for their future careers. In our own futures, we hope to continue the process of learning about public health emergency preparedness, and as we learn more, we will share more.

Tanya Telfair LeBlanc, PhD, MS

SPRINGER PUBLISHING CONNECT™

A robust set of instructor resources designed to supplement this text is located at **http://connect.springerpub.com/content/book/978-0-8261-4903-9.** Qualifying instructors may request access by emailing **textbook@springerpub.com.**

ACKNOWLEDGMENTS

The coeditors gratefully acknowledge the chapter authors who, during the greatest public health infectious disease challenge in over 100 years, generously offered their time and intellectual acumen to write about the challenges and approaches to public health emergencies they have faced—and are currently facing—in their distinguished careers as an act of generativity to the next generation of public health professionals.

The coeditors are profoundly appreciative of David D'Addona, Senior Editor, and Jaclyn Shultz, Associate Editor, of Springer Publishing Company for their brilliant ideas, incredible advice based on years of experience, patience, and tireless backing of the work of the coeditors and chapter authors to bring this book from conception to reality.

INTRODUCTION

ESSENTIAL PUBLIC HEALTH SERVICES AND FOUNDATIONAL COMPETENCIES FOR PUBLIC HEALTH EMERGENCIES

This textbook provides a unique case study approach to public health emergencies through the combined perspectives of both the 2020 10 Essential Public Health Services and the 2021 Master of Public Health (MPH) Foundational Competencies.

The focus of this introductory chapter is on how both students and public health practitioners can use the textbook to develop and strengthen their practical knowledge and skills in addressing the complex task of preparing for, mitigating, responding to, and recovering from a variety of public health emergencies ranging from natural to man-made disasters. It also includes recognizing the commonalities, such as epidemiologic surveillance and the incident command system (ICS) structure, in preparing and responding across all types of public health emergencies.

First, the purposes of the three parts of the book, namely, (1) Fundamentals of Public Health Emergency Preparedness, (2) Lessons Learned From Actual Incidents, and (3) Special Considerations are outlined to orient the reader toward the content structure. After that, the details of the 2020 10 Essential Public Health Services and the 2021 MPH Foundational Competencies are provided, which serve as the framework for the reader in approaching the case studies to glean the lessons learned from the actual planning for, or responding to, public health emergencies. It also details the levels at which the emergency preparedness and response actions are actually performed (e.g., frontline staff, managerial, and/or executive leadership). Finally, the book's learning objectives are summarized to provide a clear path for the reader to maximize their learning, knowledge, and skills developed through both study of the book as well as through deliberations on the discussion questions at the end of each case study chapter.

An important feature of the book is that both the coeditors and the chapter authors are all public health professionals who have spent significant portions, if not all, of their public health careers in the field of public health emergency preparedness and response, tackling many of the significant types of disasters that have challenged the public health system in both this nation and globally. This book is not a theoretical exploration of public health emergencies—it is rather the distillation of practical advice and experience from the hard-learned lessons forged from the actual trials these public health professionals have faced and who are now eager to pass along the wisdom they have gained to the next generation.

PURPOSES OF THE THREE PARTS OF THE BOOK

For the ease of the reader to approach learning about the roles that they may be called upon to play in addressing public health emergencies, this book is logically arranged into three major parts.

In the first part, "Fundamentals of Public Health Emergency Preparedness," the reader gains an overall perspective of public health emergencies. Specifically, the introduction and some important historical examples of public health emergencies provide insights into the scope and magnitude of impact that such emergencies present in our communities and society. The chapters on *what is emergency preparedness* and *community preparedness: a challenge for the ages* provide insights into the terms and aims of public health emergency preparedness and is consistent with the goal of this book to prepare the reader to assume responsibilities in preparing and responding to disasters. A framework for an "all-hazards" design and approach to public health emergencies helps to show the commonalities behind planning and responses to all forms of disasters yet recognizes the unique aspects of each type of disaster that need to be addressed in distinctive ways. The chapter on disaster risk assessment helps the reader learn how to be proactive in planning for possible public health emergencies and to prioritize the use of limited resources to prepare for disasters given their likelihood of occurrence and magnitude of impact as measured by morbidity, mortality, the impact on the economy and infrastructure, and societal disruption. Finally, the methodology of developing and executing emergency operation plans is shown to be a critical aspect of an effective and efficient response to public health emergencies, especially within the context of an ICS stood up to address specific emergencies.

The second part, "Lessons Learned From Actual Incidents," is the "heart" of the book in the sense that it provides case studies that clearly demonstrate the application of the Essential Public Health Services using Foundational Competencies through activities undertaken by public health workers at different levels, namely, frontline staff, program managers and supervisors, and executive directors and leaders. By the articulation of specific activities to address disasters using the competencies needed to prepare and respond to actual public health emergencies in the case studies, the reader can gain knowledge and insights and then incorporate the lessons learned into their own learning. In the future, when they are working in public health settings and confronted with public health disasters, readers will be able to better respond knowing the vocabulary, ICS, and approaches best suited to the public health emergency as learned in this book.

In the third part of the book, "Special Considerations," the reader is provided with some of the crosscutting issues confronting public health workers in disaster settings. Public health law, for example, serves as the basis for public health action and supports public health officers in issuing health officer orders for quarantine, isolation, travel restrictions, curtailment or limitation of business and restaurant operations, and vaccination prioritization—all of which have been used in the COVID-19 pandemic. Vulnerable populations and the special considerations that need to be taken into account to address their unique needs, across many disaster scenarios, are covered in the chapter on preparedness for persons with access and functional needs as well as the chapter on children in disasters. Finally, the chapters on *evolving and emerging threats* and *going forward: other emergencies and future challenges* look to issues and threat scenarios that the readers of today may be facing in their public health emergency preparedness and response work roles in the future.

THE 2020 10 ESSENTIAL PUBLIC HEALTH SERVICES

The first of the two components of the framework for the reader in approaching the case studies and to utilize in their current or future roles in planning and responding to public health emergencies is the 2020 10 Essential Public Health Services (EPHS).

Originally developed in 1994 by a federal working group, the 10 EPHS were recently revised on September 9, 2020, as part of *The Futures Initiative: The 10 Essential Public Health Services*, the de Beaumont Foundation, Public Health National Center for Innovations, and a Task Force of public health experts. This revision "now centers equity and incorporates current and future public health practice" (The Public Health National Center for Innovations, 2021a).

A graphic providing a diagram of the 10 EPHS and their interrelationships with the three core functions of public health (Assessment, Policy Development, Assurance), together with a brief description of each service, is found in Figure I.1.

Specifically, the EPHS Framework incorporates the following elements within each essential service, many of which are applied in planning and responding to public health emergencies and are illustrated in the case studies throughout this book (The Public Health National Center for Innovations, 2021b).

CORE FUNCTION 1—ASSESSMENT: The first two EPHS fall under the Core Function of Assessment—the collecting and analyzing information about health problems and hazards affecting the population.

EPHS #1: Assess and monitor population health status, factors that influence health, and community needs and assets.

- Maintaining an ongoing understanding of health in the jurisdiction by collecting, monitoring, and analyzing data on health and factors that influence health to identify threats, patterns, and emerging issues, with a particular emphasis on disproportionately affected populations

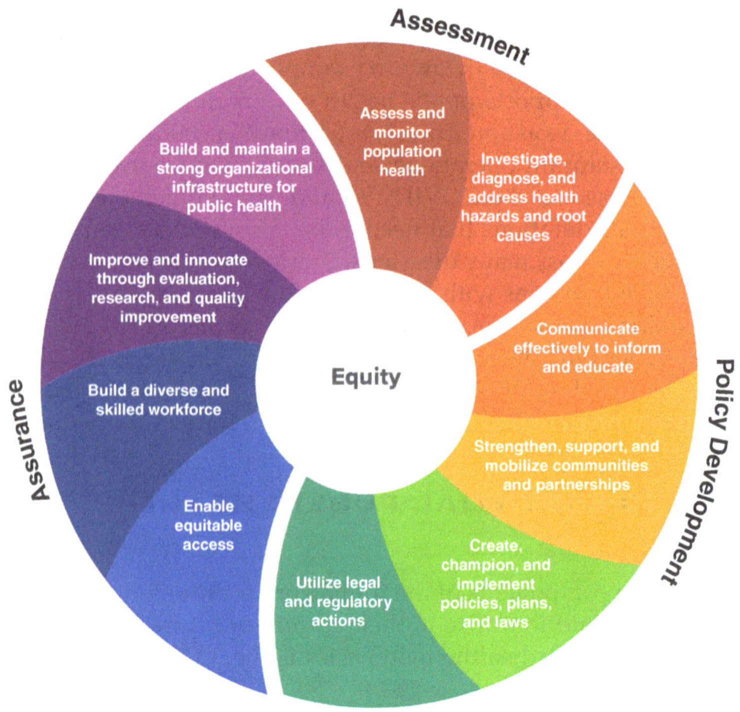

Figure I.1 The 10 Essential Public Health Services.

Source: https://phnci.org/uploads/resource-files/Alignment-between-the-10-Essential-Public-Health-Services-and-the-Core-Competencies-for-Public-Health-Professionals.pdf

- Using data and information to determine the root causes of health disparities and inequities
- Working with the community to understand health status, needs, assets, key influences, and narrative
- Collaborating and facilitating data sharing with partners, including multisector partners
- Using innovative technologies, data collection methods, and data sets
- Utilizing various methods and technology to interpret and communicate data to diverse audiences
- Analyzing and using disaggregated data (e.g., by race) to track issues and inform equitable action
- Engaging community members as experts and key partners

EPHS #2: Investigate, diagnose, and address health problems and hazards affecting the population.

- Anticipating, preventing, and mitigating emerging health threats through epidemiologic identification
- Monitoring real-time health status and identifying patterns to develop strategies to address chronic diseases and injuries
- Using real-time data to identify and respond to acute outbreaks, emergencies, and other health hazards

- Using public health laboratory capabilities and modern technology to conduct rapid screening and high-volume testing
- Analyzing and utilizing inputs from multiple sectors and sources to consider social, economic, and environmental root causes of health status
- Identifying, analyzing, and distributing information from new, big, and real-time data sources

CORE FUNCTION 2—POLICY DEVELOPMENT: The next four EPHS fall under the Core Function of Policy Development—the collaboration and consultations with communities and other stakeholders to be able to identify and develop policies, plans, and laws that impact and improve health and to effectively communicate with the public.

EPHS #3: Communicate effectively to inform and educate people about health, factors that influence it, and how to improve it.

- Developing and disseminating accessible health information and resources, including through collaboration with multisector partners
- Communicating with accuracy and necessary speed
- Using appropriate communication channels (e.g., social media, peer-to-peer networks, mass media, and other channels) to effectively reach the intended populations
- Developing and deploying culturally and linguistically appropriate and relevant communications and educational resources, which includes working with stakeholders and influencers in the community to create effective and culturally resonant materials
- Employing the principles of risk communication, health literacy, and health education to inform the public, when appropriate
- Actively engaging in two-way communication to build trust with populations served and ensure accuracy and effectiveness of prevention and health promotion strategies
- Ensuring public health communications and education efforts are asset-based when appropriate and do not reinforce narratives that are damaging to disproportionately affected populations

EPHS #4: Strengthen, support, and mobilize communities and partnerships to improve health.

- Convening and facilitating multisector partnerships and coalitions that include sectors that influence health (e.g., planning, transportation, housing, education, etc.)
- Fostering and building genuine, strengths-based relationships with a diverse group of partners that reflect the community and the population
- Authentically engaging with community members and organizations to develop public health solutions
- Learning from, and supporting, existing community partnerships and contributing public health expertise

EPHS #5: Create, champion, and implement policies, plans, and laws that impact health.

- Developing and championing policies, plans, and laws that guide the practice of public health
- Examining and improving existing policies, plans, and laws to correct historical injustices
- Ensuring that policies, plans, and laws provide a fair and just opportunity for all to achieve optimal health
- Providing input into policies, plans, and laws to ensure that health impact is considered
- Continuously monitoring and developing policies, plans, and laws that improve public health and preparedness and strengthen community resilience
- Collaborating with all partners, including multisector partners, to develop and support policies, plans, and laws
- Working across partners and with the community to systematically and continuously develop and implement health improvement strategies and plans, and evaluate and improve those plans

EPHS #6: Utilize legal and regulatory actions designed to improve and protect the public's health.

- Ensuring that applicable laws are equitably applied to protect the public's health
- Conducting enforcement activities that may include, but are not limited to, sanitary codes, especially in the food industry; full protection of drinking water supplies; and timely follow-up on hazards, preventable injuries, and exposure-related diseases identified in occupational and community settings
- Licensing and monitoring the quality of healthcare services (e.g., laboratory, nursing homes, and home healthcare)
- Reviewing new drug, biologic, and medical device applications
- Licensing and credentialing the healthcare workforce
- Including health considerations in laws from other sectors (e.g., zoning)

CORE FUNCTION 3—ASSURANCE: The final four EPHS fall under the core function of Assurance—to ensure that public health legal, regulatory, and programmatic actions and authority are utilized to protect and continually improve the population's health through effective and equitable systems provided by a skilled public health workforce, strong organizational infrastructure, and collaboration with public health's partners to reach agreed upon goals.

EPHS #7: Assure an effective system that enables equitable access to the individual services and care needed to be healthy.

- Connecting the population to needed health and social services that support the whole person, including preventive services

- Ensuring access to high-quality and cost-effective healthcare and social services, including behavioral and mental health services, that are culturally and linguistically appropriate
- Engaging health delivery systems to assess and address gaps and barriers in accessing needed health services, including behavioral and mental health
- Addressing and removing barriers to care
- Building relationships with payers and healthcare providers, including the sharing of data across partners to foster health and well-being
- Contributing to the development of a competent healthcare workforce

EPHS #8: Build and support a diverse and skilled public health workforce.

- Providing education and training that encompasses a spectrum of public health competencies, including technical, strategic, and leadership skills
- Ensuring that the public health workforce is the appropriate size to meet the public's needs
- Building a culturally competent public health workforce and leadership that reflects the community and practices cultural humility
- Incorporating public health principles in non–public health curricula
- Cultivating and building active partnerships with academia and other professional training programs and schools to assure community-relevant learning experiences for all learners
- Promoting a culture of lifelong learning in public health
- Building a pipeline of future public health practitioners
- Fostering leadership skills at all levels

EPHS #9: Improve and innovate public health functions through ongoing evaluation, research, and continuous quality improvement.

- Building and fostering a culture of quality in public health organizations and activities
- Linking public health research with public health practice
- Using research, evidence, practice-based insights, and other forms of information to inform decision-making
- Contributing to the evidence base of effective public health practice
- Evaluating services, policies, plans, and laws continuously to ensure they are contributing to health and not creating undue harm
- Establishing and using engagement and decision-making structures to work with the community in all stages of research
- Valuing and using qualitative, quantitative, and lived experience as data and information to inform decision-making

EPHS #10: Build and maintain a strong organizational infrastructure for public health.

- Developing an understanding of the broader organizational infrastructures and roles that support the entire public health system in a jurisdiction (e.g., government agencies, elected officials, and nongovernmental organizations)
- Ensuring that appropriate, needed resources are allocated equitably for the public's health
- Exhibiting effective and ethical leadership, decision-making, and governance
- Managing financial and human resources effectively
- Employing communications and strategic planning capacities and skills
- Having robust information technology services that are current and meet privacy and security standards
- Being accountable, transparent, and inclusive with all partners and the community in all aspects of practice

The central importance of these EPHS for public health practitioners and public health departments is manifested by their being used by the Public Health Accreditation Board, which accredits public health departments, as the basis for their Standards and Measures used for the accreditation process.

The EPHS encompass the totality of the services of public health departments, not only those services related to preparing and responding to public health emergencies. However, because of the complexity of public health emergencies, many if not all these services are often brought to bear in disaster settings depending upon the type and scope of a particular public health emergency. This book highlights and often uses "callouts," as well as tables at the end of each case study chapter, to illustrate and identify the specific EPHS being used when responding to a particular disaster in each of the case studies.

As part of the learning process, the reader learns to use the 10 EPHS components of this book's framework to clearly understand how the case study examples utilize EPHS in disaster settings and recognizes that they are specific applications of the EPHS that are used broadly across all the services delivered by public health.

THE 2021 MPH FOUNDATIONAL COMPETENCIES

The second of the two components of the framework for the reader in approaching and learning from the case studies, as well as to utilize in their current or future roles in planning and responding to public health emergencies, is the 2021 MPH Foundational Competencies.

It should be noted that there are other competency frameworks for public health. One specifically worth mentioning, and that the reader may wish to explore as a further source of information on competencies, is the one developed by the Council on Linkages Between Academia and Public Health Practice (Council on Linkages), which identifies a set of Core Competencies organized into eight domains reflecting skill areas within public health (Analytical/Assessment

Skills, Policy Development/Program Planning Skills, Communication Skills, Cultural Competency Skills, Community Dimensions of Practice Skills, Public Health Sciences Skills, Financial Planning and Management Skills, and Leadership and Systems Thinking Skills), and three tiers representing career stages (Tier 1—Frontline Staff/Entry Level; Tier 2—Program Management/ Supervisory Level; and Tier 3—Senior Management/Executive Level) (The Public Health National Center for Innovations, 2021b).

We have chosen to use the 22 2021 MPH Foundational Competencies developed by the Council on Education for Public Health (CEPH) and used in the CEPH accreditation, process for schools of public health and public health programs. These are ideal to serve as the basis for the understanding of the competencies used to provide the EPHS in public health emergency settings because many readers will be students in such schools and programs. We have, however, adapted the Council on Linkages approach to identifying the tiers, or levels (as noted earlier), at which the competencies are applied so that the reader will better understand the context in which the competencies would be used. The EPHS cannot be properly performed unless public health workers have the competencies to perform them.

As noted by CEPH, these competencies are informed by the traditional public health core knowledge areas (biostatistics, epidemiology, social and behavioral sciences, health services administration, and environmental health sciences) as well as crosscutting and emerging public health areas. Specifically, the MPH Foundational Competencies Framework incorporates the following elements, grouped under eight major areas, many of which are applied in planning and responding to public health emergencies and are illustrated in the case studies throughout this book (The Council on Education for Public Health, 2021). Readers wishing to further explore the use of these Foundational Competencies in settings other than public health emergencies may wish to refer to the book *Master of Public Health Competencies: A Case Study Approach* (Santella, 2020).

Evidence-Based Approaches to Public Health

1. Apply epidemiological methods to settings and situations in public health practice.
2. Select quantitative and qualitative data collection methods appropriate for a given public health context.
3. Analyze quantitative and qualitative data using biostatistics, informatics, computer-based programming and software, as appropriate.
4. Interpret results of data analysis for public health research, policy or practice.

Public Health and Healthcare Systems

5. Compare the organization, structure, and function of healthcare, public health, and regulatory systems across national and international settings.
6. Discuss the means by which structural bias, social inequities, and racism undermine health and create challenges to achieving health equity at organizational, community, and systemic levels.

Planning and Management to Promote Health

7. Assess population needs, assets, and capacities that affect communities' health.
8. Apply awareness of cultural values and practices to the design, implementation, or critique of public health policies or programs.
9. Design a population-based policy, program, project, or intervention.
10. Explain basic principles and tools of budget and resource management.
11. Select methods to evaluate public health programs.

Policy in Public Health

12. Discuss the policymaking process, including the roles of ethics and evidence.
13. Propose strategies to identify stakeholders and build coalitions and partnerships for influencing public health outcomes.
14. Advocate for political, social, or economic policies and programs that will improve health in diverse populations.
15. Evaluate policies for their impact on public health and health equity.

Leadership

16. Apply leadership and/or management principles to address a relevant issue.
17. Apply negotiation and mediation skills to address organizational or community challenges.

Communication

18. Select communication strategies for different audiences and sectors.
19. Communicate audience-appropriate (i.e., nonacademic, nonpeer audience) public health content, both in writing and through oral presentation.
20. Describe the importance of cultural competence in communicating public health content.

Interprofessional and/or Intersectoral Practice

21. Integrate perspectives from other sectors and/or professions to promote and advance population health.

Systems Thinking

22. Apply a systems thinking tool to visually represent a public health issue in a format other than a standard narrative.

As is the case with the 10 EPHS, this book highlights and often uses "call-outs," as well as tables at the end of each case study chapter, to illustrate and identify specific Foundational Competencies being used when responding to a particular disaster in each of the case studies.

LEVELS OF APPLICATION

Another lens used in this book, in addition to teaching about the 10 EPHS and the 22 Foundational Competencies, is that of the level at which the essential services and competencies are applied in the actions taken to prepare for, and respond to, public health emergencies. Adapted from the Council on Linkages, they included the following three tiers, or levels, that can also mirror the career stages that a public health worker may traverse during their public health career.

TIER/LEVEL 1—FRONTLINE STAFF/ENTRY LEVEL

Frontline staff are typically found in local public health departments since it is the responsibility of such local public health departments to directly work with individuals in the communities that they serve as well as the community-based organizations, the healthcare systems, other governmental agency partners, and community leaders within their jurisdictions. Such staff may include community health workers, epidemiology analysts, environmental sanitarians, and public health nurses. However, during public health emergencies, state- and even federal-level public health workers may be reassigned and deployed to serve as frontline staff when local human resources are overwhelmed by the magnitude and extent of the disaster at the local level. Also, in the course of a public health career, many will start out after their education in a frontline staff entry-level position.

TIER/LEVEL 2—PROGRAM MANAGEMENT/SUPERVISORY LEVEL

Program managers (e.g., directors of emergency preparedness and response programs; acute communicable disease control programs; environmental health programs; maternal, child, and adolescent health programs) may be found at local, state, and federal public health departments and agencies. Typically, they may have more advanced degrees in public health (e.g., MPH, MSPH, PhD, or DrPH) and/or greater lengths of service and experience in the field of public health. They usually supervise and/or manage groups of public health workers in programs and offices that carry out specific public health services. During public health emergencies, such managers and supervisors may be reassigned and deployed from different program areas and called on to manage specific units under an ICS structure set up to respond to a disaster in a coordinated manner.

TIER/LEVEL 3—SENIOR MANAGEMENT/EXECUTIVE LEVEL

Senior managers and executive-level staff may include job categories ranging from bureau directors (e.g., Disease Control Bureau, Health Protection Bureau, Health Promotion Bureau) to health officers and public health department directors. Typically, in addition to more advanced degrees in public health and greater lengths of service, such persons will often have had many years of higher level experience serving as program managers and supervisors. During a public health emergency, such senior managers and executive-level staff will be the decision-makers and may serve as the Incident Commander or as Section Leaders in the ICS structure. These high-level staff are the ones who provide the overall vision, lead, and oversight to the public health programs within the public health department; approve policies, strategies, and legislative proposals; and are in direct contact with the elected leaders and officials of county, state, or federal governments.

LEARNING OBJECTIVES

The learning objectives for the reader of this book are focused on identifying the EPHS needed to both address all-hazards public health emergency preparedness and response as well as those EPHS required in specific types of disasters that will require a unique mix of the application of the EPHS. Importantly, the learning objectives are also focused on the Foundational Competencies needed to carry out the EPHS used in public health emergencies. Finally, when the actions needed to prepare and respond to disasters are further framed considering the level of staff who are needed to carry out these actions, the reader will gain a fuller understanding, provided within the context of specific case studies of public health emergencies, of the tools and skills they need to learn to ultimately undertake their own roles in public health emergency preparedness and response.

Overall learning objectives for the book are as follows:

1. Understanding what constitutes a public health emergency
2. Determining what is meant by community readiness and community resilience
3. Gaining knowledge of the major agencies, organizations, and programs at local, state, and federal levels that have important roles to play in disaster settings
4. Knowing the approach to designing an all-hazards preparedness plan as well as the ancillary plans for specific hazards. This includes recognizing the commonalities, such as epidemiologic surveillance and ICS structure, that exist across all types of emergency preparedness and response activities
5. Acquiring an understanding of the approach of how to assess disaster risks
6. Understanding how to develop emergency operations plans during a disaster
7. Knowing how and when to apply public health law and legal authority to respond to a public health emergency
8. Recognizing the unique needs of vulnerable populations (e.g., persons with access and functional needs as well as children) in disaster settings
9. Knowing the 10 EPHS and the role they play in disaster situations
10. Understanding the 22 Foundational Competencies and the relation of these competencies in performing the EPHS during public health emergency preparedness and response
11. Determining the level of staff (frontline, program managers and supervisors, senior management and executives) needed to be utilized to exercise

the Foundational Competencies to perform the required EPHS during a disaster

12. Gaining a level of confidence in being able to serve in a public health disaster through an understanding of the vocabulary, structures, and functions of public health workers in disaster settings gleaned through study and application of the principles of this book

CONCLUSION

In summary, this introduction provides and details the framework for studying the 10 Essential Public Health Services, 22 Foundational Competencies, and public health staff levels needed to prepare for, and respond to, public health emergencies. The reader is now ready to explore the actual case studies presented in Part II, "Lessons Learned From Actual Incidents," to learn exactly how these services are performed in disaster settings by staff at all levels using these competencies. By consciously identifying the services and competencies, the reader will, themselves, be developing the knowledge needed to prepare and respond to public health emergencies in their current or future roles in public health agencies and organizations, including serving as active members of an ICS that stood up to respond to disasters.

Robert J. Kim-Farley, MD, MPH

REFERENCES

The Council on Education for Public Health. (2021). *Accreditation criteria: Schools of public health & public health programs.* https://media.ceph.org/documents/D2_guidance.pdf

The Public Health National Center for Innovations. (2021a). *Celebrating 25 years and launching the revised 10 Essential Public Health Services.* http://phnci.org/national-frameworks/10-ephs

The Public Health National Center for Innovations. (2021b, March). *The futures initiative: The 10 essential public health services.* https://phnci.org/uploads/resource-files/Alignment-between-the-10-Essential-Public-Health-Services-and-the-Core-Competencies-for-Public-Health-Professionals.pdf

Santella, A. J. (Ed.). (2020). *Master of public health competencies: A case study approach.* Jones & Barlett Learning.

PART I

FUNDAMENTALS OF PUBLIC HEALTH EMERGENCY PREPAREDNESS

CHAPTER 1

WHAT IS EMERGENCY PREPAREDNESS?

TANYA TELFAIR LEBLANC

KEY TERMS

Aedes Aegypti Mosquito
Bubonic Plague
CARES Act
Cold War
COVID-19
Ebola Virus Disease
Gig Worker
Guillain-Barré Syndrome
Medical Countermeasures
Metropolitan Statistical Area
Microcephaly
Mitigation
Public Health Emergency Preparedness
Sarin Gas
Social Vulnerabilities
Stafford Act
Strategic National Stockpile
World Health Organization

WHAT IS PREPAREDNESS?

What is preparedness? It depends on who you ask. Identifying a definition of preparedness is akin to the fable of the blind men and the elephants, with each defining the beast based on the particular part encountered. The Literature has multiple definitions of *preparedness*, based on specific missions of various governmental and private entities, but has fallen short in defining, in practical terms, what true preparedness actually means, writ large for the country, a state, or a community. Common definitions follow.

FEDERAL EMERGENCY MANAGEMENT AGENCY

Preparedness is defined by DHS [Department of Homeland Security]/FEMA [Federal Emergency Management Agency] as "a continuous cycle of planning, organizing, training, equipping, exercising, evaluating, and taking corrective action in an effort to ensure effective coordination during incident response" (DHS, 2012, para. 1). This cycle is one element of a broader National Preparedness System to prevent, respond to, and recover from natural disasters, acts of terrorism, and other disasters.

The Red Cross

According to the Red Cross, disaster preparedness refers to activities and measures used to prepare for and reduce the harmful effects of disasters on human populations. The main goals are to predict and, where possible, prevent disasters; mitigate their impact on vulnerable populations; and respond to and effectively cope with consequences. Disaster preparedness is complex, requiring contributions of many stakeholders and activities that range from training and logistics to healthcare, recovery, restoring access to employment, and returning to pre-disaster life conditions (International Federation of Red Cross and Red Crescent Societies, n.d.).

Centers for Disease Control and Prevention

As a component of a larger preparedness capability framework, the Centers for Disease Control and Prevention (CDC, 2019) has defined community preparedness as follows:

> Community preparedness is the ability of communities to prepare for, withstand, and recover from public health incidents in both the short and long term. Through engagement and coordination with a cross-section of state, local, tribal, and territorial partners and stakeholders, the public health role in community preparedness is to
>
> - Support the development of public health, health care, human services, mental/behavioral health, and environmental health systems that support community preparedness
> - Participate in awareness training on how to prevent, respond to, and recover from incidents that adversely affect public health
> - Identify at-risk individuals with access and functional needs that may be disproportionately impacted by an incident or event
> - Promote awareness of and access to public health, health care, human services, mental/behavioral health, and environmental health resources that help protect the community's health and address the access and functional needs of at-risk individuals
> - Engage in preparedness activities that address the access and functional needs of the whole community as well as cultural, socioeconomic, and demographic factors
> - Convene or participate with community partners to identify and implement additional ways to strengthen community resilience
> - Plan to address the health needs of populations that have been displaced because of incidents that have occurred in their own or distant communities, such as after a radiological or nuclear incident or natural disaster. (p. 11)

However, due to the complexity of the multiple variables, governmental agencies, and private sectors that are involved in preparedness and response activities; the waxing, waning, and reorganization of bureaucratic structures; and the unpredictability of public health emergencies, consistent and effective notions of preparedness/response design have eluded the country. This chapter describes the state of public health emergency preparedness and management and sheds light on past and current challenges to stimulate a new generation of thinkers toward development of more effective strategies that take into account the complexities of our nation and its states, including economics/resources, sociopolitical environments, government organizational structures, institutions, laws, regulations, diverse populations, and communication channels.

HISTORY OF CATASTROPHIC EVENTS/HISTORY OF PREPAREDNESS

Since prehistoric times, humans have attempted to respond to disaster events to protect lives and reduce illness caused by such events as floods, fires, famine, and pestilence (Haddow et al., 2014). In 430 BC, a yet unidentified infectious disease plague in Athens, Greece, lasted some 4 to 5 years and killed 25% of its population (Littman, 2009). The Black Death of 1347 caused by **bubonic plague**, a vector-borne disease spread by flea bites of infected rodents, ravaged Europe, killing an estimated 90% of the population (Beran, 2008). In 1854, the cholera epidemic in London's Soho district is credited with launching the field of disease epidemiology by Dr. John Snow, who linked the disease to fecal-contaminated water, but not before 578 people succumbed during the period between July and September of that year (Walford, 2020).

Natural (e.g., earthquakes, famine, floods, and infectious disease outbreaks) and man-made (e.g., riots, wars, bioterrorist attacks, and political unrest) disasters have always been a part of the human experience. In the past, the effect of such disasters on human populations was often more geographically restricted requiring small-scale, local responses.

In the United States, some of the earliest national responses to disasters involved providing funds for rebuilding and recovery after fires, earthquakes, and floods (Haddow et al., 2014; Roberts, 2006). In 1950, Congress passed the Federal Disaster Relief Act (Public Law 81–875). This legislation is invoked after the president of the United States declares a major disaster in a state or territory. It allows governors to request and receive federal assistance for mitigating catastrophic event damage (FEMA, 2003).

After the end of World War II in 1945, tensions between those allied with the Soviet Union (Russia) and those allied with the United States grew as the nuclear arms race escalated between the two factions. Known as the **Cold War**, this period, characterized by fears of communist expansion and aggression, raised concerns for national security and civilian protection (History.com Editors, 2009).

In response, President Harry S. Truman organized the Federal Civil Defense Administration (FCDA) in 1951 to protect life and property in the United States in the event of an enemy nuclear assault (History.com Editors, 2009; Subcommittee Hearings on H.R. 9798, 1950). The federal role in civil defense was viewed as provision of policy and guidance to support activities at the local level (Homeland Security National Preparedness Task Force, 2006).

Partnering with state and local government officials, the FCDA initiated a national program for civil defense against a potential nuclear bomb attack, emphasizing local, community, and family preparedness. Shelter-building programs, an attack warning system, stockpiled supplies, and an education campaign targeting adults and schoolchildren were developed and implemented. Millions of pamphlets containing safety and survival information were developed, printed, and distributed (Homeland Security National Preparedness Task Force, 2006). Many Americans who were financially able built backyard bomb shelters (History.com Editors, 2009). Popular among the children's education programs were the nine "Duck and Cover" movies produced by FCDA featuring Bert the Turtle, shown in classrooms across the nation (Homeland Security National Preparedness Task Force, 2006). Many people living today can still recall school drills in which children were required to "duck under desks and cover their heads!"

Federal approaches to civil defense varied during the Cold War period; for example, during the Eisenhower administration (1953–1961), a massive federal highway development program connecting major cities was undertaken to support mass evacuation during a nuclear attack (Homeland Security National Preparedness Task Force, 2006). As fears of communist aggression continued, fueled by the Soviet Union's successful nuclear bomb testing and efforts to put a man in space, the nation stood united in the focus on planning and conducting community protection strategies (Homeland Security National Preparedness Task Force, 2006). However, devastating earthquakes and hurricanes in the 1960s and 1970s demonstrated the need for a broader approach to emergency preparedness and management (Roberts, 2006). By the mid-1970s, it was clear that more coordinated national plans were required to provide aid to states facing disasters. In response to the need, in 1974, President Richard Nixon signed the Disaster Relief Act of 1974, which expanded federal emergency assistance to states and localities to include provision of rebuilding funds for public utilities, assistance to persons rendered unemployed by a disaster, relocation, temporary rent or mortgage assistance, food coupons, legal services, and crisis counseling, as well as grants and loans to state governments. But even with these added resources and initiatives, the management of disasters lacked central coordination, with multiple and diverse state, local, and federal agencies unsure who was responsible for what (Roberts, 2006).

President Jimmy Carter created FEMA in 1979 with the goal of establishing a central entity for coordination and communication with the White House, states, the National Guard, and other national and state agencies during an emergency and providing a streamlined process for sending resources to the location of the event (Roberts, 2006). From the beginning, there were challenges in that the focus was the response and not preparedness or **mitigation** in advance of an emergency (Roberts, 2006). The agency under President Ronald Reagan expanded its activities to flood and fire prevention programs, as well as nuclear attack evacuation and preparedness initiatives (Roberts, 2006).

In a continuing effort to improve emergency management and response, the Robert T. Stafford Disaster Relief and Emergency Assistance Act, amending the Disaster Relief Act of 1974, was passed by Congress and signed into law on November 23, 1988. The **Stafford Act** is foundational to subsequent legislation for national disaster responses. Its provisions authorize, upon request from a governor in an affected state, the president of the United States to declare a major disaster or emergency in situations in which local or state resources are inundated and depleted (Association of State and Territorial Health Officials

[ASTHO], 2012) and then direct comprehensive federal aid, administered by FEMA (ASTHO, 2012), to the affected area. The Stafford Act also allows the president to declare an emergency without a governor's request, if the event involves a federal facility, such as the 1995 bombing of the Murrah Federal Building in Oklahoma City (ASTHO, 2012).

As the tensions of the Cold War began to wane in 1989 with the collapse of the Berlin Wall, and in 1991 with the dissolution of the Soviet Union, the concern for preparedness, including peacetime natural disaster preparation, became less prominent in public policy debates (Homeland Security National Preparedness Task Force, 2006). The concept of preparedness for natural disasters—which covers a wide range of possibilities, including earthquakes, floods, hurricanes, oil and chemical spills, and events that are often more locally focused—faded in the national mindset since they did not constitute a central threat facing the nation. In 1992, the Federal Response Plan was enacted to provide a road map and systematic structure for delivery of aid for disasters declared under the Stafford Act (Escott, 2011).

However, life in the late 20th and early 21st centuries and, with it, changes in rapid transportation availability and world travel, centralized methods to produce and distribute food, political and civil upheavals contributing to mass migrations, and the proliferation of organized terrorism have all expanded the potential and possibility of large-scale, mass public health emergencies affecting thousands of persons per event. In addition, the long-term, unforeseen consequences of medical interventions in the past 60-plus years have contributed to the natural evolution of microorganisms producing hardy pathogenic strains resistant to available treatments. Thus, advances in technology have also advanced the potential for natural and man-made disasters that can extend beyond borders (Subbarao et al., 2008).

Going further, international and domestic terrorist activities during the 1990s altered the course of public health and perceptions of national vulnerability to deliberate threats (Stern, 1999). The release of toxic **sarin gas** in a Tokyo subway in 1995 that killed 12 and injured many; the threat of bubonic plague, which a lone potential extremist was able to purchase in 1995 (Stern, 1999); the Oklahoma City bombings that killed 168 people and injured over 680 others, linked to extremists (Sharpe, 2000); and threats to assassinate the president (President Bill Clinton) with biological agents received from an extremist group in 1998 (Stern, 1999) exposed potential vulnerabilities in national security. Particularly, the public health systems needed to become increasingly prepared for large-scale attacks that require rapid provision of medication and medical emergency services to impacted populations (Hamburg, 1999). The idea that terrorists could take deliberate action to potentially deploy biological weapons against civilian targets crystalized the need to integrate public health into the national security apparatus (Clarke, 1999). In 1998, President Clinton initiated a national biodefense program creating critical roles for agencies within the U.S. Department of Health and Human Services (HHS) (Clarke, 1999). Components of the program included investments in pathogen genome sequencing, vaccine and therapeutics research, improved diagnostics, detection strategies and disease surveillance systems (including syndromic surveillance), and creation of a national civilian stockpile of medicines and equipment (e.g., ventilators and personal protective equipment) [PPE] to fight biological pathogens (Clarke, 1999; Cruz et al., 2007). As fortification against acts of bioterrorism, in 1999 Congress appropriated $51 million to the

HHS/CDC to mobilize the public health system for protection against harmful biological agents (Cruz et al., 2007). This expansion of public health into national security allowed for the development of the National Pharmaceutical Stockpile (NPS), led by the CDC, to acquire and maintain caches of medicines and equipment readily available to mount a national response to a biological public health threat. The NPS was also in charge of rapidly dispensing and deploying pharmaceutical agents, vaccines, medical supplies, and equipment to support state and local resources in the event of a large-scale public health emergency (Cruz et al., 2007; Esbitt, 2003).

The horrific events of September 11, 2001, and the use of commercial jets as weapons of mass destruction changed the way emergency preparedness was perceived again. The response efforts mounted during the aftermath of 9/11 revealed that states required expertise and resources in place for improved capacity for response for large-scale terrorist events that extended beyond biological agents.

The country unified its concern for national security awareness and preparedness, resulting in President George W. Bush declaring the War on Terrorism. Within weeks, the War on Terrorism launched a military campaign to tamp down insurgents suspected of radicalizing and training terrorists in Afghanistan (Homeland Security National Preparedness Task Force, 2006). Under President George W. Bush, the DHS was created under the Homeland Security Act of 2002 and a comprehensive National Response Plan was developed in 2004 (Escott, 2011). The plan was designed as a set of instructions for the federal government in the event of a presidential disaster declaration. In 2004, FEMA initiated the National Incident Management System (NIMS), which was heralded as a national template for collaboration among agencies, entities, and partners with the goal of preventing, preparing for, and responding to man-made or natural disasters of varying sizes and scopes (FEMA, 2003).

On March 1, 2003, the NPS was renamed the **Strategic National Stockpile** (SNS) program, managed jointly by the newly created DHS and the HHS. In 2004, the Cities Readiness Initiative (CRI) launched efforts to provide medical countermeasure preparation, coverage, and practice in the form of drills in the largest cities and metropolitan areas in the United States where more than 50% of the nation's population resides. The CRI enabled public health departments in states and large metropolitan areas to develop specific plans, tailored to community requirements, for dispensing antibiotics and other medicines to the entire population of a metropolitan area within 48 hours. By 2006, the CRI had expanded to 72 **Metropolitan Statistical Areas** (MSAs) with at least one MSA in every state. These 72 MSAs included over 500 counties and cities and represented more than 57% of the U.S. population (LeBlanc et al., 2018; Nelson et al., 2010; Stewart & Cordell, 2007). The SNS was deployed successfully in multiple medical emergencies, including Hurricanes Rita and Katrina in 2005 and Gustav and Ike in 2008, the H1N1 pandemic in 2009, Hurricane Alex and the North Dakota flooding in 2010, Hurricanes Irene in 2011 and Isaac and Sandy in 2012, the Ebola outbreak in 2014 and 2015, Zika in 2016, and Hurricanes Harvey, Irma, and Maria in 2017 (LeBlanc et al., 2018). In 2018, the SNS transitioned away from the CDC to the Assistant Secretary of Preparedness and Response (ASPR), another agency within the HHS located in Washington, DC (LeBlanc et al., 2018).

A SAMPLE OF MAJOR DISASTERS SINCE 9/11

The following brief examples are provided to help gain a perspective and grasp a better understanding of the range, scope, and magnitude of public health emergencies occurring in recent times.

HURRICANE KATRINA

In 2005, Hurricane Katrina exposed multiple challenges for preparedness and response to a large-scale disaster affecting millions of residents. The impact was especially acute in New Orleans, with its flawed flood control system that rendered 80% of the city and surrounding parishes underwater for weeks. Transportation systems were halted, and thousands of persons were left stranded in flooded neighborhoods, without food and safe water. Approximately 1.5 million people evacuated their homes. Some sought refuge in inadequately supplied and staffed shelters, which could not accommodate or protect the deluge of people seeking help. Many persons in shelters had chronic conditions requiring medication and medical services that could not be provided. However, thousands were unable to evacuate the city and were trapped in flooded homes, resorting to climbing on rooftops to avoid drowning. Hospitals and nursing home operations were disrupted. Approximately 1,800 people were killed, and many others injured. Families were separated. Thousands of persons were displaced, some permanently (Zimmermann, 2015). The storm also exposed complications associated with social and economic vulnerabilities among residents in high-poverty areas. People displaced by Hurricane Katrina were predominantly African American (76%), largely unemployed or underemployed (53%), did not own homes (66%), lacked healthcare insurance (47%), and had chronic health conditions (56%). Approximately half of these evacuees lacked medications at the time of displacement (Brunkard, 2005; Honoré, 2020; Lichtveld et al., 2020).

Thousands of children were affected by the storm, by temporary or permanent displacement from homes or caregivers, through truncated education trajectories, and by long-lasting posttraumatic stress disorder symptoms associated with personal losses and uncertainty of survival. The National Commission on Children and Disasters (NCCD, 2010), formed in 2007 in response to Katrina's impact on persons living along the Gulf Coast, published recommendations in 2010 to improve national child protection during emergencies.

Furthermore, according to the National Council on Disabilities, Hurricane Katrina affected approximately 155,000 persons older than age 5 with physical, developmental, and cognitive disabilities in impact zones. Deaf and blind persons suffered from communication issues and could not receive information regarding evacuation procedures. Neither evacuation transportation nor shelters were equipped to accommodate many persons requiring wheelchairs, walkers, and service animals. Many hurricane survivors with disabilities' basic needs were also complicated during these emergencies by chronic health conditions and functional impairments. Persons with disabilities accounted for a disproportionate number of fatalities associated with the storm (G. W. White et al., 2007).

The storm and its aftermath highlighted the intricate dynamics of **social vulnerabilities** and the effects of poverty on survival, recovery, and resilience in large-scale natural disasters. Response to Katrina challenged the public health and public safety systems, social services, and local, state, and federal governmental agencies and revealed significant gaps in preparedness and recovery for populations with specific access and functional needs.

Hurricane Katrina, when viewed from the perspective of some 15 years later, continues to teach us that we cannot afford to neglect the effects of systemic racism that are still resulting in the disproportionate impact on lives in communities of color through greater attack, hospitalization, and mortality rates in the current pandemic of **COVID-19** (Kim-Farley, 2020).

H1N1 Influenza of 2009

Starting in March 2009, with airline travel as the primary spreader, the H1N1 influenza virus spread from Mexico to places around the world. The first known case in the United States occurred on April 11, 2009 (Hajjar & McIntosh, 2010). The virus was novel in that it was more highly transmissible and affected children more than older adults (as expected with seasonal influenza viruses). In addition, a notable majority of infected persons had one or more underlying medical conditions, including asthma, diabetes, heart or lung disease, neurological disease, pregnancy, morbid obesity, or immune disorders (Hajjar & McIntosh, 2010).

The United States mounted a comprehensive, multifaceted response to the pandemic, with the CDC leading the effort. Scientists at the CDC sequenced the genetic structure of the virus and uploaded it to a publicly accessible international influenza database that enabled scientists around the world to use the sequenced information for public health research and vaccine development. In addition, the CDC (2010) activated its Emergency Operations Center (EOC) on April 22, 2009, to coordinate a national response, including surveillance and detection, contact tracing, laboratory response, communications, identifying at-risk populations, distributing antiviral medications, developing and distributing vaccine, and disseminating traveler's health advisories.

On April 26, 2009, the U.S. government declared H1N1 a national emergency and engaged the CDC's SNS, which began providing 25% of the supplies in the stockpile for protection against transmission and to treat influenza. The supplies included 11 million regimens of antiviral drugs and PPE with over 39 million respiratory protection devices (masks and respirators), gowns, gloves, and face shields dispatched to states (allocations were based on each state's population). As part of the nation's pre-pandemic planning efforts, by April 2009 the federal government had purchased 50 million treatment courses of antiviral drugs—oseltamivir and zanamivir—for the SNS, and states had purchased 23 million antiviral regimens (CDC, 2010). In addition, the CDC provided viral laboratory testing kits starting on May 1, 2009, and by May 14, 2009, laboratories in 40 states were validated to conduct H1N1 testing. On June 11, 2009, the **World Health Organization** (WHO) declared H1N1 an international pandemic, the first such declaration in 40 years. By that time, mitigation efforts in the United States were well underway (CDC, 2010).

On July 9, 2009, the HHS, the DHS, the Department of Education, and the White House met with federal, state, local, and tribal officials to discuss existing pandemic plans, lessons learned, and preparedness priorities to urgently plan for an H1N1 influenza immunization program. On July 22, 2009, the National Institutes of Health (NIH) began a series of clinical trials to pilot test vaccines developed by two manufacturers (CDC, 2010). By September 15, 2009, the Food and Drug Administration (FDA) had approved four H1N1 vaccines, and by October 9, all states and the District of Columbia had placed orders for supplies of vaccines. By late December, vaccines were available for anyone desiring one (CDC, 2010). On August 10, 2010, the WHO declared that the H1N1 pandemic was over. From April 12, 2009, to April 10, 2010, there were 60.8 million cases, 274,304 hospitalizations, and 12,469 deaths in the United States attributed to H1N1 (CDC, 2010, n.d.-c).

EBOLA

Ebola virus disease (EVD), named for a nearby river, was at first characterized as a rare but deadly and highly contagious zoonotic infection originally recognized in 1976 in rural Central Africa (Alexander et al., 2015). It was associated with high mortality, remote locations, and low population density, which, at the time, curtailed extensive exposure (Alexander et al., 2015). However, the 2014 EVD outbreaks in West Africa (Guinea, Liberia, Sierra Leone) occurred primarily in urban areas and resulted in widespread hemorrhagic fever morbidity and mortality due to the virus (Molinari et al., 2018). An unprecedented number of cases (more than 28,600) were reported since the first confirmed case in March 2014 and, among infected persons, two in five died (Molinari et al., 2018). With thousands of persons at-risk for EVD and an overwhelmed healthcare system, the WHO declared the West African outbreak an epidemic in March 2014 and then, in August 2014, a Public Health Emergency of International Concern. In an international effort to assist affected countries and reduce the likelihood of disease spread, a number of countries supplied humanitarian aid, including volunteers, medical aid, and sanitation equipment, to affected countries. Clinicians, epidemiologists, and other healthcare providers, as well as business and personal travelers to and from the epidemic epicenters, heightened the concern for global transmission of EVD. In response, the WHO, the HHS, the CDC, and other international partners implemented measures to rapidly screen, detect, and treat travelers entering nonepidemic countries. The risk of EVD exposure in persons returning home after serving in outbreak endemic areas fueled fears of an epidemic in the United States (Venkat et al., 2015). A total of 11 people in the United States were treated for EVD between 2014 and 2016. Of that number, eight were healthcare workers who contracted the disease while serving the response in Africa and were airlifted to the United States for treatment; only one succumbed to the disease (CDC, n.d.-a).

Despite best efforts to screen persons entering the United States from affected West African countries, a person infected with EVD entered the United States from Liberia on September 20, 2014. The patient presented at a Dallas, Texas, hospital emergency department on September 25, 2014, and was treated for sinusitis and released. Several days later, the patient returned to the hospital; an EVD diagnosis was confirmed on September 30, and the patient died on October 8, 2014 (Chevalier et al., 2014). Two nurses providing direct care for the patient also were confirmed with EVD in that same October (Chevalier et al., 2014; Venkat et al., 2015).

Zika

The Zika virus was discovered in the blood of a febrile monkey in 1947 in the Zika Forest of Uganda and was first noted in a few humans in 1952. It was not until March of 2015 that large outbreaks in Brazil were observed—eventually affecting 1.3 million persons and later spreading to other countries in the Americas, including the United States (White et al., 2016). The Zika virus was associated with **Guillain-Barré syndrome** (which includes muscle weakness and sometimes paralysis) in adults. However, the greatest risk of exposure was to developing fetuses in pregnant women. In utero, exposure to the Zika virus was associated with fetal deaths and birth anomalies, principally **microcephaly** (White et al., 2016). Most cases were determined to be vector-borne through the bite of an infected ***Aedes aegypti* mosquito**, but the virus was also found in semen, making sexual transmission a possibility (CDC, n.d.-b). At the peak of the U.S. epidemic in 2016, a total of 5,168 symptomatic Zika virus cases were reported, with 4,897 cases among travelers returning from affected areas, 224 cases acquired through local mosquito-borne transmission, and 47 cases acquired by other means, including 45 through sexual transmission, one due to laboratory transmission, and one via an unknown person-to-person route. Larger transmission was observed in the territory of Puerto Rico, with 35,395 cases (CDC, n.d.-d). By 2017, due to rapid and aggressive mitigation strategies targeting affected areas, including mosquito control and community outreach, travel advisories, and efforts to raise national awareness through an informational media campaign, Zika in the United States declined dramatically. By 2020 only three cases were reported in the mainland and 48 cases reported in U.S. territories (CDC, 2021).

A COVID-19 Chronology of 2020—The Year That Changed Everything

On December 31, 2019, the government in China confirmed to the WHO that healthcare providers were treating a cluster of cases with severe respiratory infections of unknown etiology in Wuhan City, Hubei Province, associated with exposures in a live animal and seafood market. By January 7, 2020, Chinese scientists had sequenced the genome of the virus, identified it as a novel coronavirus, and then, on January 12, made the sequencing publicly available for producing diagnostic tests. The first known death associated with the disease occurred on January 11. On January 21, Chinese health officials confirmed human-to-human transmission. On January 23, with 17 reported deaths, Wuhan, a metropolitan area of 11 million people, was put under a strict quarantine that precluded travel to or from the city, and halted local travel among residents by buses and subways (WHO, 2020). On January 30, the WHO issued a Global Health Emergency. The first known case in the United States was observed and confirmed on January 20, 2020, in a Seattle, Washington, man in his 30s returning from a trip to Wuhan (Holshue et al., 2020). On February 3, 2020, the United States declared COVID-19 a national emergency (Taylor, 2021). In a press conference on February 25, 2020, Dr. Nancy Messonnier, of the CDC's National Center for Immunization and Respiratory Diseases, heralded the dangers of rapid viral spread in the United States, suggesting the implementation of comprehensive, nationwide strategies for prevention. She urged businesses, healthcare sectors, communities, and schools to anticipate potential disruptions to everyday life and immediately plan for alternatives (Zeballos-Riog, 2020). The warnings were echoed by the secretary of HHS, Alex Azar (Zeballos-Riog, 2020). However, the administrative branch of the government downplayed the threat of increasing viral spread, and some members of the public did not take the disease seriously. The first U.S. death attributed to COVID-19 was noted on February 29, but later information revealed that two additional people had succumbed to the disease days earlier (Taylor, 2021). On March 11, 2020, the WHO officially declared the disease to be a global pandemic (Peirlinck et al., 2020; WHO, 2020).

A large outbreak outside China was confirmed on February 1, among 3,700 passengers and crew of the *Diamond Princess* cruise ship. The cruise ship had departed Yokohama, Japan, on January 20 for a 16-day cruise. An 80-year-old male passenger with symptoms of pneumonia disembarked on January 25 and was later tested for, and confirmed to have, COVID-19. Aboard the ship were 380 Americans and their families who, after spending 14 days quarantined on the *Princess*, were repatriated to the United States via State Department flights to California, with some passengers continuing on to Texas (Li & Bhattacharya, 2020). Likewise, 3,000 passengers on another cruise ship, the *Grand Princess*, disembarked in San Francisco on February 21, 2020, to enjoy a holiday through March 7. By March 6, 19 crew members and two passengers were confirmed to have COVID-19 (Moriarty et al., 2020; McCormick, 2021). The ship was not allowed to dock anywhere until March 9, when passengers were gradually allowed to leave en route to quarantine quarters for 14 days. Some passengers reported unsafe conditions, including being crowded onto a bus to the Travis Airforce Base in Fairfield, California, and into a breakfast room with self-service coffee and inadequate sanitation supplies (McCormick, 2021). Both cruises had more than 800 COVID-19 cases and 10 reported deaths. During the period from February 3 to March 13, 2020, 17% of U.S. COVID-19 cases were attributed to returned cruise ship passengers (Moriarty et al., 2020). On March 13, the Cruise Lines International Association announced a 30-day voluntary suspension of cruise ship operations in the United States and, on March 17, the CDC recommended that all worldwide cruise travel be deferred (Moriarty et al., 2020). Additionally, on that same date, the president of the United States declared a national emergency. In mid-March, governors began issuing stay-at-home orders as well as school and business closings.

By March 26, 2020, the United States became the country with the most COVID-19 infections with over 81,000 cases and 1,000 reported deaths—exceeding the original outbreaks in Wuhan, China, and in Europe (Taylor, 2021). Viral spread continued and hospitals became inundated with surges of patients, PPE became scarce, ventilators were in short supply, medical staff were overwhelmed, and there were not enough respiratory therapists to meet the demand in healthcare facilities (Slavitt, 2020). Despite the burgeoning crisis, the national response lacked centrality, was minimally focused on science, and eschewed clarity of protection messaging to the public. Coordination among various agencies tasked with **public health emergency preparedness** (e.g., FEMA, the CDC, the ASPR) was lacking. The role for the SNS, which had served efficiently in prior medical emergencies, lacked transparency. Policies regarding mitigation strategies, including wearing masks for protection and practicing social distancing, became politicized, with large swaths of the population linking mitigation with culture wars and refusing to comply. State governors were put in the unenviable position of competing with other states for protective equipment. Some states fostered consortiums with others to ease competition and increase access to vital supplies (Gross, 2020). Inevitably, price gouging of medical equipment was common. Complicating matters, the federal government was reported to be competing against states for the purchase of supplies (Soergel, 2020). Against the backdrop of the pandemic, schools closed; businesses shuttered, with millions of people losing their jobs; and small businesses were forced to close due to a dwindling customer base.

Acceleration of the disease continued exponentially, with 1.77 million confirmed cases and over 100,000 people reported dead due to the virus on May 27, 2020 (Taylor, 2021). However, even in the face of these numbers, people in some states organized protests to any restrictions on mobility, school closings, mask wearing, and social distancing (Kahane, 2021; Madrigal et al., 2020).

From the start of the pandemic in the United States, it was clear that the disease was not an equal opportunity phenomenon. Poorer outcomes, morbidity, and mortality clustered among the most vulnerable in society, the aged and the economically stressed. The disease and who it affected were in some regards consistent with the current bifurcation in the economy brought on by market shifts. For the past 50 years, the U.S. economy has drifted toward an hourglass structure, with dominant tiers at the top and the bottom and a smaller tier in the center. The top tier, or careers in the information and knowledge-based economy, and investment classes are rewarded with high salaries, flexible work environments, substantial health and other benefits, and generous vacation time and sick leave policies. The scientists, communications professionals, writers, publishers, high level government office workers, investment brokers, and others were not adversely affected by stay-at-home orders. In most cases, people in these careers could work from home on their computers. The bottom tier, or careers in the basic services sector (e.g., restaurant staff, grocery clerks, sanitation workers and janitorial staff, meat and poultry processors, transportation workers, and others), did not have the luxuries of the top tier. These workers, even under pandemic conditions, had to report to work to get paid. Many of these workers receive low hourly wages, have few health benefits, and often receive no paid time off, even for sick leave. Some so-called **gig workers** (i.e., independent contractors or freelancers who work on demand for specific functions and are paid per job) also fit in this bottom tier. Paradoxically, these basic service workers proved to be absolutely essential during the lockdowns. They kept the country operating, albeit on reduced capacity, risking their own lives and the lives of their families. Essential workers are disproportionately people of color; thus, exposure to the COVID-19 virus was exceptionally high for them, and logically, they were disproportionately affected by the disease from the start (Lancet, 2020).

Sandwiched between these two dominant tiers are other essential workers, teachers, firefighters, police officers, all healthcare professionals, and many others who provide services with which community life could not exist. This part of the hourglass is smaller and metaphorically could serve as a connector between the top and bottom tiers, as all citizens depend on this important sector. Their wages and benefits are adequate, but the work demands reporting in person, and thus, this entire segment was at risk for exposure to COVID-19 as well. This was especially true for those employed in hospital emergency departments and infectious disease wards.

Severe morbidity and mortality associated with COVID-19 clustered among the middle and bottom tiers, with the greatest toll inflicted upon those in the lowest paid service sector work. At the beginning of the pandemic, American Indian/Alaska Native, Black, and Hispanic people were hardest hit. As of May 2, 2020, rates per 100,000 population indicated clear disparities in those groups. But as the pandemic wore on, cases among Whites began to accelerate, peaking in early January 2021. Overall, American Indians/Alaska Natives, Hispanics, and

Blacks were disproportionately affected by the disease and related deaths due to several factors. First, the initial large outbreaks of COVID-19 in the United States occurred in coastal large metropolitan areas, homes to large numbers of racial/ethnic minorities. Second, racial and ethnic minorities are disproportionately employed in the tiers of the economy requiring high social contact to do their jobs (Hawkins, 2020). Third, in the case of American Indians/Alaska Natives, they may be isolated in communities with limited access to medical care and even basic resources, such as water for handwashing (Hatcher et al., 2020; Hathaway, 2021). Fourth, deaths among racial ethnic minorities may be linked to a lack of access to care, or receiving suboptimal care, and related to underlying health conditions (e.g., diabetes, hypertension, heart disease), and other challenges to recovery (Bambra et al., 2020).

COVID-19 Rates Per 100,000 Population, United States, Selected Dates, May 2020-January 2021

	AI/AN	Asian/PI	Black	Hispanic	White
2-May-20	49.29	20.32	41.14	55.6	16.17
21-Nov-20	195.12	72.82	86.31	132.03	136.79
9-Jan-21	342.87	161.88	149.99	171.64	169.07

AI/AN, American Indian/Alaska Native; PI, Pacific Islander.

CDC DATA Tracker, 2021

Death Rates Attributed to COVID-19 Per 100,000 Population, Selected Dates, April 2020-January 2021

	AI/AN	Asian/PI	Black	Hispanic	White
11-Apr-20	2.5	3.55	7.2	4.04	3.73
21-Nov-20	3.76	1.46	1.87	1.45	3.53
9-Jan-21	4.23	3.29	2.64	1.44	3.22

AI/AN, American Indian/Alaska Native; PI, Pacific Islander.

CDC Data Tracker, 2021

Irrespective of race/ethnicity, contracting COVID-19 is related to occupational risks. Persons employed in congregate settings (e.g., schools, nursing and other care homes, homeless shelters, correctional facilities), high exposure occupations (e.g., healthcare staff, medical transport, mortuary staff, laboratory professionals), and customer-facing occupations (e.g., grocery store staff, retail workers, cab drivers) have been faced with the dilemma of going to work or not getting paid (Sinclair et al., 2021). Going further, as government-mandated COVID-19 restrictions shuttered restaurants, hair and nail salons and other personal services, and other businesses to reduce risks, millions of people lost their jobs. Among small businesses, which employ almost half of the private-sector workforce, revenue was reduced 20% by mid-year 2020 (Bauer et al., 2020). Low-income families, particularly racial ethnic minorities, were adversely impacted (Bauer et al., 2020). The COVID-19 pandemic and its associated repercussions have contributed to housing and food insecurity for thousands of persons nationwide (Bauer et al., 2020).

On the other side of this gloomy picture, workers employed in the upper tier of the economy were able to continue their careers, uninterrupted, by working from home; ordering food, supplies, and services online, due to the support of the lower tiers. The information/knowledge tier has also increased their accrued savings rate, surpassing any other time in the history of the country during the pandemic with reduced spending in hospitality and travel (Pinsker, 2020).

At the end of March 2020, the Congress appropriated a $2.2 trillion funding package to provide aid to the unemployed and struggling businesses, and direct payments to citizens earning below a defined threshold. The **CARES Act** (Coronavirus Aid Relief and Security Act) also included $10 billion to accelerate development of a vaccine to combat the virus. Deemed "Operation Warp Speed," a partnership between private and federal agencies, including HHS and the Department of Defense, it funded six companies (Johnson & Johnson, Astra Zeneca from the University of Oxford, Moderna, Nora Vax, Merck, and Sanofi/GlaxoSmithKline), which greatly reduced the time required for developing, testing, and conducting clinical trials and by truncating bureaucratic hurdles for approval and dissemination (FDA, 2021). Pfizer-BioTech was a company also engaged in developing a COVID-19 vaccine but did not receive Operation Warp Speed funds. In the fall of 2020, two companies successfully developed vaccines that demonstrated safety and effectiveness in clinical trials. On December 11, 2020, the Pfizer vaccine received emergency use authorization (EUA) from the FDA for distribution (FDA, 2021). EUA is a rapid approval system used in national emergency situations that require the administration of **medical countermeasures** or vaccines to meet an emerging medical crisis (FDA, 2021). The EUA requires rigorous testing and solid evidence of safety and effectiveness. The Moderna vaccine received EUA by the FDA on December 18, 2020 (FDA, 2021). From that point onward, a mass vaccination campaign began, reminiscent of the administration of polio vaccines in the 1950s. The first doses of the Pfizer vaccines were administered to healthcare workers on December 14, 2020 (Loftus & West, 2020).

At this writing, the United States has exceeded 49 million cases of COVID-19, with over 787,000 confirmed deaths attributable to the disease. Vaccination campaigns have been accelerated, especially in developed countries with better access to vaccines, but globally the pandemic has continued.

DISCUSSION

What have we learned? Although we may have learned many things, we are not putting the lessons learned into practice!

For the past five decades, global scientists and public health professionals have been concerned about calamitous worldwide disasters such as the influenza pandemic of 1918, which infected over one-third of the earth's population and resulted in over 50 million deaths (Parmet & Rothstein, 2018). Government and public health agencies in the United States have devoted millions of dollars in resources for constructing response infrastructures and developing structural frameworks/models for mobilizing and coordinating the multiple stakeholders across city and state bureaucracies, as well as emergency and healthcare systems for mounting responses (Katz et al., 2017). After the events of September 11, 2001, public health efforts to prepare for emergencies received renewed focus, energy, and resources (Khan, 2011) and stimulated scientists from a plethora of disciplines to study disasters from various perspectives. Henry Fischer, a sociologist studying disasters' effect on social groups, offered a linear model for understanding the natural course of a catastrophe suggesting that parts or all of an existing social structure first experience the mass emergency, followed by disruption of the social structure, then the mass emergency is mitigated, and finally an adjusted social structure carries on after the event—with severity of disruption measured on a 10-point scale based on the size, scope, and duration of the emergency (Fischer, 2003).

In February 2020, as COVID-19 spread globally, it became clear that disaster models/structural frameworks developed by public health and social scientists were based on a number of unwritten assumptions. Before a mass emergency, a social structure is assumed to be sound and cohesive, with individuals acting in ways to mutually support the whole; a healthcare system is assumed to work reasonably well, with most people able to access care; and a society's communication system is efficient for delivering unambiguous, lifesaving messages to the majority of an affected population. Disaster responses in recent years, particularly to COVID-19, have unmasked the persistent structural flaws in organizational capacity, untackled social/economic inequities, and discovered systemic flaws in communication channels.

It is important to note here that, in parallel with the buildup of efforts to address emerging threats requiring large-scale mitigation and scientific inquiry to understand the potential impact on human populations over the past 50 years, the way people communicate, receive, and understand information has markedly changed. The internet and its contentious offspring, social media, have become ubiquitous features of everyday life through computers in homes, in the workplace, and on mobile devices, which may obfuscate receipt of accurate messaging (LeBlanc et al., 2019; Terrasse et al., 2019; Wang et al., 2019).

The results of the current pandemic call for a reexamination and strengthening of social/economic, medical, and public health systems before the onset of the next emergencies.

Threats to Preparedness—Tangible and Intangible—The Structure of Society Itself

People

The people in a society or nation state must have a sense of mutual identity and cooperation for a national emergency response to be successful. After the events of 9/11, the country appeared united, as Americans, against foreign terrorism. In the years since that time, the ability of Americans to view themselves as one population, willing to help each other during a crisis, has eroded. Divisiveness was apparent in several responses, Hurricane Katrina is but one example in which poor minority evacuees were met with armed police officers and were refused entry to suburban areas to escape flooding. During the COVID-19 response, the politicization of mitigation strategies that emerged among some segments of the American population likely contributed to viral spread, as mask wearing and social distancing were adamantly resisted as markers of "defense of freedom" or "patriotism." In an emergency of the magnitude of COVID-19, mutual cooperation is a fundamental requirement for an adequate response. Long before an emergency occurs, a society must achieve a sense of unity for the betterment of all citizens. We must rise to our higher selves, change hearts, endeavor to live harmoniously, and be willing to help the most vulnerable among us. Everyone in our country should have access to optimal life chances, and be fully prepared for and ready to respond to future public health emergencies, such as Katrina and COVID-19, that will inevitably arise (Kim-Farley, 2020).

The people in a society or nation-state must receive basic education on how the governing bodies work and the basics of science. Education and knowledge may serve to build trust and understanding when an emergency is thrust upon the population and decisions are made by officials that will affect their lives. If the people in a society or nation-state are not able to unite in compliance with requirements for a response, or lack a fundamental understanding of why compliance is necessary to mitigate the conditions present during a disaster, serious threats to preparedness are present.

Government

Governments are groups of leaders and workers, drawn from a population, who provide structure for the organization and protection of a society and mechanisms for maintaining order through rules and regulations. The government also provides services that ordinary people cannot provide for themselves, for instance, military defense, fire and police, education, social services, and environmental protection. In recent years, the important roles of government have been called into question and, in some segments of the population, rejected as an enemy of freedom. A lack of trust in the government is a major threat to preparedness. If people do not trust government officials and their decisions during an emergency response, they are likely to resist mitigation strategies.

On the other side of that issue, governmental leaders must be competent and knowledgeable regarding the complexity and organizational structures of agencies involved in components of emergency responses. They must be "on the same page" as their public health agencies, articulate the same guidance with "one voice," and emulate the practices requested of the population (e.g., mask wearing and practicing physical distancing as needed during the COVID-19 pandemic). Sometimes the organizational structures themselves, and lack of coordination among them, can be a threat to preparedness. The "alphabet soup" of federal agencies (e.g., the ASPR, CDC, DHS, FEMA, and the NIH), the military and private entities (e.g., Red Cross, Salvation Army), and state and local governmental structures all have fragmented portions of response activities. Who does what? How is that information conveyed to states? What do all these entities do, and how do they work together during an emergency? How are strategic plans operationalized and articulated to first responders? Where are the weak links in the chain? Which frameworks for preparedness/models of preparedness are the most efficient and effective? A lack of comprehension and "unity of vision" among the multifaceted components of governmental and private-sector actors involved in a response can pose serious threats to effectiveness and contribute to a lack of trust in the government.

Factual, Believable Communication

A serious threat to preparedness is the lack of credible, believable information available to the public. In past years, radio and television were useful tools for dissemination of information of vital importance for national protection. However, as early as Orson Welles's 1938 radio drama broadcast adaptation of H. G. Wells' *War of the Worlds*, presenting a fictional Martian invasion that used a "breaking news" format, the power of misinformation to confuse the public was evident. In 2021, the phenomenon of segmented media markets is a fixture among all media outlets and platforms. One can choose the "truths," lenses, or perspectives in which to filter the events of the day. Misinformation and disinformation "silos" in online media and in all forms of audio and video broadcasting have posed a threat to not only everyday life information but especially information related to health and public safety as well. What has come to be known as "truth decay" (in which wide swaths of the population are led to believe false information or conspiracy theories that could lead to uptake of unsafe practices and in some cases lead to violence) serves as an enormous challenge to providing accurate information to people during an emergency event. This threat will be a major concern for public health in the 21st century.

PUBLIC HEALTH'S ROLE

Most disasters put lives in peril. A strong public health system should be in place, nationwide, well before a catastrophic event—with an emphasis on provision of services equitably to all members of the population, without prejudice based on gender, race/ethnicity, national origin, or religion. A strong social contract to assist persons who have fallen on hardships (especially those who are homeless) and a healthcare system to provide medical care, regardless of employment status, are among the many required building blocks of preparedness. The content of this volume is guided by the current essential services of public health (revised in September 2020). We believe that the structure of public health should routinely provide these services and they should be integrated components of medical emergency responses.

Essential Public Health Service #1
Assess and monitor population health status, factors that influence health, and community needs and assets.

Essential Public Health Service #2
Investigate, diagnose, and address health problems and hazards affecting the population.

Essential Public Health Service #3
Communicate effectively to inform and educate people about health, factors that influence it, and how to improve it.

Essential Public Health Service #4
Strengthen, support, and mobilize communities and partnerships to improve health.

Essential Public Health Service #5
Create, champion, and implement policies, plans, and laws that impact health.

Essential Public Health Service #6
Utilize legal and regulatory actions designed to improve and protect the public's health.

Essential Public Health Service #7
Assure an effective system that enables equitable access to the individual services and care needed to be healthy.

Essential Public Health Service #8
Build and support a diverse and skilled public health workforce.

Essential Public Health Service #9
Improve and innovate public health functions through ongoing evaluation, research, and continuous quality improvement.

Essential Public Health Service #10
Build and maintain a strong organizational infrastructure for public health.

CONCLUSION

With each disaster, more evidence of the unsustainable nature of American society has been uncovered. Examples include the communication/coordination issues during 9/11, the economic and social disparities of Katrina, and the many problematic issues of the COVID-19 response. Thus, preparedness is not bureaucratic notions of artificially defined capabilities. Preparedness depends upon having an existing strong system in place to protect and sustain life under normal circumstances that can be resilient under strained circumstances. Thus, the society itself must be strong and salvageable. The building blocks of preparedness are represented in the very fabric of society itself. Despite thousands of after-action reports filed, we have not developed a sustainable strategy to learn from specific events—especially to remember and apply that learning to create systems and supports for strengthening future responses.

We want to train a cadre of public health leaders who not only understand the complexities of emergency preparedness but also comprehend the complexities of society itself to meet the challenge of building and maintaining local, state, tribal, and national security.

DISCUSSION QUESTIONS

1. How does the history of disasters and the multiple reactionary decisions by decision-makers impact current functioning? Can reactionary decisions ever be prevented? How can we think more holistically about preparedness?
2. Discuss the impact of the events of September 11, 2001, on preparedness efforts.
3. As a group project or discussion, describe as many of the societal disruptions caused by COVID-19 as you are able and predict the long-term consequences of them for American society. Develop plans or strategies to improve.
4. Discuss the impact of misinformation and disinformation with examples you have personally witnessed. How can poor communication be dangerous in an emergency situation? What role does the media play?

DISCLAIMER

This chapter was prepared by Tanya Telfair LeBlanc in his/her personal capacity. The opinions expressed in this article are the author's own and do not reflect the view of the Centers for Disease Control and Prevention, the Department of Health and Human Services, or the United States government.

REFERENCES

Alexander, K. A., Sanderson, C. E., Maranthe, M., Lewis, B. L., & Rivers, C. M. (2015). What factors might have led to the emergence of Ebola in West Africa? *PLOS Neglected Tropical Diseases, 9*(6), e0003652. https://doi.org/10.1371/journal.pntd.0003652

Association of State and Territorial Health Officials. (2012). *Robert T. Stafford Disaster Relief Act and Emergency Assistance Fact Sheet.* https://www.astho.org/Programs/Preparedness/Public-Health-Emergency-Law/Emergency-Authority-and-Immunity-Toolkit/Robert-T--Stafford-Disaster-Relief-and-Emergency-Assistance-Act-Fact-Sheet

Bambra, C., Riordan, R., Ford, J., & Matthews, F. (2020). The COVID-19 pandemic and health inequalities. *Journal of Epidemiology Community Health, 74*, 964–968. https://doi.org/10.1136/jech-2020-214401

Bauer, L., Broady, K., Edelberg, W., & O'Donnell, J. (2020). *Ten facts about COVID-19 and the US economy.* The Hamilton Project. https://www.brookings.edu/wp-content/uploads/2020/09/FutureShutdowns_Facts_LO_Final.pdf

Beran, G. W. (2008). Disease and destiny – mystery and mastery. *Preventive Veterinary Medicine, 86*, 198–207. https://doi.org/10.1016/j.prevetmed.2008.05.001

Brunkard, J., Namulanda, G., & Ratard, R. (2005). Hurricane Katrina deaths, 2005. *Disaster Medicine and Public Health Preparedness, 2*, 215–223. https://doi.org/10.1097/DMP.0b013e31818aaf55

Centers for Disease Control and Prevention. (n.d.-a). *2014–2016 Ebola outbreak in West Africa: Ebola in the United States.* https://www.cdc.gov/vhf/ebola/history/2014-2016-outbreak/index.html#anchor_1515001446180

Centers for Disease Control and Prevention. (n.d.-b). *Questions about Zika.* https://www.cdc.gov/zika/about/questions.html

Centers for Disease Control and Prevention. (n.d.-c). *2009 H1N1 pandemic (H1N1pdm09 virus).* https://www.cdc.gov/flu/pandemic-resources/2009-h1n1-pandemic.html

Centers for Disease Control and Prevention. (n.d.-d). *2016 case counts in the US.* https://www.cdc.gov/zika/reporting/2016-case-counts.html

Centers for Disease Control and Prevention. (2010). *The 2009 H1N1 pandemic: Summary highlights, April 2009–April 2010.* https://www.cdc.gov/h1n1flu/cdcresponse.htm

Centers for Disease Control and Prevention. (2019). *Public health emergency preparedness and response capabilities: National standards for state, local, tribal, and territorial public health* (Rev. ed.). U.S. Department of Health and Human Services. https://www.cdc.gov/cpr/readiness/00_docs/CDC_PreparednesResponseCapabilities_October2018_Final_508.pdf

Centers for Disease Control and Prevention. (2021). *2020 case counts in the US.* https://www.cdc.gov/zika/reporting/2020-case-counts.html

Chevalier, M. S., Chung, W., Smith, J., Weil, L. M., Hughes, S. M., Joyner, S. N., Hall, E., Srinath, D., Ritch, J., Thathiah, P., Threadgill, H., Cervantes, D., & Lakey, D. L. (2014). Ebola virus disease cluster in the United States–Dallas County, Texas, 2014. *Morbidity and Mortality Weekly, 63*(46), 1087–1088. https://www.ncbi.nlm.nih.gov/pmc/articles/PMC5779510

Clarke, R. A. (1999). Finding the right balance against bioterrorism. *Emerging Infectious Diseases, 5*(4), 497. https://doi.org/10.3201/eid0504.990405

Cruz, M. A., Burger, R., & Keim, M. (2007). The first 24 hours of the World Trade Center attacks of 2001—The Centers for Disease Control and Prevention emergency phase response. *Prehospital and Disaster Medicine, 22*(6), 473–477. https://doi.org/10.1017/S1049023X00005288

Department of Homeland Security. (2012). *Plan and prepare for disasters.* https://www.dhs.gov/plan-and-prepare-disasters

Disaster Relief Act of 1974. (1974). Homeland Security Digital Library. https://www.hsdl.org/c/tl/disaster-relief-act-1974

Esbitt, D. (2003). The Strategic National Stockpile: Roles and responsibilities for health care professionals for receiving the stockpile assets. *Disaster Management and Response, 1*(3), 68–70. https://doi.org/10.1016/s1540-2487(03)00044-0

Escott, M. E. A. (2011). National response plan. In G. B. Kapur & J. P. Smith (Eds.), *Emergency public health* (pp. 45–62). Jones & Bartlett Learning.

Federal Emergency Management Agency. (2003). *A citizen's guide to disaster assistance* (pp. 3-1–3-32). Author. https://training.fema.gov/emiweb/downloads/is7unit_3.pdf

Fischer, H. W. (2003). The *sociology of* disaster: Definitions, research questions, & measurements: Continuation of the discussion in a post-September 11 environment. *International Journal of Mass Emergencies and Disasters, 21*(1), 91–107. http://www.ijmed.org/articles/82/download/

Gross, E. L. (2020). Pritzker says the Trump administration forced states to compete for PPE in a 'sick Hunger Games'. *Forbes.* https://www.forbes.com/sites/elanagross/2020/07/09/pritzker-says-the-trump-administration-forced-states-to-compete-for-ppe-in-a-sick-hunger-games

Haddow, G., Bullock, J., & Coppola, D. (2014). *Introduction to emergency management* (5th ed., pp. 1–30). Butterworth–Heinemann.

Hajjar, S. A., & McIntosh, K. (2010). The first influenza pandemic of the 21st century. *Annals of Saudi Medicine, 30*(1), 1–10. https://doi.org/10.5144/0256-4947.59365

Hamburg, M. A. (1999). Addressing bioterrorist threats: Where do we go from here? *Emerging Infectious Diseases, 5*(4), 564–565. https://doi.org/10.3201/eid0504.990421

Hatcher, S., Agnew-Brune, A., Anderson, M., Zambrano, L. D., Rose, C. E., Jim, M. A., Baugher, A., Liu, G. S., Patel, S. V., Evans, M. E., Pindyck, T., Dubray, C. L., Rainey, J. J., Chen, J., Sadowski, C., Winglee, K., Penman-Aguilar, A., Dixit, A., Claw, E., . . . McCollum, J. (2020). COVID-19 among American Indian and Alaska Native persons — 23 states, January 31–July 3, 2020. *Morbidity and Mortality Weekly, 69*(34), 1166–1169. https://doi.org/10.15585/mmwr.mm6934e1

Hathaway, E. D. (2021). American Indian and Alaska native people: Social vulnerability and COVID-19. *Journal of Rural Health, 37*, 256–259. https://doi.org/10.1111/jrh.12505

Hawkins, D. (2020). Differential occupational risk for COVID-19 and other infection exposure according to race and ethnicity. *American Journal of Industrial Medicine, 63*, 817–820. https://doi.org/10.1002/ajim.23145

History.com Editors. (2009, October 27). *Cold War history*. https://www.history.com/topics/cold-war/cold-war-history

Holshue, M., Debolt, C., Lindquist, S., Lofy, K. H., Wiesman, J., Bruce, H., Spitters, C., Ericson, K., Wilkerson, S., Tural, A., Diaz, G., Cohn, A., Fox, L., Patel, A., Gerber, S. I., Kim, L., Tong, S., Lu, X., Lindstrom, S., . . . Pillai, S. K. (2020). First case of novel 2019 corona virus in the United States. *New England Journal of Medicine, 382*(10), 929–936. https://doi.org/10.1056/nejmoa2001191

Homeland Security National Preparedness Task Force. (2006). *Civil defense and homeland security: A short history of national preparedness efforts*. Department of Homeland Security. https://training.fema.gov/hiedu/docs/dhs%20civil%20defense-hs%20-%20short%20history.pdf

Honoré, R. (2020). Speaking truth to power on how Hurricane Katrina beat us. *American Journal of Public Health, 110*(10), 1463–1465. https://doi.org/10.2105/ajph.2020.305778

International Federation of Red Cross and Red Crescent Societies. (n.d.). *Disaster preparedness*. https://media.ifrc.org/ifrc/what-we-do/disaster-and-crisis-management/disaster-preparedness

Kahane, L. (2021). Politicizing the mask: Political, economic and demographic factors affecting mask wearing behavior in the USA. *Eastern Economics Journal, 47*, 163–183. https://doi.org/10.1057/s41302-020-00186-0

Katz, R., Attal-Juncqua, A., & Fischer, J. (2017). Funding public health emergency preparedness in the United States. *American Journal of Public Health, 107*(Suppl. 2), S148–S152. https://doi.org/10.2105/AJPH.2017.303956

Khan, A. (2011). Public health preparedness and response in the USA since 9/11: A national security imperative. *The Lancet, 378*, 953–956. https://doi.org/10.1016/S0140-6736(11)61263-4

Kim-Farley, R. J. (2020). Sow the wind, reap the whirlwind: Katrina 15 years after. *American Journal of Public Health, 110*(10), 1448–1449. https://doi.org/10.2105/AJPH.2020.305881

Lancet. (2020). The plight of essential workers during the COVID-19 pandemic. *The Lancet, Editorial, 395*, 1587. https://www.thelancet.com/action/showPdf?pii=S0140-6736%2820%2931200-9

LeBlanc, T. T., Ekperi, L., Avchen, R., & Kosmos, C. (2018). Medical countermeasure actions – A historical perspective. *American Journal of Public Health, 108*(Suppl. 3), S175–S176. https://doi.org/10.2105/AJPH.2018.304707

LeBlanc, T. T., Ekperi, L., Kosmos, C., & Avchen, R. N. (2019). The virtual village: A 21st-century challenge for community preparedness. *American Journal of Public Health, 109*(Suppl. 4), S258–S259. https://doi.org/10.2105/AJPH.2019.305277

Li, S., & Bhattacharya, S. (2020, February 20). U.S. to repatriate some Americans from coronavirus cruise ship. *Wall Street Journal*. https://www.wsj.com/articles/u-s-to-evacuate-some-americans-from-diamond-princess-cruise-ship-11581733214?mod=e2tw

Lichtveld, M., Covert, H., El Dahr, J., Grimsley, L. F., Cohn, R., Watson, C. H., Thornton, E., & Kennedy, S. (2020). A community-based participatory research approach to Hurricane Katrina: When disasters, environmental health threats, and disparities collide. *American Journal of Public Health, 110*(10), 1485–1489. https://doi.org/10.2105/AJPH.2020.305759

Littman, R. (2009). The plague of Athens: Epidemiology and paleopathology. *Mount Sinai Journal of Medicine, 76*, 456–467. https://doi.org/10.1002/msj.20137

Loftus, P., & West, M. G. (2020). First COVID-19 vaccine given to U.S. public. *The Wall Street Journal*. https://www.wsj.com/articles/covid-19-vaccinations-in-the-u-s-slated-to-begin-monday-11607941806

Madrigal, A. C., & Meyer, R. (2020, June 7). America is giving up on the pandemic. *The Atlantic*. https://www.theatlantic.com/science/archive/2020/06/america-giving-up-on-pandemic/612796

McCormick, E. (2021, March 10). Grand Princess passengers grapple with COVID nightmare one year after ill-fated cruise. *The Guardian*. https://www.theguardian.com/us-news/2021/mar/10/grand-princess-cruise-ship-coronavirus-one-year-later

Molinari, N. M., LeBlanc, T. T., & Stephens, W. (2018, March 10). The impact of a case of Ebola virus disease on emergency department visits in Metropolitan Dallas-Fort Worth, TX, July, 2013–July, 2015: An interrupted time series analysis. *PLOS Currents Outbreaks, 10*. https://doi.org/10.1371/currents.outbreaks.e62bdea371ef5454d56f71fe217aead0

Moriarty, L. F., Plucinski, M. M., Marston, B. J., Kurbatova, E. V., Knust, B., Murray, E. L., Pesik, N., Rose, D., Fitter, D., Kobayashi, M., Toda, M., Cantey, P. T., Scheuer, T., Halsey, E. S., Cohen, N. J., Stockman, L., Wadford, D. A., Medley, A. M., Green, G., . . . Solano County COVID-19 Team. (2020). Public health responses to COVID-19 outbreaks on cruise ships—worldwide, February–March 2020. *Morbidity and Mortality Weekly, 69*(12), 347–352. https://doi.org/10.15585/mmwr.mm6912e3

National Commission on Children and Disasters. (2010). *2010 Report to the president and Congress* (AHRQ Publication No. 10-M037). Agency for Healthcare Research and Quality. https://www.acf.hhs.gov/sites/default/files/documents/ohsepr/nccdreport.pdf

Nelson, C. D., Willis, H. H., Chan, E. W., Shelton, S. R., & Parker, A. M. (2010). Federal initiative increases community preparedness for public health emergencies. *Health Affairs, 29*(12), 2286–2293. https://doi.org/10.1377/hlthaff.2010.0189

Parmet, W. E., & Rothstein, M. A. (2018). The 1918 influenza pandemic: Lessons learned and not—Introduction to the special section. *American Journal of Public Health, 108*(11), 1435–1436. https://doi.org/10.2105/ajph.2018.304695

Peirlinck, M., Linka, K., & Costabal, F. S. (2020). Outbreak dynamics of COVID-19 in China and the United States. *Biomech Model Mechanobiol, 19*(6), 2179–2193. https://doi.org/10.1007/s10237-020-01332-5

Pinsker, J. (2020, September 3). The pandemic has created a class of super-savers. *The Atlantic*. https://www.theatlantic.com/family/archive/2020/09/saving-money-pandemic/615949

Roberts, P. S. (2006). FEMA after Katrina. *Policy Review, 137*, 15–33. https://www.hoover.org/research/fema-after-katrina

Sharpe, T. T. (2000). The identity Christian movement: Ideology of domestic terrorism. *Journal of Black Studies, 30*(4), 604–623. https://www.jstor.org/stable/2645906

Sinclair, R., Probst, T., Watson, G., & Bazolli, A. (2021). Caught between Scylla and Charybdis: How economic stressors and occupational risk factors influence workers' occupational health reactions to COVID-19. *Applied Psychology: An International Review, 70*(1), 85–119. https://doi.org/10.1111/apps.12301

Slavitt, A. (2020). *The COVID-19 pandemic underscores the need to address structural challenges of the US health care system*. JAMA Network Health Forum. https://jamanetwork.com/channels/health-forum/fullarticle/2768097

Soergel, A. (2020). States competing in 'global jungle' for PPE. *U.S. News and World Report*. https://www.usnews.com/news/best-states/articles/2020-04-07/states-compete-in-global-jungle-for-personal-protective-equipment-amid-coronavirus

Stern, J. (1999). The prospect of domestic bioterrorism. *Emerging Infectious Diseases, 5*(4), 517–522. https://doi.org/10.3201/eid0504.990410

Stewart, A., & Cordell, G. A. (2007). Pharmaceuticals and the strategic national stockpile program. *Dental Clinics of North America, 51*, 857–869. https://doi.org/10.1016/j.cden.2007.06.001

Subbarao, I., Lyznicki, J., Hsu, E., Gebbie, K. M., Markenson, D., Barzansky, B., Armstrong, J. H., Cassimatis, E. G., Coule, P. L., Dallas, C. E., King, R. V., Rubinson, L., Sattin, R., Swienton, R. E., Lillibridge, S., Burkle, F. M., Schwartz, R. B., & James, J. J. (2008). A consensus based educational framework and competency set for the discipline of disaster medicine and public health preparedness. *Disaster Medicine and Public Health Preparedness, 2*(1), 58–68. http://doi.org/10.1097/DMP.0b013e31816564af

Subcommittee hearings on H.R. 9798, to authorize a federal civil defense program, House of Representatives, Committee on Armed Services, Special Subcommittee on Civil Defense. (1950). U.S. Government Printing Office #224. https://catalog.hathitrust.org/Record/100682557

Taylor, D. B. (2021). A timeline of the corona virus pandemic. *New York Times*. https://www.nytimes.com/article/coronavirus-timeline.html

Terrasse, M., Gorin, M., & Sisti, D. (2019). *Social media, e-health, and medical ethics*. Hastings Center Report. https://onlinelibrary.wiley.com/doi/epdf/10.1002/hast.975

U.S. Food and Drug Administration. (2021). *Emergency preparedness and response: COVID-19 vaccines*. https://www.fda.gov/emergency-preparedness-and-response/coronavirus-disease-2019-covid-19/covid-19-vaccines

Venkat, A., Asher, S. L., Wolf, L., Geiderman, J. M., Marco, C. A., McGreevy, J., Derse, A. R., Otten, E. J., Jesus, J. E., Kreitzer, N. P., Escalante, M., & Levine, A. C. (2015). Ethical issues in the response to Ebola virus disease in the United State emergency departments: A position paper of the American College of Emergency Physicians, the Emergency Nurses Association, and the Society for Academic Medicine. *Academic Emergency Medicine, 22*, 605–615. https://doi.org/10.1111/acem.12642

Walford, N. S. (2020). Demographic and social context of deaths during the 1854 cholera outbreak in Soho, London: A reappraisal of Dr John Snow's investigation. *Health and Place, 65*, 102402. https://doi.org/10.1016/j.healthplace.2020.102402

Wang, Y., McKee, M., Torbica, A., & Stuckler, D. (2019). Systematic literature review on the spread of health-related misinformation on social media. *Social Science Medicine, 240*, 112552. https://doi.org/10.1016/j.socscimed.2019.112552

White, G. W., Fox, M. H., Rooney, C., & Cahill, A. (2007, January). *Assessing the impact of Hurricane Katrina on persons with disabilities. Final report.* The University of Kansas, The Research and Training Center on Independent Living. https://www.hsdl.org/?abstract&did=470742

White, M., Wollebo, H., Beckman, J. D., Tyler, K. L., & Khalili, K. (2016). Zika virus: An emergent neuropathological agent. *Annals of Neurology, 80*(4), 479–489. https://doi.org/10.1002/ana.24748

World Health Organization. (2020). *Situational reports on the COVID-19 pandemic.* https://www.who.int/emergencies/diseases/novel-coronavirus-2019/situation-reports

Zeballos-Riog, J. (2020, February 25). *Top health officials are warning coronavirus will spread in the US—challenging Trump's claim the virus is contained.* Business Insider. https://markets.businessinsider.com/news/stocks/health-officials-coronavirus-spread-us-trump-says-contained-china-2020-2-1028938088#

Zimmermann, K. A. (2015). *Katrina: Facts, damage and aftermath.* Live Science. https://www.livescience.com/22522-hurricane-katrina-facts.html

CHAPTER 2

COMMUNITY PREPAREDNESS

A CHALLENGE FOR THE AGES

TANYA TELFAIR LEBLANC

KEY TERMS

Advanced Marginality
Coalition
Community Health Resilience (CHR)
Community Resilience
Disinformation
Misinformation
Social Capital
Whole Community Approach to Public Health Emergency Preparedness

INTRODUCTION

Acknowledging the challenges of past responses and recognizing that governments cannot effectively prepare the nation for the ever-increasing variety and complexity of emerging disasters, over a decade ago the Federal Emergency Management Agency (FEMA) published a framework for building preparedness at the community level. Though not prescriptive, *A Whole Community Approach to Emergency Management: Principles, Themes, and Pathways for Action* (FEMA, 2011) offers guidance to emergency managers for recognition of the important role of communities and engagement of communities in preparing for disasters and building resilience to rebound after disasters:

> As a concept, Whole Community is a means by which residents, emergency management practitioners, organizational and community leaders, and government officials can collectively understand and assess the needs of their respective communities and determine the best ways to organize and strengthen their assets, capacities, and interests. By doing so, a more effective path to societal security and resilience is built. In a sense, Whole Community is a philosophical approach on how to think about conducting emergency management. (FEMA, 2011, p. 3)

Communities are based on place, interests, beliefs, circumstances, and other important characteristics and form the social structure in which people live, work, worship, and play. Without engagement of these formal and informal institutions, plans to respond and recover from emergencies are fragmentary, at best. The goals of jurisdictional preparedness include protecting as many people as possible from looming threats, to pre-identify resources required to protect people from bodily harm, and to have strategies in place to recover from adverse events.

The **Whole Community Approach to Public Health Emergency Preparedness** advocates for understanding the human components that make up a community and available resources, engaging its private and public sectors, including businesses; faith-based organizations; academia; local, territorial, tribal, and state governments; citizens; nonprofit organizations; disability advocates; and many others, and providing a seat at the preparedness table for representatives of groups within a community. In practice, the Whole Community Approach is built upon a number of strategic themes:

- understanding community complexity
- recognizing community capabilities and needs
- fostering relationships with community leaders
- building and maintaining partnerships
- empowering local action
- leveraging and strengthening social infrastructure, networks, and assets

These strategies are important for application in public health emergency preparedness for communities. Historically, local health departments have been tasked with provision of medical, dental, nursing, engineering, scientific, epidemiological, and technical services to protect communities from infectious diseases, prevent unsanitary living conditions, guard food safety, track the spread of diseases, and perform a plethora of other functions (American Journal of Public Health, 1950). Currently, threats to the health of a community have expanded to include man-made and natural disasters that are occurring in increasing frequency and severity (U.S. Department of Health and Human Services [HHS], n.d.).

WHOLE COMMUNITY APPROACH

Developing public health emergency operations plans must utilize a whole-community approach to be effective. The community's capacity to prepare and respond to medical emergencies is strongest when it is built upon existing structures and relationships. Understanding diversity and community complexity begins with conducting risk assessments of communities that not only identify likely hazards that could cause medical emergencies but also identify geographic distributions of individuals with disease risks or special conditions that may complicate a response or require additional services or equipment during a response. In the public health sphere, diversity and community complexity include knowledge of diseases, conditions and disability prevalence, racial/ethnic disparities in diseases and conditions in a community, vaccination rates, insured versus uninsured, and barriers to healthcare. Disasters impact persons with disease risks and can interrupt vital testing and treatment services during interruption of routine life activities. Ekperi et al. (2018) found that, during Hurricane Sandy in 2012, which impacted the tristate New York area, HIV testing was severely interrupted in zones with high hurricane devastation, potentially delaying diagnoses and medical care for persons at risk for HIV disease. Courtney et al. (2021) found that, during COVID-19 pandemic conditions, blood lead testing decreased significantly among children, which could possibly result in missed opportunities for prevention of cognitive impairment among those at risk for exposure to lead. Comprehensive knowledge of community hazards and health concerns will contribute to planning ahead to develop Continuity of Operations (COOP) plans for continuation of vital medical services during periods of social and economic disruption.

Recognizing community capabilities and needs in the public health sphere includes knowing the availability and capacity of hospitals and clinics, doctors, nurses, and other medical staff; medical and emergency equipment stockpiles; disease surveillance systems; diagnostic testing; laboratory capacity and rapid disease detection ability; and the availability of medical transportation, pharmacies, and medical information translated into required languages or knowledge of and access to available translators.

Fostering relationships with community leaders to collaborate on preparedness efforts involves public health officials partnering with civic and social leaders in a community with the goal of building preparedness and community resilience. An example of such a partnership is New York City's Department of Health and Mental Hygiene's Office of Emergency Preparedness and Response Community Preparedness Program (CPP), launched in 2016. The CPP engaged community leaders in two sectors, human services and faith-based organizations, to galvanize support for preparedness in their respective communities and to generate interest in participation in preparedness awareness and trainings sessions among constituents (Rivera, Pagaoa, Molinari, et al., 2019; Rivera, Pagaoa, Morgenthau, et al., 2019).

Boards of education and school principals are also community leaders with connections to resources that could be tapped for use during emergencies, including using school buses for emergency transport and schools as shelters.

Building and maintaining partnerships among diverse and varied stakeholders are essential for community preparedness and critical for emergency response planning. The disparate systems, organizations, groups, and individuals that make up communities must be galvanized to build community strength and resilience. In addition to law enforcement, fire and rescue, and emergency medical services, emergency managers and public health officials should foster and sustain relationships with public utilities; hospitals; social service agencies and volunteer organizations; local media; universities and colleges; local, state, territorial, and tribal government officials; aviation and port authorities; hazard mitigation planners; medical examiners and coroners; public and private laboratories; transportation companies; and many other organizations (FEMA, State and Local Guide 101, 2010). **Coalitions** with local small businesses (e.g., barber shops and beauty salons), public health community-based organizations, and nonprofit organizations that serve microcommunities, addressing specific community needs, such as homeless and runaway youth, as well as social organizations and clubs (sororities, fraternities, alumni associations, boys and girls clubs, 4-H groups, etc.) may be able to assist emergency planners in identifying hidden community needs and assets that could be otherwise missed without their vital input to planning efforts. Establishing relationships with universities and colleges can enlist the help of cadres of health and behavioral scientists, data analysts, and other experts who can provide technical support for developing health assessment surveys, conducting evaluations of responses using after-action reports, synthesizing data from various sources, conducting risk assessments, and producing and interpreting statistics.

Empowering Local Action

Local people—those who live, work and worship in communities—have institutional and historical knowledge of neighborhoods and an understanding of needs among the people with whom they live. People representing neighborhoods, tribes, racial/ethnic groups, socioeconomic groups, faith-based organizations, and many others should be encouraged to participate in emergency preparedness planning and be given roles and responsibilities for protecting their communities and responding in emergencies. This will encourage support and "buy-in" for preparedness, response, and recovery activities and will provide vital information to planners from an insider perspective.

In establishing relationships with local people and community members, public health officials should strive for new frames of reference for encountering and interacting with diverse populations. Emergency planners should avoid using outdated concepts of cultural competency which sort individuals into broad racial/ethnic/gender or religious groups which oversimplify the complexity and micro-diversity, socioeconomic, language and cultural differences within the broad and frequently artificial groupings (Kirmayer, 2012). For appropriate communication and actions with racial, ethnic, gender, and religious diverse people, public health preparedness officials should consider simply applying the golden rule, "Do unto others as you would have them do unto you." Avoid expecting minorities to accept treatment that you would not accept. As public servants, endeavor to reduce, or at least put in check, inherent biases, and respect and acknowledge the dignity of every human being, regardless of social status. In addition, acknowledge that local people are the experts in understanding their respective communities and can aid in solving unique problems requiring insider knowledge.

An example of a successful program includes the 2014 collaborative partnership among university occupational health researchers, a labor union, and seven community-based organizations serving Latino immigrant communities in New York and New Jersey that created the Immigrant Worker Disaster Resilience Workgroup to strengthen community relationships and engage workers in preparedness awareness and training activities. Through the efforts of this program, some 5,000 workers were trained, with 25 of this number trained as specialized emergency response trainers to build capacity for continuing the work (Cuervo et al., 2017).

Building upon existing social capital, the public health sphere can leverage and strengthen social infrastructure, networks, and assets. **Social capital** is a concept in the social sciences defined as resources to which people and groups have access through social connections and networks (S. Moore & Kawachi, 2017). Social capital is characterized by interconnected networks of relationships among individuals and groups (social ties or social participation), levels of trust among people in the networks, and resources that are both gained and shared through social participation. Social capital is a primary driver of disaster resilience (Gero et al., 2020). Societies with strong social capital are better able to withstand the impact of a disaster with shared resources and trusted communication.

Public health practitioners can build social capital for public health emergency preparedness and response, as well as broaden healthcare coverage for hard-to-reach populations or populations with weaker social capital. One example to consider is the work accomplished by Project ECHO (Extension for Community Health Outcomes) of the University of New Mexico. In New Mexico, many citizens live in remote rural areas, without access to hospitals and specialty medical care in close geographic proximity. In 2003, Sanjeev Arora, MD, a social entrepreneur and liver disease specialist at the University of New Mexico Health Sciences Center in Albuquerque, developed a community of practice strategy to reach and teach primary care physicians serving remote areas to provide high-quality specialty care through "telementoring." Project ECHO delivers best-practice training in specialized medical treatments to primary care providers in rural areas through videoconferencing technology. Since 2003, Project ECHO has grown to cover a wide range of program specialties, including treatment for mental health disorders, substance abuse, education, infectious and chronic diseases, Indian country programs, miner's wellness, and emergency preparedness. Project ECHO is a guided-practice model that makes care available in underserved and remote areas of the state, nation, and world through knowledge sharing in which expert teams lead virtual clinics, expanding the capacity for providers to deliver best-in-practice care. Project ECHO builds social capital and partnerships among doctors, nurses, community health workers, case managers, medical assistants, pharmacists, and many other healthcare workers, who, in turn, confer direct health benefits to people in remote geographic areas (Project ECHO, 2020).

COMMUNITY RESILIENCE VERSUS COMMUNITY HEALTH RESILIENCE

According to the Assistant Secretary for Preparedness and Response, **community resilience** is the sustained ability of communities to withstand, adapt to, and recover from adversity (HHS, n.d.). **Community health resilience (CHR)** is the ability of a community to use its assets to strengthen public health and healthcare systems and to improve the community's physical, behavioral, and social health to withstand, adapt to, and recover from adversity (HHS, n.d.). Resilience must be built into a community long before adverse conditions occur that threaten day-to-day life. Resilient communities must have building blocks of resiliency, which include (a) a sound and cohesive social structure, characterized by trust, with individuals acting to mutually support the best interest of the whole; (b) a healthcare system that works reasonably well, with most people able to access medical care when they require it; and (c) an efficient communication system able to convey clear and unambiguous lifesaving messages to people most at risk for the impact of a disaster (LeBlanc, 2021). Thus, only one arm of community resilience, albeit an important one, is actually a factor of social cohesion. The structure of the entire society and its willingness to provide protective assets to populations are essential also.

CHALLENGES TO COMMUNITY PREPAREDNESS

THE CHANGING REALITIES OF "COMMUNITY"

Communities are second only to family among the most ancient of human institutions. Beginning with the earliest times, humans have banded together for mutual aid, companionship, economic survival, and protection from threats (A. Moore, 1993). Evidence of human communities living together are replete throughout prehistory and history. Since the beginning of the Industrial Revolution, social scientists expressed concerns about changes observed in the human experience as populations retreated from rural areas and traditional close-knit communities built on family units prevalent in agrarian societies in favor of impersonal employment in factory work and life in cities among strangers. In addition to communities organized around agriculture or industries, other communities were forged from people living in the same geographic area, sharing cultural or religious characteristics, occupations, and interests, or some other quality that bound people together (Halsall, 2014; Putnam, 2000). By the latter part of the 20th century, the way people experienced life began to shift dramatically. First Coleman (1988), and later Putnam (2000), observed that, in America, social isolation was becoming acute, with people not knowing their neighbors, dwindling church and club membership, and declining civic participation (Putnam, 2000).

In *Bowling Alone,* Putnam (2000) argues that changes in the economy and work, family structure, age, suburban life, women's roles, and the prominence of television and computers in daily life, among other factors, have contributed to a decline in American community life and deprive people of needed connections with each other. Many of the social norms that held societies together have eroded. For example, changes in the family structure with the decline in marriage and birthrates and increases in the number of people living alone is altering what we think of as foundational to traditional communities (Putnam, 2000). But despite these changes, communities were forged around occupation in the manufacturing industries, as well as some formidable institutions, such as churches, temples, and synagogues, which were available for huge swaths of the American population.

Demography and Economy

Communities in the United States have significantly changed in the past 50-plus years and the realities of current life in communities do not match the old paradigms and assumptions for community needs. In short, the communities of today are not the communities of the 1950s and public health preparedness efforts should also take this into account. Changes include economic and population growth in disaster vulnerable areas (FEMA, 2011), with coastal areas, floodplain areas, and barrier islands consistently attracting an influx of residents, leading to housing development sprawl and sparking tourism in these areas. Population aging, growth in persons with mental and physical disabilities living in residences rather than in singular institutions, and the plethora of persons in the general population living with chronic diseases (e.g., hypertension, asthma, obesity, kidney disease) add additional considerations for protection planning. Demographic shifts have also changed the makeup of some communities, with racial/ethnic minorities becoming more numerous in some areas due to immigration and fecundity trends (FEMA, 2011). Additional trends challenging preparedness plans include the dwindling of populations in the northeastern and midwestern states (Pew Charitable Trust, 2016), adults living alone, single parents with young children (U.S. Census Bureau, 2020), persons living in group homes or institutional settings (nursing homes, those in detention centers; U.S. Census Bureau, 2021a), unhoused persons, persons living in poverty, and persons living on the margins of society. For the past 50-plus years, economic, social, and political systems that formerly provided mechanisms for family stability and upward mobility in America have retracted, leaving a large segment of the population vulnerable to extreme poverty and social exclusion. Principally, deindustrialization eliminated millions of living-wage factory jobs available for persons without specific skills or clear career paths. Accompanying the reduction in jobs was a philosophical shift away from corporate responsibility and loyalty toward workers. The economy rapidly moved toward a bifurcated structure characterized by a high-end information technological-financial sector at the top requiring advanced education, and a low-end service sector at the bottom requiring minimal education. The buildup in low-level service sector jobs in this new economy provided neither the compensation nor benefits required for workers' life stability, safety, healthcare, or protection during emergency situations requiring resources. For more than three generations now, the poor have been overwhelmingly made up of very young, undereducated single mothers and their children trapped in decaying pockets first within inner cities, and now often isolated in rural areas. At the same time, political movements driven by perceptions of unworthiness of female-headed households retracted Lyndon Johnson's Great Society provisions to aid and train the poor, and reduced welfare benefits. High school completion rates in inner-city and rural poverty areas are some of the lowest in the nation, further diminishing chances to occupy high-level sector jobs. Persons born into such environments have been left out of the American social contract that assumes that through education and hard work, anyone can succeed. Thus, the changed opportunity structure in the country has contributed to the rise of increasingly intractable social inequality and the notion of **advanced marginality**. Advanced marginality differs from poverty in a number of ways. First, poverty can be a temporary state, whereas advanced marginality is viewed as multigenerational, long term, and perhaps even permanent. Second, pockets of people experiencing advanced marginality are geographically isolated from mainstream people and institutions that could provide access to opportunities for improved life chances. Third, the structure of society itself reinforces advanced marginality through fear, stigma, and media misrepresentations that fuel political judgments against efforts to assist people affected by the conditions that define the concept—poor educational outcomes, unemployment, homelessness, incarceration, substance use, geographic isolation, single parent female-headed household status, a lack of health insurance, and being a public assistance recipient (Wacquant, 2007). Public health emergency preparedness practitioners should at least be aware that many of these people are likely to live in their communities and present unique issues of isolation, are likely not connected to social institutions, may not be able to receive public health emergency warning or evacuation messages, and may be hidden in plain sight.

Technology and Imagined Communities

Although the term "community" is used extensively in the popular lexicon, its meaning has become murky, at best. In 1983, Benedict Anderson's treatise described the spread of imagined communities through wide distribution of print media. Currently, the concept of community itself is also challenged and conflicted by rapidly changing global economies, shifting population trends, social change, evolving cultural norms, and expanding technologies. In today's world, the internet has opened a Pandora's box for connecting people around the globe and sorting them into like-minded silos, where encounters with differing opinions are rare (Garber, 2017). Mobile devices, which many rely on to access the internet and use for both business and social activities, have become indispensible around the planet. People are becoming more isolated from real human interaction and spending more time in screen-based social or business networks and sharing and reinforcing ideas in cloistered internet-based groups. Thus, communities are increasingly becoming symbolic and based on a real or imagined affinity with an ideology and forming among people who may be geographically distant from each other. In short, communities are becoming more virtual than physical. Going further, with its easy access, unregulated nature, and anonymity, the internet makes it possible for almost anyone to have a forum to rapidly spread conspiracy theories and information not based on facts. Layered on top of this is the dramatic shift in the global economic structure, discussed earlier, which has been further challenged by the technological and information industries, which favor cognitive and collaborative job skills to support the expanding availability of information services, supplanting jobs that require physical dexterity. Jobs in information technology require higher education and specialized training. An unforeseen consequence of this trend is the millions of young and some not-so-young persons, primarily male, who do not possess the skills required in 21st-century career opportunities. Jobless and marginalized males often seek refuge in the dark corners of certain internet "communities" that offer rationalization for their plight based on some imaginary common enemy. Another deeply disturbing 21st-century complication is the retrenchment of science and rejection of scientific evidence in some virtual communities.

These phenomena have spawned a number of complex social problems that have spilled over onto government, public health, and other institutions and challenge efforts to galvanize communities for preparedness efforts. First, the anonymity of the internet and social media has opened the door for widespread misrepresentation of personas who purport to be authorities and may convince some audiences that they are reputable sources of information. Second, the self-selection cloistering effect of social media reinforces perspectives of the cloister to the exclusion of new information or differing opinions. Third, the internet and all forms of social media have opened doors for efficient conveyance of radical propaganda that may be used to spread and legitimize deviant behaviors and violence among marginalized and isolated individuals. Fourth, with deliberate **misinformation** and **disinformation**, the distinction between fact and fiction is blurred. A good example of this involves the rise of the anti-vaccination movement, which has been especially prominent during the recent COVID-19 pandemic. Fifth, the purveyors of faulty information have become particularly skilled in having spurious information "trend" widely, and we guardians of public health have catching up to do. Imagined communities, coupled with the spread of misinformation and disinformation, create unique and perhaps insurmountable barriers for building a true community response to a large-scale medical emergency.

Sustainability of Community Coalition Building

Coalitions equal community strength for building and sustaining effective preparedness programs that provide security for the maximum number of people in a neighborhood, village, or city. Building sustainable community coalitions can be challenging. Multistakeholder partnerships, with diverse constituents, can be difficult to manage, given competing priorities and varied perspectives on how activities should be undertaken and accomplished. Population mobility (U.S. Census Bureau, 2021b), attrition in public health careers (Leider et al., 2016), and personality mismatches can all contribute to strained or dissolving partnerships. Public health leaders and practitioners should invest in trainings and learn how to develop strategies for communicating with, and leading, diverse groups of people toward preparedness goals. In addition, public health leaders should understand that community coalitions are rarely static and are generally ever-changing. Thus, coalition building is never completed and must be a constant priority and activity for public health officials. To accomplish the task of building coalitions, one must understand the communities, the people who live in them, and the community's needs. Understanding who is in a community, what their circumstances are, what is required to respond to an emergency, and how to communicate with all or most of the stakeholders is central to implementing a successful preparedness and response program. Unfortunately, in many instances, only the people with connections have knowledge of community preparedness activities, with marginalized groups left behind.

CONCLUSION

In summary, to achieve robust levels of community resilience, public health professionals must first understand the people they serve and acknowledge that communities have changed. Preparedness planning and activities must include representation of the whole community to be effective. In addition, public health professionals must ensure wide distribution of factual information using appropriate messaging and channels to save lives during an emergency event. These are our challenges in preparing communities for emergencies; we must navigate the diversity divide and the communication technology terrain, break through the barriers, and identify the best ways to convey lifesaving information based on known facts and best evidence. This book provides practical examples and real-life case studies to demonstrate how foundational public health competencies may be applied to meet these and other challenges.

DISCUSSION QUESTIONS

1. Despite efforts to build community coalitions, some groups are inevitably omitted from preparedness and response activities. Discuss a strategy to reach hidden populations in your community.
2. Discuss how to conduct an assessment to find out who is living in your community, identify resources, and develop a plan to reach out to all or most.
3. Develop a community communication strategy to reach everyone in your community. Can this be done? Why or why not?
4. Discuss reasons why some people do not desire to participate in community efforts. Can you think of ways to encourage people who resist involvement to participate?

DISCLAIMER

This chapter was prepared by Tanya Telfair LeBlanc in his/her personal capacity. The opinions expressed in this article are the author's own and do not reflect the view of the Centers for Disease Control and Prevention, the Department of Health and Human Services, or the United States government.

REFERENCES

American Journal of Public Health. (1950). Local health department services and responsibilities: Official statement of the American Public Health Association. *American Journal of Public Health, 40*(1), 67–72. https://www.ncbi.nlm.nih.gov/pmc/articles/PMC1528496/

Anderson, B. (1983). *Imagined communities: Reflections on the origins and spread of nationalism.* Version.

Coleman, J.S. (1988). Social capital and the creation of human capital. *American Journal of Sociology, 94* (Suppl.), S95– S120. https://www.jstor.org/stable/2780243

Courtney, J., Chuke, S., Dyke, K., Credle, K., LeCours, C., Egan, K., & Leonard, M. (2021). Decreases in young children who received blood lead level testing during COVID-19–34 jurisdictions, January–May 2020. *Morbidity and Mortality Weekly, 7*(5), 155–161. https://doi.org/10.15585/mmwr.mm7005a2

Cuervo, I., Leopold, L., & Baron, S. (2017). Promoting community preparedness and resilience: A Latino immigrant community-driven project following Hurricane Sandy. *American Journal of Public Health, 107*(Suppl. 2), S161–S164. https://doi.org/10.2105/AJPH.2017.304053

Ekperi, L. I., Thomas, E., LeBlanc, T. T., Adams, E. E., Wilt, G. E., Molinari, N. A., & Carbone, E. G. (2018). The Impact of Hurricane Sandy on HIV Testing Rates: An Interrupted Time Series Analysis, January 1, 2011–December 31, 2013. *PLoS Currents, 10.* https://doi.org/10.1371/currents.dis.ea09f9573dc292951b7eb0cf9f395003

Federal Emergency Management Agency. (2010). *Guide for all-hazard emergency operations planning: State and local guide (SLG) 101.* https://www.fema.gov/pdf/plan/slg101.pdf

Federal Emergency Management Agency. (2011, December). *A whole community approach to emergency management: Principles, themes, pathways for action* (FDOC 104-008-1). https://www.fema.gov/sites/default/files/2020-07/whole_community_dec2011__2.pdf

Garber, M. (2017, July 3). What does 'community' mean? *The Atlantic.* https://www.theatlantic.com/entertainment/archive/2017/07/what-does-community-mean/532518

Gero, K., Hikichi, H., Aida, J., Kondo, K., & Kawachi, I. (2020). Associations between community social capital and preservation of functional capacity in the aftermath of a major disaster. *American Journal of Epidemiology, 189*(11), 1369–1378. https://doi.org/10.2105/AJPH.2017.304053

Halsall, J. R. (2014). The re-invention of sociology of community. *International Review of Social Sciences and Humanities, 8*(1), 91–98. http://eprints.hud.ac.uk/id/eprint/22382

Kirmayer, L. J. (2012). Rethinking cultural competence. *Transcultural Psychology, 49*(2), 149–164. https://doi.org/10.1177/1178632920970580

LeBlanc, T. T. (2021). Strengthening social and economic, medical, and public health systems before disasters strike. *American Journal of Public Health, 111*(5), 842–843. https://doi.org/10.2105/AJPH.2021.306247

Leider, J. P., Harper, E., Shon, J. W., Sellers, K., & Castrucci, B. (2016). Job satisfaction and expected turnover among federal, state and local public health practitioners. *American Journal of Public Health, 106*, 1782–1788. https://doi.org/10.2105/AJPH.2016.303305

Moore, A. (1993). *Cultural anthropology: The field study of human beings* (pp. 109–127). Collegiate Press.

Moore, S., & Kawachi, I. (2017). Twenty years of social capital and health research: A glossary. *Journal of Epidemiology and Community Health, 71*, 513–517. https://doi.org/10.1136/jech-2016-208313

Pew Charitable Trust. (2016, March 27). *Many Northeast, Midwest states facing dwindling workforce.* https://www.pewtrusts.org/en/research-and-analysis/blogs/stateline/2016/05/27/many-northeast-midwest-states-face-shrinking-workforce

Putnam, R. D. (2000). *Bowling alone.* Simon & Schuster.

Rivera, L., Pagaoa, M., Molinari, N., Morgenthau, B., & LeBlanc, T. T. (2019). Preassessment of community-based organization preparedness in two sectors, human services and faith-based, New York City 2016. *American Journal of Public Health, 109*(S4), S290–S296. https://doi.org/10.2105/AJPH.2019.305141

Rivera, L., Pagaoa, M., Morgenthau, B., Paquet, C., Molinari, N., & LeBlanc, T. T. (2019). Participation in community preparedness programs in human services organizations and faith-based organizations—New York City, 2018. *Morbidity and Mortality Weekly, 68*(35), 757–761. https://doi.org/10.15585/mmwr.mm6835a2

University of New Mexico. (n.d.). *Project Echo*. https://hsc.unm.edu/echo

U.S. Census Bureau. (2020). *Historical household tables*. https://www.census.gov/data/tables/time-series/demo/families/households.html

U.S. Census Bureau. (2021a). 2020 census *group quarters*. https://www.census.gov/newsroom/blogs/random-samplings/2021/03/2020-census-group-quarters.html

U.S. Census Bureau. (2021b). *CPS historical migration/geographic mobility tables*. https://www.census.gov/data/tables/time-series/demo/geographic-mobility/historic.html

U.S. Department of Health and Human Services. (n.d.). *Community resilience*. https://www.phe.gov/Preparedness/planning/abc/Pages/community-resilience.aspx

Wacquant, L. (2007). *Urban outcasts: A comparative sociology of advanced marginality*. Polity Press.

Community Preparedness Resources

https://www.ready.gov/community-preparedness-toolkit

https://www.fema.gov/emergency-managers/individuals-communities/faith-preparedness

https://www.fema.gov/emergency-managers/individuals-communities/voluntary-organizations

https://www.fema.gov/emergency-managers/individuals-communities/children

https://www.fema.gov/sites/default/files/2020-07/developing-maintaining-emergency-operations-plans.pdf

https://www.fema.gov/emergency-managers/practitioners/resilience-analysis-and-planning-tool

https://www.fema.gov/sites/default/files/2020-06/fema-tribal-planning-handbook_05-2019.pdf

https://www.naccho.org/programs/public-health-preparedness

https://www.naccho.org/programs/public-health-preparedness/community-resilience

https://assets.publishing.service.gov.uk/government/uploads/system/uploads/attachment_data/file/552867/pfe_guide_for_communities.pdf

https://www.gov.uk/government/publications/preparing-for-emergencies/preparing-for-emergencies#community-resilience

https://www.london.gov.uk/sites/default/files/community_preparedness_report.pdf

https://www.phe.gov/about/aspr/Pages/default.aspx

https://www.phe.gov/Preparedness/planning/abc/Pages/community.aspx

https://asprtracie.hhs.gov

https://hsc.unm.edu/echo/institute-programs/covid-19-response/nm-covid19/first-responder

Resources for Coalition Building

https://www.amazon.com/Crucial-Conversations-Talking-Stakes-Second/dp/1469266822

CHAPTER 3

ALL-HAZARDS PREPAREDNESS DESIGN

A Systems Approach

Glen P. Mays

KEY TERMS

Backbone Organization
Cooperative Agreement
Emergency Preparedness Capabilities
Emergency Support Function #8
Moratoria
Underrepresented and Marginalized Communities

INTRODUCTION

> By failing to prepare, you are preparing to fail.
>
> — *Benjamin Franklin*

Emergency preparedness depends upon a broad collection of resources and practices that help communities prepare for and respond to the health consequences of hazardous events. These capabilities demand contributions from a wide array of stakeholders operating in both the public and private sectors, including public health but also medical care, emergency management, transportation, business, and social services sectors. This chapter examines key principles and practices in designing emergency preparedness systems that can address a wide variety of health threats, using an all-hazards perspective. A clear understanding of the desired functions and capabilities of the preparedness system is required, along with a detailed map of the stakeholders who perform these functions and their relationships. Preparedness systems vary widely across the United States in their design and in their performance, revealing significant opportunities for improvement.

DEFINING EMERGENCY PREPAREDNESS SYSTEMS

An emergency preparedness system comprises the institutions that participate in preparing for and responding to hazardous events for a defined population of residents, along with the relationships that connect these institutions and help them work together (Centers for Disease Control and Prevention [CDC], 2018). These interorganizational systems operate at multiple levels of geographic scale, beginning at the local community level such as a county or city. Systems also operate at larger units of geography, including regional multi-county districts, states and territories, and multistate regions, as well as at national and international levels. A wide variety of institutions participate in emergency preparedness systems, including public health agencies, emergency management agencies, hospitals and other healthcare providers, public safety agencies, social service providers, businesses and employers, public utilities, and faith-based organizations.

FEDERAL, STATE, AND LOCAL ROLES

Given the structural complexity of these systems, it becomes important to identify how roles and responsibilities are distributed across stakeholders within each system. The federated structure of government in the United States distributes responsibilities for emergency preparedness across federal, state, territorial, tribal, and local (STLT) governments, with significant responsibilities delegated to the state/territorial and local levels (Figure 3.1; Nowell et al., 2018). At the federal level, the Federal Emergency Management Agency (FEMA) within the U.S. Department of Homeland Security has responsibility for the National Preparedness System that includes plans and protocols for responding to events that threaten national security. Within this federal system, the U.S. Department of Health and Human Services (HHS) and the CDC have lead responsibility for managing public health and medical support functions at the national level. The HHS preparedness activities are coordinated through the Assistant Secretary of Preparedness and Response (ASPR), with responsibilities that include planning, resource management, and research.

Federal agencies rely heavily on STLT governments and their community partners to implement emergency preparedness plans and protocols at all levels of geography across the United States. Correspondingly, federal agencies provide funding, technical assistance, data, and decision tools to STLT governments to inform and support their activities. For example, FEMA's National Incident Management System (NIMS) defines a clear chain of command for making decisions during emergency events, along with protocols and processes followed by all levels of government and the private sector in preparing for and responding to these events (Jensen & Youngs, 2015). FEMA also provides funds to state and local emergency management agencies and their partners to support adoption of NIMS and related work in hazard assessment, planning, mitigation, response, and recovery. Similarly, the CDC's Public Health Preparedness and Response Capabilities identify the core responsibilities of governmental public health agencies and their community partners in preparing for and responding to hazardous events and includes processes for assessing and improving these capabilities (CDC, 2018). The CDC distributes funds to STLT governments and their partners to support the development and improvement of these capabilities. The ASPR carries out activities that span the public health and medical care responsibilities of HHS, including development of a comprehensive preparedness and

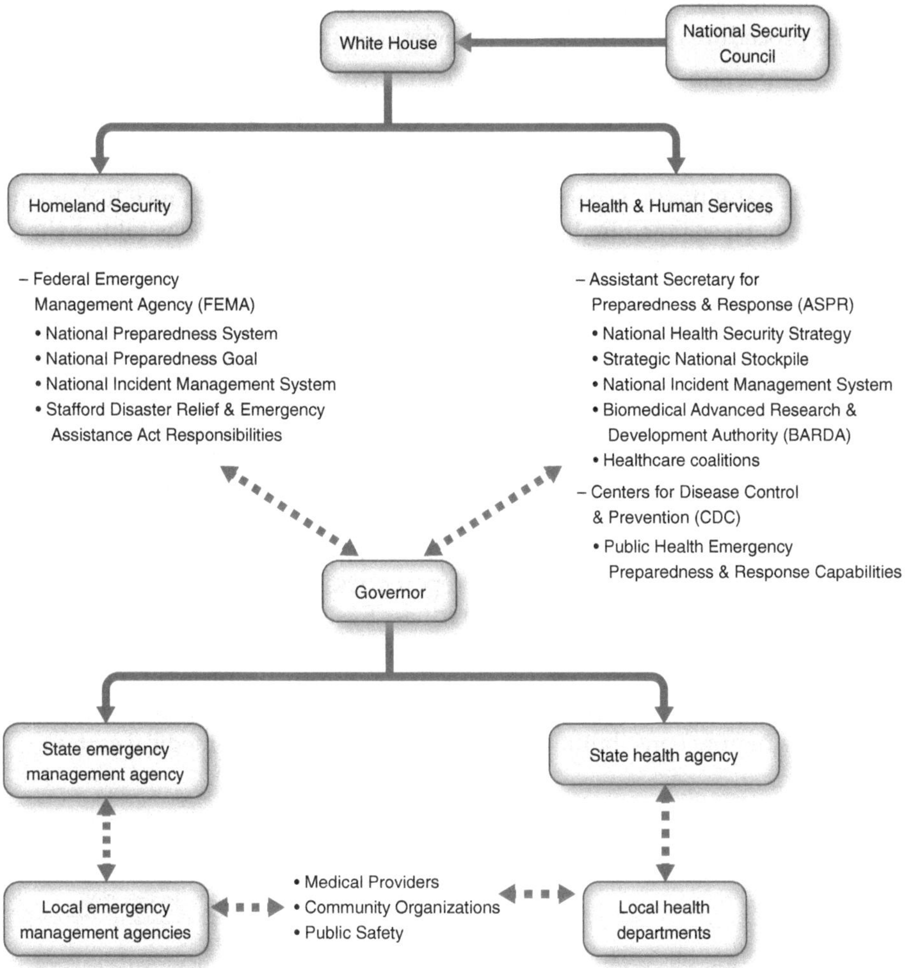

Figure 3.1 Institutions that shape the design of emergency preparedness systems.

response strategy called the National Health Security Strategy; management of the Strategic National Stockpile containing protective medical therapies, vaccines, supplies, and equipment; and oversight of the Biomedical Advanced Research and Development Authority (BARDA) that develops new medical and pharmaceutical products that offer protection against major health threats (ASPR, 2018).

State governments have broad legal powers in preparing for and responding to hazardous events, including the regulation of medical practices, businesses, local governments, and personal behavior (Gostin, 2000). Some of these powers are implemented and enforced through state public health agencies, such as quarantine and isolation orders and vaccination requirements, while other powers are exercised by other state agencies or by the governor directly. Additionally, state governments delegate some of these powers to local governments, where they are implemented by local health departments and other city and county agencies. The COVID-19 pandemic during 2020 and 2021 required the activation of many of these powers at both state and local levels, including business closures, worksite restrictions, mask requirements, restrictions on public and private gatherings, hospital restrictions on elective medical procedures, and **moratoria** on evictions (Gostin & Wiley, 2000).

CORE FUNCTIONS AND CAPABILITIES

A critical first step in designing any system involves identifying the desired functions and capabilities to be performed. These capabilities determine which institutions need to be engaged in the system and how roles and responsibilities should be allocated among these institutions. Federal agencies have taken the lead in identifying core functions and capabilities for U.S. emergency preparedness systems through an interconnected series of federal frameworks that have developed and improved over time (Figure 3.2). At the highest level, FEMA's National Preparedness System identifies core functions for emergency preparedness systems as a whole, including all levels of government and nongovernmental institutions operating within all relevant sectors (Institute of Medicine [IOM], 2015). One element of this system, known as **Emergency Support Function #8 (ESF #8)**, focuses specifically on functions to address the public health and medical needs of populations before, during, and after hazardous events (FEMA, 2019). A related framework, FEMA's National Preparedness Goal, specifies 32 capabilities to be performed by the National Preparedness System, spanning the five mission areas of prevention, protection, mitigation, response, and recovery (Obama, 2011). One of these 32 capabilities focuses specifically on the implementation of public health, healthcare, and emergency medical services, while many of the other capabilities require contributions from the public health and medical sectors.

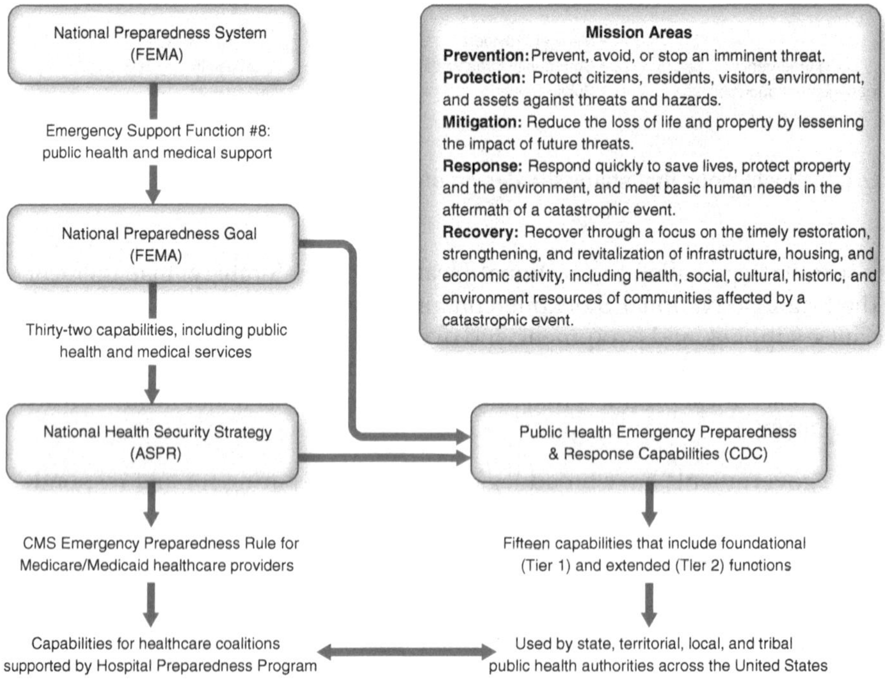

Figure 3.2 Federal frameworks that define emergency preparedness functions and capabilities.

ASPR, Assistant Secretary for Preparedness and Response; CDC, Centers for Disease Control and Prevention; CMS, Centers for Medicare and Medicaid Services; FEMA, Federal Emergency Management Agency.

A third framework, the ASPR's National Health Security Strategy, identifies functions to be performed by sectors that contribute broadly to health protection activities, including especially the public health and medical care sectors (ASPR, 2018). This strategy identifies key roles for numerous federal agencies and programs that carry out public health and medical care responsibilities, including the CDC, Medicare and Medicaid, the National Institutes of Health, the Veterans Health Administration, the Substance Abuse and Mental Health Services Administration (SAMHSA), the U.S. Department of Defense, the Environmental Protection Agency, the U.S. Department of Agriculture, and many others. Informed by this strategy, the ASPR identifies emergency preparedness functions that healthcare providers are required to carry out as a condition of their participation in the federal Medicare and Medicaid programs. These requirements are specified in a federal regulation known as the Centers for Medicare and Medicaid Services (CMS) Emergency Preparedness Rule (Ramsey Hamilton & Miller, 2017). Similarly, the ASPR defines **emergency preparedness capabilities** to be performed by hospitals and other community partners that participate in the federal Hospital Preparedness Program (HPP). The HPP provides funding and technical assistance to support a national network of regional healthcare coalitions focused on emergency preparedness and response, with coalition membership that includes local hospitals, public health agencies, emergency medical services agencies, emergency management agencies, and other community organizations (Ramsey Hamilton & Miller, 2017).

Informed by these larger frameworks, the CDC plays the leading federal role in defining capabilities performed by the public health sector within the nation's emergency preparedness systems. These elements, known as Public Health Emergency Preparedness and Response (PHEPR) Capabilities, are tightly integrated with capabilities defined for other sectors and stakeholders, including those articulated in the FEMA and ASPR frameworks (CDC, 2018). The CDC PHEPR framework defines a total of 15 capabilities, which fall within two tiers (Exhibit 3.1). Tier 1 capabilities function as foundational elements for public health agencies, while Tier 2 capabilities build upon and extend the Tier 1 capabilities in collaboration with external partners and collaborators. The capabilities reflect six crosscutting domains of activity for public health agencies: community resilience (Capabilities #1 and #2), incident management (Capability #3); information management (Capabilities #4 and #6), countermeasures and mitigation (Capabilities #8, #9, #11, and #15), surge management (Capabilities #5, #7, #10, and #14), and surveillance (Capabilities #12, and #13). The CDC supports implementation of these capabilities by providing funding and technical assistance to state, territorial, local, and

EXHIBIT 3.1 Capabilities for Public Health Emergency Preparedness and Response Defined by the CDC

1: Community Preparedness (Tier 1): Identify risks and hazards that threaten the health of the jurisdiction, strengthen community partnerships to support preparedness for hazardous events, coordinate with partners and share information through community social networks, and coordinate training and provide guidance to support community involvement with preparedness efforts.
2: Community Recovery (Tier 2): Identify and monitor community recovery needs that result from a hazardous event; support recovery operations for public health, healthcare, human services, and related systems in the community; and implement corrective actions to mitigate damage from future incidents.

(continued)

EXHIBIT 3.1 Capabilities for Public Health Emergency Preparedness and Response Defined by the CDC (*continued*)

3: Emergency Operations Coordination (Tier 1): Coordinate with emergency management to implement public health emergency operations protocols by establishing a standardized, scalable system of oversight, organization, and supervision that is consistent with jurisdictional standards and practices and the National Incident Management System.
4. Emergency Public Information and Warning (Tier 1): Develop, coordinate, and disseminate information, alerts, warnings, and notifications to the public and to incident management personnel.
5. Fatality Management (Tier 2): Support the recovery and preservation of remains; the identification of the deceased; the determination of cause and manner of death; the release of remains to authorized individuals; and the provision of mental/behavioral health assistance for the grieving.
6: Information Sharing (Tier 1): Conduct multijurisdictional and multidisciplinary exchange of health-related information and situational awareness data among federal, state, local, tribal, and territorial levels of government and the private sector.
7: Mass Care (Tier 2): Coordinate with and support partner agencies to address the public health, healthcare, mental/behavioral health, and human services needs of those impacted by an incident using large-scale congregate delivery modalities. This capability includes coordinating ongoing surveillance and public health assessments to ensure that health needs are met as the incident evolves.
8: Medical Countermeasure Dispensing and Administration (Tier 1): Provide medical countermeasures to targeted population(s) to prevent, mitigate, or treat the adverse health effects of a public health incident, according to public health guidelines. This capability focuses on dispensing and administering medical countermeasures such as vaccines, antiviral drugs, antibiotics, and antitoxins.
9: Medical Material Management and Distribution (Tier 1): Acquire, manage, transport, and track medical material during a public health incident or event, and recover and account for unused medical material, such as pharmaceuticals, vaccines, gloves, masks, ventilators, or medical equipment after an incident.
10: Medical Surge (Tier 2): Provide adequate medical evaluation and care during events that exceed the limits of the normal medical infrastructure of an affected community. Functions include assisting the healthcare system in coping with a hazard impact, maintaining or rapidly recovering operations that were compromised, and supporting the delivery of medical care and associated public health services, including disease surveillance, epidemiological inquiry, laboratory diagnostic services, and environmental health assessments.
11: Nonpharmaceutical Interventions (Tier 2): Implement actions that people and communities can use to slow the spread of illness or reduce the adverse impact of public health emergencies, including isolation, quarantine, restrictions on movement and travel, social distancing, external decontamination, hygiene, and other precautionary protective behaviors.
12: Public Health Laboratory Testing (Tier 1): Implement methods to detect, characterize, and confirm public health threat agents in multiple matrices, including clinical specimens, food, water, soil, and other environmental samples. Functions include the ability to securely acquire and transport samples, report timely data, provide investigative support, and use partnerships to address actual or potential exposures.
13: Public Health Surveillance and Epidemiological Investigation (Tier 1): Create, maintain, support, and strengthen routine surveillance and detection systems and epidemiological investigation processes. This function includes the ability to expand surveillance systems and processes in response to incidents of public health significance.
14: Responder Safety and Health (Tier 2): Protect public health and other emergency responders during predeployment, deployment, and postdeployment phases of incident response.
15: Volunteer Management (Tier 1): Coordinate with emergency management and partner agencies to identify, recruit, register, verify, train, and engage volunteers to support the public health agency's preparedness, response, and recovery activities during predeployment, deployment, and postdeployment phases of incident response.

CDC, Centers for Disease Control and Prevention.

Source: Data from Centers for Disease Control and Prevention. (2018). *Public Health Emergency Preparedness and Response Capabilities: National standards for state, local, tribal and territorial public health*. https://www.cdc.gov/cpr/readiness/00_docs/CDC_PreparednesResponseCapabilities_October2018_Final_508.pdf tribal public health authorities across the United States through the PHEPR **Cooperative Agreement** Program and related initiatives.

The concept of all-hazards preparedness is central to all the federal frameworks used by FEMA, the ASPR, and the CDC. This concept means that emergency preparedness capabilities should be designed to address a wide range of potential hazardous events, including those involving biological, chemical, radiological, nuclear, explosive, environmental, technological, and psychological threats (Marcozzi & Lurie, 2012). Federal frameworks require preparedness systems to conduct hazard vulnerability assessments on a regular basis in order to identify the likelihood and severity of various types of hazards in the geographic areas served and to identify the population subgroups most vulnerable to each type of hazard. FEMA, for example, recommends that communities use the Threat and Hazard Identification and Risk Assessment protocol, which helps users identify community-specific threats and hazards, set capability targets for each core capability identified in the National Preparedness Goal, and estimate resources needed to meet the capability targets (IOM, 2015). Using this type of information, preparedness system stakeholders can tailor their capabilities to the specific types of risks and vulnerabilities found within their service areas.

SYSTEM DESIGN FEATURES

A fundamental challenge facing emergency preparedness systems operating at all levels of geography involves coordination across institutions and sectors. These systems comprise diverse government and private-sector organizations that operate with different missions, incentives, and resources. Many organizations do not specialize solely in emergency preparedness, and they often face difficult trade-offs between investing time and money in preparedness capabilities as compared to investing in other mission areas often considered to be of more immediate priority. Emergency preparedness is largely a public good that benefits the entire community, so the economic phenomenon of free-rider problems can lead institutions to underinvest in these capabilities under the assumption that other community stakeholders will address the needs (Carande-Kulis et al., 2007; Olson, 1971). Additionally, the costs of developing and maintaining preparedness capabilities are immediate and ongoing for contributing organizations, while the benefits of these capabilities may be observable only over the longer term when future hazardous events occur. Such time inconsistencies can lead institutions to delay or forego investing in preparedness, particularly when confronting more immediate resource needs. Because hazardous events are uncertain as to their location and severity, the costs and the benefits of preparedness capabilities may not accrue equitably across community organizations, causing some organizations to bear a disproportionate share of costs while others experience disproportionate benefits. This economic phenomenon, known as the wrong-pocket problem, can also lead organizations to underinvest in preparedness.

Emergency preparedness systems are particularly vulnerable to free-riding, time-inconsistency, and wrong-pocket problems because of the heavy dependence on collective actions within these systems (Carande-Kulis et al., 2007; Olson, 1971). These problems may diminish the performance of emergency preparedness systems significantly by eroding contributions from selected community partners. Several strategies, described in the following, can help to mitigate these problems and facilitate multisector coordination.

Backbone Institutions

Multisector partnerships and networks benefit when at least one organization performs key convening and coordinating roles for the entire system (Kania & Kramer, 2011). These backbone institutions typically provide a wide variety of administrative functions for the system, including recruiting and retaining participating institutions; maintaining rosters of participants and key contacts; operating communication channels such as email lists, websites, and phone trees; scheduling and managing recurring meetings; planning key events such as training sessions and exercises; and serving as the repository for key documents and resources such as assessments, strategic plans, and operating protocols. **Backbone organizations** often play roles in distributing funding or other key resources throughout the system, managing financial resources and human resources that are shared by the system, maintaining contracts and agreements among participating institutions, and administering grants and other shared funding vehicles that support the work of the system. These organizations also perform key leadership functions such as helping participants reach consensus on key decisions, resolving conflicts, establishing a culture of trust and transparency, and promoting the mission, vision, and values of the system.

State and local public health agencies often function as backbone institutions for emergency preparedness systems because of their legal authorities and administrative capabilities relevant to emergencies. State and territorial health agencies, along with several large metropolitan local health departments, serve as the lead recipients for federal funding programs such as the CDC PHEPR Cooperative Agreement program and the ASPR HPP and are responsible for distributing federal funds to other community partners within these programs (IOM, 2015). Similarly, state and local emergency management agencies provide these roles for emergency preparedness funding programs administered by FEMA, and as such these agencies are also strongly positioned for the backbone institution role. This mix of emergency preparedness funding streams and recipient agencies has the potential to create confusion and conflicts regarding designated backbone institutions. To prevent or resolve conflicts, some jurisdictions divide this role between two or more agencies with clearly developed lines of responsibility and coordination mechanisms (Nowell et al., 2018). Other jurisdictions create multiagency councils or separate not-for-profit organizations to perform the backbone institution roles on behalf of the government agencies.

Governance and Decision-Making Structures

Multisector networks require effective governance structures to provide oversight and strategic direction for the collaborative. State and local emergency preparedness systems are no different from other types of networks in this need for effective governance. State and local laws determine both the existence of governing bodies as well as their composition and duties. Some governments create independent governing boards to oversee emergency preparedness activities, while others delegate these oversight responsibilities to other entities, such as state and local boards of health, or to subdivisions of elected bodies such as county commissioners and city councils. Governing bodies often benefit when they include representation from all the major sectors engaged in emergency preparedness activities, in order to facilitate buy-in and ensure that a full range of perspectives inform key decisions. Additionally, governing bodies often benefit by including stakeholders from outside the formal emergency preparedness system in order to bring in additional areas of expertise and obtain independent perspectives.

Governing bodies that oversee emergency preparedness systems at state and local levels vary widely in their powers and duties as defined in law (Nowell et al., 2018). Some are empowered with strong decision-making authority such as the ability to approve budgets, allocate resources, hire and fire leadership, evaluate system performance, and adopt policies and procedures concerning the operation of the system (Carlson et al., 2015). Alternatively, some bodies hold advisory responsibilities only, with decision-making retained by elected government officials or government agencies. Governing bodies are well positioned to promote multisector coordination in emergency preparedness when they have the following attributes: (a) include broad representation of relevant sectors, areas of expertise, and communities—including historically **underrepresented and marginalized communities**; (b) include independent voices from outside of emergency preparedness systems, such as scientific and research institutions, community-based organizations, and consumer advocacy; (c) hold at least some decision-making authority regarding resource allocation, policies, and performance evaluation; and (d) use consistent and transparent processes for making decisions (Hyde & Shortell, 2012; Varda et al., 2012).

Information Exchange and Communication

Emergency preparedness systems require robust capabilities for acquiring, exchanging, and analyzing information relevant to hazards and risks (IOM, 2015). These capabilities allow relevant stakeholders within the system to maintain situational awareness about current and potential threats, to monitor the use of resources in responding to these threats, to identify highly vulnerable population groups, and to update preparedness and response activities rapidly as circumstances change. Stakeholders require capabilities for exchanging and linking a wide variety of information sources relevant to hazard risks and responses, in near-real time, including (Gotham et al., 2007):

- public health surveillance data regarding cases of disease and injury, deaths, hospitalizations, emergency department use, vaccinations, drug overdoses, and unusual symptoms
- healthcare and electronic medical record data on real-time resource availability such as hospital and intensive care unit beds, physician and nurse staffing levels, vaccine supply, and the location of patients with electricity-dependent medical resource needs
- 911 call center data on call volume, location, and types of emergency response by police, fire, ambulance, and other first responders
- law enforcement and criminal intelligence data regarding threat-related information

- social service agency data on real-time resource availability such as temporary shelter space, emergency food assistance, housing assistance, and childcare services
- demographic and socioeconomic data describing the prevalence of social and economic characteristics that place people at elevated risk during hazardous events, including historically marginalized racial and ethnic groups as well as poverty, crowded housing, a lack of transportation, and language barriers
- environmental and weather monitoring data, including air and water quality monitoring, temperature, storm, fire, and flood stage tracking data
- facility licensing and inspection data on the locations of relevant businesses and industries, including those with potentially hazardous biological, chemical, radiological, and nuclear agents
- traffic, transportation, and mobility monitoring data, including road volumes, transportation times, evacuation routes, public transit, and cellphone mobility data

State and local jurisdictions vary widely in the availability, quality, and timeliness of these data sources and in the ability to exchange, link, and analyze data sources rapidly. The COVID-19 pandemic during 2020 and 2021 exposed these variabilities, with many jurisdictions experiencing gaps and delays in the acquisition of information regarding diagnostic testing, confirmed cases, hospitalizations, deaths, and vaccinations—particularly for racial and ethnic minority populations (Krieger et al., 2020). Some jurisdictions have access to specialized resources that facilitate these types of capabilities, including local and regional health information exchanges, social information exchanges, syndromic surveillance systems, and medical claims data repositories. But many other jurisdictions lack access to these types of resources, particularly in rural areas and low-resource communities. As one notable asset, the U.S. Department of Homeland Security and the U.S. Department of Justice support a national network of 70 Fusion Centers located in every state and in major metropolitan cities that allow the exchange of threat-related information across federal, state, and local levels (Lenart et al., 2012). Public health emergency preparedness systems can strengthen their information-sharing capabilities by helping their stakeholders become trained and authorized in using Fusion Center resources.

Performance Measurement and Reporting

One of the most important tools in promoting coordination within state and local emergency preparedness systems is a robust approach for measuring system performance and reporting this information back to both internal and external stakeholders. Measurement and reporting capabilities promote multisector coordination through several important pathways (Hyde & Shortell, 2012; Krieger et al., 2020; Varda et al., 2012). These capabilities allow stakeholders within the system to identify areas of relative strength and weakness and to detect how performance changes over time. This information can serve as a source of motivation for stakeholders, helping them to set goals, monitor progress, and document accomplishments. This information can stimulate productive peer pressure by helping collaborating organizations hold each other accountable for shared performance outcomes. When shared with external stakeholders like public officials, the media, and the public, performance information can promote broad awareness about preparedness levels that can lead to enhanced public support. Finally, comparative information about performance across state and local emergency preparedness systems allows stakeholders to identify external benchmarks, engage in friendly competition, and identify strategies used in other jurisdictions to improve performance.

Several resources exist to help state and local emergency preparedness systems engage in performance measurement and reporting. First, federal agencies maintain program-specific performance measurement initiatives, including the CDC's PHEPR Cooperative Agreement program and the ASPR's HPP (CDC, n.d.). A key strength of these initiatives is that they use measures developed specifically to reflect the objectives and capabilities emphasized in each program, ensuring that results are highly relevant to program activities and that results reveal the extent to which programs are meeting their goals. An important limitation, however, is that these initiatives often revise their measures over time to reflect changes in program priorities, thereby precluding the ability to track progress over time. These programs rely primarily on measures reported by the recipients of federal funding, which are typically not validated or independently verified and which are vulnerable to reporting biases due to their association with funding. Because each performance measurement initiative is program specific, the results cannot be easily combined across programs to examine the performance of the emergency preparedness system as a whole. Finally, these initiatives often do not publicly report comparative information on performance, thereby reducing the opportunities for peer pressure, friendly competition, and public awareness to motivate improvements.

An alternative performance measurement and reporting initiative, the National Health Security Preparedness Index, addresses some of the limitations inherent in federal program-specific initiatives. The Index uses a large collection of measures drawn from a variety of different data sources in order to assess the performance of state and local emergency preparedness systems as a whole (Mays et al., 2020; Uzun Jacobson et al., 2014). The Index uses measures derived from national data sources that are collected consistently over time, thereby allowing for valid assessments of change and progress. The Index aggregates information from a diverse collection of measures derived from multiple sources—including public health agencies, hospitals, federal inspectors, and administrative data—thereby reducing vulnerabilities due to reporting biases from a single source. Finally, the Index publicly reports comparative information on results annually, thereby encouraging peer comparisons, peer learning, friendly competition, and public awareness. The Index is well suited to explore patterns of variation and change in state and local emergency preparedness systems, as demonstrated in the next section.

ASSESSING STRENGTHS AND VULNERABILITIES IN PREPAREDNESS SYSTEMS

The National Health Security Preparedness Index provides a useful tool for assessing and comparing emergency preparedness systems across the United States. The index was created in 2013 with support from the CDC through a collaborative effort of more than 30 academic and professional organizations (Uzun Jacobson et al., 2014). Since 2015, the index has been supported by the Robert Wood Johnson Foundation and guided by an advisory committee that includes representation from the CDC, the ASPR, the U.S. Department of Defense, and state and local public health professionals.

MEASURES AND DATA SOURCES

Because no single agency or organization has the ability to support all of the protections necessary to keep people safe and healthy in the face of these events, the Index reflects preparedness as a responsibility shared by many different stakeholders in government and society. Correspondingly, the Index combines information from 130 measures derived from more than 60 different data sources and from multiple sectors in order to offer a broad view of preparedness levels achieved for the nation as a whole and for individual U.S. states and counties.

The Index measures are grouped into one of six domains representing broad areas of preparedness activity:

- *health security surveillance:* actions to monitor and detect health threats and to identify where hazards start and spread so that they can be contained rapidly
- *community planning and engagement:* actions to develop and maintain supportive relationships among government agencies, community organizations, and individual households and to develop shared plans for responding to disasters and emergencies
- *information and incident management:* actions to deploy people, supplies, money, and information to the locations where they are most effective in protecting health and safety
- *healthcare delivery:* actions to ensure access to high-quality medical services across the continuum of care during and after disasters and emergencies
- *countermeasure management:* actions to store and deploy medical and pharmaceutical products that prevent and treat the effects of hazardous substances and infectious diseases, including vaccines, prescription drugs, masks, gloves, and medical equipment
- *environmental and occupational health:* actions to maintain the security and safety of water and food supplies, to test for hazards and contaminants in the environment, and to protect workers and emergency responders from health hazards while on the job

These Index domains correspond closely to the six domains represented in the CDC PHEPR Capabilities. The Index further divides these six domains into a total of 19 subdomains reflecting specific areas of practice and policy. Individual measures are used to calculate measures for each of the 19 subdomains and then combined into summary measures for each of the six domains and an overall Index composite measure. All summary measures are scaled along a range from 0 to 10, with 10 representing the highest capability level observed in the data. The Index produces annual summary measures for each of the 50 U.S. states and the District of Columbia, along with national averages. Additionally, county-level Index estimates use a subset of 84 measures that are relevant to capabilities at the local level.

NATIONAL TRENDS AND PATTERNS IN PREPAREDNESS LEVELS

Results from the Index show that the nation's readiness for disease outbreaks, natural hazards, and other large-scale emergencies have improved by statistically significant levels since 2013. The national average Index score remained at 6.8 out of 10 in 2020, unchanged from the previous year and a 11.5% improvement since 2013 (Figure 3.3; Mays et al., 2020). These trends suggest that the United States will require at least 12 more years to reach a health security level of at least 9.0 on the 10-point scale. For the first year since 2013, 2020 did not show an increase in overall preparedness levels from the prior year, likely reflecting the fact that preparedness systems were fully occupied with COVID-19 response activities and had few resources to devote to preparedness planning and quality improvement for future emergencies.

Significant improvements in preparedness occurred since 2013 in four of the six domains monitored in the Index: surveillance, community planning, incident management, and environmental/occupational health (Figure 3.4). The highest levels of preparedness occurred in the incident and information management domain, indicating the ability to implement standardized processes and protocols in managing the acute phases of emergency events (Figure 3.4). Strong incident management can lead to faster response times, fewer errors, and more efficient use of resources when emergencies occur. Preparedness in this domain reached 8.9 in 2020, significantly higher than any other domain monitored in the Index.

The largest gains in preparedness occurred in the community planning and engagement domain, which increased by 19.5% between 2013 and 2017 to reach a national average of 5.4. Relationships that connect people and organizations together help communities become more resilient to disasters and may accelerate recovery after events occur. Historically, the United States showed widely variable performance in developing supportive relationships among

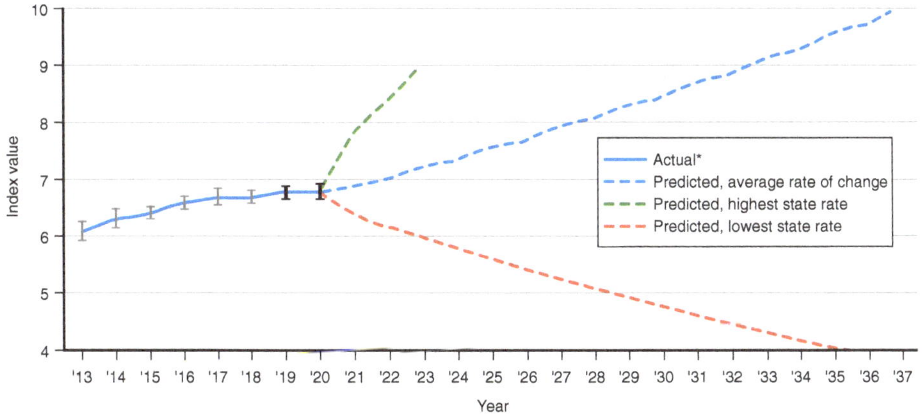

Figure 3.3 Trends over time in preparedness system performance using the National Health Security Preparedness Index.

Note: Vertical lines indicate statistical confidence intervals.
*Statistically significant trend from baseline ($p < .01$).

Source: Reproduced with permission from Colorado School of Public Health. (2021). *National Health Security Preparedness Index 2021 summary of key findings.* University of Colorado.

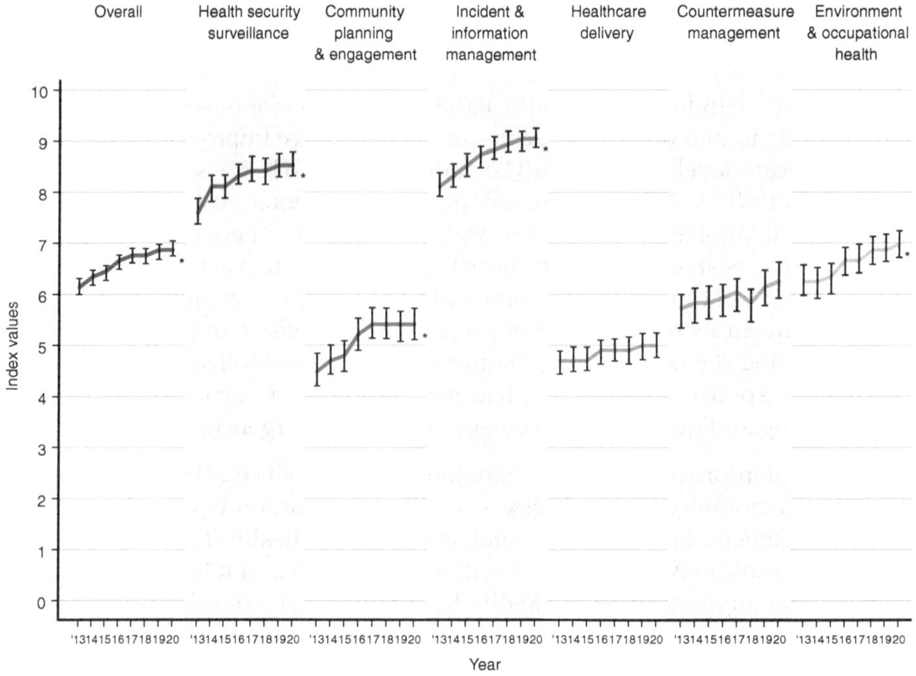

Figure 3.4 Trends over time in preparedness system domains using the National Health Security Preparedness Index.

Note: Vertical lines indicate statistical confidence intervals.
*Statistically significant trend from baseline ($p < 0.01$).

Source: Reproduced with permission from Colorado School of Public Health. (2021). *National Health Security Preparedness Index 2021 summary of key findings.* University of Colorado.

government agencies, community organizations, and individual residents and in engaging these stakeholders in planning for emergencies. This domain stood out as the nation's weakest area of preparedness in the first Index released in 2013, but it improved by more than any other domain monitored in the Index through 2017. Since that year, however, preparedness levels in this domain have remained flat.

Preparedness levels remained lowest in the healthcare delivery domain, which measures the capacities of healthcare professionals and facilities to meet surging demand for care during and after emergency events. Health security in this domain remained flat between 2013 and 2015 but trended up modestly since then. Health security levels in this domain remained at a national average of 5.0 in 2020. Specific measures within this domain that have failed to improve over time in selected states include the supply of physicians and nurses relative to population size, EMS emergency response times, hospital airborne isolation room capacity, nursing home staffing levels, nursing home infection control violations, and mental health shortage area designations.

VARIATION IN PREPAREDNESS ACROSS THE UNITED STATES

At the state level, preparedness levels improved in a total of 29 states between 2019 and 2020, while it declined in seven states, and remained largely unchanged in 15 states (Figure 3.5). A total of 10 states had health security levels that fell significantly below the national average, while 14 states had levels significantly

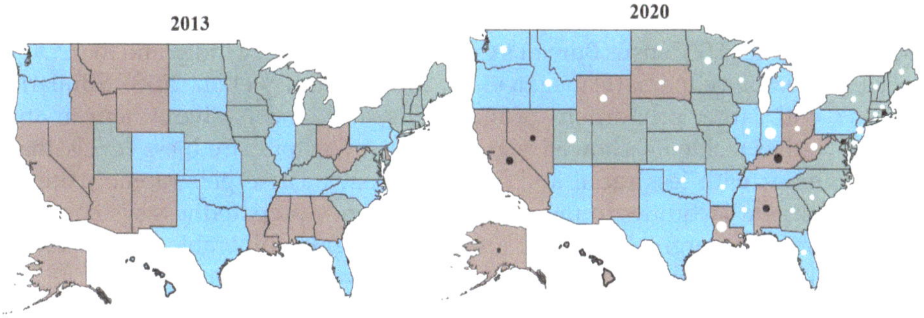

Figure 3.5 Variation across states in preparedness system performance using the National Health Security Preparedness Index.

Note: Green = above national average; Blue = within national average; Red = below national average. Dark circle = reduction from prior year; Light circle = improvement from prior year.

Source: Reproduced with permission from Colorado School of Public Health. (2021). *National Health Security Preparedness Index 2021 summary of key findings*. University of Colorado.

above the national average. Kansas joined the group of above-average states for the first time in 2020, while Minnesota and New York rejoined this group in 2020. Kentucky and Alabama moved into the group of below-average states in 2020. Large geographic differences in health security persisted across the United States, with a gap of 32% in the Index values of the highest and lowest states in 2020. States in the South-Central, Upper Mountain West, Pacific Coast, and Midwest regions experienced significantly lower health security levels and smaller gains in health security over time compared to their counterparts in other regions. Below-average regions contain disproportionate numbers of low- and moderate-income residents and rural residents who have fewer personal and community resources to draw upon in the event of an emergency.

County-level estimates of preparedness levels show that wide geographic differences exist not just across states but also within states (Figure 3.6). Across the United States, preparedness levels in rural areas were more than 8% lower than in urban areas in 2020. Counties with lower preparedness levels showed

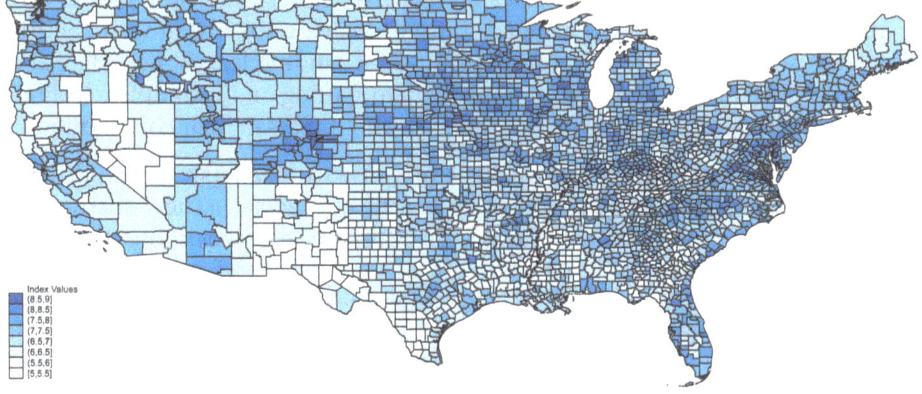

Figure 3.6 Variation across counties in preparedness system performance using the National Health Security Preparedness Index.

Source: Reproduced with permission from Colorado School of Public Health. (2021). *National Health Security Preparedness Index 2021 summary of key findings*. University of Colorado.

significantly higher rates of social and health vulnerability among residents, as measured by the U.S. Census Bureau's Community Resiliency Index and the CDC's Social Vulnerability Index (Flanagan et al., 2018; Summers et al., 2018). Similarly, counties with larger proportions of Black, Hispanic, and Native American and Alaska Native residents showed significantly lower preparedness levels than other counties with less racial and ethnic diversity. These geographic patterns reveal persistent inequities in the nation's emergency preparedness systems that leave historically marginalized communities and highly vulnerable residents with fewer health protections than their counterparts across the United States.

CONCLUSION: IMPROVING SYSTEM DESIGN AND PERFORMANCE

The nation's emergency preparedness systems comprise complex networks of public health agencies, emergency management agencies, medical providers, and other community partners working together to protect people against the health consequences of hazardous events. These systems support a core set of capabilities in preparing for, responding to, and recovering from events using an all-hazards approach. The structure and performance of these systems vary widely across the United States, leaving some communities with fewer health protections than others. The COVID-19 pandemic exposed many of these weaknesses and vulnerabilities in preparedness systems across the United States Fortunately, most systems have achieved significant improvements in capabilities in recent years despite limited resources, and considerable opportunities exist for continued improvement.

Closing current gaps and inequities in preparedness systems will require new and more coordinated actions by government and the private sector, particularly given the likelihood of continued future growth in the frequency and intensity of hazardous events. Promising steps to achieve these improvements include the following:

- **Increase investments in core public health infrastructure.** The two primary federal programs that support emergency preparedness capabilities in public health and healthcare settings—the PHEP program and the HPP—have experienced significant reductions in funding over most of the past decade, despite rising risks and costs. Recent research estimates a $4.5 billion annual shortfall in spending necessary to achieve comprehensive public health capabilities across all states and communities. Insufficient funding leaves most state and local public health agencies with inadequate staffing and incomplete technological infrastructure needed to address health threats in their communities.
- **Strengthen multisector networks and network leadership.** Multisector networks and coalitions focused on health and social issues exist across the United States, including healthcare preparedness coalitions that specialize in preparedness issues. Growth in these networks in selected states and communities has contributed to rising Index values over time, but the more recent stagnation in Index trends related to community engagement and planning indicate that new attention is needed. Regional healthcare preparedness coalitions consistently lack broad participation from sectors such as long-term care, mental health, and emergency medical services. Research demonstrates these multisector networks can achieve profound effects on population health status over time. Health security professionals should

work strategically to broaden participation in coalitions and networks and to link disparate networks together so as to focus their attention on improving preparedness capabilities. These networks are central to the capability of Community Preparedness as defined by the CDC.

- **Enhance medical surge capacity.** The National Health Security Preparedness Index has consistently identified constraints in healthcare delivery system capacity to address surges in demand for care during large-scale emergencies. The COVID-19 pandemic offered new perspectives on the extensiveness of these constraints and emphasized the need for stakeholders to test new approaches for addressing them.
- **Expand real-time data acquisition, integration, and analytic capacity.** Preparedness stakeholders rely on an array of fragmented and cumbersome data and surveillance systems to identify and respond to health risks in their populations. Electronic clinical data systems and medical information technology infrastructure remain largely disconnected from the public health surveillance systems and registries that are used for population-level monitoring and response at state and local levels. The ability to extract near-real-time information from these data systems remains extremely limited in many situations, including during the COVID-19 pandemic. Local, state, and federal stakeholders should create processes for identifying unmet needs in data systems and analytic capacity across the U.S. preparedness enterprise and for developing data acquisition and exchange platforms that can address unmet needs.
- **Expand research and evaluation on preparedness systems.** A recent review of emergency preparedness research conducted by the National Academy of Medicine found that available scientific evidence remains very limited regarding the system capabilities and practices that are most effective in improving outcomes during and after hazardous events. Increased support for preparedness research is needed to inform and guide system improvements.

These actions can help not only to improve overall levels of emergency preparedness across the United States but also to reduce and eliminate inequities in preparedness capabilities across U.S. states and communities. Using these strategies, emergency preparedness systems can bring the United States closer to the goal of equal protection for all.

DISCUSSION QUESTIONS

1. Discuss the use of the word "capability" in public health emergency preparedness. Describe some of the ways you have seen this word used and how it is defined by various entities.
2. Discuss the federal role in public health emergency preparedness and compare it with the role of state and local health departments.
3. Discuss plausible reasons for disparities in preparedness in some states. Why are some states more prepared than others?
4. Think of additional challenges to preparing a large, diverse country for response to emergencies. Google preparedness programs in other countries and compare them with the United States.

REFERENCES

Assistant Secretary for Planning and Response. (2018). *National health security strategy 2019–2022*. U.S. Department of Health and Human Services. https://www.phe.gov/Preparedness/planning/authority/nhss/Documents/NHSS-Strategy-508.pdf

Carande-Kulis, V. G., Getzen, T. E., & Thacker, S. B. (2007). Public goods and externalities: A research agenda for public health economics. *Journal of Public Health Management, 13*(2), 227–232. https://doi.org/10.1097/00124784-200703000-00024

Carlson, V., Chilton, M. J., Corso, L. C., & Beitsch, L. M. (2015). Defining the functions of public health governance. *American Journal of Public Health, 105*(Suppl. 2), S159–S66. https://doi.org/10.2105/AJPH.2014.302198

Centers for Disease Control and Prevention. (2018). *Public Health Emergency Preparedness and Response capabilities: National standards for state, local, tribal and territorial public health*. https://www.cdc.gov/cpr/readiness/capabilities.htm

Centers for Disease Control and Prevention. (n.d.). *Operational readiness review*. https://www.cdc.gov/cpr/readiness/orr.html

Federal Emergency Management Agency. (2019). *Emergency support function #8 - Public health and medical services annex*. U.S. Department of Homeland Security. https://www.fema.gov/pdf/emergency/nrf/nrf-esf-08.pdf

Flanagan, B. E., Hallisey, E. J., Adams, E., & Lavery, A. (2018). Measuring community vulnerability to natural and anthropogenic hazards: The Centers for Disease Control and Prevention's social vulnerability index. *Journal of Environmental Health, 80*(10), 34–36. https://www.ncbi.nlm.nih.gov/pmc/articles/PMC7179070/

Gostin, L. O. (2000). Public health law in a new century: Part I: Law as a tool to advance the community's health. *JAMA, 283*(21), 2837–2841. https://doi.org/10.1001/jama.283.21.2837

Gostin, L. O., & Wiley, L. F. (2000). Governmental public health powers during the COVID-19 pandemic: Stay-at-home orders, business closures, and travel restrictions. *JAMA, 323*(21), 2137–2138. https://doi.org/10.1001/jama.2020.5460

Gotham, I. J., Sottolano, D. L., Hennessy, M. E., Napoli, J. P., Dobkins, G., & Le, L. H. (2007). An integrated information system for all-hazards health preparedness and response: New York State Health Emergency Response Data System. *Journal of Public Health Management and Practice, 13*(5), 486–496. https://doi.org/10.1097/01.PHH.0000285202.48588.89

Hyde, J. K., & Shortell, S. M. (2012). The structure and organization of local and state public health agencies in the U.S.: A systematic review. *American Journal of Preventive Medicine, 42*(5, Suppl. 1), S29–S41. https://doi.org/10.1016/j.amepre.2012.01.021

Institute of Medicine. (2015). *Healthy, resilient, and sustainable communities after disasters: Strategies, opportunities, and planning for recovery*. National Academies Press. https://doi.org/10.17226/18996

Jensen, J., & Youngs, G. (2015). Explaining implementation behaviour of the National Incident Management System (NIMS). *Disasters, 39*(2), 362–388. https://doi.org/10.1111/disa.12103

Kania, J., & Kramer, M. (2011, Winter). Collective impact. *Stanford Social Innovation Review*, 36–41. https://ssir.org/articles/entry/collective_impact#

Krieger, N., Testa, C., Hanage, W. P., & Chen, J. T. (2020). US racial and ethnic data for COVID-19 cases: Still missing in action. *Lancet, 396*(10261), e81. https://doi.org/10.1016/S0140-6736(20)32220-0

Lenart, B., Albanese, J., Halstead, W., Schlegelmilch, J., & Paturas, J. (2012). Integrating public health and medical intelligence gathering into Homeland Security Fusion Centres. *Journal of Business Continuity & Emergency Planning, 6*(2), 174–179. https://pubmed.ncbi.nlm.nih.gov/23315252/

Marcozzi, D. E., & Lurie, N. (2012). Measuring healthcare preparedness: An all-hazards approach. *Israel Journal of Health Policy Research, 1*(1), Article 42. https://doi.org/10.1186/2045-4015-1-42

Mays, G. P., Childress, M. T., & Paris, B. (2020). *The National Health Security Preparedness Index: 2020 release*. Colorado School of Public Health, University of Colorado. https://nhspi.org/wp-content/uploads/2020/06/NHSPI_2020_Key_Findings.pdf

Nowell, B., Steelman, T., Velez, A-L. K., & Yang, Z. (2018). The structure of effective governance of disaster response networks: Insights from the field. *The American Review of Public Administration, 48*(7), 699–715. https://doi.org/10.1186/s12889-018-6376-7

Obama, B. (2011). *Presidential policy directive 8 - National preparedness*. White House. https://www.dhs.gov/xlibrary/assets/presidential-policy-directive-8-national-preparedness.pdf

Olson, M. (1971). *The logic of collective action public goods and the theory of groups, second printing with a new preface and appendix*. Harvard University Press.

Ramsey Hamilton, C., & Miller, D. (2017). The new CMS emergency preparedness final rule and its impact on healthcare in 2017. *Journal of Healthcare Protection Management, 33*(1), 77–81. https://pubmed.ncbi.nlm.nih.gov/30351552/

Summers, J. K., Harwell, L. C., Smith, L. M., & Buck, K. D. (2018). Measuring community resilience to natural hazards: The Natural Hazard Resilience Screening Index (NaHRSI)-Development and Application to the United States. *Geohealth, 2*(12), 372–394. https://doi.org/10.1029/2018GH000160

Uzun Jacobson, E., Inglesby, T., Khan, A. S., Rajotte, J. C., Burhans, R. L., Slemp, C. C., & Link, J. M. (2014). Design of the National Health Security Preparedness Index. *Biosecurity and Bioterrorism: Biodefense Strategy, Practice, and Science, 12*(3), 122–131. https://doi.org/10.1089/bsp.2014.0024

Varda, D., Shoup, J. A., & Miller, S. (2012). A systematic review of collaboration and network research in the public affairs literature: Implications for public health practice and research. *American Journal of Public Health, 102*(3), 564–571. https://doi.org/10.2105/AJPH.2011.300286

CHAPTER 4

DISASTER RISK ASSESSMENT

A PRIMER

KIMBERLEY SHOAF

KEY TERMS

Community Health Assessment (CHA)
Community Health Improvement Plan (CHIP)
Disaster
Hazard
Hazard Risk Assessment Instrument (HRAI)
Hazard Vulnerability Assessment (HVA) Tool
Health Hazard Assessment and Prioritization (hHAP) Tool
Pennsylvania Public Health Risk Assessment Tool (PHRAT)
Public Health Accreditation Board (PHAB)
Public Health Emergency Preparedness (PHEP) Program
Risk
Threat
Threat and Hazard Identification and Risk Assessment (THIRA)
Vulnerability

INTRODUCTION

The Core Functions of Public Health are Assessment, Policy Development, and Assurance (Institute of Medicine, Committee for the Study of the Future of Public Health, Division of Health Care Services, 1988). Over the years, these three Core Functions have evolved to include the 10 Essential Services that form the backbone of what public health does on a daily basis. Our efforts to protect the health of populations must begin with a valid, evidence-based assessment process, whether that assessment be of the public's health on a day-to-day basis or in times of emergency. Indeed, the **Public Health Accreditation Board (PHAB)** requires the completion of a **community health assessment (CHA)** prior to developing a **community health improvement plan (CHIP),** which then serves as the basis of a strategic plan for the improvement of the health of the jurisdiction as a prerequisite to public health programs applying for accreditation.

As part of the public health emergency and disaster planning process, it is similarly essential that an assessment process be utilized before planning for emergencies. Assessments ensure that the activities that follow—policies and assurances—are appropriate and sufficient by identifying which hazards are relevant to the population and how they might impact the health of the community. This chapter provides an overview of this hazard and disaster risk assessment process. Included in the chapter are a brief definition of the terminology used in risk assessment for disasters, an exploration of the history of disaster risk assessments within public health, a description of the various models available for public health, an outline of the processes involved in conducting a hazard risk assessment for public health purposes, and, finally, a discussion of the future evolutions needed in hazard assessment to deal with our changing environment.

DEFINITIONS

Both the public health world and the world of emergency management are replete with terminology that is used in very specific ways. Sometimes the same words have different meanings in different professional circles. To assist the reader in understanding the terms used in disaster preparedness and management and to ensure that terminology is not misinterpreted, we present here a number of important terms and their definitions as used in this chapter:

- **Hazard**—According to the National Association of Safety Professionals (NASP), a hazard is a "source of potential damage, harm or adverse health effects on something or someone" (Gislason, 2018, para. 6). In other words, an earthquake, a tornado, or an emerging infectious disease are hazards, but they are not necessarily a disaster. They have the potential to cause harm.
- **Disaster**—There are a number of definitions of a disaster. From a public health perspective, the World Health Organization (WHO) defines a disaster as "serious disruption of the functioning of a community or a society causing widespread human, material, economic or environmental losses which exceed the ability of the affected community or society to cope using its own resources" (WHO, n.d.). Thus, an earthquake, even though it may be a great tragedy, only becomes a disaster when it causes damages that exceed the ability of the community to cope with them.
- **Vulnerability**—This is defined as the conditions or circumstances that make a community (or individual) "susceptible to the damaging effects of a hazard" (United Nations Office for Disaster Risk Reduction [UNISDR], 2009, p. 30).
- **Risk**—According to most disaster researchers, risk is "the probability of a hazard occurrence and the interaction of that hazard with society or its elements" (Birkmann, 2013, p. 856). Hence, risk is the interaction of hazards and vulnerability in a community.
- **Threat**—The term "threat" is used in the intelligence and homeland security world. According to the U.S. Department of Homeland Security (DHS; 2010), it is defined as the likelihood that an attack (or other hazard/hazards) will occur.

HISTORY OF DISASTER RISK ASSESSMENT IN PUBLIC HEALTH

The history of disaster risk assessment within public health is tied into the broader history of the roles of public health in disaster preparedness and response, as well as the evolving understanding of the threat arising from a myriad of potential public health emergencies (e.g., natural hazards, bioterrorism). Prior to September 11, 2001, the field known today as public health preparedness or emergency public health was a small field occupied primarily by public health departments that had experienced a significant disaster in their own jurisdictions and their academic partners. For example, as a result of the bombing of the Alfred P. Murrah Federal Building in Oklahoma City in 1995 and the 1999 tornadoes in Oklahoma City, a demand for expertise in disaster injury was created. The injury section of the Oklahoma State Health Department quickly developed expertise in disaster injury and became a leader in the field. Similarly, after the 1994 Northridge earthquake in Los Angeles County, the Los Angeles County Department of Public Health and their partners at the UCLA Fielding School of Public Health developed an expertise in disaster planning specific to public health in the county.

At the national level in public health, events around the world such as Desert Storm (Iraq 1990–1991), the Oklahoma City bombing (1995), and the anthrax letters of 1998 resulted in a focus within the Centers for Disease Control and Prevention (CDC) on preparing public health departments and their partners at all levels for the need to respond to a bioterrorism event. Starting in 1999, the U.S. Department of Health and Human Services (HHS) funded state and local health departments through the CDC's Bioterrorism Preparedness and Response Program and, in 2000, the CDC established the first four Academic Centers for Public Health Preparedness. Separate funding for the UCLA Center for Public Health and Disasters (CPHD) in 2000 directed the development of an interactive training program for local health departments to respond to a disaster. This funding allowed close work between the CPHD and the Santa Barbara County Health Department and identified a specific need for a tool to conduct a hazard risk assessment prior to writing disaster response plans or training the health department staff to respond to disasters.

The CPHD conducted an exhaustive search of both the published literature and the grey literature at the time, which found a number of models for conducting a hazard risk assessment, but none were specific to the responsibility that public health holds to protect the health of the population at large. The models were primarily utilized by emergency management, particularly as a part of applying for hazard mitigation funding from the Federal Emergency Management Agency (FEMA). For many of the models in practice at the time, the outputs were often vague and broad (e.g., high, medium, low impact) or focused on those measures directly related to a disaster declaration (e.g., number of casualties and deaths, dollar amount of damage).

Working with local public health partners, there was an expressed desire to have a process that was systematic and resulted in measured results that could drive disaster planning. Over the next few years, a process was developed and tested by the CPHD and the Santa Barbara Health Department. The resultant process used components of multiple existing frameworks and focused the efforts on public health (Backman, 1996; Coburn et al., 1993;

de Boer, 1990; FEMA, n.d.; Keller, 1989; Kramer & Bahme, 1992; Malilay et al., 1997). The end product of this collaboration was the UCLA **Hazard Risk Assessment Instrument (HRAI)**, a workbook outlining a process that was focused on indicators important for public health in a lead role in the health and medical support function in response to a disaster (Shoaf et al., 2006). Following the development of HRAI, the UCLA CPHD worked with local health departments in California and Nevada to prepare a hazard risk assessment toolkit, which was later published online and widely promoted to health departments across the country.

In 2010, the CDC created a pilot project within the **Public Health Emergency Preparedness (PHEP) program** to assess the impact of a risk-based funding model. To fund the program, health departments needed to be able to assess their risk for disaster. In 2011, 10 Metropolitan Statistical Areas received funding under the program for 2 years; the first step was conducting a hazard risk assessment. In addition to the pilot project, the CDC's *PHEP Capabilities* document now listed as the first function under the first capability: Conduct a public health jurisdictional risk assessment (CDC, 2018). Funding from the CDC under the PHEP program and the requirement to conduct such an assessment created a surge in the development of models for conducting a hazard-specific public health risk assessment.

Currently, the *Public Health Emergency Preparedness and Response Capabilities* (CDC, 2018) document outlines the national standards for state, territorial, local, and tribal public health agencies regarding how they prepare and respond to public health emergencies. The first capability identified is Community Preparedness with four functions. The first of those functions is to "[d]etermine risks to the health of the jurisdiction" (CDC, 2018, p. 11). Hence, public health agencies at all levels should be conducting hazard risk assessments on a regular basis.

PUBLIC HEALTH MODELS OF HAZARD RISK ASSESSMENT

There are a number of models for conducting a hazard risk assessment that exist both within public health and in the larger emergency management field. The Assistant Secretary of Preparedness and Response TRACIE (Technical Resources, Assistance Center, Information Exchange) has evaluated several tools that are available for conducting a hazard vulnerability assessment (HHS, 2018). We explore the five models that serve as the core models utilized by public health to "determine the risks to the health of the jurisdiction" (CDC, 2018, p. 11). There are certainly other models that are utilized, but these five often serve as the basis on which these other models operate.

UCLA HAZARD RISK ASSESSMENT INSTRUMENT

The UCLA HRAI (Shoaf et al., 2006) was originally developed by the UCLA CPHD under CDC funding. It is based on the premise that risk is a function of the interaction of a hazard with a community's vulnerabilities. In this model, risk is mitigated by a community's resources.

$$\textit{Risk} = \textit{Hazard} * (\textit{Vulnerability} - \textit{Resources})$$

This model has a four-step quantitative process: (a) assess the probability of mishap, (b) assess the severity of consequences, (c) score the consequences, and

(d) analyze the risk. The tool provides step-by-step instructions for conducting the assessment, with worksheets for each step. As it was built specifically for public health, the consequences that are examined are public health–specific and include

- human impact—measured as fatalities, injuries/illness requiring emergency medical services (EMS) transport, outpatient injuries/illness, hospital emergency department (ED) injuries/illness, trauma level injuries/intensive care unit (ICU) illness;
- interruption of healthcare—measured as basic EMS, outpatient services, hospital ED services, trauma units, and ancillary health services;
- community impact—measured as water supply contamination, water supply availability, population displacement, public utilities, and transportation; and
- impact on public health infrastructure—measured as personnel, equipment loss, laboratory services, community services, internal communications, and interagency communications. For each of these measures, the impact of the hazard is weighed against the baseline capacity.

The initial model was created for natural hazards that result primarily in injury; however, later iterations of HRAI included illnesses as outcomes. In practice, additional indicators have been added such as mental health providers and dialysis centers. The toolkit also provides generic hazard models based on historic events for an earthquake, rainfall-induced flooding, riverine flooding, a hurricane, a tornado, and a terrorist bombing.

Kaiser Permanente Hazard Vulnerability Assessment (HVA) Tool

Contemporaneous with the development of the UCLA HRAI, emergency management personnel at Kaiser Permanente in California developed a **Hazard Vulnerability Assessment (HVA) tool.** This tool was developed for hospitals to be able to meet the demands of accreditation, which were beginning to require such assessments. The Kaiser HVA, as it has become known, has been adopted (and adapted) widely by healthcare systems. First published in 2000, it has been updated a number of times, most recently in 2018. It utilizes an ordinal scale of N/A, low, medium, and high for probability of occurrence and what they term severity.

Severity = (Magnitude – Mitigation)

The 2018 tool includes 61 hazards prepopulated into the tool (including zombies!). Probability is defined as the likelihood of occurrence and is augmented by the number of actual alerts and activations. Magnitude includes human impact (probability of death or injury), property impact (physical losses and damage), and business impact (interruption of services). Mitigation includes preparedness (preplanning), internal response (time, effectiveness, resources), and external response (community/mutual aid staff and supplies). These six indicators are averaged with the probability to produce a risk score defined as the relative threat of the hazard.

L.A. County Health Hazard Assessment and Prioritization (hHAP) Tool

Following funding by the CDC's risk-based pilot project in 2011, the Los Angeles County Department of Public Health developed the **Health Hazard Assessment and Prioritization (hHAP) tool.** It was developed using elements of the UCLA HRAI and Kaiser HVA models previously described (Dean et al., 2013). An advancement of this model over its predecessors is the incorporation of the hazard assessment into a larger framework of prioritization and planning. Thus, the six steps of this tool begin with forming a steering committee and defining your geographic region. Steps 3, 4, and 5 are similar to the steps in both the UCLA HRAI and the Kaiser HVA: identify possible hazards, assess risk components, and then rank and prioritize results. The final step is planning, review, and update.

The hHAP calculates a Relative Risk Score based on eight components similar to those in the UCLA HRAI:

- hazard probability
- health severity (increase in morbidity, hospitalizations, mortality)
- community impact (disruption in routine community activities, damage to communications and infrastructure, and interruption of social services)
- impact to public health, impact on healthcare
- impact on mental-behavioral health
- community agency resources (includes agreements with other agencies, coordination with governmental and nongovernmental agencies, and community preparedness)

These elements are scored on an ordinal scale and create the relative risk score as follows:

$$\textit{Relative Risk Score} = \textit{Probability} \times \textit{Health Severity} \times \textit{Impacts} \times \textit{Agency Resources}$$

The instrument includes instructions and definitions for each of the components of the tool. Furthermore, scenarios are incorporated for the 61 hazards included (no zombies!). The scenarios are designed specifically for Southern California based on the results of real events or existent scenarios (e.g., the Southern California Shakeout scenario; Jones et al., 2008), but the instructions state that they should be adapted for other locations based on their specific circumstances.

Pennsylvania Public Health Risk Assessment Tool (PHRAT) Workbook

The **Pennsylvania Public Health Risk Assessment Tool (PHRAT**; Figure 4.1) was developed in response to the CDC risk-based funding pilot project by the Drexel School of Public Health in collaboration with the Pennsylvania Department of Health (Peters et al., 2019). Like hHAP, it built off the UCLA HRAI and the Kaiser HVA. Like the UCLA HRAI, the PHRAT utilizes a quantitative approach to assessing risk and compares quantitative measurements of impact

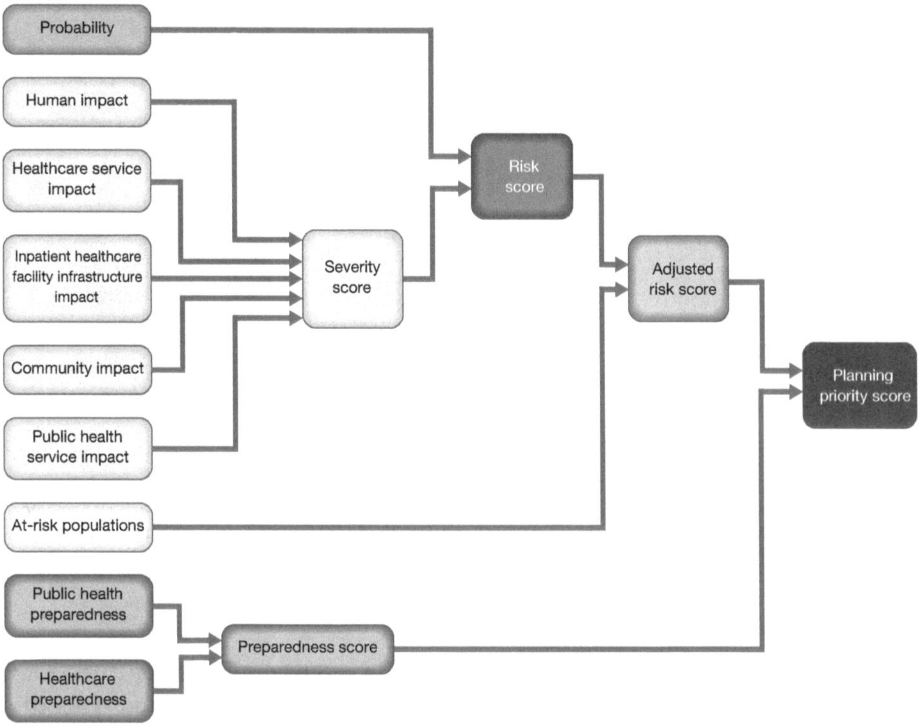

Figure 4.1 Pennsylvania public health risk assessment conceptual overview.

Source: Reproduced with permission from Esther Chernak, MD, MPH.
Pennsylvania Public Health Risk Assessment Tool (PHRAT) | Drexel Dornsife School of Public Health. (n.d.). https://drexel.edu/dornsife/research/centers-programs-projects/center-for-public-health-readiness-communication/our-projects/phrat

against baseline measures. It breaks its analyses down into a Public Health System Risk Assessment and a Healthcare System Risk Assessment and then combines them for an overall jurisdictional assessment. The individual items measured in these two assessments are very similar to the UCLA HRAI for public health and the Kaiser HVA for the healthcare impact. This tool, however, does not stop with assessing the impact; it adds a component regarding at-risk populations that are not explicitly included in previous models. It also includes, in a very defined way, preparedness measures in the form of rating the jurisdiction on each of the relevant capabilities (PHEP Capabilities, CDC, 2018, for public health and HPP capabilities, HHS, 2012, for healthcare). The PHRAT conceptual model ties all these components into a planning priority score for each hazard.

Threat and Hazard Identification and Risk Assessment

The DHS created the **Threat and Hazard Identification and Risk Assessment (THIRA**; Figure 4.2) in 2012 to provide a standard process for identifying threats and hazards to align with the National Preparedness Goal (FEMA, 2018). THIRA is a three-step process: identify threats and hazards of concern, give threats and hazards context, and establish capability targets.

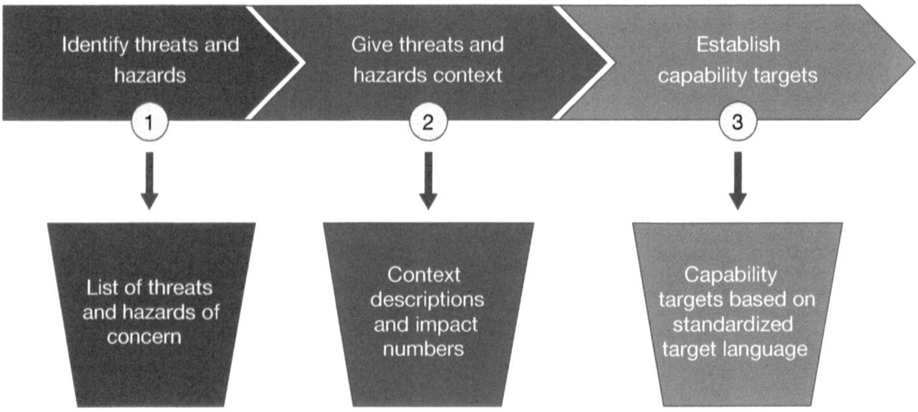

Figure 4.2 Three-step THIRA process.

Source: From Federal Emergency Management Agency. (2018). *Threat and hazard identification and risk assessment (THIRA) and stakeholder preparedness review (SPR) guide: Comprehensive preparedness guide (CPG) 201* (3rd ed.). U.S. Department of Homeland Security. https://www.fema.gov/sites/default/files/2020-04/CPG201Final20180525.pdf.

In Step 1, THIRA identifies a number of threats and hazards in three categories: natural hazards, technological hazards, and human-caused incidents. This distinction between technological and human-caused hazards is essentially a difference in intentionality, with technological being assumed to be unintentional and the human-caused (i.e., active shooter, cyberattack, explosive attack, bioterrorist attack) to be intentional. Unlike the other assessment strategies, THIRA suggests that jurisdictions select hazards that are likely to occur and, uniquely to this model, challenge at least one of the core capabilities more than any other threat.

The second step in a THIRA is to provide context to the threats and hazards selected. This involves writing "context descriptions" or scenarios that include location, magnitude, and time of incident and estimating the impacts. Within THIRA, impacts are written using a uniform set of common metrics (i.e., number of fatalities, number of structure fires, number of people requiring medical care). The example metrics provided are for the whole community and thus are broader than that required for public health planning. Furthermore, the guidelines provide examples of the standard metrics, but there is no reference for what these commonly measured impacts are. The impacts are also reported as a single number for the community.

The final step of the THIRA is to establish capability targets for the 32 FEMA-designated capabilities. For public health to use the THIRA, this step would most likely refer to the PHEP and HPP capabilities (HHS, 2012; CDC, 2018). In some respects, this step divorces the capabilities from specific hazards, but looks to identify metrics whereby the community demonstrates abilities to respond to the hazardous situations identified. These capability targets are stated using standardized target language that is similar to writing a SMART objective in public health (CDC, n.d.). An example of a standardized target statement is "Within (#) hours of an incident, provide emergency sheltering for (#) people; maintain sheltering operations for (#) days" (FEMA, 2018).

The current version of the THIRA documentation (FEMA, 2018) includes the planning step that follows the hazard assessment. The *Comprehensive Preparedness*

Guide (FEMA, 2018) combines THIRA with the *Stakeholder Preparedness Review*. This added planning piece is useful to demonstrate how the hazard assessment translates into the planning process seamlessly.

STRENGTHS AND WEAKNESSES OF THE HAZARD RISK ASSESSMENT MODELS

The hazard risk assessment process is part and parcel of the broader risk management functions of an agency. For public health, that means that the assessment of the risk to the health of the community needs to lead into plans to reduce, mitigate, and/or respond to those needs. Hence, a hazard risk assessment is a specialized needs assessment like others undertaken by public health. As such, it should be a "well-thought-out and *impartial systematic* effort to collect *objective data* or information that brings to light or enhances understanding of the need for services or programs" (Soriano, 2013, p. 4). Utilizing any one of the models described here will allow for the systematic collection of objective data. Which might an agency choose?

Three of the tools described are specific to public health—UCLA's HRAI; the PHRAT, developed by Drexel University School of Public Health; and the hHAP, developed by the Los Angeles County Department of Public Health—and result in an analysis that would enhance the understanding of the specific services needed by the public health sector to respond to an emergency. The other two models, the HVA and THIRA, would need to be adapted by the health department to provide the information about local public health needs to protect and serve their particular community. Certainly, the HVAs that hospitals are doing (often using the Kaiser model) may feed into the jurisdiction's public health hazard risk assessment, but alone, this model does not provide sufficient information for public health planning. Furthermore, any public health hazard risk assessment should serve as a resource and flow into a jurisdictional THIRA.

The fundamental difference between the three public health-specific models is the use of a quantitative analysis of the ratio of the impact of the hazard to a jurisdiction's baseline capacity. Both the UCLA HRAI and the PHRAT utilize quantitative data to describe this ratio, whereas the hHAP uses simply an ordinal scale to develop a relative risk score. For jurisdictions that may not have the capacity to develop the detailed data necessary to utilize the HRAI or the PHRAT, the hHAP provides an alternative that also meets the criteria of a systematic collection of objective data.

The PHRAT builds upon the quantitative nature of the UCLA HRAI by incorporating an at-risk population assessment and applying results to the capabilities of the jurisdiction. The PHRAT also created an Excel sheet with built-in macros to help with the calculations. This tool would readily feed into a jurisdiction's THIRA.

STEPS FOR CONDUCTING A HAZARD RISK ASSESSMENT

As described earlier, there are four basic steps that need to be taken in conducting a hazard risk assessment: (a) identify the hazards that are relevant for your jurisdiction and the likelihood that they will occur, (b) assess the impact that the relevant hazards could impose on your community's health, (c) evaluate your community's ability to meet the demands generated by the hazard, and (d) incorporate the results into the planning process. These steps are detailed in the following sections.

Identify Relevant Hazards and Their Likelihood of Occurrence

All the tools described earlier have a list of potential hazards to work from; however, it is still necessary to determine the likelihood that each hazard will actually occur. The first part of this is to identify the system life cycle you are using for planning. Ideally, the life cycle is short enough to confer urgency in planning but long enough for hazards that occur infrequently to be rated as well. Most of the models described previously suggest a life cycle of 25 years; however, as noted further in this section, it does not mean that "100 year" events are not considered within that life cycle.

Once the life cycle is identified, it is necessary to identify those hazards that exist in the jurisdiction and how likely they are to occur within the chosen life cycle. There are many sources of information about hazards, which range from scientific products from academics and government entities through historical records and media sources to anecdotal reports. It is best to use the highest level of evidence available for each hazard. For those with minimal scientific products available, using alternative sources is better than eliminating the hazard from the list or guessing.

Hazard probability products such as the National Seismic Hazard Map (NSHM) from the U.S. Geologic Survey (USGS; Figure 4.3) or FEMA's Flood Risk Maps (Figure 4.4) provide scientifically valid estimates of the probability of occurrence of certain hazards. However, such sources can be a bit difficult to interpret. For example, the NSHM includes a number of maps to demonstrate the probability of the seismic hazard in a region. The map on the left portrays the frequency of damaging earthquake shaking in 10,000 years across the country.

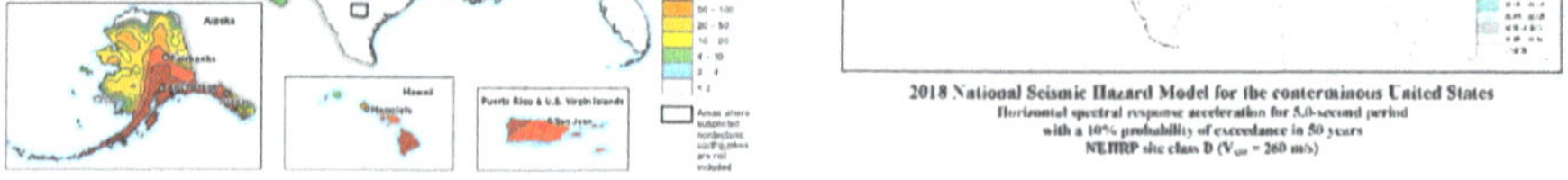

A B

Figure 4.3 The map on the left shows the frequency of damaging earthquake shaking in 10,000 years. On the right, the map shows the ground motion expected with a 10% probability of exceedance in 50 years.

Source: From Rukstales, K., & Petersen, M. (2019). *Data release for 2018 update of the U.S. National Seismic Hazard Model: U.S. geological survey data release.* https://doi.org/10.5066.P9WT5OVB

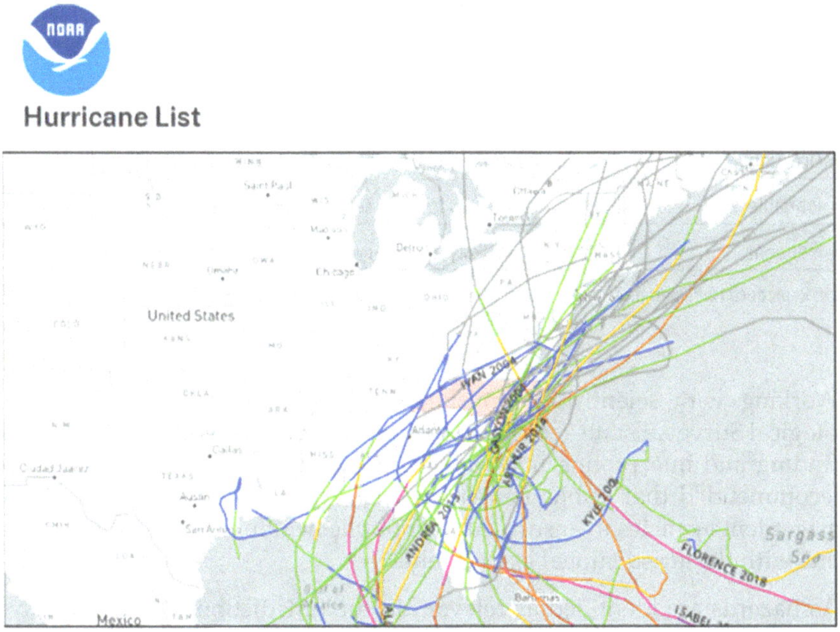

Figure 4.4 Historic hurricane tracks for North Carolina 1995–2020 (National Oceanic and Atmospheric Agency).

The map on the right is formatted to portray the level of ground motion that has a 10% probability of being exceeded in 50 years. A damaging earthquake in this instance is defined as having a Modified Mercalli Intensity of VI or a ground motion acceleration of about 8% to 15% of gravity. This level of ground motion correlates with the light yellow areas in the map on the right. Hence, those areas (and the areas in the warmer colors) have at least a 5% probability of occurring at least once in 25 years.

Other hazards have data available in a library of historic occurrences. For example, the National Oceanic and Atmospheric Agency (NOAA) has a library of historic hurricane tracks that can be mapped (coast.noaa.gov/hurricanes/#map=4/32/-80). A search for hurricane tracks that impacted North Carolina in the past 25 years resulted in the map in Figure 4.4 with 33 matching storms. It is fairly easy to surmise that North Carolina might expect to be impacted by at least one hurricane every year. It is important when looking at historic data to not ignore hazard events that do not rise to the level of a disaster. For example, some think about pandemics as occurring every 100 years or so because they only focus on the pandemic events that are the most severe, such as the 1918 influenza pandemic and the 2019 SARS-CoV-2 (which we are in the middle of at the time of this writing). By only including these very impactful pandemics, one would assume the 100-year return period. However, influenza pandemics occurred in 1957, 1968, and 2009 as well. This suggests a 20-year return period is more likely than a 100-year return period. The other tip is to think about hazards that may occur outside of the jurisdiction but would still have the ability to impact it. For example, a manufacturing plant or a nuclear power-generating facility in a neighboring jurisdiction could be problematic due to winds carrying a hazardous plume across the area.

EXHIBIT 4.1 Likelihood of Occurrence

0 = Improbable:	The probability of the occurrence of the hazard is zero.
1 = Remote:	The hazard is not likely to occur in the system life cycle, but it is possible.
2 = Occasional:	The hazard is likely to occur at least once in the system life cycle.
3 = Probable:	The hazard is likely to occur several times in the system life cycle.
4 = Frequent:	The hazard is likely to occur cyclically or annually in the system life cycle.

Source: Reproduced with permission from University of California, Los Angeles Hazard Risk Assessment Instrument.

Working with scientists from state and national agencies—like the U.S. Geological Survey, a state geological survey, or a local university—can be helpful in finding and interpreting information on hazard probability. Furthermore, it is recommended that public health agencies collaborate with local emergency management agencies to ensure that the public health hazard risk assessment is in line with the jurisdictional assessment.

As hazards are identified as relevant to the jurisdiction, it is helpful to rank them on an ordinal scale. Because they are not all measured on the same time frame (earthquakes that occur on a scale of hundreds of years vs. fires that occur annually) an ordinal scale makes it easier to compare across events. One ordinal scale that could be useful is found in the UCLA HRAI. In this way, the scientific data are translated into a scale that is easier to interpret across hazards (Exhibit 4.1).

Assess the Impact of the Relevant Hazards on the Health of the Population

There are two schools of thought on assessing the impact of the hazards on the population's health. The first is a quantitative approach to the impact, comparing the expected numbers following the hazard to a baseline, with the assumption that the baseline is indicative of capacity. This quantitative approach is utilized in the UCLA HRAI and the PHRAT. Such an approach requires the availability of data on past events and scientifically valid models of future events. For some hazards, FEMA's Hazus may be used to estimate impacts. Hazus is a standardized risk modeling methodology that is available for earthquakes, hurricanes, floods, and tsunamis for the United States. It is based in a geospatial information system and estimates impacts including values for transportation impact, casualties, damage to infrastructure, and displaced populations that are relevant for public health planning (FEMA, 2016).

There are also published scenarios for many hazards in a number of communities. These scenarios may be useful for identifying a number of parameters important to public health including casualties, displaced populations, and impact on hospitals. One example is the ShakeOut Scenario produced by the USGS for Southern California. To develop this scenario, over 100 scientists from multiple disciplines came together to produce scientifically valid projections of impact from a potential earthquake occurring on the southern portion of the San Andreas Fault. Table 4.1 shows estimated casualties from building damage in that modeled earthquake (Jones et al., 2008). These estimates come from conducting postprocessing of Hazus results so that they match the categories used in the HRAI. (See Shoaf & Seligson, 2011, for a discussion of how the processing occurred.)

TABLE 4.1 Injuries Resulting From Building Damage in the ShakeOut Earthquake Scenario

County	Fatal	Trauma	ED Visits	Outpatient	EMS transports
Los Angeles	66	16	4,100	7,700	234
Imperial	0	0	0	0	1
Kern	0	0	0	100	1
Orange	1	0	700	1,500	22
Riverside	61	15	4,100	7,400	251
San Bernardino	132	32	7,400	13,400	469
San Diego	0	0	0	0	0
Ventura	0	0	0	0	0
8 County Totals	260	63	16,300	30,100	978

Source: From Jones, B. L. M., Bernknopf, R., Cox, D., Goltz, J., Hudnut, K., Perry, S., Ponti, D., Porter, K., Reichle, M., Seligson, H., Shoaf, K., Treiman, J., & Wein, A. (2008). *The ShakeOut scenario* (USGS Open File Report 2008-1150; California Geological Survey Preliminary Report 25). U.S. Geological Survey. p. 308.

ED, emergency department; EMS, emergency medical support.

Some public health agencies may not have the expertise to utilize such models or conduct other scientifically valid models. They may be more inclined to use the approach put forth in the Kaiser HVA or the hHAP. This approach relies less on absolute numbers, and instead provides levels of impact for the different parameters that can be used to set priorities for strategic planning. However, these models lack the specificity needed to inform planning on a more tactical level.

Evaluate Your Community's Ability to Meet the Demands

This next step is designed to determine whether or not the jurisdiction has the resources available to meet the needs generated by the hazard. Both the UCLA HRAI and the PHRAT do this quantitatively by comparing the impacts of the hazard to the baseline for each indicator. This is based in the assumption that the jurisdiction's resources are sufficient to meet the baseline needs. While this provides a series of numbers of potentially unmet needs, the determination of the capacity of the community to meet these needs requires further work. It is ideal that the organizations and agencies that provide those services work with public health to evaluate the capacity for meeting such needs that exceed baseline. In the HRAI, there is a 5-point scale from 0 to 4, indicating the severity of the impact. A score of zero (0) indicates that the impact does not deviate from the baseline level in any appreciable way. On the other end, a score of four (4) indicates that impact may be catastrophic, requiring significant outside resources and potentially having a prolonged recovery. Exhibit 4.2 is an example of the impact scoring for fatalities in the HRAI. In this example, the hazard adds 0.35 deaths per 100,000 population to the baseline of 1.70 deaths per 100,000 population. The jurisdiction determined that the additional deaths would have minimal impact and could be handled by existing agency resources (Shoaf et al., 2006).

EXHIBIT 4.2 **Example of Impact Score**

UNIT OF MEASUREMENT	
Number of fatalities per 100,000 population per day	
BASELINE DATA	**HAZARD-SPECIFIC DATA**
1.70	.35
Using the scale that follows, assess your agency's current abilities to respond to the anticipated disaster impact.	
0 = Baseline	Added impact of disaster is negligible
1 = Minimal	Cases are adequately handled by agency using existing resources
2 = Moderate	Stretches capacity of existing resources; draws upon resources provided by mutual aid
3 = Severe	Needs far exceed capacity of local authority and adjacent mutual providers
4 = Catastrophic	Available resources are overwhelmed, requiring significant resources from outside affected area for response; recovery will be difficult, even with the help of mutual resources
score (0–4) (Enter this score into the Fatalities column on Worksheet 3)	

Incorporate the Results Into the Planning Process

The final step of the process is to incorporate the results into the planning for the community. This is explicitly spelled out in the hHAP model. Regardless of the model used, this is the purpose of conducting a hazard risk assessment. Results may be used to plan strategically about which resources or interventions may be necessary to respond to an emergency. They may also provide indications of the quantity of materiel or personnel that are required to meet the needs generated by the disaster. The strategic plans may then utilize several approaches to addressing the specific disaster such as prepositioning resources in the jurisdiction, developing contracts with companies or mutual aid agreements with partners for receipt of resources, and changing staffing ratios in hospitals to provide surge capacity.

FUTURE OF PUBLIC HEALTH HAZARD RISK ASSESSMENT

This chapter has covered the past and the present of hazard risk assessments for public health. What lies ahead in the future? Currently, all the models that have been described rely on manually conducting the hazard assessment. At best, some of the models have included Excel spreadsheets with macros written to move the process from one step to the next, calculating values input along the way. Automating this process would make it more accessible for smaller health departments that do not have access to academic partners or those with expertise in modeling. It would allow for data from real events to be incorporated into future iterations of the model, allowing for increasing accuracy for jurisdictions that share similar hazards (e.g., wildfires, floods, earthquakes, tornadoes, tsunamis). It would also standardize the process across jurisdictions and make their results more comparable for planning purposes. Recently, the Los Angeles County Department of Public Health, Emergency Preparedness Division under

CDC funding developed a web-based mapping project following the hHAP model. This project includes the hazard assessment piece and modules on at-risk populations. Furthermore, it feeds directly into planning templates that could be used as hazard-specific annexes to an emergency response plan. This is the direction that hazard risk assessment needs to go to enable all local health departments to have the information necessary to plan effectively.

The other area for future improvements in hazard risk assessment is incorporating the rapid changes in the climate and emerging infectious diseases. As hazard risk assessments are often based on historic records, they often do not incorporate the changing nature of the risk due to climate change. The risk tied to climate change has a significant impact on multiple hazards, both in terms of their likelihood of occurrence and the severity of their impact. Directly tied to climate, we have seen major shifts in wildfires along the West Coast of the United States and hurricanes in the Atlantic. In 2020 the country experienced historic wildfires, exceeding the previous records established in 2018. These historic wildfires also led to historic records in poor air quality. At one point in September 2020, in Portland, Oregon; Seattle, Washington; San Francisco, California; and Vancouver, British Columbia, the smoke from wildfires resulted in these cities switching from their normal status as cities with good air quality to cities with the worst air quality of any major city in the world. Similarly, the Atlantic hurricane season for 2020 had a record number of named storms, forcing a move from the normal naming system to use of the Greek alphabet. As of November 30, there were 30 named storms in the 2020 season, breaking the record of 28 named storms in the 2005 hurricane season.

In addition to the changes in these direct climate hazards, climate change also plays a role in the development and expansion of infectious diseases. Vector-borne diseases are particularly susceptible to change in climatic conditions. As median temperatures rise, the geographic spread of vectors such as mosquitoes expand and the risk of the disease they carry, such as dengue or malaria, moves into new locations. There will need to be new modeling to help future hazard risk assessment incorporate the changes in hazard probability as well as severity resulting from these climate changes.

CONCLUSION

In general, conducting a hazard risk assessment is essential to planning appropriately for potential disasters. Assessment is a key function of public health that applies to the practice of emergency public health as well as daily public health. State, territorial, local, and tribal health departments need public health professionals with the competencies to conduct such an assessment.

DISCUSSION QUESTIONS

1. Define and discuss the use of the terms *"hazard," "disaster," vulnerability," "risk," and "threat"* within the context of emergency preparedness and response.
2. Discuss the approaches and relative merits among the tools for hazard assessment, including the Hazard Vulnerability Assessment (HVA) tool; the Health Hazard Assessment and Prioritization (hHAP) tool; the Pennsylvania Public Health Risk Assessment Tool (PHRAT); the Hazard Risk Assessment Instrument (HRAI); and the Threat and Hazard Identification and Risk Assessment (THIRA).

3. Discuss some of the potential future improvements in hazard risk assessment.
4. Discuss the evolving roles of public health at local, state, and national levels in disaster preparedness and response.

REFERENCES

Backman, F. (1996, February 8–12). *The risk assessment matrix*. FDSOA Health and Safety.

Birkmann, J. (2013). Risk. In P. T. Bobrowsky (Ed.), *Encyclopedia of natural hazards* (pp. 856–862). Springer. https://doi.org/10.1007/978-1-4020-4399-4_296

Centers for Disease Control and Prevention, Center for Preparedness and Response. (2018, October). *Public health emergency preparedness and response capabilities: National standards for state, local, tribal, and territorial public health*. U.S. Department of Health and Human Services. https://www.cdc.gov/cpr/readiness/00_docs/CDC_PreparednesResponseCapabilities_October2018_Final_508.pdf

Centers for Disease Control and Prevention. (n.d.). *Develop SMART objectives*. https://www.cdc.gov/phcommunities/resourcekit/evaluate/smart_objectives.html

Coburn, A., Spence, R. S., & Pomonis, A. (1993). *Vulnerability and risk assessment*. UNDP Disaster Management Training Programme.

Dean, B., Bagwell, D. A., Dora, V., Khan, S., & Plough, A. (2013). Los Angeles County Department of Public Health's Health Hazard Assessment. *Journal of Public Health Management and Practice, 19*(5, Suppl. 2), S84–S90. https://doi.org/10.1097/PHH.0b013e3182928e63

de Boer, J. (1990). Definition and classification of disasters: Introduction of a disaster severity scale. *Journal of Emergency Medicine, 8*, 591–595. https://doi.org/10.1016/0736-4679(90)90456-6

Federal Emergency Management Agency. (n.d.). Vulnerability Analysis. In *Emergency Managment Guide for Business and Industry*.

Federal Emergency Management Agency. (2016). *HAZUS 3.2. Software*. https://www.fema.gov/flood-maps/products-tools/hazus

Federal Emergency Management Agency. (2018). *Threat and hazard identification and risk assessment (THIRA) and stakeholder preparedness review (SPR) guide: Comprehensive preparedness guide (CPG) 201* (3rd ed.). U.S. Department of Homeland Security. https://www.fema.gov/sites/default/files/2020-04/CPG201Final20180525.pdf

Gislason, E. (2018). *Types of hazards*. https://naspweb.com/blog/types-of-hazards

Institute of Medicine, Committee for the Study of the Future of Public Health, Division of Health Care Services. (1988). *The future of public health*. National Academies Press.

Jones, B. L. M., Bernknopf, R., Cox, D., Goltz, J., Hudnut, K., Perry, S., Ponti, D., Porter, K., Reichle, M., Seligson, H., Shoaf, K., Treiman, J., & Wein, A. (2008). *The ShakeOut scenario* (USGS Open File Report 2008–1150; California Geological Survey Preliminary Report 25). U.S. Geological Survey. https://pubs.usgs.gov/of/2008/1150

Keller, A. Z. (1989, September 12–13). *The Bradford Disaster Scale* [Presentation]. Disaster Prevention, Planning and Limitations: Proceedings of the First Conference, University of Bradford, England, United Kingdom.

Kramer, W. M., & Bahme, C. W. (1992). Hazard identification exercise. In *Fire officer's guide to disaster control* (2nd ed.). Penwell Publishing Company.

Malilay, J. N., Henderson, A. K., McGeehin, M., & Flanders, W. D. (1997). Estimating health risks from natural hazards using risk assessment and epidemiology. *Risk Analysis, 17*(3), 353–358. https://doi.org/10.1111/j.1539-6924.1997.tb00873.x

Pennsylvania Public Health Risk Assessment Tool (PHRAT) | Drexel Dornsife School of Public Health. (n.d.). https://drexel.edu/dornsife/research/centers-programs-projects/center-for-public-health-readiness-communication/our-projects/phrat

Peters, R., Hipper, T. J., Kricun, H., & Chernak, E. (2019). A quantitative public health risk assessment tool for planning for at-risk populations. *American Journal of Public Health, 109*(Suppl. 4), S286–S289. https://doi.org/10.2105/AJPH.2019.305181

Rukstales, K., & Petersen, M. (2019). *Data release for 2018 update of the U.S. National Seismic Hazard Model: U.S. Geological Survey data release*. https://doi.org/10.5066.P9WT5OVB

Shoaf, K. I., & Seligson, H. (2011). Estimating casualties for the Southern California Shakeout. In R. Spence, E. So, & C. R. Scawthorn (Eds.), *Human casualties in earthquakes* (pp. 125–137). Springer Netherlands. https://doi.org/10.1007/978-90-481-9455-1

Shoaf, K. I., Seligson, H. A., Stratton, S. J., & Rottman, S. J. (2006). *Hazard Risk Assessment Instrument workbook*. UCLA Center for Public Health and Disasters.

Soriano, F. I. (2013). *Conducting needs assessments: A multidisciplinary approach* (2nd ed.). Sage Publications.

United Nations Office for Disaster Risk Reduction. (2009). *Terminology on disaster risk reduction*. Author. https://www.preventionweb.net/files/7817_UNISDRTerminologyEnglish.pdf

U.S. Department of Health and Human Services. (2012). *Healthcare preparedness capabilities*. http://www.phe.gov/Preparedness/planning/hpp/reports/Documents/capabilities.pdf

U.S. Department of Health and Human Services. (2018). *ASPR TRACIE evaluation of hazard vulnerability assessment tools*. https://files.asprtracie.hhs.gov/documents/aspr-tracie-evaluation-of-hva-tools-3-10-17.pdf

U.S. Department of Homeland Security. (2010). *DHS risk lexicon* (2010 ed.).

World Health Organization. (n.d.). https://www.who.int/hac/about/definitions/en

CHAPTER 5

EMERGENCY OPERATIONS PLANS

ESSENTIAL TOOLS FOR PREPAREDNESS AND RESPONSE

GLEN P. MAYS

KEY TERMS

CDC's Operational Readiness Review (ORR) Process
CDC's Set of 15 Public Health Emergency Preparedness and Response Capabilities
Continuity of Government (COG) Plans
Continuity of Operations (COOP) Plans
Emergency Operations Center (EOC)
Emergency Operations Plans (EOPs)
Emergency Support Function #8 (ESF#8)
Federal Emergency Management Agency (FEMA)
FEMA's Comprehensive Preparedness Guide
Horizontal Alignment
Incident Command System (ICS)
National Health Security Preparedness Index (NHSPI)
National Preparedness System
National Response Framework
Threat and Hazard Identification and Risk Assessment (THIRA)
Vertical Alignment

INTRODUCTION

> Plans are worthless, but planning is everything.
> – Dwight D. Eisenhower (Garcia Contreras et al., 2020)

Emergency operations plans (EOPs) define the scope of activities and division of responsibilities for responding to hazardous emergency events. Developing and refining EOPs are essential components of emergency preparedness as practiced by individual organizations and by governmental jurisdictions at local, state, territorial, tribal, and federal levels. The utility of an EOP derives partly from the content of the plan itself but more so from the planning process. A responsive and actionable EOP requires a stakeholder-engaged process of assessment, priority setting, analysis, specification, testing, and continuous refinement. Deriving utility from the plan requires regular application and continuous updating based on lessons learned during real and simulated emergency events. Opportunities exist for transforming static and cumbersome plans into dynamic public health decision tools using the power of modern informatics, analytics, and data science.

WHO NEEDS TO PLAN?

EOPs are important tools for all stakeholders responsible for responding to hazardous events. Emergencies often develop rapidly and unfold in highly unpredictable ways, making it ineffective to rely on improvised responses or simple replication of past actions. EOPs allow organizations to identify plausible response options and assess their benefits and risks before incidents occur, carefully considering trade-offs, contingencies, roles, and other implementation issues. By helping organizations work through these issues in advance, including through experience gained by preparedness drills and exercises, EOPs prepare organizations to rapidly implement and adapt their responses during real events. Because effective emergency response requires communication and coordination among many different stakeholders, EOPs help these stakeholders develop shared mental models for how they will jointly make decisions and take actions during real events. Similarly, EOPs help organizations coordinate response activities across government jurisdictional boundaries and across the continuum of local, state, territorial, tribal, and federal emergency response agencies.

Recognizing the importance of EOPs to effective emergency decision-making, the **Federal Emergency Management Agency (FEMA)** supports state, territorial, local, and tribal (STLT) governments across the United States in developing jurisdiction-wide EOPs as part of the National Preparedness Strategy (Figure 5.1). This type of EOP broadly covers all government functions and all nongovernmental community and social systems within a government jurisdiction, including public health, mental health, and medical services (Nowell et al., 2018). For similar reasons, many federal and state agencies and professional accreditation bodies require the development of facility-level EOPs for specific types of organizations as a condition of funding, regulatory approval, licensing, and accreditation. Facilities such as hospitals, medical clinics, educational institutions, childcare facilities, housing authorities, critical infrastructure suppliers, and selected types of businesses and workplaces fall under these types of facility-specific EOP requirements. Within this planning ecosystem, public health agency EOPs serve as a bridge connecting jurisdiction-wide EOPs with facility-level EOPs, integrating public health considerations into planning at all levels (Figure 5.1).

Public health agencies play unique and multifaceted roles in emergency planning and EOP development. These agencies have primary responsibility for determining the public health risks and consequences associated with all emergency incidents that occur within their jurisdictions (Keim, 2010). In many jurisdictions and situations, public health agency leaders possess the legal authority to declare public health emergencies and activate emergency protocols within their jurisdictions. These agencies play either leading or supporting roles in jurisdiction-wide emergency response activities for hazards with significant public

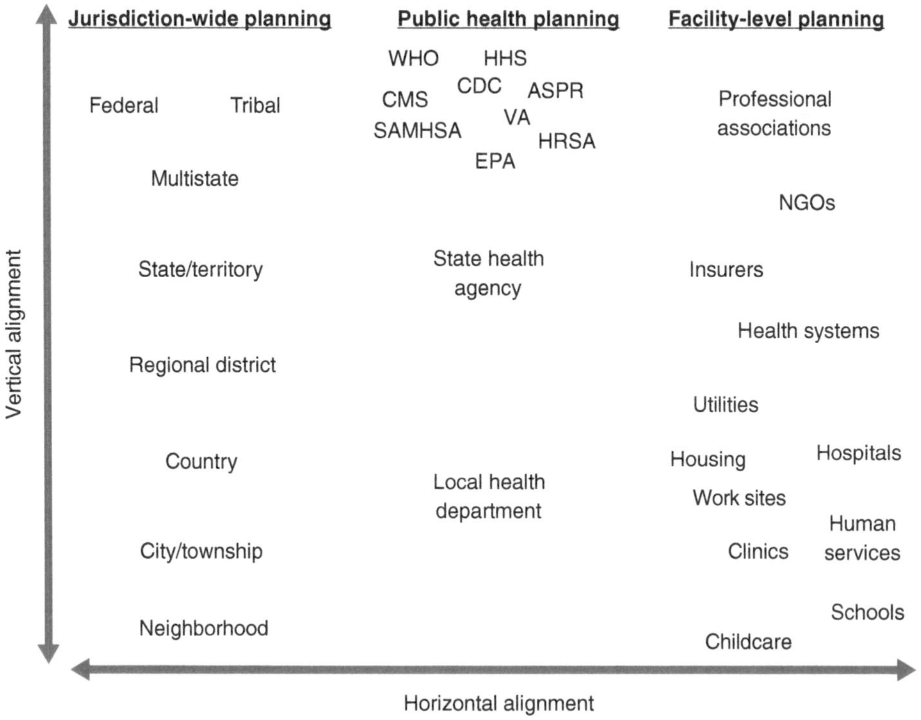

Figure 5.1 Multiple levels of emergency operations planning in the United States.

ASPR, U.S. Assistant Secretary for Preparedness and Response; CDC, Centers for Disease Control and Prevention; CMS, Centers for Medicare and Medicaid Services; EPA, U.S. Environmental Protection Agency; HHS, U.S. Department of Health and Human Services; HRSA, Health Resources and Services Administration; NGOs, nongovernmental organizations; SAMHSA, Substance Abuse and Mental Health Services Administration; VA, U.S. Department of Veterans Affairs; WHO, World Health Organization.

health consequences. Similarly, these agencies hold the authority to activate and manage a dedicated public health **emergency operations center (EOC)** for their jurisdiction or, alternatively, to manage public health functions within an EOC housed within another governmental unit. Finally, public health agencies play essential roles in helping other governmental and private-sector institutions develop and update their EOPs in ways that address public health consequences successfully. In many cases, these agencies have the responsibility to review and approve facility-level EOPs developed by other agencies and organizations within their jurisdiction, such as hospitals, schools, water and sewer authorities, regulated industries, and other institutions of public health significance. The unique public health roles in EOP development are reflected in public health emergency preparedness and response capabilities as defined by the Centers for Disease Control and Prevention (CDC, 2018). As such, it is important to incorporate public health roles and capabilities appropriately into EOPs to ensure alignment and consistency across multiple levels of emergency planning.

THE PLANNING PROCESS

Emergency preparedness stakeholders have used numerous planning theories, models, and guidelines over time to facilitate the process of EOP development (Keim, 2010, 2013). Based on experiences with these approaches,

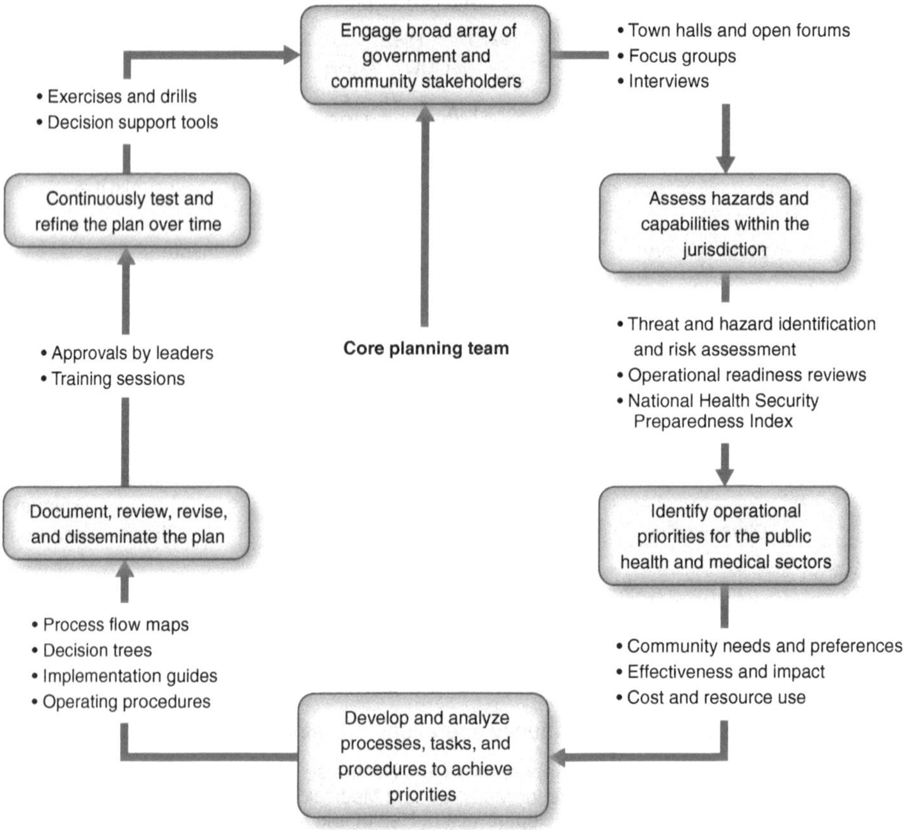
Engage broad array of government and community stakeholders
• Town halls and open forums
• Focus groups
• Interviews
Assess hazards and capabilities within the jurisdiction
• Threat and hazard identification and risk assessment
• Operational readiness reviews
• National Health Security Preparedness Index
Identify operational priorities for the public health and medical sectors
• Community needs and preferences
• Effectiveness and impact
• Cost and resource use
Develop and analyze processes, tasks, and procedures to achieve priorities
• Process flow maps
• Decision trees
• Implementation guides
• Operating procedures
Document, review, revise, and disseminate the plan
• Approvals by leaders
• Training sessions
Continuously test and refine the plan over time
• Exercises and drills
• Decision support tools
Core planning team

Figure 5.2 Key steps in the emergency operations planning process.

planners have identified a core series of steps that support effective EOP planning (Figure 5.2). These components are now incorporated into major EOP planning frameworks such as **FEMA's Comprehensive Preparedness Guide** (FEMA, 2010). The sections that follow outline core steps as they apply to EOP development for public health agencies.

Step 1: Stakeholder Engagement

A critical first step in the planning process is to identify the array of stakeholders who need to be engaged in developing and implementing the EOP. These stakeholders include all organizations who have roles and responsibilities to carry out as part of the organization's response to emergency events. For public health agencies, external stakeholders typically include representatives from relevant emergency management agencies, healthcare providers, human services organizations, public safety agencies, emergency medical services, and other organizations within the jurisdiction. Representatives from community segments within the jurisdiction that could be disproportionately affected by hazardous events should also be included, such as racial and ethnic minority populations, low-income families, the disabled, and non-English-speaking communities. Internal stakeholders include representatives from relevant operating divisions within the public health agency, such as epidemiology, laboratory, communicable disease control, environmental health, and health statistics and informatics.

As part of this first step, planners identify a core planning team composed of a small group of representatives who collectively have knowledge of, and experience with, the full array of planning stakeholders. This team develops and implements strategies for engaging larger groups of stakeholders in the planning process, such as town hall meetings, open forums, focus groups, and key informant interviews.

Step 2: Hazard and Capability Assessment

Working with the larger collection of stakeholders, the core planning team identifies the array of hazards and risks that are relevant in the jurisdiction, the likelihood of each type of incident, plausible ranges for magnitude and intensity, and the population groups anticipated to be disproportionately affected. Established assessment frameworks such as FEMA's **Threat and Hazard Identification and Risk Assessment (THIRA)** process are valuable tools in accomplishing this second core step (Fenner-Crisp & Dellarco, 2016), as are data and modeling tools such as the National Risk Index and the Hazus model (Summers et al., 2018). Disaster risk assessment and tools are further examined in Chapter 4 of this textbook. Stakeholders from the jurisdiction's emergency management agencies often have experience with these types of tools and frameworks, and as such they are valuable contributors to the hazard assessment process.

After identifying hazards and risks, the EOP planning team takes stock of the capabilities that exist within the agency and jurisdiction to address identified threats. In conducting this assessment, planners collect and review information from a wide variety of sources, including after-action reports (AARs) from recent emergency exercises and real events, results from assessments and evaluations of emergency preparedness programs, and data from external performance measurement systems. For example, the **CDC's Operational Readiness Review (ORR) process** conducted as part of the Public Health Emergency Preparedness and Response Cooperative Agreement program is a federally organized performance measurement and improvement initiative used by public health agencies for EOP capability assessment (CDC, n.d.). Using the ORR process, state, territorial, and local preparedness stakeholders conduct detailed evaluations of the functionality of their emergency preparedness and response operations using self-assessments, structured data collection and reporting, and external review by subject matter experts. As another example, the **National Health Security Preparedness Index (NHSPI)** is an external performance measurement tool that produces annual composite measures of emergency preparedness capabilities for all 50 states and the District of Columbia and for individual counties, using data from more than 60 secondary data sources (see Chapter 3; Mays et al., 2020). Information from resources like ORR and NHSPI can help EOP planning teams assess their capabilities efficiently from multiple perspectives.

Step 3: Priority Setting

A pivotal next step in the planning process involves identifying operational priorities for the public health agency during emergency events. Which operations should the agency seek to maintain and expand and which activities must be scaled back or discontinued to free up capacity for higher priority functions? Priority setting must consider the effectiveness, impact, and value of various agency operations and functions from multiple perspectives, along with the resource requirements of these functions and the consequences of reducing or discontinuing selected functions. The needs and preferences of community stakeholders should be actively solicited as part of this process and incorporated directly into priority setting. Once operational priorities are identified, the planning team develops goals and objectives for each priority area.

Step 4: Process Development and Analysis

Based on the priorities and objectives developed in Step 3, the planning team works with stakeholders to identify the sequence of actions needed to achieve each objective and the responsible institutions and individuals for each action. The team considers key implementation barriers and facilitators relevant to these actions, and the resources required for implementation. Process flow maps, implementation diagrams, and decision trees are helpful tools for analyzing alternative implementation scenarios and relevant operational contingencies. As part of this process, the planning team identifies information and data streams, as well as other intelligence resources, that will be used to support operational decision-making and actions during emergency response.

Step 5: Documentation, Review, and Dissemination

The planning team integrates results from Steps 2 through 4 of the process into a coherent written plan and circulates it broadly among key stakeholders for feedback. Multiple iterations of review and revision are beneficial during this process. A final plan is circulated for approval by operational leaders within the public health agency and other partner organizations. The approved plan is then widely disseminated among operational staff at all organizations that are implicated in the plan. The planning team organizes educational and training sessions to build EOP awareness, knowledge, and skills among relevant staff.

Step 6: Testing and Improvement

An effective EOP requires repeated cycles of testing and updating using exercises, drills, and responses to real emergency events. To enhance feasibility and minimize disruptions, agencies can use a series of focused and repeated simulations and exercises that test selected components of the plan over time. Following each test, after-action debriefing and reporting processes (AARs) allow the agency to identify areas for improvement and incorporate updates into the plan. As noted later in this chapter, opportunities exist for agencies to move their EOPs into a dynamic electronic decision support environment and integrate them with computer modeling and analysis capabilities to enhance EOP testing, utilization, and updating.

PLAN COMPONENTS

Widely used emergency planning frameworks such as FEMA's (2010) Comprehensive Preparedness Guide recommend that every EOP include a common set of components (Exhibit 5.1). These components represent a standardized approach to EOP organization and content that offers several important

EXHIBIT 5.1 Core Components of an Emergency Operations Plan

Purpose: A summary statement describing how the plan is intended to be used, and who are the intended audiences and types of users. This statement should be supported by a brief synopsis of the plan components and annexes.
Scope: A description of the types of emergency and disaster response capabilities that are covered in the plan, the range of responsible entities that are implicated in the plan (e.g., government agencies and private sector organizations), and the geographic areas to which the plan applies.
Situation Overview: A description of the overall "planning environment," including a summary of the range of hazards faced by the jurisdiction and general descriptions of how the jurisdiction expects to receive and provide assistance through its response structures. This overview includes statements about: (a) the relative probability and impact of each type of hazard; (b) geographic areas likely to be affected by particular hazards; (c) vulnerable critical facilities such as nursing homes, schools, hospitals, and infrastructure; (d) the distribution of the population across the jurisdiction, including any concentrated populations of individuals with disabilities and other social and health vulnerabilities; (e) areas where the jurisdiction is dependent upon other jurisdictions for critical resources; (f) the process used by the jurisdiction to determine its capabilities and limits in order to prepare for and respond to the defined hazards; and (g) the actions taken by the jurisdiction to minimize the impact of hazards, including short- and long-term strategies.
Planning Assumptions: A list of key assumptions regarding risks, capabilities, needs, and resources that are assumed to be true for the purposes of implementing planned activities. During emergency situations, users need to adapt the plan if assumptions are found to be inconsistent with facts of the incident.
Concept of Operations (CONOPS): A written or graphic statement that explains the overall design and intent of emergency operations. Describe how the organization will accomplish its mission and core objectives during emergency situations in order to reach a desired end state. Include a brief discussion of the activation levels identified by the jurisdiction for its emergency operations center. Briefly describe direction and control mechanisms to be used, alert and warning systems, and continuity matters that may be addressed in more detail in the plan annexes.
Organization and Assignment of Responsibilities: A description of the range of emergency functions and tasks to be performed, by position and responsible organization. Do not include full procedural details to be described in plan annexes. When two or more organizations perform the same kind of task, one should be listed with primary responsibility, with the others providing supporting roles. A matrix of organizations and areas of responsibility, including functions, should be included to summarize primary and supporting roles. Shared general responsibilities, such as developing standard operating procedures, should be included. Organization charts, especially those depicting how a jurisdiction is implementing the Incident Command Structure or Multiagency Coordination System structure, are helpful.
Direction, Control, and Coordination: A description of the framework for all direction, control, and coordination activities during emergencies. Specify which entities have tactical and operational control of response assets and resources. Explain how multijurisdictional coordination systems will operate while allowing each jurisdiction to retain its own authorities. Provide information on how individual agency and facility plans nest into the jurisdiction-wide plan (horizontal integration) and how plans for higher land lower levels of government are expected to layer on the plan (vertical integration).
Information Collection, Analysis, and Dissemination: A description of the essential types of data and information needed to execute and manage all emergency operations identified in the plan. Identify the type of information needed, the source of the information, who uses the information, how the information is shared, the format for acquiring and storing the information, and any specific times the information is needed.
Communications: A description of communication protocols and coordination procedures used between response organizations during emergencies. Identify a framework for delivering communications support and how the jurisdiction's communications functions integrate with regional or national disaster communications networks. This section may be expanded as an annex and is usually supplemented by communications standard operating procedures and field guides.

(*continued*)

EXHIBIT 5.1 Core Components of an Emergency Operations Plan *(continued)*

Administration, Finance, and Logistics: A description of general administrative support requirements and policies for managing resources. Include the following elements: (a) references to intrastate and interstate mutual aide agreements, including the Emergency Management Assistance Compact; (b) legal authorities and policies for augmenting staff by reassigning public employees and soliciting volunteers, along with relevant liability provisions; and (c) general policies on maintaining financial records, reporting, tracking resource needs, tracking the source and use of resources, acquiring ownership of resources, and compensating the owners of private property used by the jurisdiction.
Plan Development and Maintenance: A description of the planning process, participants in that process, and how development and revision of different plan components are coordinated during the preparedness phase. Assign responsibility for the overall planning and coordination to a specific position, and provide for a regular cycle of training, evaluating, reviewing, and updating of the plan.
Authorities and References: An overview of the legal basis for emergency operations and activities. This section includes (a) laws, statutes, ordinances, executive orders, regulations, and formal agreements relevant to emergencies; (b) descriptions of the extent and limits of the emergency authorities granted to the senior official, including the conditions under which these authorities become effective and when they would be terminated; (c) pre-delegation of emergency authorities; and (d) provisions for continuity of operations or continuity of government.
Supporting Annexes: This section includes additional planning documents that focus on specific emergency functions, hazards, and/or agencies. Each annex follows the same structure and content as that of the basic plan.

Source: Data from Federal Emergency Management Agency. (2010). *Developing and maintaining emergency operations plans.* U.S. Department of Homeland Security.

advantages to emergency preparedness professionals. First and foremost, the use of standard EOP components reduces the likelihood that an EOP will omit key information that users need to implement planned activities. EOP documents must convey a wide range of information needed to support successful implementation, including the following:

- a description of when to use the plan and for what purposes
- key assumptions on which the plan is based
- the set of objectives to be achieved along with specific activities that will accomplish each objective
- the assignment of activities to responsible parties
- standard operating procedures for implementing key activities
- communication strategies
- financial and logistical management

Plans that overlook some of these elements can introduce significant difficulties and delays in emergency response as users determine which activities to implement and how to implement them in the context of a specific hazardous event. A standardized set of EOP components offers the advantage of helping users quickly navigate the planning document to locate relevant information. This navigation feature is particularly important when EOP planning documents are voluminous and detail-rich, and when users face imperatives for rapid EOP implementation during emergency events. Furthermore, standardized EOP components help emergency preparedness professionals compare and coordinate EOP documents across institutions and jurisdictions, and are consistent with an all-hazards approach, thereby helping to make the planned activities consistent and interoperable across settings.

Alongside the general set of EOP components specified in FEMA planning frameworks, governmental public health agencies need to develop EOPs that reflect their agencies' unique responsibilities in implementing and coordinating emergency operations relevant to public health and medical care delivery. These unique responsibilities, referred to as public health emergency operations, are described in detail as part of the **CDC's set of 15 public health emergency preparedness and response capabilities** (CDC, 2018). In particular, Capability #3 details the functions and tasks to be performed by public health agencies in coordinating emergency operations and consists of five core functions:

- determining the need for public health emergency operations
- activating public health emergency operations, which may include administering a dedicated public health emergency operations center (EOC) and/or performing functions within an EOC based within another governmental unit
- developing and maintaining emergency action plans that address public health and healthcare needs in the jurisdiction throughout all phases of emergency response and recovery
- managing and sustaining public health emergency operations during the response and recovery phases
- discontinuing and evaluating public health emergency operations

These functions are further subdivided into a set of 21 tasks that reflect detailed actions carried out by public health agencies in coordination with emergency management agencies and other stakeholders in the jurisdiction (Exhibit 5.2). The EOPs developed by public health agencies reflect these tasks and the unique elements of public health decision-making and action that are embedded within them. Important crosscutting elements of public health emergency response and coordination, described in the following, feature prominently in the EOPs developed by public health agencies.

Emergency Declarations and Orders

Public health agency leaders in many states, territories, and local jurisdictions possess the legal authority to declare public health emergencies and to issue certain types of public health orders within their jurisdictions—such as those related to quarantine, isolation, and the regulation of commercial and public activities (see also Chapter 16 regarding Public Health Law). The specific types of emergency declaration powers and responsibilities given to public health agencies varies across jurisdictions based on state and local law. In jurisdictions that do not delegate these powers directly to public health agency leaders, the public health agency is often responsible for advising other government officials—such as governors, mayors, and county commissioners or their offices of emergency management—on the execution of

EXHIBIT 5.2 Core Functions and Tasks Required for Public Health Emergency Operations Coordination

Capability Definition: Emergency operations coordination is the ability to coordinate with emergency management and to direct and support an incident or event with public health or healthcare implications by establishing a standardized, scalable system of oversight, organization, and supervision that is consistent with jurisdictional standards and practices and the National Incident Management System (NIMS).
Function 1: Conduct preliminary assessment to determine the need for activation of public health emergency operations
Task 1: Determine the public health response role. Coordinate with emergency management officials to determine if public health will have a lead response role, a supporting role, or no role based on identified or potential public health consequences.
Task 2: Determine response activation levels based on the complexity of the incident or event. Coordinate with emergency management officials in collecting and analyzing data to assess the situation and determine emergency response operations applicable to jurisdictional needs.
Task 3: Develop the public health incident management structure. Document a flexible and scalable public health incident management structure that is consistent with NIMS and is coordinated with the jurisdictional incident, unified, or area command structure.
Function 2: Activate public health emergency operations
Task 1: Activate public health incident command and emergency management functions. Activate necessary public health functions and support mutual aid according to the public health incident management role and incident requirements.
Task 2: Identify personnel with the necessary skills to fulfill required incident command and public health incident management roles. Coordinate with emergency management agencies and other partners to develop staffing pools that include federal, regional, state, local, tribal, and territorial personnel with necessary public health expertise to serve as incident commander and other public health incident management roles.
Task 3: Designate personnel coverage for multiple operational periods. Develop continuous long-term staffing plans for required incident command and other public health incident management roles.
Task 4: Establish primary and alternate locations and virtual communication structures for the public health emergency operations center. Identify primary and backup physical space and secure necessary equipment, such as desks, lighting, power outlets, and internet access, as well as virtual communication structures to support public health emergency operations.
Task 5: Assemble designated personnel at the appropriate emergency operations center(s). Notify personnel to report either physically or virtually to the public health emergency operations center (EOC) or jurisdictional EOC.
Function 3: Develop and maintain an incident response strategy
Task 1: Develop incident action plans. Produce or contribute to (as appropriate for the public health incident management role) an incident action plan that receives approval prior to each operational period.
Task 2: Update and share incident action plans. Revise and brief personnel on the incident action plan by the start of each new operational period.
Task 3: Disseminate incident action plans. Make incident action plans available to relevant public health response personnel, volunteers, and partner agencies according to emergency operations protocols.
Function 4: Manage and sustain the public health response
Task 1: Coordinate public health and healthcare emergency management operations. Ensure coordination among public health agencies, the healthcare system, and other relevant stakeholders according to incident requirements.
Task 2: Track public health resources. Ensure systems are in place to track and account for all public health resources during the public health response.

(*continued*)

EXHIBIT 5.2 Core Functions and Tasks Required for Public Health Emergency Operations Coordination (*continued*)

Task 3: Maintain health situational awareness. Compile information gathered from public health, healthcare, and other stakeholders, such as fusion centers to support a common operating picture.
Task 4: Conduct shift change briefings. During shift changes, formally share information between outgoing and incoming public health personnel to communicate priorities, status of tasks, and safety guidance.
Task 5: Develop continuity of operations plan(s). Identify response priorities to ensure the continuation and recovery of critical public health functions.
Function 5: Demobilize and evaluate public health emergency operations
Task 1: Return public health resources and staffing to their prior "ready state" of operations. Archive records and restore systems, supplies, and staffing to pre-incident readiness.
Task 2: Conduct final incident closeout of public health operations. Turn over documentation, conduct hot washes and incident debriefings, and identify final closeout requirements with responsible agencies and jurisdiction officials.
Task 3: Produce after-action report(s). Conduct after-action processes for public health operations in partnership with other emergency operations stakeholders to identify areas of success, promising practices, and opportunities for improvement.
Task 4: Develop improvement plan(s). Document priorities and identify corrective actions assigned to public health.
Task 5: Implement and track progress on improvement plan(s). Complete the corrective actions assigned to public health and establish a system to track completion and effectiveness of corrective actions.

Source: Centers for Disease Control and Prevention. (2018). *Public health emergency preparedness and response capabilities: National standards for state, local, tribal, and territorial public health.* https://www.cdc.gov/cpr/readiness/00_docs/CDC_PreparednesResponseCapabilities_October2018_Final_508.pdf

emergency powers that have significant public health consequences. Public health EOPs must specify the circumstances that justify public health emergency declarations and public health emergency orders and delineate which government officials have responsibility for these actions.

Emergency Operations Centers

Public health agencies hold the authority to activate and manage a dedicated public health EOC for their jurisdiction or, alternatively, to manage public health functions within an EOC housed within another governmental unit. The EOC is a physical or virtual location from which coordination and support of emergency management activities is directed. Dedicated public health EOCs may be needed for hazardous events that create particularly prevalent and severe public health consequences, such as infectious disease outbreaks and environmental health disasters. For these types of events, public health control and mitigation strategies often function as the primary means of emergency response and recovery, such as the use of epidemiological surveillance, laboratory testing, regulation of risk-enhancing business and household activities, and distribution of medical and pharmaceutical countermeasures such as vaccines and therapeutics. The public health EOP specifies when and how to activate a dedicated public health EOC (including the use of the **Incident Command System**, or **ICS**, structure) and, alternatively, when and how to activate public health functions within an EOC embedded within another unit of government.

Coordination of Emergency Operations

Public health agencies play essential roles in helping other governmental and private-sector institutions develop EOPs in ways that address public health consequences successfully and ensure coordination and interoperability. In many cases, public health agencies have the responsibility to review and approve facility-level EOPs developed by other agencies and organizations within their jurisdiction, such as hospitals, schools, regulated industries, and other institutions of public health significance. This function, a form of **horizontal alignment** in emergency operations, ensures that individual facilities can interface successfully with the public health agency during emergencies for tasks such as information exchange, requests for assistance, sharing of equipment and personnel, and the implementation of emergency orders and regulations (see Figure 5.1). Horizontal coordination also requires that a jurisdiction's public health EOP is well integrated with similar plans of neighboring and peer jurisdictions. Public health agencies achieve this form of coordination through periodic peer review of other jurisdiction's EOPs, and through the development of mutual aid agreements and compacts with these peer jurisdictions. Additionally, public health agencies are responsible for coordinating their own jurisdiction's public health EOP with the EOPs developed by different levels of government across the federal, state, territorial, local, and tribal continuum. This function, a form of **vertical alignment** in emergency operations, includes protocols for requesting public health assistance from higher levels of government, as well as protocols for delivering requested assistance to lower levels of government. Effective public health EOPs include core mechanisms for achieving both horizontal and vertical coordination.

As part of their coordination responsibilities, public health agencies ensure that their jurisdiction's public health EOP is aligned and consistent with other types of emergency plans that exist for the jurisdiction. These other types of plans include the following:

- Preparedness plans for the public health agency, which describe how the agency develops and maintains capabilities in preparing for and responding to hazardous events both before and after the events occur. Preparedness plans include processes for identifying and meeting staff training needs related to carrying out the emergency actions specified in the EOP, such as through exercises and drills.
- **Continuity of operations (COOP) plans** for the public health agency, healthcare organizations, and other institutions of public health significance within the jurisdiction. These plans identify essential functions that organizations maintain during an emergency, essential facilities and staff that carry out essential functions, orders of succession if key officials are unable to perform duties, and delegations of authority to other organizational units if normal channels of direction are disrupted.
- **Continuity of government (COG) plans** for governments that operate within the jurisdiction. These plans address actions to ensure the preservation or reconstitution of essential government institutions so that constitutional, legislative, judicial, and administrative responsibilities are maintained.
- Emergency action plans for employers and worksites. These plans, required by the Occupational Safety and Health Administration (OSHA), specify procedures that employers use for reporting emergencies to relevant government

authorities; evacuating employees; sheltering in place; performing rescue, tracking, and reunifying employees; and employee training.

- Post-incident recovery plans for governmental jurisdictions. These plans identify how resources are used to guide future community development after hazardous events have occurred, including redevelopment of public health and medical care systems.
- Mitigation plans for government jurisdictions. These plans, required by the federal Disaster Mitigation Act of 2000 for jurisdictions requesting federal disaster assistance funding, outline actions for reducing future risks associated with known hazards within the jurisdiction. Like EOPs, these plans are based on a formal hazard assessment and a set of planning assumptions about future risks.

As these types of plans are updated over time, public health agencies identify how to adapt their public health EOPs to maintain alignment and consistency.

Emergency Support Functions

The federal government designates governmental public health agencies to perform specific roles in responding to emergency events as part of national preparedness. The modern legal basis for these roles includes Presidential Policy Directive 8, an executive order issued by President Obama in 2011 that authorized the development of the National Preparedness Goal and the **National Preparedness System** (Obama, 2011). The National Preparedness System includes preparedness frameworks for each of the five emergency mission areas of hazard prevention, protection, mitigation, response, and recovery. The fourth of these frameworks, the **National Response Framework**, defines processes for responding to all types of disasters and emergencies, and develops a set of 15 emergency support functions (Federal Emergency Management Agency, 2019b). **Emergency Support Function #8 (ESF #8)**, devoted specifically to the provision of public health and medical services during emergencies, provides guidance and direction for governmental public health agencies in emergency response (FEMA, 2019a). The ESF #8 policy defines core capabilities that designated public health agencies are expected to perform, including providing public information and warning about health risks, conducting health surveillance to monitor health and medical needs in the population, managing surges in demand for medical care, providing public health and medical consultation, responding to threats associated with vector-borne diseases, and addressing environmental health risks and exposures such as those related to air, water, food, and workplaces. The U.S. Department of Health and Human Services (HHS) is charged with leading the ESF #8 capabilities in coordination with state, territorial, tribal, and local partners. In turn, partner governments are responsible for designating ESF #8 supporting agencies for their jurisdictions. Public health agencies are frequently designated as the ESF #8 supporting agencies for their jurisdictions, and, as such, public health EOPs need to include strategies for performing ESF #8 capabilities.

Healthcare Oversight and Crisis Standards of Care

Public health agencies play important roles in overseeing the practice of mental health and medical care during hazardous events, and public health EOPs include these roles. Large-scale hazardous events may generate surges in patient volume that have the potential to exceed the capacity of emergency departments, hospitals, physician practices, and other local healthcare delivery sites. In these situations, departures from standard medical practices may be necessary to allow scarce medical resources to be deployed in ways that reduce morbidity and mortality. State and territorial governments have broad legal powers to regulate the practice of medical care, and therefore, state and territorial public health agencies play essential roles in determining the need for emergency orders and regulations concerning medical practice (Gostin, 2000). During the COVID-19 pandemic, for example, many states issued emergency orders that required hospitals to suspend the delivery of elective medical procedures to preserve hospital beds, staff, and personal protective equipment for COVID-19 patients. States used emergency powers to relax medical provider licensing requirements to allow retired and out-of-state professionals to practice within the jurisdiction and to allow a broader array of professionals to perform essential practices such as diagnostic testing and administering vaccinations.

As part of their emergency powers, state and territorial governments have the authority to implement crisis standards of care, which empower healthcare providers to depart from standard medical practices to allocate scarce resources in ways that minimize harm to the population at large (Margus et al., 2020). These standards allow providers to triage patients to different levels of care based on availability and assessments of potential patient benefit. The crisis standards of care may also adjust the nurse-to-patient staffing ratios and allow for other ancillary staff (e.g., emergency medical technicians, or EMTs) to provide additional services during declared emergencies (e.g., performing COVID-19 vaccination). When activated by state or territorial governments, these standards provide legal protections to healthcare providers who comply with the standards, reducing the risk of medical malpractice liability. State and territorial public health agencies are responsible for developing guidelines for healthcare providers to follow regarding ethical processes for making triage decisions and for allocating scarce medical resources and services. These guidelines are formalized in crisis standards of care plans developed by each state and territory. Using these guidelines, individual healthcare facilities develop their own crisis standards of care that define specific processes to be used in allocating scarce resources and services during emergencies. Public health EOPs developed by state and territorial public health agencies must include information about when and how crisis standards of care are implemented.

PLAN LIMITATIONS AND CONSTRAINTS

Participants in strategic and operational planning often observe that the planning process is more valuable than the plan itself (Garcia Contreras et al., 2020). This observation may apply to EOPs, particularly when these plans exhibit qualities that limit their use and utility. EOPs tend to be dense and complex documents, describing many activities with responsibilities assigned to numerous organizational units and partners, and with specific conditions and contingencies that describe when and how each action should be implemented. Only a subset of these activities and contingencies are likely to be relevant for a specific emergency event. Users often find it difficult to navigate and parse these plans to identify the most relevant components, particularly while operating in an environment of time and resource constraints created by an emergency. Even with frequent and high-quality testing and training, users may be unable to maintain comprehensive knowledge of all the plan elements due to its density and complexity, creating barriers to real-time navigation and parsing.

Relatedly, EOPs are static free-text documents that cannot specify and analyze all possible combinations of the actions and contingencies described in the plan. EOPs typically describe large numbers of discrete actions and contingencies, resulting in many possible combinations of these plan elements. Some of these combinations may be highly beneficial in the context of a specific emergency event, while other combinations may be irrelevant, infeasible, or entail high levels of risk. Due to their static written format, EOPs are unable to analyze and display the many alternative combinations of activities and contingencies. Consequently, users experience difficulties in determining which combinations of plan elements are optimal in each circumstance.

Finally, because EOPs are static documents, they are updated only periodically and incrementally. Responders are not able to update EOPs rapidly and dynamically during the emergency response. This constraint is particularly problematic in the context of a novel emergency that is not fully anticipated in the hazard assessment component of the EOP. Experiences during the COVID-19 pandemic illustrate this problem, with public health agencies unable to fully anticipate constraints in jurisdictional capacities for diagnostic testing, contact tracing, and case investigation (Lash et al., 2021). Given the difficulties of rapidly updating EOPs, users may find that these plans are limited in their utility for real-time decision support during emergency response.

MOVING FROM PLANNING TO DECISION SUPPORT

Modern approaches to informatics and decision support offer opportunities for overcoming the limitations of traditional EOPs and improving their use and utility during emergency decision-making. By moving EOPs into a dynamic electronic decision support environment, users can quickly navigate the complexity and density of plans to identify components that are most relevant to the attributes of a specific hazardous event and the current stage of the response process. By applying modern data analytics and artificial intelligence methods to the EOP, users can quickly identify specific combinations of plan activities that are most likely to address current needs and risks. Frameworks currently exist for converting a static EOP into a dynamic decision support system for public health agencies, using an approach initially proposed by Mark Keim and the CDC (Hawe et al., 2015; Keim, 2013). Key elements of EOP decision support frameworks are summarized in the following subsections.

Developing Decision Support Content

Converting a static EOP into an electronic decision support system requires breaking the EOP down into its component parts and positioning these parts within a searchable relational database (Keim, 2013). The basic building blocks for this system are the discrete actions or tasks listed in the EOP. A single EOP may include dozens or hundreds of discrete actions. Each action can be tagged (or indexed) with several important attributes, including (a) the objective(s) to be accomplished with the action, (b) the hazard(s) to be addressed by the action, (c) the circumstances or contingencies that should be present to justify and trigger the action, (d) the entity responsible for implementing the action, and (e) the resources required to implement the action. Each of these attributes can be established as a separate data table in the relational database, such that linked tables exist for actions, objectives, hazards, contingencies, responsible entities, and resources.

Once the core elements of an EOP are identified and placed into a relational database of tables, these elements can be used to construct decision rules that describe when certain actions should be taken and what consequences are likely to occur as a result. Several types of decision rules are useful within EOP decision support systems, based on the principles and methods of decision analysis (McNeil & Pauker, 1984; Owens, 2002):

- Implementation rules: These elements specify the conditions and contingencies—or triggers—that should be met to implement the action. These rules often take the form of "if, then" statements.
- Resource use rules: These elements describe the human, financial, and other resources that are used to implement the action.
- Success rules: These elements describe the likelihood of achieving an objective or desired outcome, specified as a function of the actions that are implemented and the conditions and contingencies that are present.

Each decision rule is specified as a mathematical formula that can be programmed into the relational database. Numeric parameters are used in each decision rule to quantify elements such as the threshold conditions that trigger an action, the resources consumed by an action, and the likelihood that certain outcomes occur in response to an action. These parameters can be derived from a variety of sources, including published research studies, past experience of the agency, and the professional judgments of subject matter experts (Owens, 2002). If uncertainty exists about the specific value of a numeric parameter, the decision system can be designed to use a range of plausible values and produce a range of possible results to use for sensitivity analysis and contingency planning.

Integrating Risk and Capability Data

EOP decision support systems can be enhanced significantly by integrating data about risks and capabilities that exist within the jurisdiction. Public health agencies import these types of data from a variety of sources, including previously completed hazard assessments, public health surveillance systems, electronic health information exchange systems, existing federal and state surveys, and web-based systems for requesting and reporting emergency assistance (Gotham et al., 2007). Existing national data systems such as the CDC's Social Vulnerability Index, the U.S. Census Bureau's Community Resilience Estimates, and the Robert Wood Johnson Foundation's National Health Security Preparedness Index can be used in combination with state and local data sources. Once these data are imported into the EOP decision support system, they can be used to construct additional parameters that are incorporated into decision rule formulae. For example, an implementation rule may specify that actions to suspend elective medical procedures in hospitals should be considered once available hospital bed capacity in the jurisdiction falls below 10%, using data on hospital bed utilization imported from a local or statewide health information exchange.

Incorporating Analytic Modeling and Simulation Methods

Once the elements of an EOP are extracted into a relational database, translated into decision rules, and linked with jurisdiction-specific risk and capability data, preparedness professionals can apply modern data querying, modeling, and simulation methods that enable rapid use for emergency decision-making. At the most basic level of functionality, users can query the EOP database using search criteria reflecting combinations of objectives, hazard types, and responsible entities to rapidly generate subsets of plan elements that are most relevant to specific emergency situations and stages of response. By applying more advanced methods of artificial intelligence and optimization, users can run algorithms to identify specific combinations of emergency actions that are most likely to achieve desired objectives in the EOP, taking into consideration jurisdiction-specific risks, capabilities, and available resources. These algorithms use the computational methods of decision tree analysis and regression tree analysis to predict the likelihood of achieving EOP objectives based on the implementation rules, resource use rules, and success rules specified within the EOP decision support system (Doupe et al., 2019). Artificial intelligence methods allow the computer to analyze and compare many possible combinations of emergency actions—far more combinations than could be actively considered by emergency preparedness professionals using static EOP documents. Based on these algorithms, users can generate lists of emergency actions that are rank ordered and prioritized based on their estimated likelihood of success and degree of uncertainty. Users can easily recalculate these algorithms as new risk and capability data become available during an emergency, and as decision rules and emergency actions are modified during the course of emergency response. At the most advanced levels of application, users can specify alternative assumptions about how risks and capabilities may change during the future course of an emergency event and then apply simulation methods to determine how these assumptions influence the combinations of recommended actions that are most likely to achieve success in emergency response.

The reliability and accuracy of EOP decision support systems can be validated and improved over time by applying data gathered during previous emergency events. These retrospective studies, known as calibration analyses, can be used to improve the decision rules and decision formulae used within the system (Owens, 2002). For events such as the COVID-19 response, users typically have access to retrospective data about the risk and capability levels within the jurisdiction, the combinations of emergency actions implemented, the resources used, and the objectives and outcomes achieved. By incorporating these data elements into the EOP decision model, a calibration analysis can solve for the decision rule parameter values that maximize the likelihood of achieving the objectives and outcomes that were in fact achieved during the real event. As such, the decision model is trained and optimized to predict the results from actual emergency events. Multiple calibration analyses can be conducted using data from multiple emergency events and multiple jurisdictions, allowing the EOP decision support system to achieve increasingly greater precision and less uncertainty regarding its decision rules and parameters. In this way, the decision support system can improve continuously with each application to an emergency event.

It is important to keep in mind that an EOP decision support system, like all data-driven algorithms, reflects the limitations and biases that are embedded in the data and the modeling assumptions used (Sun et al., 2020). For example, algorithms may predict that emergency actions have lower probabilities of success when implemented in low-resource and historically marginalized communities that face higher baseline levels of risk and vulnerability. Such biases in algorithm prediction may be caused by baseline risks and vulnerabilities that are imperfectly measured, and by other unmeasured structural inequalities such as differences in the amount of pre-event emergency preparedness assistance and post-event disaster recovery assistance received. As jurisdictions develop and refine their EOP decision support systems, it is critically important for developers to implement large-scale testing that can identify and correct these types of structural biases in algorithms.

CONCLUSION AND FUTURE DIRECTIONS

EOPs represent valuable tools for public health agencies to use before and during their responses to hazardous emergency events. These plans are utilized at all levels of the emergency preparedness and response enterprise, starting at the local level and scaling up to state, territorial, tribal, and national levels. The utility of an EOP derives partly from the elements included in the plan itself, but more so from the process that is used to develop the plan. A responsive and actionable plan requires a stakeholder-engaged process of assessment, priority setting, analysis, specification, testing, and continuous refinement. Public health agencies carry out unique and essential responsibilities in developing public health EOPs for their jurisdictions and in coordinating and aligning the EOPs developed by other governmental and private-sector organizations. Deriving utility from an EOP requires regular application and continuous updating based on lessons learned during real and simulated emergency events. Public health agencies have begun to take steps toward transforming static and cumbersome EOP documents into dynamic public health decision support tools using the power of modern informatics, data science, and machine learning. Continued advances in technology-supported emergency decision support systems have the potential to strengthen the ability of public health agencies to respond effectively to hazardous events and limit their adverse health consequences.

DISCUSSION QUESTIONS

1. Discuss why emergency operations plans are important tools for all stakeholders responsible for responding to hazardous events.
2. What are some of the roles that public health agencies play in emergency planning and emergency operations plan development?
3. Describe the concepts of horizontal alignment and vertical alignment in the context of coordination of emergency preparedness and response.
4. Discuss how moving emergency operations plans (EOPs) into a dynamic electronic decision support environment can help overcome the limitations of traditional EOPs.

REFERENCES

Centers for Disease Control and Prevention. (n.d.). Operational readiness review. https://www.cdc.gov/cpr/readiness/orr.html

Centers for Disease Control and Prevention. (2018). *Public health emergency preparedness and response capabilities: National standards for state, local, tribal and territorial public health.* https://www.cdc.gov/cpr/readiness/capabilities.htm

Doupe, P., Faghmous, J., & Basu, S. (2019). Machine learning for health services researchers. *Value Health, 22*(7), 808–815. https://doi.org/10.1016/j.jval.2019.02.012

Federal Emergency Management Agency. (2010). *Developing and maintaining emergency operations plans.* U.S. Department of Homeland Security. https://www.fema.gov/sites/default/files/2020-05/CPG_101_V2_30NOV2010_FINAL_508.pdf

Federal Emergency Management Agency. (2019a). *Emergency support function #8 - Public health and medical services annex.* U.S. Department of Homeland Security. https://www.fema.gov/pdf/emergency/nrf/nrf-esf-08.pdf

Federal Emergency Management Agency. (2019b). *National response framework* (4th ed.). U.S. Department of Homeland Security. https://www.fema.gov/sites/default/files/2020-04/NRF_FINALApproved_2011028.pdf

Fenner-Crisp, P. A., & Dellarco, V. L. (2016). Key elements for judging the quality of a risk assessment. *Environmental Health Perspectives, 124*(8), 1127–1135. https://doi.org/10.1289/ehp.1510483

Garcia Contreras, A. F., Ceberio, M., & Kreinovich, V. (2020). Plans are worthless but planning is everything: A theoretical explanation of Eisenhower's observation. In M. Ceberio & V. Kreinovich (Eds.), *Decision making under constraints* (pp. 93–98). Springer International.

Gostin, L. O. (2000). Public health law in a new century: Part I: Law as a tool to advance the community's health. *JAMA, 283*(21), 2837–2841. https://doi.org/10.1001/jama.283.21.2837

Gotham, I. J., Sottolano, D. L., Hennessy, M. E., Napoli, J. P., Dobkins, G., Le, L. H., Burhans, R. L., & Fage, B. I. (2007). An integrated information system for all-hazards health preparedness and response: New York State Health Emergency Response Data System. *Journal of Public Health Management and Practice, 13*(5), 486–496. https://doi.org/10.1097/01.PHH.0000285202.48588.89

Hawe, G. I., Coates, G., Wilson, D. T., & Crouch, R. S. (2015). Agent-based simulation of emergency response to plan the allocation of resources for a hypothetical two-site major incident. *Engineering Applications of Artificial Intelligence, 46*, 336–345. https://doi.org/10.1016/j.engappai.2015.06.023

Keim, M. E. (2010). O2C3: A unified model for emergency operations planning. *American Journal of Disaster Medicine, 5*(3), 169–179. https://doi.org/10.5055/ajdm.2010.0019

Keim, M. E. (2013). An innovative approach to capability-based emergency operations planning. *Disaster Health, 1*(1), 54–62. https://doi.org/10.4161/dish.23480

Lash, R. R., Moonan, P. K., Byers, B. L., Bonacci, R. A., Bonner, K. E., & Donahue, M. (2021). COVID-19 case investigation and contact tracing in the US, 2020. *JAMA Network Open, 4*(6), e2115850-e. http://doi.org/10.1001/jamanetworkopen.2021.15850

Margus, C., Sarin, R. R., Molloy, M., & Ciottone, G. R. (2020). Crisis standards of care implementation at the state level in the United States. *Prehospital and Disaster Medicine, 35*(6), 599–603. https://doi.org/10.1017/S1049023X20001089

Mays, G. P., Childress, M. T., & Paris, B. (2020). *The national health security preparedness index: 2020 release.* Colorado School of Public Health, University of Colorado. https://nhspi.org/wp-content/uploads/2020/06/NHSPI_2020_Key_Findings.pdf

McNeil, B. J., & Pauker, S. G. (1984). Decision analysis for public health: Principles and illustrations. *Annual Review of Public Health, 5*, 135–161. https://doi.org/10.1146/annurev.pu.05.050184.001031

Nowell, B., Steelman, T., Velez, A-L. K., & Yang, Z. (2018). The structure of effective governance of disaster response networks: Insights from the field. *The American Review of Public Administration, 48*(7), 699–715. https://doi.org/10.1177/0275074017724225

Obama, B. (2011). *Presidential policy directive 8 - national preparedness.* White House. https://www.dhs.gov/xlibrary/assets/presidential-policy-directive-8-national-preparedness.pdf.

Owens, D. K. (2002). Analytic tools for public health decision making. *Medical Decision Making, 22*(5 Suppl.), S3–S10. https://doi.org/10.1177/027298902237969

Summers, J. K., Harwell, L. C., Smith, L. M., & Buck, K. D. (2018). Measuring community resilience to natural hazards: The Natural Hazard Resilience Screening Index (NaHRSI)-Development and application to the United States. *Geohealth, 2*(12), 372–394. https://doi.org/10.1029/2018GH000160

Sun, W., Nasraoui, O., & Shafto, P. (2020). Evolution and impact of bias in human and machine learning algorithm interaction. *PLoS One, 15*(8), e0235502. https://doi.org/10.1371/journal.pone.0235502

PART II

LESSONS LEARNED FROM ACTUAL INCIDENTS

CHAPTER 6

HURRICANE DISASTERS AS A PUBLIC HEALTH PROBLEM

THE HURRICANE HARVEY DISASTER IN TEXAS

J. DANIELLE SHARPE AND DAVID S. RICKLESS

KEY TERMS

Chief Complaint
Environmental Hazards
Low-Pressure Center
Medically Sensitive Populations
Millibar
Social Determinants of Health
Syndromic Surveillance

HURRICANE DISASTERS AS A PUBLIC HEALTH PROBLEM

Hurricanes are defined as tropical cyclones that are characterized by strong winds, **low-pressure centers**, and heavy rainfalls. Occurring in the Atlantic Ocean, hurricanes in the United States primarily make landfall in states along the Gulf Coast and East Coast, including Florida, Texas, Louisiana, North Carolina, South Carolina, Alabama, and Georgia (Figure 6.1; Sharpe, 2019). Based on the Saffir-Simpson Hurricane Wind Scale, hurricanes can be categorized in regard to potential damage levels on the basis of central pressure, wind speed, and storm surge (Table 6.1; Saffir, 1977; Simpson, 1971). For instance, Hurricane Harvey in 2017 made landfall in Texas as a Category 4 hurricane,

---

The following icons, located in the margins throughout the chapter and within the summary tables, denote essential services of public health, CEPH competencies, and leadership levels: Essential services of public health; CEPH competencies; Leadership levels.

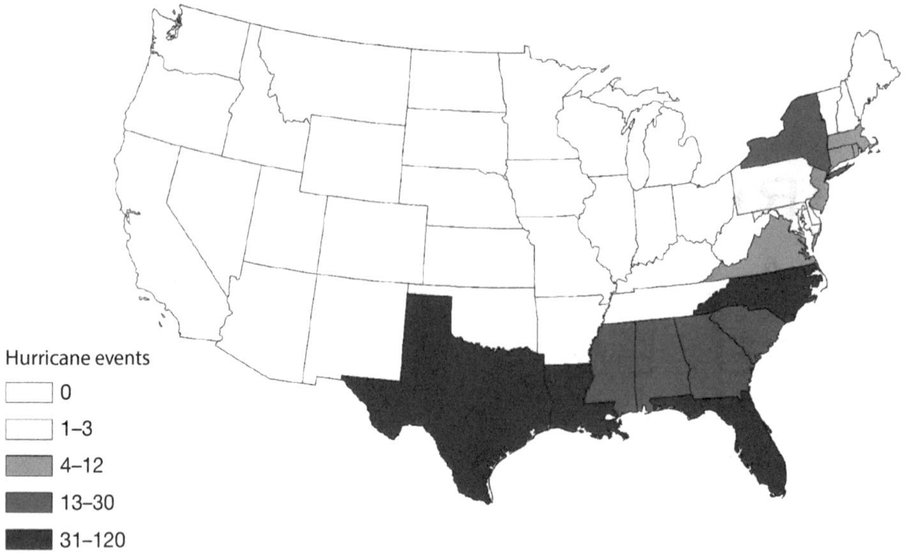

Figure 6.1 The geographic distribution of hurricanes for the contiguous United States by State, 1851–2017.

Source: Adapted with permission from Sharpe, J. D. (2019). A comparison of the geographic patterns of HIV prevalence and hurricane events in the United States. *Public Health*, *171*, 131–134. https:/doi.org/10.1016/j.puhe.2019.04.001

which is generally characterized as having a storm center of low atmospheric pressure of 920 to 944 **millibars**, wind speeds of 130 to 156 miles per hour, and up to 18 feet in storm surge. A hurricane of such magnitude can cause extreme levels of damage in impacted areas.

In the immediate aftermath of a weather-related disaster, such as a hurricane, the impacted area must often cope with extensive property destruction, infrastructure damage, and **environmental hazards** (Vick et al., 2018). In addition, mass injuries and casualties may require urgent medical attention, resulting in medical surges inundating nearby hospitals and healthcare providers (Vick et al., 2018). Moreover, hurricane disasters may interrupt operations of essential medical facilities, leaving community hospitals and healthcare providers unprepared and underprepared to handle large-scale disasters at the outset (Sharpe

TABLE 6.1 Saffir-Simpson Hurricane Scale

Category	Central Pressure (mb)	Wind Speed (mph)	Storm Surge (ft)	Damage Level
1	≥980	74-95	4-5	Minimal
2	965-979	96-110	6-8	Moderate
3	945-964	111-129	9-12	Extensive
4	920-944	130-156	13-18	Extreme
5	<920	>156	>18	Catastrophic

ft, feet; mb, millibar; mph, miles per hour.

Source: Adapted from Saffir, H. S. (1977). *Design and construction requirements for hurricane resistant construction.* American Society of Civil Engineers; Simpson, R. H. (1971). *A proposed scale for ranking hurricanes by intensity* [Conference session]. Minutes of the Eighth NOAA, National Weather Service Hurricane Conference, Miami, Florida, United States.

& Clennon, 2020; Shartar et al., 2017). These adverse impacts are especially problematic for groups that already experience disadvantage in the absence of major disasters and other hazardous events, such as older adults, people with disabilities or chronic diseases, those who are unemployed or living in poverty, and racial and ethnic minorities (Cutter et al., 2003; Cutter & Finch, 2008; Flanagan et al., 2011, 2018). During a disaster, existing inequalities in healthcare access and outcomes may be exacerbated, and **social determinants of health** are brought to the forefront (Quinn, 2006).

To approach hurricanes and floods from a public health perspective, it is helpful to first understand how a natural hazard becomes a public health emergency. Historically, severe storms and other hazardous events were considered the domain of physical scientists and engineers. More recently, however, researchers have been paying more attention to the "social" aspect of natural disasters—the political, demographic, and socioeconomic factors that turn a natural hazard into a disaster impacting a population. Today, many scientists think of natural disasters as a convergence of physical exposure (e.g., living in the path of a hurricane) and social or economic processes that influence who is impacted the most (the most vulnerable) and who is best prepared to recover (the least vulnerable; Wisner et al., 2004). These concepts came into play when Hurricane Harvey made landfall in Texas in 2017.

INTRODUCTION TO THE 2017 HURRICANE HARVEY DISASTER

On August 25, 2017, Hurricane Harvey made landfall on San José Island, Texas, developing into a 5-day event primarily affecting eastern and coastal areas in Texas (Figure 6.2; Federal Emergency Management Agency [FEMA], 2018). Hurricane Harvey was a Category 4 storm, releasing the most rainfall ever for a tropical cyclone event in the United States, resulting in over 100 direct and indirect fatalities in Texas, and costing an estimated $125 billion in damages, second only to Hurricane Katrina (Figure 6.3; FEMA, 2018). In Houston, Texas, over 60 inches of rain caused widespread flooding, covering nearly one-third of the city and damaging more than 200,000 homes (FEMA, 2018; Pines, 2018). Direct damage from flood inundation was not the only concern. Floodwaters also carried contaminants from industrial facilities and hazardous waste sites, producing a cocktail of toxic emissions, petrochemicals, sewage, and garbage (Friedrich, 2017).

Healthcare provision was another challenge during such a disastrous hurricane. Hurricane Harvey directly impacted 7.5 million Texans (FEMA, 2018), including millions of persons who were socially and economically marginalized. The combination of hazardous physical and toxic exposures and disaster-related injuries and illnesses contributed to increases in emergency department visits, both in Houston and in cities that sheltered evacuees (Liu et al., 2019). For evacuees displaced to temporary shelters, mental health needs were of concern, as this disaster disrupted both social support systems and the availability of medical services (Shultz & Galea, 2017; Taioli et al., 2018). Along the same lines, special attention was needed to ensure that patients with illnesses requiring special healthcare resources, such as diabetes, had sufficient access to essential medications and medical devices (The Lancet Diabetes & Endocrinology, 2017). Because **medically sensitive populations** also tend to have more adverse health outcomes and lower access to healthcare services, an effective public health approach to disaster response should account for

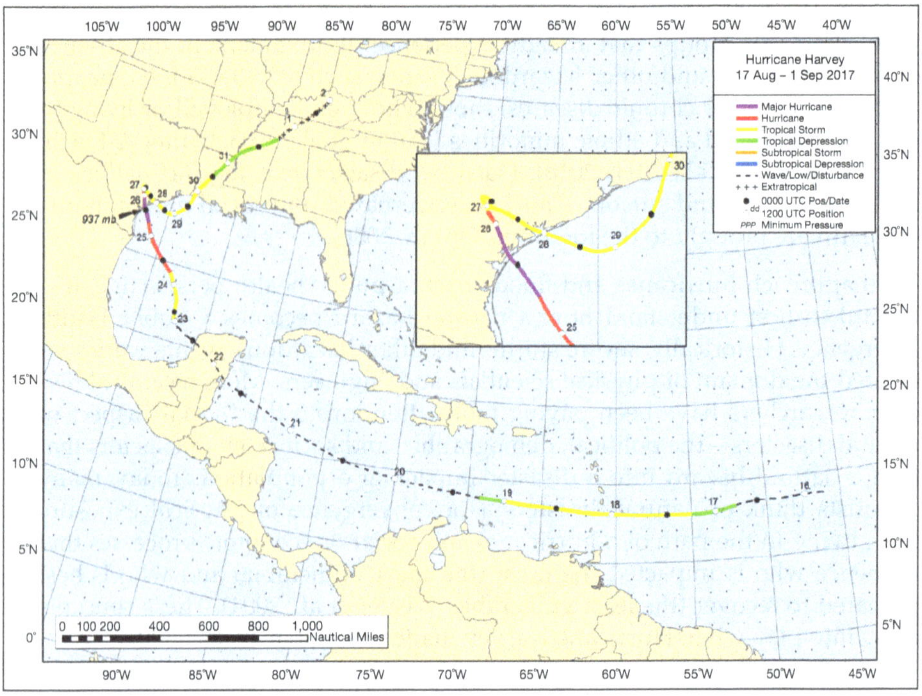

Figure 6.2 The Hurricane Harvey storm track in the United States and the Caribbean region, August 17, 2017–September 1, 2017.

Source: National Oceanic and Atmospheric Administration/National Weather Service/National Hurricane Center, 2017.

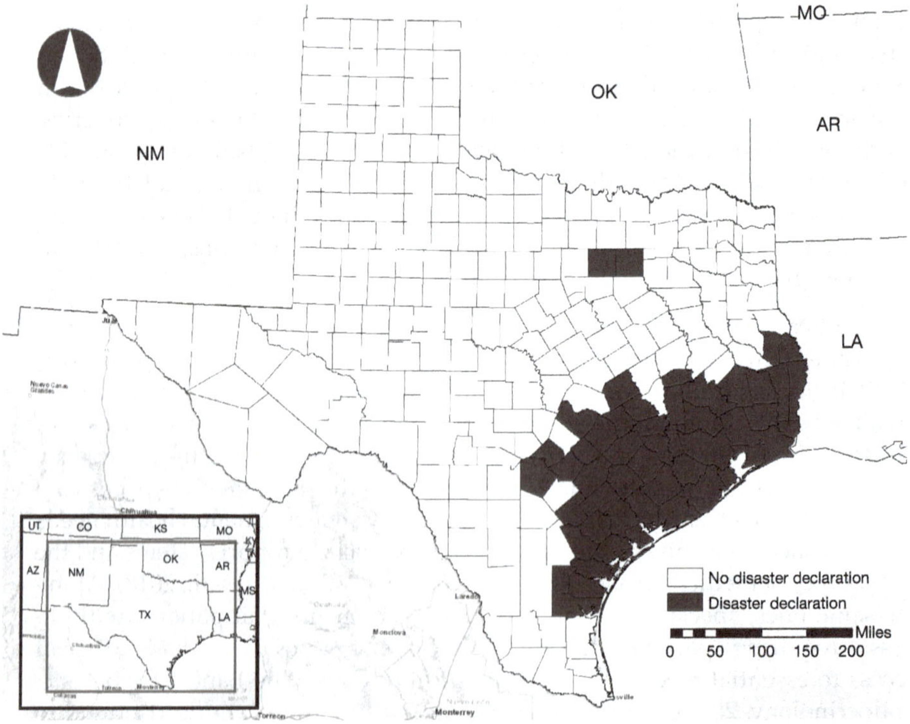

Figure 6.3 Hurricane Harvey disaster declarations in Texas, October 2017.

preexisting social vulnerabilities and inequities in hazard exposure as well as the immediate needs of populations during an emergency.

Public health professionals are well equipped to address social vulnerabilities and inequities during a hurricane disaster, such as in 2017 with Hurricane Harvey. Assessing the magnitude of a population's vulnerability highlights the varying needs, assets, and capacities of diverse communities in anticipation of disasters. Doing so may also identify programs that can assess the needs of communities, prevent negative disaster outcomes, and improve health outcomes in an emergency. The remainder of this chapter uses the 2017 Hurricane Harvey disaster in southeastern Texas as a case study to examine the following aspects of a public health response to an emergency:

- how and where a hurricane can lead to increased demand for emergency medical services and how public health practitioners can respond
- how and where socially vulnerable populations may access emergency medical care during a hurricane disaster
- what public health professionals can learn from the 2017 Hurricane Harvey disaster and apply to future public health emergency responses

DEMAND FOR MEDICAL SERVICES DURING THE 2017 HURRICANE HARVEY DISASTER

Disasters triggered by natural hazards, such as hurricanes, can cause extensive negative consequences among human populations regarding morbidity and mortality outcomes (Vick et al., 2018). Such adverse effects are of public health importance considering that increases in disaster-associated injuries and deaths in hard-hit communities can lead to complications associated with medical surge in those very communities as well as in neighboring, unaffected communities. Medical surge is the occurrence of an increased volume of individuals seeking medical care and treatment that exceeds the normal expectations and capabilities of healthcare facilities and medical infrastructure in communities directly and indirectly impacted by a disaster (Barbera & Macintyre, 2007). Medical surge is an especially important outcome of disasters that healthcare facilities need to plan for and manage, particularly as healthcare systems may be underprepared to accommodate significant increases in healthcare-seeking behavior and healthcare utilization due to a sudden, destructive, and widespread disaster.

Public health practitioners assist with managing medical surge events in a variety of capacities. Biostatisticians are needed to work with **syndromic surveillance** systems, such as ESSENCE, or the Electronic Surveillance System for the Early Notification of Community-based Epidemics, to analyze large data sets of emergency department visits and interpret inflection points indicating medical surge. Epidemiologists can assist with controlling medical surge events by quantifying the magnitude of medical surge events and determining how many additional patients hospitals and other urgent healthcare institutions are likely to encounter. Environmental health scientists and behavioral health scientists can aid with responding to medical surge events by exploring **chief complaint** data to identify potential environmental hazards in the community and predict mental healthcare needs of the community in the short term and long term, respectively.

During the 2017 Hurricane Harvey disaster in Texas, occurrences of medical surge were documented approximately 260 miles northwest of Houston, Texas, in the unimpacted region of the Dallas–Fort Worth metropolitan area (Stephens et al., 2020). Prior to Hurricane Harvey, emergency departments in the Dallas–Fort Worth area operated as usual, managing normal levels of patient traffic. During the weeks leading up to the hurricane disaster, an average of 7,499 daily visits were recorded for the emergency departments in Dallas–Fort Worth through August 24, 2017 (Stephens et al., 2020).

From the landfall of Hurricane Harvey on August 25, 2017, to the storm's dissipation from the Dallas–Fort Worth area on September 4, 2017, average daily emergency department visits increased by 1.6% to 7,615 visits (Table 6.2; Stephens et al., 2020). After the storm, evidence of medical surge became even more pronounced. Between September 5, 2017, and September 15, 2017, an increase of 5.8% to 8,056 average daily visits was recorded (Stephens et al., 2020). A majority of the medical surge–associated emergency department visits involved seeking care for signs and symptoms related to gastrointestinal illness, respiratory illness, fever, and skin rashes (Stephens et al., 2020).

Overall for the Hurricane Harvey disaster, emergency departments in the Dallas–Fort Worth metropolitan area documented a 7.4% increase in average daily visits between the pre–Hurricane Harvey and post–Hurricane Harvey time periods, highlighting that medical surge can continue to adversely affect healthcare systems long after a natural hazard has dissipated (Stephens et al., 2020). Such a sustained increase in medical surge weeks after the start of this hurricane indicates the manner in which medical surge can continue to complicate the provision of medical care and the capacity of healthcare facilities on a long-term basis in areas that are both directly and indirectly impacted by a disaster.

During Hurricane Harvey, medical surge was also documented in the Dallas–Fort Worth metropolitan area for individuals who evacuated from the Hurricane Harvey impact zone, of which 40% originated from the Harris County–Houston metropolitan area (Table 6.3; Stephens et al., 2020). Prior to the storm, emergency departments in the Dallas–Fort Worth area saw an average of 22 visits per day from individuals residing in southeastern Texas counties, based on the period from August 14, 2017, to August 24, 2017 (Stephens et al., 2020). After Hurricane Harvey made landfall, the average daily visits of evacuees from the Hurricane Harvey impact zone at Dallas–Fort Worth emergency departments increased to 80 average daily visits through September 4, 2017, a medical surge of approximately 264% in average daily emergency department visits (Stephens et al., 2020).

TABLE 6.2 Total Daily Emergency Department Visits in the Dallas-Fort Worth Metropolitan Area in Texas Before, During, and After Hurricane Harvey, August 14, 2017-September 15, 2017

	Mean	Standard Deviation	Minimum	Maximum
Before Hurricane Harvey	7,499	433	6,707	8,016
During Hurricane Harvey	7,615	466	6,665	8,413
After Hurricane Harvey	8,056	620	7,053	8,976

Note: Before Hurricane Harvey = August 14-24, 2017. During Hurricane Harvey = August 25-September 4, 2017. After Hurricane Harvey = September 5-15, 2017.

Source: Adapted from Stephens, W., Wilt, G. E., Lehnert, E. A., Molinari, N. M., & LeBlanc, T. T. (2020). A spatial and temporal investigation of medical surge in Dallas-Fort Worth during Hurricane Harvey, Texas 2017. *Disaster Medicine and Public Health Preparedness*, *14*(1), 111-118. https://doi.org/10.1017/dmp.2019.143

TABLE 6.3 Evacuee Daily Emergency Department Visits in the Dallas-Fort Worth Metropolitan Area in Texas Before, During, and After Hurricane Harvey, August 14, 2017-September 15, 2017

	Mean	Standard Deviation	Minimum	Maximum
Before Hurricane Harvey	22	4	16	27
During Hurricane Harvey	80	23	37	123
After Hurricane Harvey	39	10	23	56

Note: Before Hurricane Harvey = August 14-24, 2017. During Hurricane Harvey = August 25-September 4, 2017. After Hurricane Harvey = September 5-15, 2017.

Source: Adapted from Stephens, W., Wilt, G. E., Lehnert, E. A., Molinari, N. M., & LeBlanc, T. T. (2020). A spatial and temporal investigation of medical surge in Dallas-Fort Worth during Hurricane Harvey, Texas 2017. *Disaster Medicine and Public Health Preparedness*, *14*(1), 111-118. https://doi.org/10.1017/dmp.2019.143

As a result of the storm, emergency departments in Dallas–Fort Worth reported a significant medical surge due to the healthcare needs of Hurricane Harvey evacuees. During the storm, high and significant spatial clustering of medical surge due to evacuees was documented in Dallas–Fort Worth, with the primary spatial clusters of evacuees being from the following counties: Brazoria, Fort Bend, Galveston, Harris, and Jefferson (Figure 6.4; Stephens

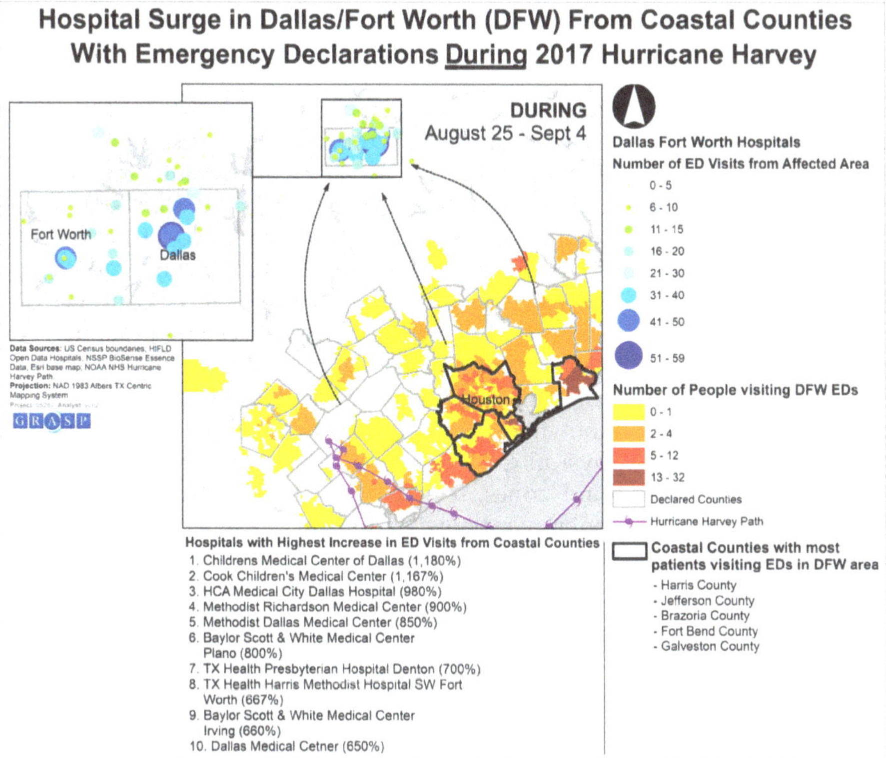

Figure 6.4 Medical surge in the daily emergency department visits of evacuees in the Dallas–Fort Worth Metropolitan area in Texas during Hurricane Harvey, August 25, 2017–September 4, 2017.

Source: Adapted with permission from Stephens, W., Wilt, G. E., Lehnert, E. A., Molinari, N. M., & LeBlanc, T. T. (2020). A spatial and temporal investigation of medical surge in Dallas–Fort Worth during Hurricane Harvey, Texas 2017. *Disaster Medicine and Public Health Preparedness*, *14*(1), 111–118. https:/doi.org/10.1017/dmp.2019.143

et al., 2020). The most common chief complaints reported during evacuee visits to emergency departments in Dallas-Fort Worth included:

- gastrointestinal illness (25% of visits)
- respiratory illness (22% of visits)
- fever (19% of visits)
- injuries (14% of visits), including traffic-related injuries

After Hurricane Harvey, emergency department visits by evacuees decreased to near pre-disaster baseline levels, reducing by over 50% to 39 average daily emergency department visits from Hurricane Harvey evacuees. Overall, evacuee-associated emergency department visits contributed to significant medical surge at emergency departments in the Dallas–Fort Worth metropolitan area during Hurricane Harvey, overwhelming emergency departments in the area and hindering the timely and adequate provision of medical care (Chambers et al., 2020) and related services for the usual patient populations of emergency departments in the Dallas–Fort Worth area in the long term.

SOCIAL VULNERABILITY AND ACCESS TO MEDICAL CARE DURING THE 2017 HURRICANE HARVEY DISASTER

The concept that populations experience hazards and disasters differently depending on demographic factors and socioeconomic status is known as social vulnerability, and the overall impact of a disaster can be exacerbated for communities that are more socially vulnerable than others (Wisner et al., 2004). Social vulnerability is not an inherent quality of a population but a construct used to represent the concrete effects of structural racism, uneven economic development, income inequality, and other underlying social and historical processes that produce inequality. Natural hazards scholars have developed quantitative methods to measure and estimate social vulnerability. In 2000, a research group led by Susan L. Cutter, PhD, introduced a place-based vulnerability model, a social vulnerability index known as SoVI (Cutter et al., 2000). They combined layers representing both physical exposure (flood risk zones, hurricane storm surge extents, hurricane wind zones, technological hazard zones, and earthquake frequency) with sociodemographic data to generate a geographic map of the overall vulnerability score. The SoVI formula has been updated since then (Hazards and Vulnerability Research Institute, 2017) and is widely used.

In 2007, a team of social scientists at the Centers for Disease Control and Prevention (CDC) led by Barry E. Flanagan, PhD, developed the CDC Social Vulnerability Index (CDC SVI) to support locating the most socially vulnerable communities in the United States (Flanagan et al., 2011, 2018). CDC SVI incorporates 15 variables from U.S. Census Bureau databases, grouped into four themes: socioeconomic status, household composition and disability, minority status and language, and housing type and transportation (Figure 6.5).The index includes a percentile rank for the 15 individual variables, the four themes, and an overall measure of social vulnerability. Quantitative models of social vulnerability, including SoVI and CDC SVI, allow for efficient comparison between geographical units (e.g., census tracts or counties). This is useful for public health practitioners,

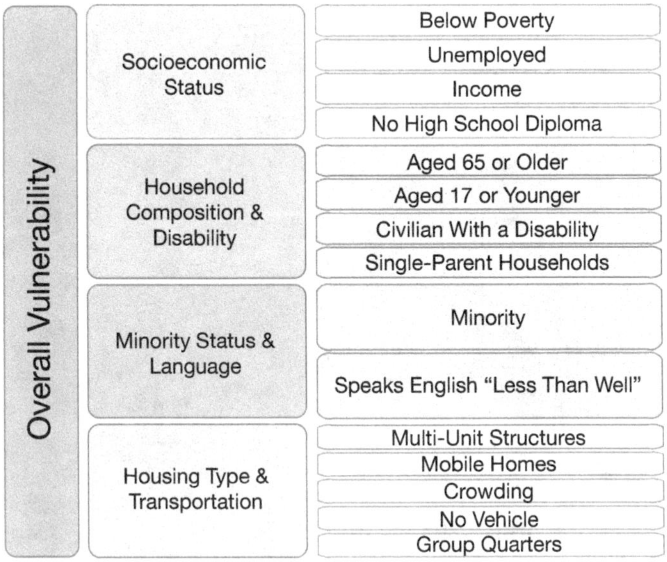

Figure 6.5 Components of the Centers for Disease Control and Prevention Social Vulnerability Index.

emergency managers, and other professionals who need to quantify the vulnerability of communities in their jurisdictions, locate populations most in need, and efficiently allocate resources before, during, and after disasters. Their use comes with a caveat: The impacts of natural disasters are felt unevenly because of existing socioeconomic inequalities, meaning that while quantifying a community's immediate needs is essential, practitioners may also wish to consider how structural inequities in various social systems can be addressed.

Public health practitioners are essential to mitigating the adverse outcomes that populations experiencing disproportionate levels of social vulnerability may experience after disaster events and public health emergencies. Epidemiologists may collaborate with geographers to conduct descriptive geographic mapping of CDC SVI or another social vulnerability tool using geographic information system (GIS) software in order to understand the distribution of vulnerable populations across communities. Epidemiologists and geographers may also work together to conduct advanced spatial analyses to determine the factors contributing to adverse outcomes across varying levels of social vulnerability for communities directly and indirectly impacted by a disaster. Public health policy and disaster management professionals can also use CDC SVI to target the allocation of disaster resources, such as food, water, medicine, shelters, or emergency funding, to communities experiencing higher levels of social vulnerability that may need assistance and support before, during, and after disaster events.

The concept of social vulnerability played a vital role in where persons in the hurricane impact zone accessed emergency medical care during Hurricane Harvey (Figure 6.6; Rickless et al., 2021). During and after Hurricane Harvey, an estimated 11,243 emergency care visits occurred in the impact zone at emergency departments in Houston, Texas, and 2,602 emergency care visits occurred at facilities managed by Disaster Medical Assistance Teams (DMATs), which are multidisciplinary groups of physicians, nurses, and paramedics providing additional medical resources during federally declared disasters (Mace et al., 2007). When using GIS to visualize the proportion of persons

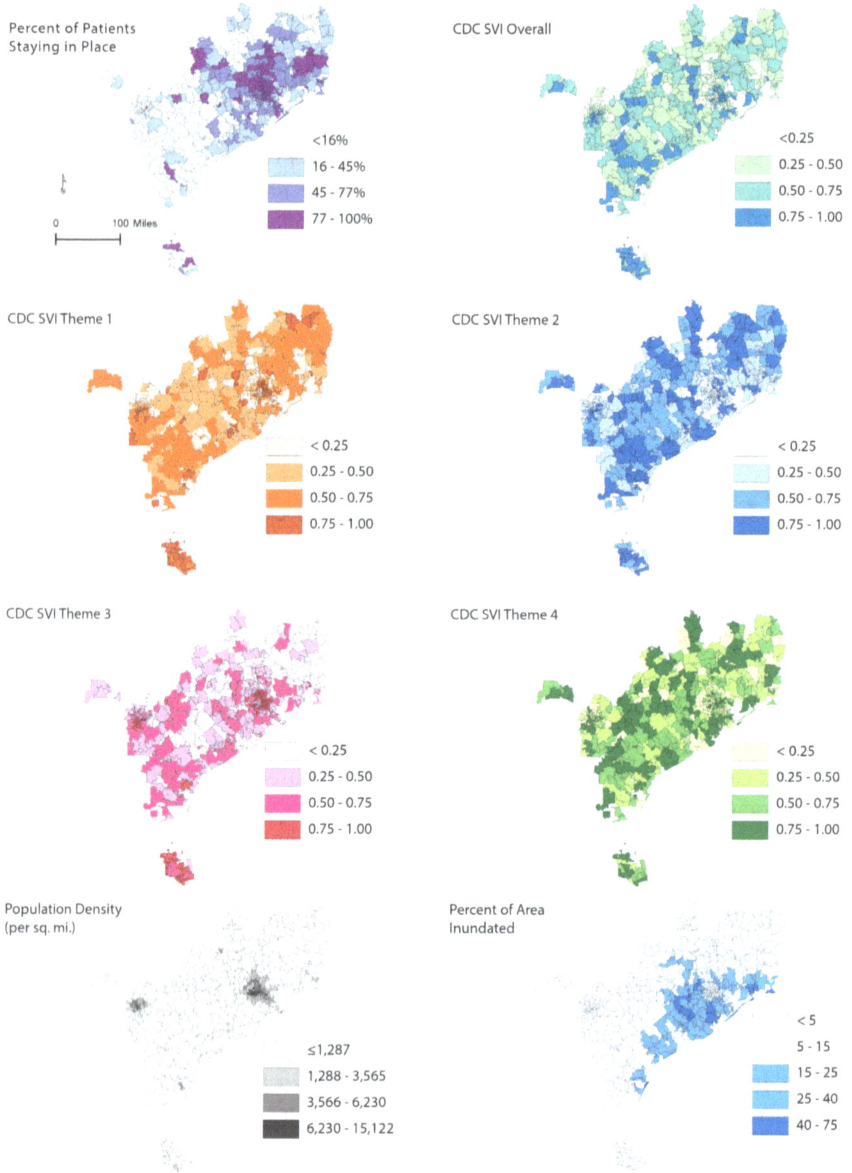

Figure 6.6 The spatial distribution of medical care access, social vulnerability components, population density, and flooding inundation in southeastern Texas during Hurricane Harvey, August 24, 2017–September 29, 2017.

Source: Reproduced with permission from Rickless, D. S., Wilt, G. E., Sharpe, J. D., Molinari, N., Stephens, W., & LeBlanc, T. T. (2021). Social vulnerability and access of local medical care during Hurricane Harvey: A spatial analysis. *Disaster Medicine and Public Health Preparedness*. Advanced online publication. https://doi.org/10.1017/dmp.2020.421

accessing medical care at emergency departments and DMATs in the hurricane impact zone, a spatial cluster of persons accessing care was evident in communities near Houston, Texas. Flood inundation and population density were spatially clustered in the Houston, Texas, metropolitan area as well.

During Hurricane Harvey, components of social vulnerability directly impacted the ability of individuals to access medical care in an area where disaster effects were minimal (Table 6.4). Of the four CDC SVI themes, socioeconomic

TABLE 6.4 Estimated Impact of Social Vulnerability, Population Density, and Flooding Inundation on Medical Care Access in Houston, Texas, and the Dallas-Fort Worth Metropolitan During Hurricane Harvey, August 24, 2017-September 29, 2017

Variable	Short Time Period (August 24-September 8, 2017) Total Effect (*p* value)	Long Time Period (August 24-September 29, 2017) Total Effect (*p* value)
Socioeconomic Status	0.701 (0.006)	0.652 (0.003)
Household Composition & Disability	−0.348 (0.064)	−0.341 (0.047)
Minority Status & Language	−0.216 (0.292)	−0.246 (0.171)
Housing Type & Transportation	−0.079 (0.607)	0.029 (0.756)
Population Density (per square mile)	0.000 (0.012)	0.000 (0.001)
Flooding Inundation	0.639 (0.019)	0.664 (0.010)

Source: Adapted from Rickless, D. S., Wilt, G. E., Sharpe, J. D., Molinari, N., Stephens, W., & LeBlanc, T. T. (2021). Social vulnerability and access of local medical care during Hurricane Harvey: A spatial analysis. *Disaster Medicine and Public Health Preparedness*. Advanced online publication. https://doi.org/10.1017/dmp.2020.421

status vulnerability had the greatest impact on whether persons seeking emergency healthcare services during Hurricane Harvey accessed care in the impact zone or in an unaffected area. Particularly, a 10 percentage point increase in socioeconomic status vulnerability in an area led to a 7.01% increase in the proportion of persons accessing healthcare within the hurricane impact zone immediately after the landfall of Hurricane Harvey (Rickless et al., 2021). A similar association was maintained weeks after the storm dissipated, as a 10 percentage point increase in an area's socioeconomic status vulnerability led to a 6.52% increase in the proportion of persons accessing care in the impact zone (Rickless et al., 2021). In other words, the population utilizing medical care in the impact zone tended to have lower socioeconomic status.

Vulnerability due to household composition and disability status also impacted whether people were able to access emergency medical care outside the hurricane impact zone. Greater household composition vulnerability, indicated by high numbers of young children, older adult persons, or persons living with disabilities, was associated with seeking healthcare in an area that was not directly affected by Hurricane Harvey. In the immediate aftermath of Hurricane Harvey, a 10 percentage point increase in household composition and disability vulnerability led to a 3.48% decrease in the proportion of persons accessing medical care in the hurricane impact zone (Rickless et al., 2021). A similar magnitude of a 3.41% decrease in proportion of persons accessing care in hard-hit areas was also found approximately 4 weeks after the landfall of Hurricane Harvey (Rickless et al., 2021). This means the Dallas–Fort Worth medical surge events discussed earlier in this chapter (Stephens et al., 2020) likely included patients with higher levels of social vulnerability due to household composition.

Beyond factors of social vulnerability, widespread flooding during and after Hurricane Harvey also had a substantial impact on where persons affected by the disaster were able to access emergency medical care. Extensive flooding forced more persons to restrict their access of healthcare services to medical facilities located within the Hurricane Harvey impact zone as opposed to in an unaffected area. Specifically, a 10% increase in flood inundation had a total impact of a 6.39% increase and a 6.64% increase in the proportion of persons accessing care in the impact zone immediately and up to 1 month after Hurricane Harvey, respectively (Rickless et al., 2021). The extent of flooding was just as critical to where Hurricane Harvey–impacted populations accessed care as was social vulnerability related to socioeconomic status.

APPLYING CHAPTER PRINCIPLES TO FUTURE HURRICANE DISASTERS

In summary, during and in the aftermath of Hurricane Harvey, more persons accessed emergency medical care in the unimpacted metropolitan area of Dallas–Fort Worth, Texas, than emergency departments in the area could manage; people who accessed emergency medical care in the Dallas–Fort Worth area had a higher vulnerability based on household composition and disability, while people who accessed emergency medical care in the Hurricane Harvey impact zone had a higher vulnerability based on socioeconomic status and experienced more extensive flooding. This chapter demonstrates that public health practitioners can and should incorporate GIS tools, their understanding of the medical surge capacity for healthcare facilities in their respective jurisdictions, and a social vulnerability framework to better characterize the health status and movement of persons seeking emergency medical care during a public health emergency triggered by disasters of great magnitude, such as Hurricane Harvey (Table 6.5; Table 6.6). For future hurricanes, public health practitioners should be able to use the frameworks and tools introduced in this chapter to do the following:

- *Monitor the health status* of communities and *diagnose and investigate* community health problems in areas directly and indirectly impacted by hurricanes through the use of syndromic surveillance data and the identification of medical surge events.
- *Mobilize community partnerships*, such as with DMATs, to more completely identify and solve health problems in areas directly and indirectly impacted by hurricanes.
- *Evaluate* the effectiveness, accessibility, and quality of personal and population-based health services, such as the spatial patterns of medical surge and healthcare access in areas directly and indirectly impacted by hurricanes.
- *Research* the social vulnerability of disproportionately affected populations in a hurricane impact zone and how such vulnerability may impact healthcare-seeking behaviors in order to gain new insights to health problems and better contextualize emerging public health issues in the long term for areas directly and indirectly impacted by hurricanes.

DISCUSSION QUESTIONS

1. Suppose an imminent hurricane warning was issued for Miami, Florida, in a large geographic area with several nursing homes, day-care centers, and government housing projects. How would the health department use the CDC Social Vulnerability Index to prepare an evacuation strategy?

2. Discuss a plan for identifying and activating community members in preparing for a hurricane. What kinds of organizations, officials, and community members would you include? What kind of communication strategy would you consider to keep community members informed?
3. In a medical surge situation, how would you use syndromic surveillance to identify health hazards? What kinds of data would you consider?
4. Propose an evaluation of a response to a hurricane. What kinds of questions would you ask? What kinds of data would you use?

SUMMARY

TABLE 6.5 **Select Essential Services of Public Health Demonstrated in the 2017 Hurricane Harvey Emergency**

Essential Service # and Definition	Context in Chapter Case	Competency # It Ties to	Importance for Emergency Preparedness, Response, or Recovery
1. Assess and monitor population health status, factors that influence health, and community needs and assets (Assessment)	Monitor community health problems through syndromic surveillance data and the identification of medical surge events.	*1, 7*	Comprehension of the extent of health problems in a community before, during, and after an emergency is essential for preparing, response, and recovery.
2. Investigate, diagnose, and address health problems and hazards affecting the population (Assessment)	Monitor community health problems through syndromic surveillance data and the identification of medical surge events.	*1, 2, 3, and 4*	Specific health problems or hazards during emergencies may be detected quickly with syndromic surveillance to aid in rapid response.
4. Strengthen, support, and mobilize communities and partnerships to improve health (Policy Development)	Mobilize community partnerships, such as with Disaster Medical Assistance Teams, to identify and solve health problems.	*6, 13, 15, 16, and 17*	Strong community partnerships enhance awareness of hazards, communication, and response during emergencies.
9. Improve and innovate public health functions through ongoing evaluation, research, and continuous quality improvement (Assurance)	Evaluate the effectiveness, accessibility, and quality of population-based health services, such as the spatial patterns of healthcare access and medical surge.	*1, 2, 3, 4, 12, 14, 15*	Learning from emergencies through research and evaluation efforts provides valuable lessons for future emergencies and helps identify mistakes or gaps in preparedness.
10. Build and maintain a strong organizational infrastructure for public health (Assurance)	Research the social vulnerability of populations in a hurricane impact zone and how such vulnerability impacts healthcare-seeking behaviors.	*1, 2, 3, 4*	Before emergency situations occur, maintaining a strong preparedness system to include knowledge of existing social vulnerabilities aids in mounting an effective, efficient response.

TABLE 6.6 Select CEPH Competencies Needed for Frontline Health Workers, Managers, and Leaders for Hurricane Emergency Preparedness, Response, and Recovery

Competency # and Definition	Context in Case/Chapter	Level	Importance for Emergency Preparedness, Response, and Recovery
2. Select quantitative and qualitative data collection methods appropriate for a given public health context.	Use syndromic surveillance data and the identification of medical surge events.	Level 1	Epidemiologists and health scientists use knowledge of research and evaluation methods to develop appropriate data collection strategies for solving public health problems related to emergencies.
3. Analyze quantitative and qualitative data using biostatistics, informatics, computer-based programming, and software, as appropriate.	Research the social vulnerability of potentially hard-hit populations in a hurricane impact zone.	Level 1	Epidemiologists and health scientists use analytical skills to learn from data collected during an emergency response. Patterns of health hazards that emerge from the data may inform future readiness efforts.
7. Assess population needs, assets, and capacities that affect communities' health.	Evaluate the effectiveness, accessibility, and quality of personal and population-based health services (spatial patterns of healthcare access and medical surge in areas impacted by hurricanes).	Level 2	Administrators, policy makers, and decision-makers use data collected on emergencies and reports provided by epidemiologists and health scientists to inform public health policies, identify population needs, and direct resources toward activities that will best benefit the community.
13. Propose strategies to identify stakeholders and build coalitions and partnerships for influencing public health outcomes.	Partner with disaster medical assistance teams to identify and solve health problems in areas impacted by hurricanes.	Level 2	Administrators, policy makers, and decision-makers use data collected on emergencies and reports provided by epidemiologists and health scientists to convey health problem concerns to community stakeholders for obtaining "buy in" and support for addressing specific health concerns.

Key: Essential services of public health; CEPH competencies; Leadership levels.

ACKNOWLEDGMENTS

We thank Dr. Noelle-Angelique M. Molinari (CDC), Grete Wilt (CDC), Erica Lehnert (CDC), William Stephens (Tarrant County Public Health), and Dr. Tanya LeBlanc (CDC) for their significant roles in supporting the work presented in this chapter.

DISCLAIMER

This chapter was prepared by J. Danielle Sharpe and David S. Rickless in his/her personal capacity. The opinions expressed in this article are the author's own and do not reflect the view of the Centers for Disease Control and Prevention, the Department of Health and Human Services, or the United States government.

REFERENCES

Barbera, J. A., & Macintyre, A. G. (2007). *Medical surge capacity and capability handbook: A management system for integrating medical and health resources during large-scale emergencies*. U.S. Department of Health and Human Services, Office of the Assistant Secretary for Preparedness and Response. https://www.phe.gov/Preparedness/planning/mscc/handbook/chapter1/Pages/default.aspx

Chambers, K. A., Husain, I., Chathampally, Y., Alan, V., Cardenas-Turanzas, M., Cardenas, F., Sharma, K., Prater, S., & Rogg, J. (2020). Impact of Hurricane Harvey on healthcare utilization and emergency department operations. *The Western Journal of Emergency Medicine, 21*(3), 586–594. https:/doi.org/10.5811/westjem.2020.1.41055

Cutter, S. L., Boruff, B. J., & Shirley, W. L. (2003). Social vulnerability to environmental hazards. *Social Science Quarterly, 84*(2), 242–261. http://doi.org/10.1111/1540-6237.8402002

Cutter, S. L., & Finch, C. (2008). Temporal and spatial changes in social vulnerability to natural hazards. *Proceedings of the National Academy of Sciences, 105*(7), 2301–2306. https:/doi.org/10.1073/pnas.0710375105

Cutter, S. L., Mitchell, J. T., & Scott, M. S. (2000). Revealing the vulnerability of people and places: A case study of Georgetown County, South Carolina. *Annals of the Association of American Geographers, 90*(4), 713–737. https://doi.org/10.1111/0004-5608.00219

Federal Emergency Management Agency. (2018). *2017 hurricane season FEMA after-action report*. https://www.fema.gov/media-library-data/1531743865541-d16794d43d3082544435e1471da07880/2017FEMAHurricaneAAR.pdf

Flanagan, B. E., Gregory, E. W., Hallisey, E. J., Heitgerd, J. L., & Lewis, B. (2011). A social vulnerability index for disaster management. *Journal of Homeland Security and Emergency Management, 8*(1), 1–22. https://doi.org/10.2202/1547-7355.1792

Flanagan, B. E., Hallisey, E. J., Adams, E., & Lavery, A. (2018). Measuring community vulnerability to natural and anthropogenic hazards: The Centers for Disease Control and Prevention's Social Vulnerability Index. *Journal of Environmental Health, 80*(10), 34–36. https://www.neha.org/sites/default/files/jeh/JEH6.18-Column-Direct-From-ATSDR.pdf

Friedrich, M. J. (2017). Determining health effects of hazardous materials released during Hurricane Harvey. *Journal of the American Medical Association, 318*(23), 2283–2285. https://doi.org/10.1001/jama.2017.15558

Hazards and Vulnerability Research Institute. (2017). *Social Vulnerability Index for the United States - 2010–2014*. https://artsandsciences.sc.edu/geog/hvri/sovi%C2%AE-0

The Lancet Diabetes & Endocrinology. (2017). South Asian floods and Hurricane Harvey: Diabetes in crisis. *Lancet Diabetes & Endocrinology, 5*(10), 757. https://doi.org/10.1016/S2213-8587(17)30291-7

Liu, E. L., Morshedi, B., Miller, B. L., Miller, R., Marshal Isaacs, S., Fowler, R. L., Chung, W., Blum, R., Ward, B., Carlo, J., Hennes, H., Webster F., Perl, T., Noah, C., Monaghan, R., Tran, A. H., Benitez, F., Graves, J., Kibbey, C., . . . Swienton, R. E. (2019). Dallas MegaShelter medical operations response to Hurricane Harvey. *Disaster Medicine and Public Health Preparedness, 13*(1), 90–93. https:/doi.org/10.1017/dmp.2017.123

Mace, S. E., Jones, J. T., & Bern, A. I. (2007). An analysis of disaster medical assistant team (DMAT) deployments in the United States. *Prehospital Emergency Care Journal, 11*(1), 30–35. https:/doi.org/10.1080/10903120601023396

Pines, J. M. (2018). Freestanding emergency department visits and disasters: The case of Hurricane Harvey. *The American Journal of Emergency Medicine, 36*(8), 1513–1515. https:/doi.org/10.1016/j.ajem.2018.01.016

Quinn, S. C. (2006). Hurricane Katrina: A social and public health disaster. *American Journal of Public Health, 96*(2), 204. https:/doi.org/10.2105/AJPH.2005.080119

Rickless, D. S., Wilt, G. E., Sharpe, J. D., Molinari, N., Stephens, W., & LeBlanc, T. T. (2021). Social vulnerability and access of local medical care during Hurricane Harvey: A spatial analysis. *Disaster Medicine and Public Health Preparedness*. Advanced online publication. https:/doi.org/10.1017/dmp.2020.421

Saffir, H. S. (1977). *Design and construction requirements for hurricane resistant construction*. American Society of Civil Engineers.

Sharpe, J. D. (2019). A comparison of the geographic patterns of HIV prevalence and hurricane events in the United States. *Public Health, 171*, 131–134. https:/doi.org/10.1016/j.puhe.2019.04.001

Sharpe, J. D., & Clennon, J. A. (2020). Pharmacy functionality during the Hurricane Florence disaster. *Disaster Medicine and Public Health Preparedness, 14*(1), 93–102. https:/doi.org/10.1017/dmp.2019.114

Shartar, S. E., Moore, B. L., & Wood, L. M. (2017). Developing a mass casualty surge capacity protocol for emergency medical services to use for patient distribution. *Southern Medical Journal, 110*(12), 792–795. https:/doi.org/10.14423/SMJ.0000000000000740

Shultz, J. M., & Galea, S. (2017). Preparing for the next Harvey, Irma, or Maria - Addressing research gaps. *The New England Journal of Medicine*, *377*(19), 1804–1806. https:/doi.org/10.1056/NEJMp1712854

Simpson, R. H. (1971). *A proposed scale for ranking hurricanes by intensity. Minutes of the Eighth NOAA*, National Weather Service Hurricane Conference, Miami, Florida, United States.

Stephens, W., Wilt, G. E., Lehnert, E. A., Molinari, N. M., & LeBlanc, T. T. (2020). A spatial and temporal investigation of medical surge in Dallas-Fort Worth during Hurricane Harvey, Texas 2017. *Disaster Medicine and Public Health Preparedness*, *14*(1), 111–118. https:/doi.org/10.1017/dmp.2019.143

Taioli, E., Tuminello, S., Lieberman-Cribbin, W., Bevilacqua, K., Schneider, S., Guzman, M., Kerath, S., & Schwartz, R. M. (2018). Mental health challenges and experiences in displaced populations following Hurricane Sandy and Hurricane Harvey: The need for more comprehensive interventions in temporary shelters. *Journal of Epidemiology and Community Health*, *72*(10), 867–870. https:/doi.org/10.1136/jech-2018-210626

Vick, D. J., Wilson, A. B., Fisher, M., & Roseamelia, C. (2018). Assessment of community hospital disaster preparedness in New York. *Journal of Emergency Management*, *16*(4), 213–227. https://doi.org/10.5055/jem.2018.0371

Wisner, B., Blaikie, P., Cannon, T., & Davis, I. (2004). *At risk: Natural hazards, people's vulnerability, and disaster* (2nd ed.). Routledge.

CHAPTER 7

TORNADOES AND RELATED PUBLIC HEALTH RISKS

THE JOPLIN TORNADO PUBLIC HEALTH RESPONSE

ZHEN CONG, ZHIRUI CHEN, AND AARON HAGEDORN

KEY TERMS

Built Environment
Cognitive Behavioral Therapy
Enhanced Fujita Scale
ESSENCE
FEMA's Whole Community Approach
Posttraumatic Stress Disorder (PTSD)
YouTube Channels

INTRODUCTION

Tornadoes pose a serious threat to public health. Over the last 10 years, tornadoes have caused the highest number of fatalities of any weather-related natural hazard in the United States. In addition, tornadoes produce the highest wind speeds recorded on Earth and suddenly destroy the infrastructure on which people depend for shelter, clean water, safe food, and medical care. Moreover, tornadoes can cause short- and long-term psychological stress as survivors deal with the loss of their most valuable assets, injuries to themselves or others, and the possible loss of loved ones and livelihoods. This chapter describes the extent to which tornadoes are a serious and persistent threat across several regions, as well as areas where tornadoes most often occur, the immediate and long-term health hazards of tornadoes, and finally

---

The following icons, located in the margins throughout the chapter and within the summary tables, denote essential services of public health, CEPH competencies, and leadership levels: Essential services of public health; CEPH competencies; Leadership levels.

a case study of the 2011 Joplin tornado, including the public health response and lessons learned to reduce health risks associated with tornadoes.

TORNADOES AND RELATED PUBLIC HEALTH RISKS

Categorization and Frequency of Tornadoes

A tornado appears as a rotating and funnel-shaped cloud, touching the ground and usually attached to a thunderstorm. It comes with whirling winds with a speed as high as 300 mph and could wipe a path that is more than one mile in width and 50 miles in length. The **Enhanced Fujita Scale**, implemented by the National Weather Service (NWS) since 2007, classifies tornadoes into six categories (EF0 to EF5) according to their wind speeds and the degree of damage they cause (McDonald et al., 2010). Each category is associated with a certain wind speed range. For example, an EF0 tornado has an estimated wind speed of 65 to 85 mph (3-second gust) and causes minor damage to buildings or trees, whereas an EF5 tornado has a 3-second gust speed of over 200 mph and causes incredible damage.

The NWS Storm Prediction Center has a database of tornadoes that provides tornado properties such as the intensity of the tornado, the date and time when the tornado occurred, the number of induced injuries and fatalities, the latitude and longitude for the touchdown and lift-off points, estimated property damage, and the path length and width as well as additional information. Figure 7.1 presents the total number of tornadoes observed in the United States since 1950. Although tornadoes are observed worldwide, the United States has the most tornadoes, averaging over 1,000 recorded tornadoes each year (National Center for Environmental Information, 2019).

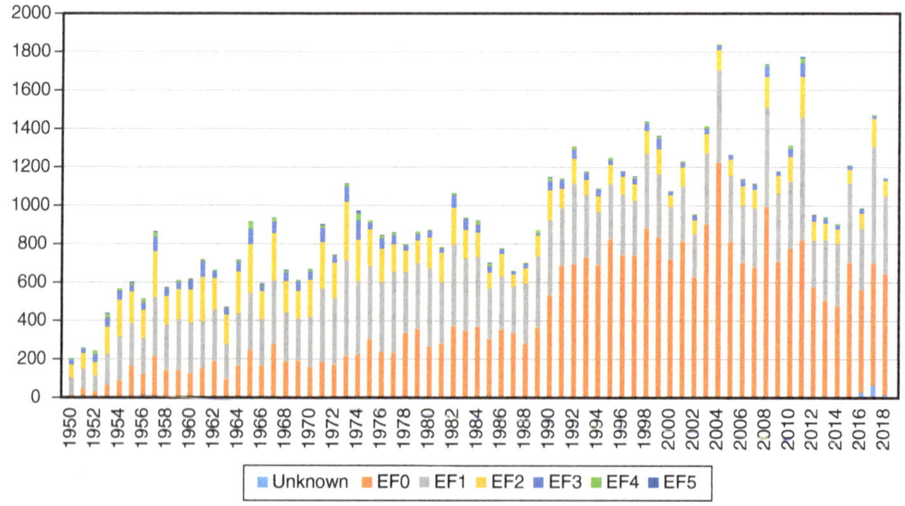

Figure 7.1 Annual numbers of tornadoes reported in the United States from 1950 to 2018.

Source: Calculated based on Severe Weather Database Files (1950–2018) from the Storm Prediction Center of the National Weather Service; National Weather Service. (2020). *Severe weather database files (1950-).* Storm Prediction Center WCM Page. http://www.spc.noaa.gov/wcm

Areas Where Tornadoes Occur Frequently

While tornadoes are possible anywhere, Figure 7.2 presents the geographic distributions of tornadoes between 1950 and 2011. Two large and distinct regions have a particularly high frequency of tornadoes and account for the majority of severe wind events. The most obvious region is the so-called Tornado Alley, which ranges from Texas to Alabama in the south-central region, extending as far north as South Dakota in the west, and Indiana in the east. Second, Florida is known for especially high risks for tornadoes. Florida's uniquely high risk is a result of the high frequency of thunderstorms and suitable weather conditions (National Center for Environmental Information, 2019; National Research Council of the National Academies, 1993).

Tornadoes do not always occur with a single touchdown; multiple tornadoes could happen together and cause even higher damages. The term "tornado outbreak" is defined as "the occurrence of several tornadoes over a region, usually all by thunderstorms embedded in the same extratropical cyclone" (National Research Council of the National Academies, 1993). Outbreaks do not occur frequently, but once they happen, they have a high impact and could result in shocking casualties. For example, the tornado super outbreak that happened on April 27, 2011, resulted in 199 tornadoes in 24 hours and led to 316 deaths and over 2,700 injuries (National Weather Service, 2011b). This record number of fatalities reveals the vulnerability of human society despite modern advances in tornado forecasting, advanced warning times, and extensive media coverage of warnings.

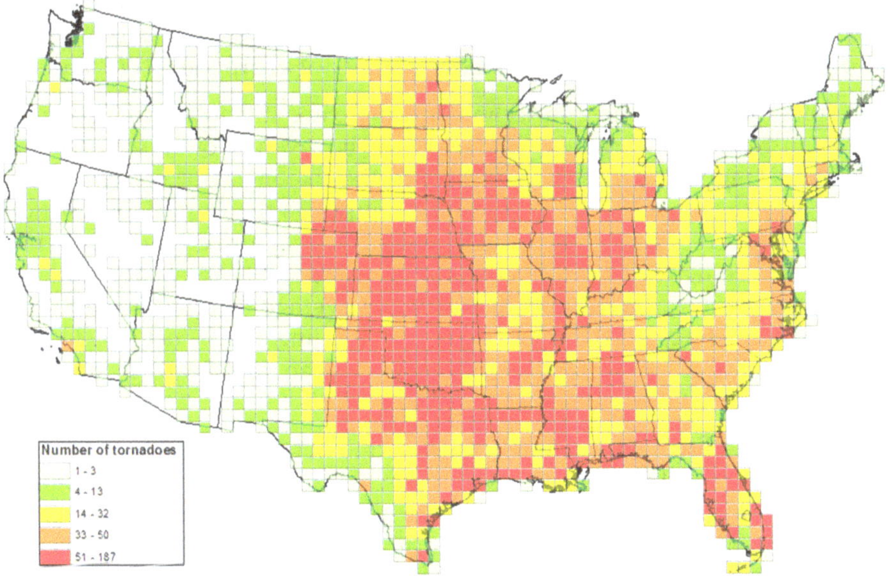

Figure 7.2 Number of tornado events in 60 km × 60 km grids for 1950–2011.

Source: Reproduced with permission from Luo, J. (2014). *Impacts, assessments, and responses: Interdisciplinary perspectives on tornadoes* [PhD dissertation]. Texas Tech University. https://ttu-ir.tdl.org/handle/2346/58910. Calculated based on Severe Weather Database Files (1950–2011) from the Storm Prediction Center of National Oceanic and Atmospheric Administration's National Weather Service. (2012). *Severe weather database files (1950-): Storm Prediction Center WCM page.* https://www.spc.noaa.gov/wcm

Tornado Warning and Protective Action

Tornadoes are a type of rapid-onset disaster. The national average lead time of tornado warnings has been relatively stable since 1986 with different calculations and reports suggesting warnings are issued between 13 to 18.8 minutes before a tornado strikes, though the lead time has increased slightly since 2012 (Brooks & Correia, 2018; Hoekstra et al., 2011). With continuous improvements in technology allowing for multiple warning information channels and longer lead times, a better understanding of social mechanisms and individual behaviors centering on receiving warnings and response to warnings is especially important (Brooks & Correia, 2018; Coleman et al., 2011; Hoekstra et al., 2011; Luo et al., 2015; Simmons & Sutter, 2008).

Due to the very quick development of tornadoes, reliable warning systems are of vital significance and an optimal warning could considerably reduce fatalities and injuries (Simmons & Sutter, 2011). Tornado warnings are issued by the NWS, and the warning system mainly includes outdoor warning sirens, local television and radio stations, cable television systems, cell phone apps, severe weather text messages, and an NWS weather radio. Public warning sirens are utilized in many cities; however, rural areas and smaller towns are not well equipped with sirens. Not everyone may hear warning sirens when they are inside a building, particularly those with hearing loss or in noisy environments because public warning sirens are an outdoor system (NWS, n.d.-b). Those already concerned about ominous-looking clouds can find more details through National Oceanic and Atmospheric Administration (NOAA) Weather Radio, local radio and television stations, and cable television systems (NWS, n.d.-b). Some smartphone apps can offer convenient and timely warning notifications, perhaps the most universal being the Wireless Emergency Alerts provided through the Federal Emergency Management Agency (FEMA) and sent at no cost to users from cell towers in the vicinity of a tornado (NWS, n.d.-b).

Despite the development in technology, there are still substantial social disparities in receiving warnings. Studies have shown that lower socioeconomic status and language barriers could reduce the likelihood of receiving warnings (Aguirre et al., 1991; Luo et al., 2015). A study on the April 2011 Tuscaloosa tornado revealed racial/ethnicity differences among three ethnic and racial groups concerning their risk perception, preparedness, and shelter lead time; particularly, African American respondents on average had the shortest shelter time (Senkbeil et al., 2014). Other barriers to warning access include electricity outages, rurality, a lack of a storm radio, deep sleep, and hearing impairment (Kuligowski et al., 2016; Walters et al., 2020).

Furthermore, ignoring warnings could lead to devastating consequences. For example, high casualties from the 2011 Joplin tornado were in part attributed to people ignoring tornado warnings (Paul & Stimers, 2012). Taking proper protective action upon receiving tornado warnings, such as taking shelter, is a key factor in reducing casualties (Hammer & Schmidlin, 2002; Paul & Stimers, 2012). Different from the contexts of hurricanes, taking protective action for tornado warnings does not necessarily mean evacuate; it is more likely to take shelter in place appropriately. Because of the short lead time of tornado warnings, compliance to warnings quickly is critical.

Consistent with the social vulnerability approach, individuals' likelihood for taking protective action is different by gender, education level, whether respondents were at home, whether they had access to a basement in the house, whether they heard warning sirens, the number of warning sources they noticed, past tornado exposure, and household plan of tornado response (Balluz et al., 2000; Luo et al., 2015; Paul et al., 2015). Besides, high false-alarm rates have been identified as a major reason that people did not respond properly to warnings (Simmons & Sutter, 2011).

Public Health Concerns

Tornadoes present a great threat to health and lives because the high wind speeds could destroy the **built environment**, injure or kill people, pollute the environment with hazardous materials, destroy telecommunication equipment needed for seeking help, and lead to long-term exposure to mold and fungus; the harm is indiscriminate, often with little or no warning to those affected (Deng et al., 2018; National Institute of Standards and Technology [NIST], 2014; Simmons & Sutter, 2011, 2013). Even the weak tornadoes (i.e., EF0 or EF1, the majority of tornadoes) can cause some damage and fatalities (Simmons & Sutter, 2011), let alone tornadoes with higher ratings. For example, Figure 7.3 shows a building damaged by the EF3 Dallas tornado on October 20, 2019. Tornadoes with a rating of EF4 and EF5 are regarded as violent tornadoes. Essentially no structures can withstand this force, exposing occupants to flying debris, spreading hazardous chemicals and building materials including poisons and carcinogens, destroying electrical and telecommunication infrastructure, and potentially making water sources unsafe for some time.

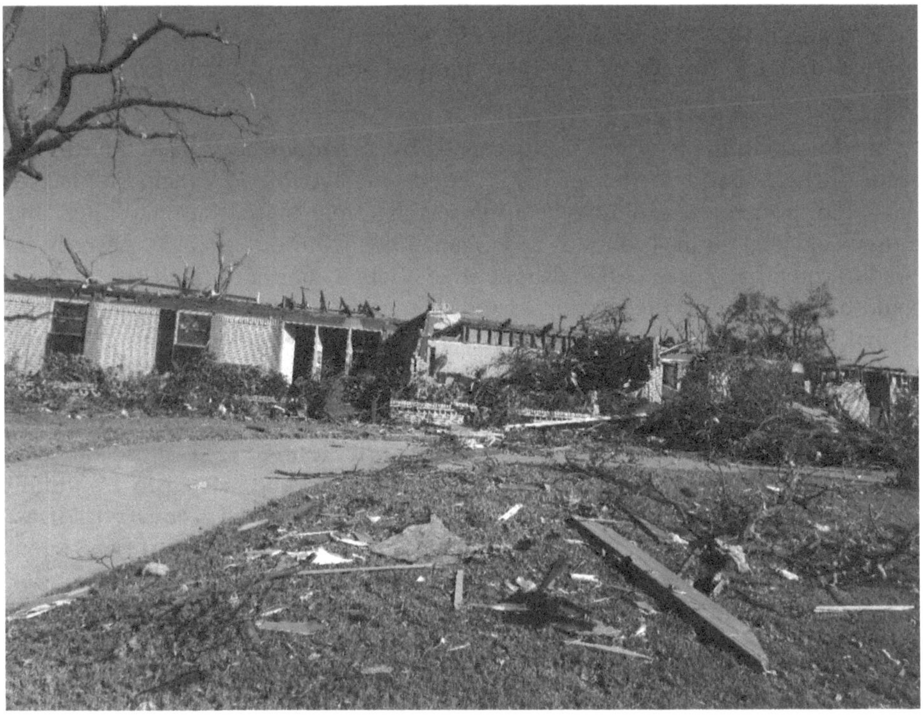

Figure 7.3 A building damaged by the EF3 Dallas tornado on October 20, 2019.

Deaths and Injuries

Between 1950 and 1994, more than 4,115 deaths and 70,063 injuries were identified as directly related to tornadoes in the United States (Bohonos & Hogan, 1999). More recent data show that over the 22-year span between 1995 to 2016 there were 472 killer tornadoes that resulted in 1,730 fatalities as well as 2,121 injury-producing tornadoes that produced 24,229 injuries (Fricker, 2020). The over 5,000 total fatalities caused by tornadoes from 1950 to 2011 exceeds the number of deaths caused by hurricanes and earthquakes combined (NIST, 2014). Half of the deadly tornadoes were rated EF4 or EF5 and were responsible for nearly 90% of the deaths (Centers for Disease Control and Prevention [CDC], 2012).

Tornadoes can lead to a rise in serious physical injuries, not only as a result of events that occur during the tornado but also from dangers that remain after. The majority of serious injuries and deaths occurred on the same day as the tornado struck, caused by airborne collisions and falls, impact from airborne solid objects, or structural collapse (Bohonos & Hogan, 1999; CDC, 2012; Chiu et al., 2013). Most tornado deaths are attributed to multisystem trauma, including a substantial proportion of head injuries, the most common cause of death associated with tornadoes (CDC, 2012; Chiu et al., 2013; Zhao et al., 2019). There were also deaths related to power outages because of house fires or medical conditions that rely on critical equipment and devices such as oxygen concentrator machines and refrigeration for insulin (Chiu et al., 2013).

Soft tissue wounds are the most commonly reported cause of injury as debris can quickly accelerate to ballistic rates by the winds (Bohonos & Hogan, 1999; Fricker et al., 2017). Bone fractures account for more than 30% of those sent to hospitals, making fractures the most frequently reported cause of admission to hospitals (Bohonos & Hogan, 1999; Deng et al., 2018). Chest and head regions were most affected in terms of severe injuries (Niederkrotenthaler et al., 2013; Zhao et al., 2019). Minor strains, lacerations, blunt trauma, organ damage, body surface, and lower-limb injuries also happen frequently (Bohonos & Hogan, 1999; Deng et al., 2018; Zhao et al., 2019).

In addition to the injuries directly caused by tornadoes, additional injuries can occur during the rescue and recovery period after the tornado, including lacerations, foot punctures, sunburn, heat injuries, hammer injuries, animal bites, and musculoskeletal strain (Bohonos & Hogan, 1999; Chiu et al., 2013). A study by Niederkrotenthaler et al. (2013) also reported about a quarter of all tornado injuries could have been prevented by increasing safety protocol during cleanup. Because of that, future emergency preparedness planning and public health initiatives would also benefit from focusing on safety during the cleanup, such as enhancing public health messaging regarding the safe use of tools and proper protective wear.

The social vulnerability approach has been widely used to relate social characteristics to predisposing vulnerability to disasters and has been a guiding approach in examining people's preparedness, response, and recovery to disasters (Boruff et al., 2003). Concerning deaths and injuries, a variety of risk factors contribute to higher risks of dying or being injured in tornadoes, such as gender, age, vulnerable home construction, a lack of underground shelter options, and people who are outside or in mobile homes (Deng et al., 2018; Niederkrotenthaler et al., 2013). For example, older adults were more likely to be killed or injured in tornadoes (Legates & Biddle, 1999; NIST, 2014; Schmidlin et al., 1998). Data also show that women, adults over 45 years old, and those under 18 years old are also disproportionately injured in tornadoes (Deng et al., 2018). For instance, in a study on the 2011 Joplin EF5 tornado, it was found that while people over age 65 accounted for 15% of the population, they represented 38% of the tornado fatalities and females were more likely to be injured than males (NIST, 2014). Niederkrotenthaler et al. (2013) discovered a high risk of injury during violent tornadoes for persons who were not in a storm shelter or tornado safe room, which are scarce in the Southeast and other parts of the country. The highest odds of fatalities and injuries existed in mobile home residents who usually have lower socioeconomic status (Niederkrotenthaler et al., 2013; Simmons & Sutter, 2011).

Mental Health

Tornadoes can also cause short-term and long-term mental health problems. **Posttraumatic Stress Disorder (PTSD)** and depression are the two most commonly assessed and reported mental health problems in disaster studies (Norris et al., 2002), as well as in research about tornadoes (Yuan et al., 2018). Niederkrotenthaler et al. (2013) used telephone surveys to screen for PTSD after a tornado in Alabama in April 2011, in which 22% of the sample screened positive, pointing out a need for long-term psychosocial support, and 66% of affected individuals required crisis counseling. Houston et al. (2015) examined the prevalence of PTSD and depression among Joplin adults, reporting the probable PTSD relevance was 12.6% 6 months after the tornado and 26.7% 2.5 years after the tornado; and the prevalence for depression was 20.8% 6 months after and 13.3% 2.5 years after. In a Chinese investigation about the prevalence of PTSD and depression among 247 adolescent survivors after the 2016 Yancheng tornado, Xu et al. (2018) reported that 57.5% of respondents reported symptoms of PTSD, while 58.7% of the respondents reported suspected depression. Furthermore, age, female gender, ethnic minority status, poverty, less education, more tornado experience, low level of social support, pre-tornado trauma exposure, and pre-disaster psychiatric problems have been found to be risk factors of experiencing PTSD and depression after a tornado strikes (Adams et al., 2014; Houston et al., 2015; Xu et al., 2018). Additionally, fears and worries could result from tornadoes. For example, Polusny et al. (2011) reported that 37% of adolescents who experienced tornadoes in rural Minnesota were afraid they would be injured and 22% of them worried that they would be killed in the storm. In the long-term recovery from tornadoes, mental health distress was also reported to be related to great resource loss and debt (Clay & Greer, 2019).

It is worth noting that children and teenagers are considered to have a higher risk of having mental health problems after disasters than do older adults (Norris et al., 2002) because their perceptions, thoughts, and feelings are more sensory-oriented, and their coping skills are easily overwhelmed (Miller et al., 2018). In the context of tornadoes, it was also found that the child population between ages 4 to 10 displayed more difficulty than did older children, with symptoms such as stomachaches, headaches, or scaring easily (Houston et al., 2015). Adams et al. (2014) examined 2,000 adolescents and caregivers after the Spring 2011 tornado outbreak, reporting that 6.7% of adolescents met the diagnostic criteria of PTSD, and 7.5% of them met the criteria for a major depressive episode. Among the youth population, the risk factors included female gender, prior trauma exposure, greater tornado exposure, lower household income, an injured family member, lower levels of social support, and older age, among others (Houston et al., 2015; Paul et al., 2015).

Although these mental health problems can lead to substantial strain on family and communities in the recovery journey, studies have found that many people are resilient or have posttraumatic growth, which enables them to quickly return to pre-disaster functioning (Adams et al., 2014; Yuan et al., 2018). However, research also indicates a need for mental health services following natural disasters, while low mental health service utilization among disaster-affected individuals was identified in some studies (Houston et al., 2015; Wang et al., 2008). The reasons for low mental health service utilization after tornadoes are understudied, but perceived barriers of mental health service could include concerns about stigma and reexperiencing the traumatic event, shame and rejection, low mental health literacy, a lack of knowledge and treatment-related doubts, fear of negative social consequences, limited resources, time, and expenses (Kantor et al., 2017). Mental health problems can last long after tornadoes depart; thus, mental health services should be provided over an extended time to treat trauma related to the disaster and psychiatric disorders (Niederkrotenthaler et al., 2013).

Other Health Problems

Tornadoes can lead to the spread of infectious conditions that support mold and other hazards and endanger the safety of the food supply. One infectious challenge after tornadoes is caused by mucormycosis, a fungal infection that can be inhaled, leading to serious health issues for those with weakened immune systems. Cutaneous mucormycosis can infect the body through injuries to the skin and has a fatality rate ranging between 29% to 83% (Kouadio et al., 2012). Researchers investigated a cluster of cases of cutaneous mucormycosis among persons injured during the Joplin tornado in 2011 and found 13 people were identified in the zone that sustained the most severe damage during the tornado, five of whom (38%) died (Austin et al., 2014; Neblett Fanfair et al., 2012). The victims had a median of five wounds (ranging between 1 to 7); 11 victims (85%) had at least one fracture, while nine (69%) had blunt trauma and five (38%) had penetrating trauma. There was also an increase in respiratory illness associated with the Joplin tornado because of the huge amount of debris produced. During the cleanup process, people had excessive exposure to dust and mold, but few wore protective masks or took other protective measures (Forshee-Hakala, 2015).

Tornadoes During COVID-19

Caused by the 2019 novel coronavirus (SARS-CoV-2), the number of confirmed cases of coronavirus disease 2019 (COVID-19) worldwide is over 26 million as of September 2020. On March 11, 2020, the World Health Organization (WHO, 2020b) identified COVID-19 as a pandemic, which has posed a serious threat to human health and profoundly changed different aspects of our lives, forcing us to adjust to a new normal of living. As a typical slow-onset disaster, COVID-19 has spread through the United States since the first diagnosed case in January 2020 (Holshue et al., 2020) and may persist for a long time in the absence of widespread vaccination for coronavirus.

Meanwhile, some disasters resulting from extreme weather events have overlapped with COVID-19 (Quigley et al., 2020). According to the U.S. Storm Prediction

Center (2020), more than 1,100 tornadoes occurred between January to September 2020, with a peak in April. Some of these tornado events caused many deaths and injuries. For example, a violent EF4 tornado attacked Putnam County, Tennessee, in the early morning hours of March 3, 2020, leading to 19 fatalities, 87 injuries, and approximately $100 million in property damage (National Center for Environmental Information, 2020). From April 12 to 13, 2020, cold fronts swept across the southeast of the United States, bringing about strong winds and tornadoes (Quigley et al., 2020). This devastating weather system, which affected Alabama, Georgia, Mississippi, South Carolina, and Tennessee, killed more than 30 people and destroyed a plethora of homes (Fentress & Fausset, 2020).

The occurrence of both tornado and COVID-19 has brought additional challenges to individuals, communities, governments, and health authorities. On the one hand, the impacts of tornadoes may be worse in such a multi-hazard scenario. For fear of COVID-19 transmission attributed to the gathering of displaced people, individuals may be reluctant to evacuate to public shelters when receiving tornado warnings (Jenkins, 2020). Some public transit agencies have had to reduce or cease services as a result of a significant drop in ridership and the fear of COVID-19 infection in urban areas (Garcia, 2020; J. E. Smith, 2020), which may cause trouble to low-income and marginalized groups who are most dependent on public transportation (Wilbur et al., 2020) and prevent them from evacuating to shelters in tornadoes. Moreover, many communities have declared that they will not open or operate public shelters during COVID-19 (American Meteorological Society, 2020). In addition to the problems with evacuation and shelters, there has also been a shortage of manpower and resources to respond to tornadoes during the epidemic. COVID-19 may reduce the number of domestic volunteers because many volunteers are retired older adults who are at a higher risk of infection. Other volunteers may be deterred by mobility restrictions. In addition, there could be a decrease in the amount of relief goods available for tornado-related victims due to panic buying and supply problems (Waldrop, 2020). At the same time, COVID-19 can also limit the global humanitarian response mechanism in terms of the rapid mobilization of humanitarian staff, volunteers, and resources due to the worldwide epidemic and travel restrictions (Quigley et al., 2020). Furthermore, governmental and health authorities may face special challenges. Governments were caught off guard with few preexisting plans for such a multi-hazard scenario (Jenkins, 2020), and their ability to immediately respond to tornadoes and promote community recovery was also impaired due to restrictions on movement and transportation, as well as a lack of funding and resources attributed to COVID-19 (Quigley et al., 2020). With limited medical staff, hospital beds, personal protective equipment (PPE), and medical equipment, different levels of health systems that have already been overwhelmed by COVID-19 may struggle to cope with the increasing demands for medical services and assistance resulting from tornadoes. On the other hand, the outbreaks of tornadoes may promote the additional spread of COVID-19. Urgent evacuation, crowding of shelters, and search and rescue could expose people to risks of being in close contact with each other, which would significantly increase the community transmission possibilities (Law, 2020). Moreover, in the face of life threats and property losses caused by tornadoes, individuals seem to rarely think about COVID-19 (Waldrop, 2020), which makes them relax mitigative measures, such as wearing masks and practicing social distancing.

To promote human health and well-being in a multi-hazard scenario of both tornado and COVID-19, disaster risk management and COVID-19 preparedness and response should be well coordinated to comprehensively improve tornado preparedness, response, and recovery processes (WHO, 2020a). In terms of preparedness, individuals should be well informed of the importance of tornado preparedness via online public education and be provided with resources about how to prepare during COVID-19. For example, Ready Campaign (2020) specifically called on people to bring hand sanitizer and disinfecting wipes, and maintain social and physical distancing, when they go to a public shelter, in addition to other routine preparations for tornadoes. Tornado sheltering guidelines during COVID-19 were published online to teach people the safe use of public storm shelters during the epidemic (American Meteorological Society, 2020). Public shelters that are open during the epidemic should be identified and advertised through their websites or social media to enable individuals to fully understand the alternative shelters and specific conditions of shelters. Moreover, public shelters should develop specific plans to ensure human safety and health according to their actual situations and the guidelines of the CDC and local health authorities and prepare relevant materials, such as masks, hand sanitizer, and thermometers, as well as relief goods. Governments at all levels need to integrate disaster risk management and response plans with COVID-19 plans to ensure the rational allocation and optimal use of available human, financial, and material resources, with a priority of protecting vulnerable groups and ensuring inclusiveness and equity (WHO, 2020a). Medical institutions should enhance the capacity of medical staff to respond to tornadoes during a pandemic through specialized training, preparing adequate PPE and medical equipment in advance (Quigley et al., 2020), and developing field triage and casualty management and referral guidelines with a focus on prevention of COVID-19 (WHO, 2020a).

When it comes to tornado response, early warnings from multiple sources should be issued with COVID-19 risk communications to alert people of the risks of transmission (WHO, 2020a). Individuals need to be careful to identify the nearby shelters that are operating and strictly follow the guidelines about safety and health on the way out. When public shelters resettle tornado-related victims, strict measures should be taken to reduce the risk of COVID-19 transmission, such as wearing masks, practicing social distancing, handwashing, and ensuring sanitation and hygiene measures, waste disposal, temperature monitoring, and nucleic acid testing, if necessary. Well-trained search and rescue teams should be provided with PPE and monitor for the transmission of coronavirus during the rescue operation. Medical response staff members need to be equipped with PPE and infection prevention and control measures when providing mobile outpatient services and referral; they also need to conduct effective triage for suspected cases and contacts with COVID-19 precautions, including isolation (WHO, 2020a). Importantly, governments can, in a timely manner, surveil the post-disaster situations and develop health emergency information management systems to make sure information on tornadoes and COVID-19 can be received by communities, health facilities, shelters, and other relevant settings (WHO, 2020a). This can promote tornado response, reduce the transmission of COVID-19, and may help people relieve feelings of insecurity and uncertainty.

In the recovery process of tornadoes, public and private sectors need to work together to assist tornado-related residents in resettlement and recovery from damage and loss, which aims to help them get back to a normal life. Specifically, the mental health of tornado-related victims, emergency personnel, and medical staff is a conspicuous issue in the context of the epidemic. Surveillance for their emotional well-being (e.g., loneliness, frustration, dread) and mental disorders (e.g., anxiety, depression, posttraumatic stress disorder [PTSD]) should be conducted promptly. Evidence-based psychological interventions, such as **cognitive-behavioral therapy,** art therapy, emotion-focused therapy, and prolonged exposure therapy, can be provided for individuals, families, and communities in safe forms such as cybercounseling, hotlines, and smartphone-based support (Shi & Hall, 2020).

CASE STUDY OF THE 2011 JOPLIN TORNADO PUBLIC HEALTH RESPONSES

BACKGROUND OF THE JOPLIN TORNADO

Late in the afternoon of May 22, 2011, one of the deadliest tornadoes in U.S. history landed in Joplin, a city located in the southwestern corner of Missouri. The Joplin tornado, rated EF5 on the Enhanced Fujita Scale with a maximum wind of more than 200 mph, touched down southwest of Joplin at 5:34 p.m. CDT and proceeded to last 38 minutes. Its entire path across the city was 22.1 miles long and 1 mile in width (NWS, 2011a; see Figure 7.4). This tornado was estimated to affect 41% of Joplin's population, killed 161 people, injured 1,000, damaged nearly 8,000 structures including critical health and utility infrastructure, and resulted in an estimated loss of $3 billion (FEMA, 2011b; NIST, 2014). It is the costliest and seventh deadliest tornado in U.S. history; it is also the single deadliest tornado in the United States since 1950 when modern record keeping started (NWS, n.d.-a; Paul & Stimers, 2012). The high level of casualties in Joplin shocked the community and experts alike; it has raised wide concerns of society's vulnerability to disasters when we generally expect

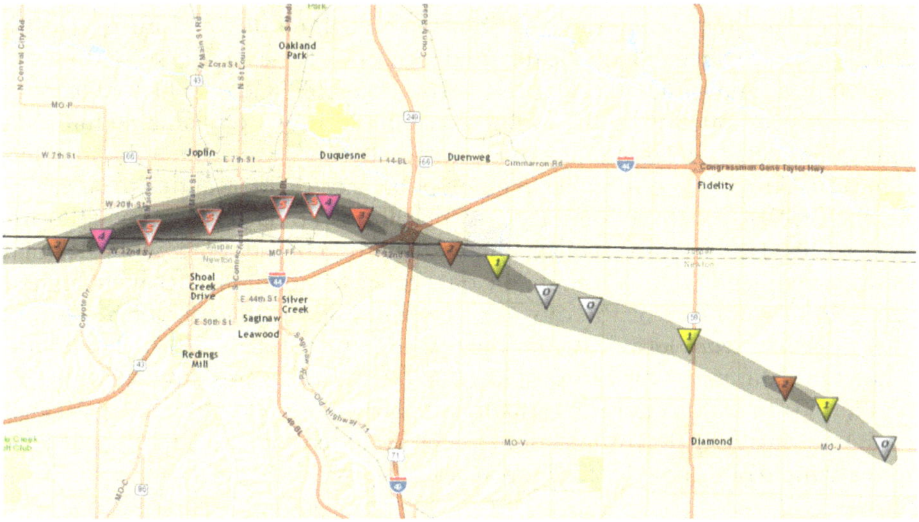

Figure 7.4 Track map of Joplin tornado from 5:34 p.m. to 6:12 p.m. on May 22, 2011 (numbers in the triangle note EF scales in the corresponding areas).

Source: Reprinted from National Weather Service. https://www.weather.gov/sgf/news_events_2011may22. Copyright 2011 by NWS.

our society to be relatively safe with the advancement of technology, especially for a well-warned tornado (Simmons & Sutter, 2013).

Assess and Monitor Population Health

Before the tornado, monitoring weather conditions and issuing tornado warnings are regarded as critical public health issues, because taking proper protective actions upon receiving tornado warnings, such as taking shelter, is a key factor to reduce fatalities and injuries. Despite the astounding fatalities, the Joplin tornado was actually well warned and was closely monitored before the touch-down. At 1:30 p.m. CDT, the NWS issued a tornado watch for Southwest Missouri. At 5:17 p.m. CDT, the NWS Forecast Office in Springfield issued a tornado warning for Joplin. Before the initial touchdown at 5:34 p.m. CDT, there was approximately a 17-minute window of opportunity when residents were sent warnings from broadcasts on television and radio; online NWS watches, alerts, and warnings; activation of a first and second siren; text messages; posts on social media; NOAA Weather Radio; observation of the physical environment; and messages spread between acquaintances (NWS, 2011a).

After the tornado, monitoring the deaths and injuries is critical for the community to provide timely and targeted health services. In Joplin, bodies were recovered from collapsed buildings, and the Missouri Highway Patrol was requested to take charge of the missing person list and identify both survivors and those who died. The task was completed by June 4 (FEMA, 2011b). Joplin's mass fatalities following the tornado presented a great challenge for those monitoring deaths. Although the Disaster Mortuary Operational Response Team was deployed to help with fatality management within 2 days after the tornado, it was overwhelmed. In addition to response personnel, volunteers and others without fatality management training also participated in body recovery operations (FEMA, 2011b).

In addition to monitoring deaths, there were multiple measures taken to monitor people with injuries as well as health conditions and mental health conditions. To monitor injuries, the Division of Community and Public Health of Missouri Department of Health and Senior Service (MDHSS, n.d.) used **ESSENCE**, a syndromic surveillance system. The ESSENCE data included about 762 records compiled from the Joplin tornado and provided valuable information about tornado-related injuries. However, the data were limited and could be improved to be more valuable to guide public health interventions. For example, the ESSENCE data set only focused on those who used emergency department services; thus, those who were injured but did not seek emergency hospital services were omitted. In addition, the data collected about injuries were limited with a brief summary of the causes of injuries and no information regarding where persons were located when they were injured (NIST, 2014). These limitations in data collection can provide a reference for future data collection to monitor health status after the tornado. Similarly, the CDC provided a data set for monitoring fungal skin infection, which included injury and personal data from a sample of 87 people (Kuligowski et al., 2016).

Furthermore, additional efforts were made at surveillance regarding the health conditions and to provide solutions to reduce public health concerns. According to a summary of the CDC, residents were checked door-to-door on their medical needs, and the health department prioritized power restoration for ventilator-dependent patients. There were also coordinated efforts in childhood lead surveillance and cleaning up of lead-contaminated properties (CDC, 2017). These monitoring and surveillance services adopted appropriate methods to depict a community health profile of Joplin residents that was useful for diverse audiences, leading to subsequent health investigation and improvement programs.

Frontline public health staff play an important role in collecting data and information in monitoring efforts. Frontline workers need to be informed and trained on issues that range from initial research design, questionnaire/ interview outline design and test, sampling, informed consent, and confidentiality to data collection and preservation for the purpose of ensuring a comprehensive and valid data set (National Association of County & City Health Officials, 2013). In the case of the ESSENCE data set for the Joplin tornado, public health frontline workers mainly focused on individuals who visited the emergency department or used emergency department services of a hospital and collected data regarding gender, age range, and category of the chief complaint (e.g., the reason for going to the hospital; NIST, 2014). In the example of a data set created by the CDC to monitor fungal skin infection, frontline public health staff collected injury and personal data from individuals randomly selected from the ESSENCE data set. The data included both medical record chart abstraction and face-to-face interviews (NIST, 2014). The interviews provided a qualitative description of what happened from the time when the tornado started until the time the injured individual sought medical care (NIST, 2014). These data collection efforts by frontline workers were the basis for subsequent data analysis and application. From the public health supervisory level, professionals usually take on the leading role of surveillance service after a tornado. Program managers are expected to properly apply epidemiological methods in practice, especially observational study designs, due to their responsibilities for designing and scheduling a comprehensive survey to ensure that the data collected are useful to present health conditions and problems, identify community resources, and finally help address health concerns. It is also important for public health program managers to actively promote cooperation with other agencies to make full use of the collected data. For example, after collecting data, both the MDHSS Division of Community and Public Health and the CDC provided data sets to NIST by describing the detailed design, sampling, covered topics, and results of data collection, which promotes the cooperation with the NIST on the technical investigation of the Joplin tornado (NIST, 2014).

Investigate, Diagnose, and Address Health Hazards and Root Causes

Diagnosing and investigating health concerns can effectively identify key issues and investigate public health threats and responses after tornadoes. Although deaths and injuries were major public health concerns of tornadoes, other health issues also presented health hazards. After the Joplin tornado, staff from Missouri's local public health agencies, the CDC, and the MDHSS worked together to identify, investigate, and respond to mucormycosis fungal infection found in tornado-affected victims (MDHSS, 2011). Initially, two patients hospitalized with tornado injuries were suspected of necrotizing fungal soft-tissue infections. The MDHSS launched immediate surveillance for such infections at hospitals and laboratories that served patients injured in the tornado. With the support of the CDC, a total of 18 suspected cases of cutaneous mucormycosis were identified, among which 13 were confirmed (CDC, 2011). Meanwhile, public health staff suggested that victims in the tornado area who had unhealed wounds seek immediate medical attention (Cable News Network, 2011). The case of fungal infection in the Joplin tornado showed the importance of identifying and investigating health threats in a timely manner to reduce their impact on public health (Austin et al., 2014).

In addition to physical health, diagnosing mental health issues is important to guide the provision of mental healthcare. Houston et al. (2015) conducted two surveys at approximately 6 months and 2.5 years postdisaster to examine the prevalence of posttraumatic stress and depression among Joplin adults and emphasized the importance of long-term community health monitoring, assessment, referrals, outreach, and services after the Joplin tornado. These diagnoses provided guidance for a variety of counseling services to help tornado-affected victims emotionally recover in the long term (Dods, 2016). For example, for children and teenagers who were considered to be at higher risk of mental health issues, professional counselors provided school-based, small-group counseling services for students in some Joplin schools, and children with more severe disorders were referred to community mental health providers (Kanter & Abramson, 2014). However, even though there was a high need for mental health services and services were made accessible, the actual use of supportive services after the Joplin tornado was quite low (Houston et al., 2015), which raises questions about how to best approach survivors and the need for special consideration to broach the subject of post-tornado mental health service promotion and implementation.

The training of frontline workers was important for diagnosing health issues. For example, after the tornado, the Substance Abuse and Mental Health Services Administration (SAMHSA) updated stress and grief materials and distributed them to state and local agencies, preparing frontline workers to better identify those who were in need and to provide timely and appropriate services (Public Health Emergency, 2011).

Communicate Effectively to Inform and Educate

Health and risk communications help to increase awareness of health risks, promote healthy behaviors, and create support for health policies, programs, and practices (National Association of County & City Health Officials, 2013). Those services allow tornado-affected residents to make an optimal decision about their health and well-being. After the Joplin tornado, the health and risk communication systems faced unique challenges. The communication systems were damaged, compromising communication among institutions and residents. Lots of efforts were made to recover the communication. Communication was improved via a trailer in Joplin with satellite uplink and an 800-MHz radio; in addition, ambulance radios became the communication infrastructure during the initial response (MDHSS, 2011). The phone line systems were also damaged and overwhelmed during and after the tornado, but texting, social media, and the internet still worked and helped victims share and receive health information (South Dakota Department of Health, 2011).

Many different institutions contributed to communicating health risks and the availability of health services. For example, the website of the Office of Assistant

Secretary for Preparedness and Response published public health emergency information to the public; information about Medicare, Medicaid, and the Children's Health Insurance Plan benefits was disseminated by the Centers for Medicare and Medicaid Services after the disaster, and stress management information was also offered by the website of SAMHSA (Department of Health and Human Services, 2012). The CDC was able to publish the whole process and results of the monitoring of mucormycosis infection on its website in a timely manner (CDC, 2011), assisting the public to understand the fungal infection, alleviate panic, and remind tornado-affected residents to take precautions to prevent and treat any evidence of disease. Meanwhile, some institutions and residents helped disseminate information regarding emergency public health and warning, available health resources, and the needs of tornado-affected victims by launching Facebook pages or releasing videos on **YouTube channels**.

Notably, educating the public to take precautionary actions was an important public task faced by Joplin health officials. The education mission was especially important when access to clean drinking water and safe food became an issue. Because of the damage to the water supply, 4,000 customer service lines leaked; the pressure of two elevated storage towers dropped in 10 minutes and went to zero within 2 hours. Due to the impossibility of maintaining system pressure, a boil water order was issued by the Missouri Department of Natural Resources (Barnhart, 2011). In order to cooperate with the implementation of governmental order, and to assist residents in tornado areas to drink clean water, the Joplin Health Department conducted water system boil advisory educational activities to the community and regulated facilities during the period of low water pressure (MDHSS, 2011). Residents were also provided information concerning reasons for contaminated water after the tornado, how to purify water and disinfect drinking water containers, and techniques to disinfect wells or private water sources (MDHSS, 2011). Similarly, power outage education was provided to the community due to massive electric outage in the tornado area, especially to remind residents of food safety after a power failure (MDHSS, 2011).

Public health frontline staff are usually responsible for conducting educational activities and disseminating health-related information. For example, within the first hours after the Joplin tornado, the staff from the local health department started to adopt timely field visits to provide infection control procedures, disease monitoring, and education programs for shelter staff of the Red Cross Shelters (MDHSS, 2011). Moreover, in the first 24 hours, health staff started to visit and educate volunteer food providers at temporary food sites, and within the first 72 hours, they visited more than 400 food establishments to control spoiled food due to tornado damage and power outages (MDHSS, 2011). The effectiveness of information communication requires strong communication skills of frontline staff. Cultural competency is especially important when communicating with people of different races, ethnicities, or nations. The responsibilities of public health program managers could include formulating health promotion policies, coordinating health information, organizing and training staff, and promoting cooperation with other health agencies to effectively communicate health risks and implement educational programs.

Strengthen, Support, and Mobilize Communities and Partnerships

Different from many other public health problems, the public health of tornadoes is built upon the preparedness and recovery of the community, infrastructure, and health system. FEMA recognized the importance of collaboration between public sectors and private sectors to respond to public health issues in its **Whole Community approach**, which highlights innovative ways to collaborate and gain access to nontraditional resources to respond to disasters (FEMA, 2011b). In the aftermath and recovery of the Joplin tornado, the private and public sectors collaborated closely and coordinated to contribute material and emotional resources to respond to the disaster and rebuild the whole community.

The public sector primarily focused on restoring public services, enabling the city to return to normal operation and order (D. J. Smith & Sutter, 2013). From the municipal level, the main job of city officials was to organize debris removal and to waive some building regulations, simplify procedures, and reevaluate local zoning laws immediately after the tornado, which helped accelerate rebuilding. The state government and FEMA provided massive financial assistance for city recovery (FEMA, 2011a). FEMA installed more than 600 temporary housing units, paid for most debris removal costs, and built temporary school facilities (D. J. Smith & Sutter, 2013). In FEMA's report on their response to the Joplin tornado, strengths and limitations of the Whole Community approach were discussed with details in different areas. It was suggested that the capacities of the City of Joplin and Jasper County were overwhelmed, but the preparedness partnerships that developed among different entities proved to be mainly successful. For example, the Whole Community approach mobilized volunteers in recovering bodies and provided mental health counseling to support the personnel who might not have been trained in the past; although two fire stations were damaged, they still functioned because of the mutual aid provided by other areas (FEMA, 2011b). With the support of the CDC's Public Health Emergency Preparedness (PHEP) cooperative agreement program, many residents, particularly those injured, were evacuated to neighboring states; in addition, health departments in those states helped to provide and administer tetanus vaccinations based on the existing partnership (CDC, 2017).

The post-disaster contributions from the private sector were enormous and phenomenal, which not only assisted residents to feel some relief from their immediate challenges but also supported recovery (D. J. Smith & Sutter, 2013). The private sector, including charities, the business community, Joplin residents, and volunteers from all over the country, provided immediate and basic care and attention to the affected residents (D. J. Smith & Sutter, 2013). It was estimated that by November 2011, more than 92,000 volunteers from diverse churches, charities, businesses, hospitals, and school groups contributed more than 528,000 person-hours in the disaster-affected area (D. J. Smith & Sutter, 2013). Nonprofit organizations provided food, clothes, clean water, and shelters to residents and helped to remove debris and establish resource centers to coordinate services and resources (FEMA, 2011a; The Salvation Army, 2016). Counseling services were arranged to assist victims who needed support for emotional recovery (Dods, 2016), free day care was provided to support survivors, and millions of donations were collected to rebuild the city (D. J. Smith & Sutter, 2013). Insurance companies wrote advance checks to enable families to obtain immediate shelter and nourishment and to assist residents to make plans for rebuilding (Kennedy, 2011). Many businesses across the nation organized large donations of money and in-kind services, enabling local businesses to reopen and pay their employees who were faced with homelessness or heavy damage to their homes. Public health frontline workers are responsible for building a relationship with the affected community and exploring and reflecting on the health-related problems and needs of tornado-related residents. Meanwhile, they will actively empower residents to take part in their work with both the public and private sectors. For public health program managers, they need to place a strategic emphasis on community partnership and coordinate the division of labor and cooperation between the public and private sectors.

Create, Champion, and Implement Policies, Plans, and Laws

Local policies and plans are developed in both governmental and private sectors to guide the practice of public health and improve community-level health. In response to the Joplin tornado, the Joplin City Health Department formulated a plan for vital services in the first 100 days following the tornado. This local service planning covered a long list of public health services in preparation for conducting and coordinating health administrative operations, environmental and epidemiological services, public health medical services, and animal control, with the collaboration of many public and private institutions (MDHSS, 2011). The local health department staffed the Emergency Operation Center (EOC) to direct health administrative operations with the help of some other medical service partners, including the Jasper County Health Department Access Family Care and St. John's Regional Medical Center (Joplin Health Department, 2011). The EOC also worked with the Environmental Protection Agency to monitor air quality in the tornado-affected area, and after this monitoring ended in August, the Joplin Health Department further conducted asbestos air monitoring services to ensure continued air safety (MDHSS, 2011). Mosquito fogging appeared about 10 days after the tornado, and the health department inspected a total of 36 miles of ditches and 72 acres of depressions and utilized larvicide to control mosquitoes in the tornado-affected area (Joplin Health Department, 2011). As for animal control, the Joplin City Health Department animal control staff worked with other animal control agencies and the Humane Society of Missouri to transport 1,308 pets to the emergency pet shelter, set up a temporary pet triage clinic to care for animals, develop animal rescue operations and animal trapping programs to capture animals hiding in debris, and deal with deceased animals (Joplin Health Department, 2011). Supported by local government and the private sector and led by qualified agencies, this local health emergency response plan played an important role in protecting the public health of the community.

Frontline staff members were mainly responsible for implementing policies and plans and collecting feedback and evidence to improve plans and services. As revealed from the Joplin health emergency response planning earlier, many partners are often involved in enforcing policy-related services, including both governmental and private sectors. Staff should identify the division of tasks among different stakeholders and pay attention to building partnerships with them for providing more efficient services. At the supervisory level, public health program managers should discuss multiple dimensions of the policymaking process and coordinate across agencies in the implementation of services. In the case of the planning of the vital services, the health program managers took diverse aspects into consideration and coordinated many agencies' efforts (MDHSS, 2011). Each health agency was clear about its tasks and worked collectively in an efficient way.

Utilize Legal and Regulatory Actions

This service includes reviewing, evaluating, improving, and enforcing laws, regulations, and ordinances on federal, state, and local levels to prevent health problems and protect public health (National Association of County & City Health Officials, 2013). During the response to the Joplin tornado, due to the emergency medical situation, several state laws and regulations that were deemed impediments to rapid public health services were waived by the Missouri governor, to assist recovery and promote community well-being. For example, the director of MDHSS and the State Board of Pharmacy had the full discretionary authority by Executive Order 11-10 on May 24, 2011, to temporarily waive or suspend administration rules and regulations to prioritize public health and safety (Missouri Secretary of State, 2011a). This order improved restrictions on prescribing by pharmacists during tornado response and recovery, enabling tornado-affected victims to obtain a 30-day supply of medicines (D. J. Smith & Sutter, 2013). Similarly, the state gave St. John's Hospital a 2-year waiver to operate a psychological unit out of a wooden building because this hospital was severely damaged by the tornado and had to move operations to tents and modular units (D. J. Smith & Sutter, 2013). This regulation allowed the hospital to get through the licensing procedures quickly and to provide timely health services for residents in the tornado-affected area.

The main task of frontline staff is to enforce policies and evaluate their impact on public health and health equity leadership. For example, the Missouri State Executive Order 11-17 was issued after the Joplin tornado, which set up a permanent state Resource, Recovery & Rebuilding Center to provide convenient and centralized services and information to tornado-affected residents (Missouri Secretary of State, 2011b). In order to implement this order, the staff from at least 13 state departments were brought together to function as a one-stop shop for Joplin residents who were affected by the tornado and who needed assistance (Office of Missouri Governor Jeremiah W. (Jay) Nixon, 2012). The staff was encouraged to actively communicate with tornado-affected residents, government agencies, or other organizations tasked with enforcement responsibilities, be updated on the progress and effects of law enforcement, and make an objective evaluation. The frontline staff mainly provided services regarding temporary housing, unemployment assistance, and driver's licenses and other identification cards, which assisted residents with bureaucratic processes and helped them recover better; they also need to organize and provide feedback to public health program managers, who can help improve the existing laws and regulations and promote their enforcement to meet the unmet needs of public health (Office of Missouri Governor Jeremiah W. (Jay) Nixon, 2012; D. J. Smith & Sutter, 2013).

Enable Equitable Access

In this service, the local public health system will work with the local health department and other partners, such as hospitals, managed care providers, and community health agencies, to identify the specific needs of different groups of the population and barriers to receiving public health services. After that, the collaboration of public health, primary care, oral health, social services, mental health systems, and some organizations, which are unconventional parts of the health service system (e.g., housing, transportation, and grassroots organizations), will coordinate the delivery of targeted, ongoing, and culturally and linguistically appropriate health service for tornado-affected residents, especially some vulnerable population groups (National Association of County & City Health Officials, 2013).

One critical healthcare need following the Joplin tornado was to treat a large number of residents with serious injuries that occurred during the tornado or in the process of removing debris and rebuilding from the catastrophic damage the tornado caused to many residential and nonresidential buildings (NIST, 2014). One big challenge in delivering healthcare was that the tornado also damaged, sometimes severely, healthcare facilities, including the St. John's Regional Medical Center, Freeman Health System, and the Ozark Center. St. John's and Freeman Health System operated the emergency medical service system in Joplin and the Ozark Center provided services for behavioral health and autism. The damage to St. John's Regional Medical Center caused six deaths. There were gas leaks, flooding, and both St. John's Regional Medical Center and Freeman Health System lost power after the tornado (FEMA, 2011b; South Dakota Department of Health, 2011). The damages to these facilities presented additional challenges in providing healthcare services promptly to victims of a mass disaster that resulted in mass casualties.

When the Joplin tornado struck the city, St. John's Regional Medical Center had 183 patients inside the building. Those patients were evacuated in 90 minutes. Not aware of the damage to the facility, new victims continued to present themselves or were transported to St. John's Regional Medical Center. Similarly, immediately after the tornado, 130 patients self-presented to the Freeman Health System, even though their emergency department had only a capacity of 40 beds (South Dakota Department of Health, 2011). Those overwhelming demands had to be addressed by triage.

Triage operations were set up in the parking lot of St. John's Regional Medical Center. Patients in critical condition were transported to Freeman Health System and St. John's Hospital in Springfield (FEMA, 2011b; South Dakota Department of Health, 2011). Medical personnel and volunteers used any undamaged vehicles such as ambulances and pickup trucks to transport patients (FEMA, 2011b). It was reported that 713 injured individuals were also transported to 42 hospitals in four adjacent states (CDC, 2017). Field triage locations were set up across Joplin to treat injuries. About 200 people received medical treatment in these temporary centers including Memorial Hall, McAuley Catholic High School, and the parking lots of Home Depot and Lowe's stores (FEMA, 2011b). Moreover, some ambulances were parked strategically in areas with significant damages and provided treatment on-site.

The Freeman Health System relied on emergency generators to treat approximately 400 victims in the first few hours after the tornado, including 22 lifesaving surgeries in the first 12 hours (FEMA, 2011b; South Dakota Department of Health, 2011). Eventually, about 1,000 patients were treated at the Freeman Emergency Department and the Alternate Care Site (South Dakota Department of Health, 2011). The Missouri 1 Disaster Medical Team of the State of Missouri deployed a mobile field hospital covering 8,000 square feet with 60 beds. This enabled the St. John's medical staff to start treating patients in this facility 1 week after the tornado (FEMA, 2011b). In addition, the MDHSS deployed a Mobile Medical Unit and treated 157 patients with its 24-bed emergency room (CDC, 2017). In addition to physical injuries, the CDC enabled mental health providers to provide support at family assistance shelters (CDC, 2017). The CDC's PHEP cooperative agreement program also made efforts to address the needs of dialysis and ventilator-dependent patients and reduced risks in lead exposure as well as fungal and mosquito-borne diseases after the tornado (CDC, 2017).

Furthermore, after identifying the need for preventing tetanus among the tornado-affected community, Joplin City and Jasper County Health Departments' medical services workers, state and local health departments, clinics, and hospitals worked together to formulate a tetanus vaccine administration plan for both residents and workers. In a few weeks, over 17,000 tetanus vaccinations were administered by several medical partners in the community. Because affected residents were placed in different shelters and there was still lots of debris on the roads, vaccine distribution was conducted in both stationary and roving locations moving through tornado-affected neighborhoods, ensuring that this health service could be well delivered to people with limited mobility or transportation (MDHSS, 2011).

Public health frontline staff members must work on identifying the needs of different population groups and delivering health-related services. They should be good at observing and discovering specific needs, structural biases, social inequities, and racism that undermine health and impact health equity at the organizational, community, and societal levels (National Association of County & City Health Officials, 2013). At the supervisory level, public health program managers should design relevant services and implementation plans according to specific assessment of needs and service delivery (National Association of County & City Health Officials, 2013).

Improve and Innovate Through Evaluation, Research, and Quality Improvement

The main target objects of evaluation are population-based health services, personal health services, and local public health system performance. After evaluation, information can be collected to improve health-related services by allocating resources and reshaping relevant programs (National Association of County & City Health Officials, 2013). Different federal agencies provided assessments on services and responses relevant to the Joplin tornado. FEMA published *The Response to the 2011 Joplin, Missouri, Tornado Lessons Learned Study* in December 2011, summarized responses including public health responses, and reflected on areas for improvements based on interviews and data analysis (FEMA, 2011b). The assessment recognized the strength of responses from different departments and suggested areas for improvement. The strengths included a timely response from emergency responders to address the needs of survivors, effective communication of emergency information to support recovery, good preparation with national-level exercise, and successful coordination between federal and local agencies. It also identified areas of improvement focusing on better coordination and the need for trained and deployable staff in a time of emergency (FEMA, 2011b). Similarly, the NWS published *NWS Central Region Service Assessment Joplin, Missouri, Tornado - May 22, 2011* in July 2011 as a response to this rare and high impact event. It conducted more than 100 interviews with different stakeholders including survivors, NWS staff, emergency management, media, city officials, and local businesses. The purpose was to examine the warning services, how the warnings were disseminated, and the community's preparedness and responses to warnings. It found that the warnings were issued on time and critical information was effectively communicated and received. The responses of the weather service, media, and emergency management were professional and saved many lives. Particularly, the NWS Springfield Weather Forecast Office was found to be well prepared and provided exemplary services. However, the assessment revealed complexity in community responses as related to many factors such as false alarms, the credibility of warnings, and public compliance. For example, the majority of residents did not take protective action immediately when warnings were received as a result of the lost credibility of initial siren activations. The NWS provided several suggestions on improving the warnings and response system, including a system that could provide impact-based rather than phenomenon-based risk assessment because the former could help to increase clarity and encourage compliance to warnings (NWS, 2011a). The NIST also published *Technical Investigation of the May 22, 2011, Tornado in Joplin, Missouri,* which adopted ethnographic methods and techniques to understand how the residents' perception and response affected the consequences by describing residents' opinions about receiving and understanding the tornado warning, perception and personalizing of the threat of the tornado, triggers for a decision to act, and protective action taking. The NIST further investigated the wind environment and technical conditions; the performance of the emergency communication system and the public response; the performance of residential, commercial, and critical buildings that were associated with fatalities and injuries; and made suggestions for subsequent tornado prevention, response, and recovery (NIST, 2014).

Other entities such as hospitals and researchers also conducted evaluations of their services and intervention programs after the tornado. A brief assessment of the various medical responses to the Joplin tornado covered immediate response considerations, evacuation, special immediate concerns, and the recovery process of the Mercy St. Johns' Hospital and Freeman Health System (South Dakota Department of Health, 2011). After analyzing the processes, outcomes, effectiveness, and limitations of the responses, the report provided suggestions for future improvement. Some key lessons learned included the importance of dependable communication, having sufficient supplies, and that the disaster planning and exercises are much more important than the disaster plan itself, among others (South Dakota Department of Health, 2011). Kanter and Abramson (2014) conducted an informal evaluation of the school-based intervention for promoting the mental health of students and staff 6 months after the tornado. In the program, teachers and relevant staff were trained to master techniques for practical classroom mental health interventions to support students and staff who suffered from anxiety or depression (Kanter & Abramson, 2014). Professional counselors provided school-based, small-group counseling services for students and referred children with more severe disorders to community mental health providers (Kanter & Abramson, 2014). The evaluation supported the importance of such school-based mental health services to the community's recovery.

At the level of frontline staff, most efforts are focused on data collection in coordination with analysts who evaluate public health services and policies.

Public health program managers are responsible for leading the evaluation and improving the current services and policies. The combination of quantitative and qualitative data led to a thorough evaluation of population-based public health programs. These evaluation services help identify gaps and limitations in current health-related services at both the personal and community level, as well as problems in public health systems, which can facilitate future service improvement to better promote recovery after the tornado.

Build and Maintain a Strong Organizational Infrastructure for Public Health

Research and reflections on public health services around tornadoes will summarize the lessons learned and provide insights and guidance for future preparation, response, and recovery processes. One major area of research regarding the Joplin tornado public health is why it resulted in such a high level of casualties. Considering the highly developed communications technologies and extensive knowledge of atmospheric conditions regarding the formation of tornadoes, numerous studies have tried to address how such a death toll could still happen (Simmons & Sutter, 2012). It was found that one important reason for high casualties was that many residents ignored tornado warnings and failed to take protective actions in time or did not take appropriate protective action (Kuligowski et al., 2016; NWS, 2011b; Paul & Stimers, 2012). Some residents were unaware of the warning due to falling asleep, impaired hearing, or being disconnected from tornado-related emergency communications (Paul & Stimers, 2012). A majority of people did not perceive personal risk even though they received signals, because they were unable to confirm the existence of a tornado or were confident that the tornado would not damage their local area (Kuligowski et al., 2016). To make things worse, there were several false alarms of warnings in Joplin weeks before, which disarmed residents of the possibility of a real tornado touchdown (NWS, 2011a). Some residents even believed that there was a "protective bubble" around and "storms [are] always blowing over and missing Joplin" (NWS, 2011a). Therefore, many residents failed to take protective actions in time. Even those who were able to seek shelter may not have reached an optimal location before being affected by the tornado (Kuligowski et al., 2016). In addition, previous building codes and a lack of basements also contributed to excessive damages and casualties (Prevatt et al., 2012). Other factors accounting for such a high death toll included the sheer magnitude of the tornado, the tornado's path through commercial and densely populated residential areas, and the relatively long path of the damaged area (Paul & Stimers, 2012).

Cong and colleagues (Cong et al., 2014, 2017; Luo et al., 2015) conducted a series of studies to compare the Joplin tornado with another devastating tornado that happened 1 month earlier. In April 2011 an EF4 tornado struck Tuscaloosa, Alabama, and caused over 60 fatalities and 1,500 injuries, making it the second costliest tornado in U.S. history. These two cities had different previous experiences with tornadoes. At the time when these tornadoes happened, only 10 tornado events had been reported in the Joplin area since 1995, and only one tornado was EF2 or above; in contrast, 35 events of tornadoes were reported in Tuscaloosa County, and eight were EF2 or above during the same period of time (National Center for Environmental Information, n.d.). Although having an emergency plan in place was important for residents to take protective action in both cities (Cong et al., 2014), some significant differences were identified. Cong et al. (2017) examined predictors for the likelihood of receiving warnings and the number of warning channels in these two places. The study found that Joplin residents were much less likely to receive warnings and had fewer sources of warnings than Tuscaloosa residents due to less preparation in Joplin. In Joplin, gender, marital status, education, and having an emergency plan affected the likelihood of receiving warnings (Cong et al., 2017). In contrast, very few respondents were unwarned in Tuscaloosa; thus, social disparity was not reflected in the likelihood of receiving warnings. Additionally, the number of warning sources increased the respondents' likelihood of taking protective action in Joplin but not in Tuscaloosa because Tuscaloosa residents tended to take action immediately when warnings were received, whereas Joplin residents needed more confirmation of the imminent tornado to take any action (Luo et al., 2015). These findings suggest that public health and recovery concerning tornadoes should be situated in the social and historical contexts. In insufficiently prepared places, the social disparity may present more risks for not receiving warnings, and the number of warning sources may be more consequential in mobilizing protective action. Therefore, places at risk for tornadoes but with few experiences of them, and therefore less preparation, such as Joplin, should be prioritized by emergency management agencies and public health officials.

Data collection and sharing will promote and support coordinated research efforts. In the example of diverse research exploring the reasons for the high death toll after the Joplin tornado, the NIST received cooperation and information from many Joplin citizens; federal, state, and local authorities; businesses; organizations; professional associations; individuals representing building designers; building owners; utilities; media; disaster researchers; and disaster responders (NIST, 2014). Similarly, Paul and Stimers (2014) shared data and information from the Jasper County Emergency Operation Center, Jasper County, the Missouri Department of Public Safety, and the *Joplin Globe* (local daily newspaper) to analyze the damage zone and location of victims. All this research and the investigations identified some innovative points regarding the causes of the high death toll in the Joplin tornado and suggested many ways to improve relevant services and facilities to reduce the damage of future tornadoes and protect public health as well. Public health frontline workers need training in research methods, skills, and ethics, which can enable them to be proficient in collecting, analyzing, and reporting research data using both quantitative and qualitative approaches. Likewise, public health program managers should have some research background, be proficient at applying for funding and designing research projects, and be able to effectively allocate human, financial, and material resources to conduct research activities that aim to promote public health.

CONCLUSION

Tornadoes occur frequently in the United States and can cause many fatalities, injuries, infections, exposure to toxic chemicals, mental health problems, and other health problems along with massive damage. Today, nearly all areas of the United States are covered by the NOAA's Doppler weather radars for broadcasting warnings with a reasonable lead time. However, access to warnings and taking appropriate protective action are still among the biggest public health challenges. Despite the heavy damage that occurs to structures due to tornadoes, deaths and injuries are the most salient public health issues, and social disparities in those areas have attracted broader attention. The 2011 EF5 Joplin tornado was the costliest and deadliest tornado in modern history. The case study of Joplin and its public health response described challenges in its warning, response, and recovery process and summarized lessons learned. The damaged healthcare and critical utility infrastructure presented unique public health challenges after the tornado. The case study highlights the coordination of a variety of public and private sectors in delivering critical services.

DISCUSSION QUESTIONS

1. Review the geographic area nicknamed "Tornado Alley" and consult census data to identify pockets of poverty and persons with disabilities or other health disparities as a class project. Discuss your findings.
2. What kinds of warning messages would you provide for persons residing in mobile homes? Is this a hard-to-reach community? What are some barriers to messaging, and how would you overcome them?
3. What advice would you provide for homebuilders and construction companies in areas prone to tornadoes?
4. As a public health professional, how would you use after-action reports and other data sources to inform policies for tornado preparedness?
5. Review tornado patterns for the past 20 years. Discuss your conclusions.

SUMMARY

TABLE 7.1 **Select Essential Services of Public Health Demonstrated in the 2011 Joplin Tornado Public Health Response**

Essential Service # and Definition	Context in Chapter Case	Competency # It Ties to	Importance for Emergency Preparedness, Response, or Recovery
1. Assess and monitor population health status, factors that influence health, and community needs and assets (Assessment)	• Monitoring weather conditions and issuing tornado warnings • Monitoring the deaths and injuries (physical and mental)	2, 3, 4	Monitoring of weather conditions, as well as disparities in living conditions of local populations, are essential for preparing for and issuing early warnings for tornadoes.
2. Investigate, diagnose, and address health problems and hazards affecting the population (Assessment)	Local public health agencies, the CDC, and MDHSS worked together to identify, investigate, and respond to infections found in tornado-affected victims.	1, 3, 4	Identification of health hazards exposed after a tornado with syndromic surveillance and other data sources is essential for treating persons in impact zones. Potential electrical and chemical exposure and other environmental hazards should be addressed in preparedness plans.
3. Communicate effectively to inform and educate people about health, factors that influence it, and how to improve it (Policy Development)	Institutions came together to communicate health risks and the availability of health services.	18, 19	Early warning systems must reach populations at risk and strive for reaching the most vulnerable with appropriate, actionable messages including families with children, older persons, people who speak different languages, and the visual or hearing impaired.
4. Strengthen, support, and mobilize communities and partnerships to improve health (Policy Development)	Private and public sectors collaborated and coordinated to contribute material and emotional resources.	6	Communities must work together well in advance of tornado season to mobilize resources and be prepared to act immediately after an event. Local organizations, schools, day-care centers, universities, businesses, and so on should be involved in community preparedness planning.
5. Create, champion, and implement policies, plans, and laws that impact health (Policy Development)	Joplin City Health Department formulated a plan for vital services in the first 100 days following the tornado.	12, 13, 15	Community leaders and elected officials should develop policies for preparing for and responding to tornadoes in advance of events. Comprehensive policies should be anticipatory of future events but flexible for modification based on specific impact zones.
6. Utilize legal and regulatory actions designed to improve and protect the public's health (Policy Development)	State laws and regulations waived by the Missouri governor to assist recovery and promote community well-being.	13, 14, 15, 22	Public health professionals use data and after-action reports to advocate for governmental policies that contribute to the health of the overall community.
7. Assure an effective system that enables equitable access to the individual services and care needed to be healthy (Assurance)	Local public health system worked with local health department and other partners to identify specific needs of different groups and barriers to receiving services.	7, 12, 13, 14, 15,	The impoverished persons living in trailer parks, the disabled, and persons with access and functional needs should be prioritized for enhanced strategies for early warning and response.

(*continued*)

TABLE 7.1 **Select Essential Services of Public Health Demonstrated in the 2011 Joplin Tornado Public Health Response (*continued*)**

Essential Service # and Definition	Context in Chapter Case	Competency # It Ties to	Importance for Emergency Preparedness, Response, or Recovery
9. Improve and innovate public health functions through ongoing evaluation, research, and continuous quality improvement (Assurance)	Different federal agencies provided assessments on services and responses relevant to the Joplin tornado.	2, 3, 4, 13, 14	Public health professionals utilize information from evaluations conducted on responses and research conducted on responses to improve the quality of preparedness for future events.
10. Build and maintain a strong organizational infrastructure for public health (Assurance)	Research and reflections on public health services around tornadoes summarize lessons learned and provide insights and guidance for preparation, response, and the recovery process.	2, 3, 4, 5	Before emergency events, the resources, response capacity, warning systems, and community partnerships must be in place, and plans for response should be practiced in advance. Tabletop exercises and mock events ensure that stakeholders are aware of responsibilities and roles. Building the infrastructure is of extreme importance for effective responses.

CDC, Centers for Disease Control and Prevention; MDHSS, Missouri Department of Health and Senior Service.

TABLE 7.2 **Select CEPH Competencies Needed for Frontline Health Workers, Managers, and Leaders for Tornado Emergency Preparedness, Response, and Recovery**

Competency # and Definition	Context in Case/Chapter	Level	Importance for Emergency Preparedness, Response, and Recovery
1. Apply epidemiological methods to settings and situations in public health practice.	MDHSS Division of Community and Public Health and CDC provided data sets to NIST by describing the detailed design, sampling, covered topics, and results of data collection to promote the cooperation with NIST on the technical investigation of the Joplin tornado.	Level 2	Mid-level public health managers should be skilled in epidemiological methods to design and lead data collection efforts. These managers are critical for crafting methodologies for solving complex public health problems. They supervise the collectors of data and the statisticians and guide interpretation of data and ensure reporting quality.
2. Select quantitative and qualitative data collection methods appropriate for a given public health context.	Workers need to be informed and trained on issues from initial research design, questionnaire/interview outline design and test, sampling, informed consent, and confidentiality to data collection and preservation.	Level 1	Data collectors and statisticians should be skilled at research design and analytical methods, as well as ethical issues related to science. Under supervision of managers, they serve as yeomen in the organizational framework to put data collection methods into practice and are key to learning from emergency events.
4. Interpret results of data analysis for public health research, policy, or practice.	At 1:30 CDT, the NWS issued a tornado watch for Southwest Missouri.	Level 3	Public health leaders are the decision-makers, reviewing data findings, interpreting, and translating the findings into actionable practice. They also liaise with governments to advocate for directing resources toward solving problems and informing long-term policies to protect the public.
7. Assess population needs, assets, and capacities that affect communities' health.	Mosquito fogging appeared about 10 days after the tornado, and the health department utilized larvicide to control mosquitoes in the tornado-affected area.	Level 1	Public health professionals at this level may be called upon to provide direct services to communities and have direct contact with affected communities to ascertain damage to health and life, and serve to convey information about imminent needs, dislocated households, and disease exposures.
16. Apply leadership and/or management principles to address a relevant health issue.	SAMHSA updated stress and grief materials and distributed them to state and local agencies.	Level 3	Public health leaders must have a broad comprehensive knowledge of public health principles, including critical knowledge of social determinants of health and health equity. Leaders make decisions that will impact the conduct of a response. Persons at this level must work across governments and communities to ensure that decisions made actually serve the people.
21. Integrate perspectives from other sectors and/or professions to promote and advance population health.	Staff from Missouri's local public health agencies, the CDC, and the MDHSS worked together to identify, investigate, and respond to mucormycosis fungal infection found in tornado-affected victims.	Level 2	Persons at this level serve as team leaders in various public health investigative work and functions, including data collection, analysis, and interpretation; intervention implementation; response to emergencies; and supervision of boots on the ground professionals.

CDC, Centers for Disease Control and Prevention; CEPH, Council on Education for Public Health; MDHSS, Missouri Department of Health and Senior Service; NIST, National Institute of Standards and Technology; NWS, National Weather Service; SAMHSA, Substance Abuse and Mental Health Services Administration.

Key: Essential services of public health; CEPH competencies; Leadership levels.

REFERENCES

Adams, Z. W., Sumner, J. A., Danielson, C. K., McCauley, J. L., Resnick, H. S., Grös, K., Paul, L. A., Welsh, K. E., & Ruggiero, K. J. (2014). Prevalence and predictors of PTSD and depression among adolescent victims of the Spring 2011 tornado outbreak. *Journal of Child Psychology and Psychiatry, 55*(9), 1047–1055. https://doi.org/10.1111/jcpp.12220

Aguirre, B. E., Anderson, W. A., Balandran, S., Peters, B. E., & White, H. M. (1991). *Saragosa, Texas, tornado, May 22, 1987: An evaluation of the warning system.* National Academies Press. https://doi.org/10.17226/1766

American Meteorological Society. (2020). *Tornado sheltering guidelines during the COVID-19 pandemic.* https://www.ametsoc.org/index.cfm/ams/about-ams/ams-statements/statements-of-the-ams-in-force/tornado-sheltering-guidelines-during-the-covid-19-pandemic

Austin, C. L., Finley, P. J., Mikkelson, D. R., & Tibbs, B. (2014). Mucormycosis: A rare fungal infection in tornado victims. *Journal of Burn Care & Research, 35*(3), e164–e171. https://doi.org/10.1097/bcr.0b013e318299d4bb

Balluz, L., Schieve, L., Holmes, T., Kiezak, S., & Malilay, J. (2000). Predictors for people's response to a tornado warning: Arkansas, 1 March 1997. *Disasters, 24*(1), 71–77. https://doi.org/10.1111/1467-7717.00132

Barnhart, M. (2011). *Missouri American Water Joplin Tornado Response at American Water Works Association National Conference.* http://tristatewater.org/wp-content/uploads/2011/11/Matt-Barnhardt-Mo-American-Joplin-Tornado-Response.pdf

Bohonos, J. J., & Hogan, D. E. (1999). The medical impact of tornadoes in North America. *The Journal of Emergency Medicine, 17*(1), 67–73. https://doi.org/10.1016/s0736-4679(98)00125-5

Boruff, B. J., Easoz, J. A., Jones, S. D., Landry, H. R., Mitchem, J. D., & Cutter, S. L. (2003). Tornado hazards in the United States. *Climate Research, 24*(2), 103–117. https://doi.org/10.3354/cr024103

Brooks, H. E., & Correia Jr, J. (2018). Long-term performance metrics for National Weather Service tornado warnings. *Weather and Forecasting, 33*(6), 1501–1511. https://doi.org/10.1175/waf-d-18-0120.1

Cable News Network. (2011). Aggressive fungal infection striking Joplin victims. *ABC News.* https://abcnews.go.com/Health/rare-fungal-infection-hitting-joplin-tornado-victims/story?id=13812164

Centers for Disease Control and Prevention. (2011). Notes from the field: Fatal fungal soft tissue infections after a tornado—Joplin, Missouri, 2011. *Morbidity and Mortality Weekly Report, 60*(29), 992. https://www.cdc.gov/mmwr/preview/mmwrhtml/mm6029a5.htm

Centers for Disease Control and Prevention. (2012). Tornado-related fatalities—five state, Southeastern United States, April 25–28, 2011. *Morbidity and Mortality Weekly Report, 61*(28), 529–533. https://www.cdc.gov/mmwr/preview/mmwrhtml/mm6128a3.htm

Centers for Disease Control and Prevention. (2017). *Public Health Emergency Preparedness (PHEP) program stories from the field: Tornado in Joplin, Missouri.* https://www.cdc.gov/cpr/readiness/00_docs/PHEP_Stories_Missouri.pdf

Chiu, C. H., Schnall, A. H., Mertzlufft, C. E., Noe, R. S., Wolkin, A. F., Spears, J., Casey-Lockyer, M., & Vagi, S. J. (2013). Mortality from a tornado outbreak, Alabama, April 27, 2011. *American Journal of Public Health, 103*(8), e52–e58. https://doi.org/10.2105/AJPH.2013.301291

Clay, L. A., & Greer, A. (2019). Association between long-term stressors and mental health distress following the 2013 Moore tornado: A pilot study. *Journal of Public Mental Health, 18*(2), 124–134. https://doi.org/10.1108/jpmh-07-2018-0038

Coleman, T. A., Knupp, K. R., Spann, J., Elliott, J. B., & Peters, B. E. (2011). The history (and future) of tornado warning dissemination in the United States. *Bulletin of the American Meteorological Society, 92*(5), 567–582. https://doi.org/10.1175/2010bams3062.1

Cong, Z., Liang, D., & Luo, J. (2014). Family emergency preparedness plans in severe tornadoes. *American Journal of Preventive Medicine, 46*(1), 89–93. https://doi.org/10.1016/j.amepre.2013.08.020

Cong, Z., Luo, J., Liang, D., & Nejat, A. (2017). Predictors for the number of warning information sources during tornadoes. *Disaster Medicine and Public Health Preparedness, 11*(2), 168–172. https://doi.org/10.1017/dmp.2016.97

Deng, Q., Lv, Y., Xue, C., Kang, P., Dong, J., & Zhang, L. (2018). Pattern and spectrum of tornado injury and its geographical information system distribution in Yancheng, China: A cross-sectional study. *BMJ Open, 8*(6), e021552. https://doi.org/10.1136/bmjopen-2018-021552

Department of Health and Human Services. (2012). *HHS public health and medical services emergency support preparedness.* https://oig.hhs.gov/oei/reports/oei-04-11-00260.pdf

Dods, L. (2016). *Not all wounds are visible: Recovery in Joplin, MO*. https://macematfcc.wordpress.com/2016/10/26/not-all-wounds-are-visible-recovery-in-joplin-mo

Federal Emergency Management Agency. (2011a). *One month after the Joplin tornado: Disaster recovery efforts in Missouri continue*. https://reliefweb.int/report/united-states-america/one-month-after-joplin-tornado-disaster-recovery-efforts-missouri

Federal Emergency Management Agency. (2011b). *The response to the 2011 Joplin, Missouri, tornado lessons learned study*. https://kyem.ky.gov/Who%20We%20Are/Documents/Joplin%20Tornado%20Response,%20Lessons%20Learned%20Report,%20FEMA,%20December%2020,%202011.pdf

Fentress, E. A., & Fausset, R. (2020). Dozens are killed as tornadoes and severe weather strike southern states. *New York Times*. https://www.nytimes.com/2020/04/13/us/tornado-storm-south.html

Forshee-Hakala, B. A. (2015). Pneumonia cases following an EF-5 tornado. *American Journal of Infection Control, 43*(7), 682–685. https://doi.org/10.1016/j.ajic.2015.02.027

Fricker, T. (2020). Evaluating tornado casualty rates in the United States. *International Journal of Disaster Risk Reduction, 47*, 101535. https://doi.org/10.1016/j.ijdrr.2020.101535

Fricker, T., Elsner, J. B., Mesev, V., & Jagger, T. H. (2017). A dasymetric method to spatially apportion tornado casualty counts. *Geomatics, Natural Hazards and Risk, 8*(2), 1768–1782. https://doi.org/10.1080/19475705.2017.1386724

Garcia, S. (2020). *Carson officials ask Metro to suspend transit service throughout LA county*. https://abc7.com/city-of-carson-suspended-transit-service-prevent-spread-covid-19/6071422

Hammer, B., & Schmidlin, T. W. (2002). Response to warnings during the 3 May 1999 Oklahoma City tornado: Reasons and relative injury rates. *Weather and Forecasting, 17*(3), 577–581. https://doi.org/10.1175/1520-0434(2002)017<0577:rtwdtm>2.0.co;2

Hoekstra, S., Klockow, K., Riley, R., Brotzge, J., Brooks, H., & Erickson, S. (2011). A preliminary look at the social perspective of warn-on-forecast: Preferred tornado warning lead time and the general public's perceptions of weather risks. *Weather, Climate, and Society, 3*(2), 128–140. https://doi.org/10.1175/2011WCAS1076.1

Holshue, M. L., DeBolt, C., Lindquist, S., Lofy, K. H., Wiesman, J., Bruce, H., Spitters, C., Ericson, K., Wilkerson, S., Tural, A., Diaz, G., Cohn, A., Fox, L., Patel, A., Gerber, S. I., Kim, L., Tong, S., Lu, X., Lindstrom, S., . . . Pillai, S. K. (2020). First case of 2019 novel coronavirus in the United States. *New England Journal of Medicine, 382*(10), 929–936. https://doi.org/10.1056/NEJMoa2001191

Houston, J. B., Spialek, M. L., Stevens, J., First, J., Mieseler, V. L., & Pfefferbaum, B. (2015). 2011 Joplin, Missouri tornado experience, mental health reactions, and service utilization: Cross-sectional assessments at approximately 6 months and 2.5 years post-event. *PLoS Currents, 7*. https://www.ncbi.nlm.nih.gov/pmc/articles/PMC4639320

Jenkins, L. M. (2020). *Considering COVID-19 makes people less inclined to seek community help, shelter during a natural disaster*. https://morningconsult.com/2020/06/15/natural-disasters-coronavirus-shelters-community-resources-poll

Joplin Health Department. (2011). *2011 Annual report*. http://joplinmo.org/DocumentCenter/View/3102/Annual-Report-2011?bidId=

Kanter, R. K., & Abramson, D. M. (2014). School interventions after the Joplin tornado. *Prehospital and Disaster Medicine, 29*(2), 214–217. https://doi.org/10.1017/s1049023x14000181

Kantor, V., Knefel, M., & Lueger-Schuster, B. (2017). Perceived barriers and facilitators of mental health service utilization in adult trauma survivors: A systematic review. *Clinical Psychology Review, 52*, 52–68. https://doi.org/10.1016/j.cpr.2016.12.001

Kennedy, W. (2011). Insurance payout from tornado to be largest in state history. *The Joplin Globe*. https://www.joplinglobe.com/news/local_news/insurance-payout-from-tornado-to-be-largest-in-state-history/article_3556cdc9-5f09-53f9-875f-9f65bbe76d88.html

Kouadio, I. K., Aljunid, S., Kamigaki, T., Hammad, K., & Oshitani, H. (2012). Infectious diseases following natural disasters: Prevention and control measures. *Expert Review of Anti-Infective Therapy, 10*(1), 95–104. https://doi.org/10.1586/eri.11.155

Kuligowski, E. D., Lombardo, F. T., & Phan, L. T. (2016). Human response to and consequences of the May 22, 2011, Joplin tornado. In S. Steinberg & W. Sprigg (Eds.), *Extreme weather, health, and communities* (pp. 311–350). Springer.

Law, T. (2020). The tornadoes that rocked the south show how much more dangerous natural disasters will be in the coronavirus era. *Time*. https://time.com/5821436/coronavirus-disasters

Legates, D. R., & Biddle, M. D. (1999). *Warning response and risk behavior in the Oak Grove-Birmingham, Alabama, tornado of 8 April 1998*. Natural Hazards Center.

Luo, J., Cong, Z., & Liang, D. (2015). Number of warning information sources and decision making during tornadoes. *American Journal of Preventive Medicine, 48*(3), 334–337. https://doi.org/10.1016/j.amepre.2014.09.007

McDonald, J. R., Mehta, K. C., Smith, D. A., & Womble, J. A. (2010). The Enhanced Fujita Scale: Development and implementation. In S. Chen, A. Diaz de Leon, A. M. Dolhon, M. J. Drerup, & M. K. Parfitt (Eds.), *Forensic engineering 2009: Pathology of the built environment* (pp. 719–728). American Society of Civil Engineers.

Miller, P. A., Tao, C., & Burleson, M. H. (2018). Classroom intervention with young children after a tornado disaster. In J. Szente (Ed.), *Assisting young children caught in disasters* (pp. 157–170). Springer.

Missouri Department of Health and Senior Service. (n.d.). *ESSENCE*. https://health.mo.gov/data/essence

Missouri Department of Health and Senior Service. (2011). *Public Health Emergency Preparedness and response*. https://clphs.health.mo.gov/lphs/pdf/emergencypreparedness%20%20.pdf

Missouri Secretary of State. (2011a). *Executive Order 11-10*. https://www.sos.mo.gov/library/reference/orders/2011/eo11_010

Missouri Secretary of State. (2011b). *Executive Order 11-17*. https://www.sos.mo.gov/library/reference/orders/2011/eo11_017

National Association of County & City Health Officials. (2013). *National public performance standards: Local assessment instrument*. https://www.naccho.org/uploads/card-images/public-health-infrastructure-and-systems/2013_1203_FINAL_NPHPS_LocalAssessmentInstrument.pdf

National Center for Environmental Information. (n.d.). *Storm events database*. https://www.ncdc.noaa.gov/stormevents

National Center for Environmental Information. (2019). *U.S. tornado climatology*. https://www.ncdc.noaa.gov/climate-information/extreme-events/us-tornado-climatology

National Center for Environmental Information. (2020). *Storm events database*. https://www.ncdc.noaa.gov/stormevents/eventdetails.jsp?id=883016

National Institute of Standards and Technology. (2014). *National Institute of Standards and Technology (NIST) technical investigation of the May 22, 2011, tornado in Joplin, Missouri*. https://nvlpubs.nist.gov/nistpubs/NCSTAR/NIST.NCSTAR.3.pdf

National Research Council of the National Academies. (1993). *Wind and the built environment: U.S. needs in wind engineering and hazard mitigation*. National Academics Press. https://doi.org/10.17226/1995

National Weather Service. (n.d.-a). *Severe weather database files (1950-). Storm Prediction Center WCM Page*. http://www.spc.noaa.gov/wcm

National Weather Service. (n.d.-b). *Severe weather preparedness: Warning systems*. https://www.weather.gov/unr/Warning_Systems

National Weather Service. (2011a). *NWS central region service assessment Joplin, Missouri, tornado – May 22, 2011*. https://www.weather.gov/media/publications/assessments/Joplin_tornado.pdf

National Weather Service. (2011b). *Service assessment-the historic tornadoes of April 2011*. https://www.weather.gov/media/publications/assessments/historic_tornadoes.pdf

Neblett Fanfair, R., Benedict, K., Bos, J., Bennett, S. D., Lo, Y.-C., Adebanjo, T., Etienne, K., Deak, E., Derado, G., Shieh, W-J., Drew, C., Zaki, S., Sugerman, D., Gade, L., Thompason, E. H., Sutton, D. A., Engelthaler, D. M., Schupp, J. M., Brandt, M. E., . . . Park, B. J. (2012). Necrotizing cutaneous mucormycosis after a tornado in Joplin, Missouri, in 2011. *New England Journal of Medicine, 367*(23), 2214–2225. https://doi.org/10.1056/NEJMoa1204781

Niederkrotenthaler, T., Parker, E. M., Ovalle, F., Noe, R. E., Bell, J., Xu, L., Morrison, M. A., Mertzlufft, C. E., & Sugerman, D. E. (2013). Injuries and post-traumatic stress following historic tornados: Alabama, April 2011. *PLoS One, 8*(12), e83038. https://doi.org/10.1371/journal.pone.0083038

Norris, F. H., Friedman, M. J., & Watson, P. J. (2002). 60,000 disaster victims speak: Part II. Summary and implications of the disaster mental health research. *Psychiatry: Interpersonal and biological processes, 65*(3), 240–260. https://doi.org/10.1521/psyc.65.3.240.20169

Office of Missouri Governor Jeremiah W. (Jay) Nixon. (2012). *After the storm: Missouri's commitment to Joplin*. https://sema.dps.mo.gov/newspubs/publications/AfterTheStormMissouriCommitmentToJoplin.pdf

Paul, B. K., & Stimers, M. (2012). Exploring probable reasons for record fatalities: The case of 2011 Joplin, Missouri, tornado. *Natural Hazards, 64*(2), 1511–1526. https://doi.org/10.1007/s11069-012-0313-3

Paul, B. K., & Stimers, M. (2014). Spatial analyses of the 2011 Joplin tornado mortality: Deaths by interpolated damage zones and location of victims. *Weather, Climate, and Society, 6*(2), 161–174. https://doi.org/10.1175/wcas-d-13-00022.1

Paul, B. K., Stimers, M., & Caldas, M. (2015). Predictors of compliance with tornado warnings issued in Joplin, Missouri, in 2011. *Disasters, 39*(1), 108–124. https://doi.org/10.1111/disa.12087

Polusny, M. A., Ries, B. J., Meis, L. A., DeGarmo, D., McCormick-Deaton, C. M., Thuras, P., & Erbes, C. R. (2011). Effects of parents' experiential avoidance and PTSD on adolescent disaster-related posttraumatic stress symptomatology. *Journal of Family Psychology, 25*(2), 220. https://doi.org/10.1037/a0022945

Prevatt, D. O., van de Lindt, J. W., Back, E. W., Graettinger, A. J., Pei, S., Coulbourne, W., Gupta, R., James, D., & Agdas, D. (2012). Making the case for improved structural design: Tornado outbreaks of 2011. *Leadership and Management in Engineering, 12*(4), 254–270. https://doi.org/10.1061/(asce)lm.1943-5630.0000192

Public Health Emergency. (2011). *2011 Joplin, Missouri tornadoes.* https://www.phe.gov/emergency/news/sitreps/Pages/missouri-tornado2011.aspx

Quigley, M. C., Attanayake, J., King, A., & Prideaux, F. (2020). A multi-hazards earth science perspective on the COVID-19 pandemic: The potential for concurrent and cascading crises. *Environment Systems & Decisions, 40*, 199–215. https://doi.org/10.1007/s10669-020-09772-1

Ready Campaign. (2020). *Tornadoes.* https://www.ready.gov/tornadoes

Schmidlin, T. W., King Paul, S., Hammer, B. O., & Ono, Y. (1998). *Risk factors for death in the 22-23 February 1998 Florida tornadoes.* Natural Hazards Center.

Senkbeil, J. C., Scott, D. A., Guinazu-Walker, P., & Rockman, M. S. (2014). Ethnic and racial differences in tornado hazard perception, preparedness, and shelter lead time in Tuscaloosa. *The Professional Geographer, 66*(4), 610–620. https://doi.org/10.1080/00330124.2013.826562

Shi, W., & Hall, B. J. (2020). What can we do for people exposed to multiple traumatic events during the coronavirus pandemic? *Asian Journal of Psychiatry, 51*, 102065. https://doi.org/10.1016/j.ajp.2020.102065

Simmons, K. M., & Sutter, D. (2008). Tornado warnings, lead times, and tornado casualties: An empirical investigation. *Weather and Forecasting, 23*(2), 246–258. https://doi.org/10.1175/2007waf2006027.1

Simmons, K. M., & Sutter, D. (2011). *Economic and societal impacts of tornadoes.* American Meteorological Society.

Simmons, K. M., & Sutter, D. (2012). The 2011 tornadoes and the future of tornado research. *Bulletin of the American Meteorological Society, 93*(7), 959–961. https://doi.org/10.1175/bams-d-11-00126.1

Simmons, K. M., & Sutter, D. (2013). *Deadly season: Analysis of the 2011 tornado outbreaks.* American Meteorological Society.

Smith, D. J., & Sutter, D. (2013). Response and recovery after the Joplin tornado: Lessons applied and lessons learned. *The Independent Review, 18*(2), 165–188. https://doi.org/10.2139/ssrn.2261353

Smith, J. E. (2020). MTS to cut service as bus driver tests positive for coronavirus. *The San Diego Union-Tribune.* https://www.sandiegouniontribune.com/news/transportation/story/2020-04-07/mts-to-cut-service-as-bus-driver-tests-positive-for-coronavirus

South Dakota Department of Health. (2011). *August 2, 2011 medical response to Joplin tornado May 22. 2011.* https://doh.sd.gov/documents/Providers/Prepare/Joplin.pdf

Storm Prediction Center. (2020). *Annual severe weather report summary 2020.* https://www.spc.noaa.gov/climo/online/monthly/2020_annual_summary.html#

The Salvation Army. (2016). *Five years later, the Salvation Army continues to serve Joplin after the costliest tornado in American history.* https://www.salvationarmyusa.org/usn/news/joplin_five_years_later

Waldrop, T. (2020). Coronavirus pandemic adds to disaster of Southeast tornado destruction. *CNN.* https://www.cnn.com/2020/04/13/us/tornadoes-coronavirus-aftermath/index.html

Walters, J. E., Mason, L. R., Ellis, K., & Winchester, B. (2020). Staying safe in a tornado: A qualitative inquiry into public knowledge, access, and response to tornado warnings. *Weather and Forecasting, 35*(1), 67–81. https://doi.org/10.1175/waf-d-19-0090.1

Wang, P. S., Gruber, M. J., Powers, R. E., Schoenbaum, M., Speier, A. H., Wells, K. B., & Kessler, R. C. (2008). Disruption of existing mental health treatments and failure to initiate new treatment after Hurricane Katrina. *American Journal of Psychiatry, 165*(1), 34–41. https://doi.org/10.1176/appi.ajp.2007.07030502

Wilbur, M., Ayman, A., Ouyang, A., Poon, V., Kabir, R., Vadali, A., Pugliese, P., Freudberg, D., Laszka, A., & Dubey, A. (2020). Impact of COVID-19 on public transit accessibility and ridership. *arXiv.* Advanced online publication. https://arxiv.org/abs/2008.02413

World Health Organization. (2020a). *Preparedness for cyclones, tropical storms, tornadoes, floods and earthquakes during the COVID-19 pandemic: Health advisory, 29 April 2020.* http://apps.who.int/iris/bitstream/handle/10665/332408/WHO-2019-nCoV-Advisory-Preparedness-2020.1-eng.pdf

World Health Organization. (2020b). *WHO characterizes COVID-19 as a pandemic.* https://www.who.int/emergencies/diseases/novel-coronavirus-2019/events-as-they-happen

Xu, W., Yuan, G., Liu, Z., Zhou, Y., & An, Y. (2018). Prevalence and predictors of PTSD and depression among adolescent victims of the Summer 2016 tornado in Yancheng City. *Archives of Psychiatric Nursing, 32*(5), 777–781. https://doi.org/10.1016/j.apnu.2018.04.010

Yuan, G., Xu, W., Liu, Z., & An, Y. (2018). Resilience, posttraumatic stress symptoms, and posttraumatic growth in Chinese adolescents after a tornado: The role of mediation through perceived social support. *The Journal of Nervous and Mental Disease, 206*(2), 130–135. https://doi.org/10.1097/NMD.0000000000000778

Zhao, F., Hu, C., Xu, Z., Deng, Q., Wu, Y., & Zhang, L. (2019). Injury patterns and medical evacuation of patients in Chifeng Tornado in China, August 11, 2017. *Disaster Medicine and Public Health Preparedness, 14*(5), 590–595. https://doi.org/10.1017/dmp.2019.100

CHAPTER 8

EARTHQUAKES

PUBLIC HEALTH AND MEDICAL RESPONSE—THE CALIFORNIA MODEL

HOWARD D. BACKER

KEY TERMS

California Emergency Medical Services Authority (EMSA)
Community Assessment for Public Health Emergency Response (CASPER)
Crisis Standards of Care (CSC)
Department Operations Center (DOC)
Disaster Medical Assistance Teams (DMAT)
Emergency Operations Center (EOC)
Emergency Support Functions (ESF)
Emergency System for Advance Registration of Volunteer Health Professionals (ESAR-VHP)
Essential Community Lifelines
Incident Command System (ICS)
Joint Information Center (JIC)
Medical Reserve Corps
Mitigation and Preparedness
National Disaster Medical System (NDMS)
National Incident Management System (NIMS)
National Preparedness Goal
National Response Framework (NRF)
Patient Unified Lookup System for Emergencies (PULSE)
Prediction Science
Stafford Act (Robert T. Stafford Disaster Relief and Emergency Assistance Act)

The following icons, located in the margins throughout the chapter and within the summary tables, denote essential services of public health, CEPH competencies, and leadership levels: Essential services of public health; CEPH competencies; Leadership levels.

INTRODUCTION

Earthquakes are complex disasters that occur without prior notice and require a response across many programs within public health departments as well as every other response agency. An immediate, organized, effective medical and public health response is critical to save lives and reduce suffering. Similar to other disasters, effective mitigation and planning, rapid situation status assessment, effective communication, response mobilization according to emergency management system standards, and responding to healthcare surge are at the core of an effective response. An understanding of planning and responding to an earthquake provides a comprehensive foundation for disaster medicine.

OVERVIEW OF EARTHQUAKES

Earthquakes present unique challenges to disaster planning and response. An earthquake is a no-notice event, unlike storms, floods, and most fires that have some advanced warning. There are now some early warning devices that send notifications, but these provide seconds, not hours or days—potentially providing time to "drop, hold, and cover" but not time to evacuate the area. Impact from an earthquake is highly variable and depends on the geology, geographic location, infrastructure and architecture in the shake zone, and the magnitude and duration of the shaking. Earthquakes can cause broad damage to infrastructure, including water and sewer lines, power lines, communication, and transportation, as well as buildings. Earthquakes also disrupt critical services such as government, healthcare, and supply chains while displacing people from home and work.

Earthquakes occur in many parts of the world. In the United States, the best-known faults occur on the West Coast (San Andreas Fault; Figure 8.1), but in the central United States, the New Madrid Seismic Zone, which is capable of generating major earthquakes, threatens parts of eight American states (Illinois, Indiana, Missouri, Arkansas, Kentucky, Tennessee, Oklahoma, and Mississippi; Figure 8.2). Earthquakes occur with surprising frequency, but **prediction science** is not yet reliable to determine when minor quakes are precursors of a large event. The U.S. Geological Service (USGS) estimates globally that each year 10,000–15,000 light earthquakes occur (magnitude 4–4.9), 1,000 to 1,500 moderate earthquakes (magnitude 5–5.9), 100–150 strong earthquakes (magnitude 6–6.9), 10–20 major earthquakes (magnitude 7–7.9), and one great earthquake (magnitude 8 or more). The last great earthquake in the United States was off the coast of Alaska (1964, magnitude 9.2). Earthquakes in other areas of the world provide stark reminders of the frequency and potential of major and great earthquakes: Chile (2010, magnitude 8.8), Japan (2011, magnitude 9.1), Haiti (2010, magnitude 7.0), Nepal (2015, magnitude 7.8), and the Indian Ocean earthquake and tsunami (2004, magnitude 9.1–9.3). Much of the earthquake disaster literature is generated from these events. Several lesser magnitude earthquakes in California, as well as some of the international earthquakes and other types of disasters, are used to inform this discussion (Table 8.1).

Magnitude is measured on several scales, including the familiar Richter scale, a modification called the Moment Magnitude Scale, and the Mercalli Intensity Scale. In general, the units of the scales are based on the magnitude of shaking waves that corresponds to the energy released. The units are logarithmic, with an

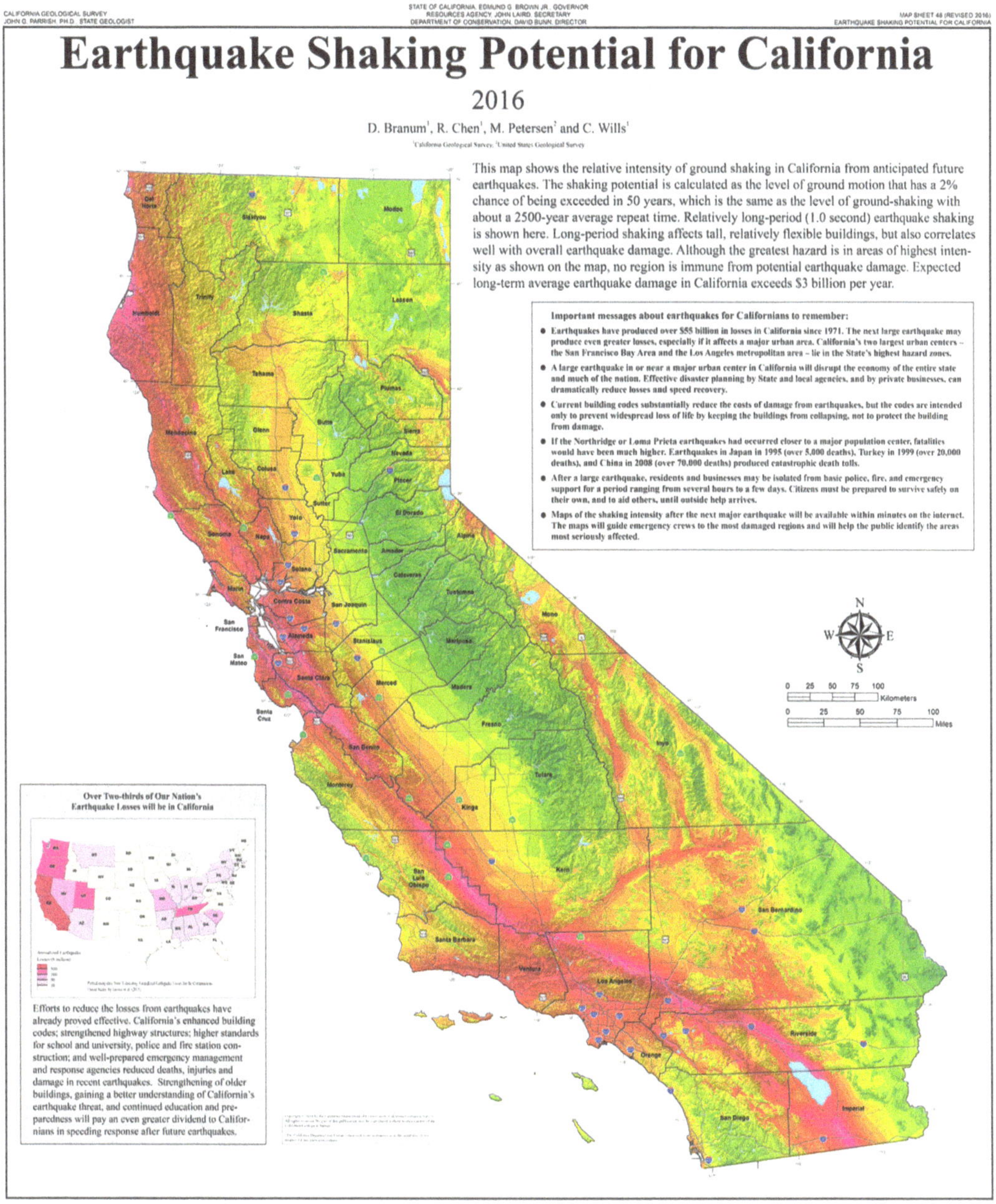

Figure 8.1 San Andreas Fault and seismic potential in California.

Source: This figure was originally created by USGS but has been published by many organizations, including California Geologic Survey (https://www.conservation.ca.gov/cgs/Documents/Publications/Map-Sheets/MS_048.pdf) and the California Department of Conservation (https://www.conservation.ca.gov/cgs/psha).

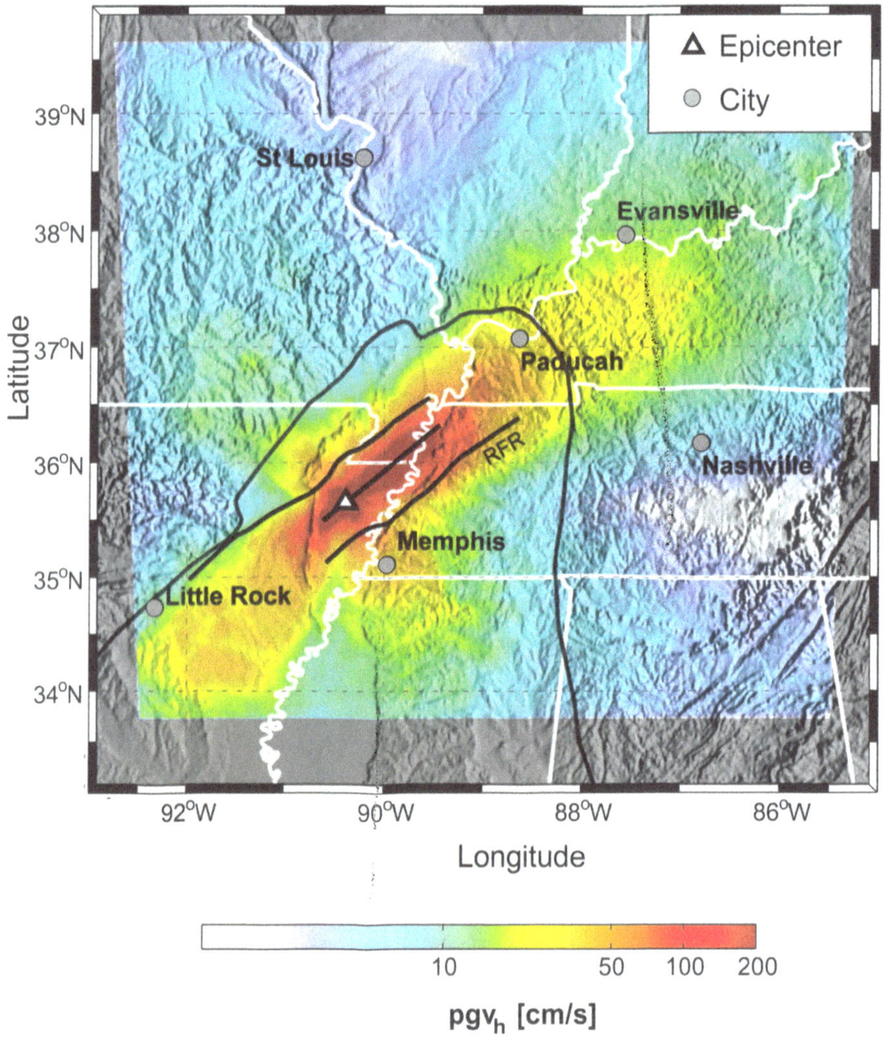

Figure 8.2 New Madrid Fault location and risk.

Source: U.S. Geological Survey. (n.d.). *Peak ground-motion variability for a magnitude 7.7 earthquake* [Image]. https://www.usgs.gov/media/images/graph-peak-ground-motion-variability-magnitude-77-earthquake

increase of 0.2 roughly indicating a doubling of energy released. The geographic location and depth of the earthquake are important factors; for example, a shallow moderate earthquake in a densely populated area may cause more damage than a major earthquake that occurs deep under the surface in a remote area.

PUBLIC HEALTH ROLE

Public health has a key role in preparing and responding to disasters in general, including earthquakes, that is outlined in the requirements of the Public Health Emergency Preparedness (PHEP) Cooperative Agreement administered by the Centers for Disease Control and Prevention (CDC) and

TABLE 8.1 Recent California Earthquakes and Other Incidents Used for Information in This Chapter

Location	Date	Magnitude	Hospitals Affected	Injured	Deaths	Notes
Northridge CA (Los Angeles) (C. H. Schultz et al., 2003; U.S. Dept Housing and Development, 1995)	1/17/1994	6.7	8 evacuated; 11 sustained some damage	8,700 1,600 hospitalized	61	Major freeways closed due to collapse. More than 2,500 aftershocks, two 6.0; at least 65,000 residential buildings sustained damage; estimated total damage between $18 billion and $20 billion (1994 value).
Napa	8/24/2014	6.0	1 partial	200	1	Many ED visits for wounds. Experimental earthquake warning system provided 5-second advanced warning.
Loma Prieta near Santa Cruz (Bay Area)	1989			3,757	57 direct, 6 indirect	Liquifaction in San Francisco caused structural damage. The highest number of deaths, 42 (Greenberg et al., 2013), occurred in Oakland because of the collapse of double decker freeways on Interstate 880. One 50-foot (15-m) section of the San Francisco–Oakland Bay Bridge collapsed with a single fatality but major traffic disruption ensued for months.
Ridgecrest (southeastern CA)	7/4–5/2019	7.1	1		1	Rural area, so little damage or injury/deaths. The Ridgecrest earthquake sequence included a magnitude-6.4 foreshock on July 4, followed by a magnitude 7.1 mainshock nearly 34 hours later, and more than 100,000 aftershocks.
Chile	2/27/2010	8.8	14 hospitals evacuated and replaced by field hospitals	525 dead; 25 missing		Tsunami devastated several coastal towns; 9% of people in affected areas lost their homes. Extensive looting in some areas.
Camp fire	11/8/2018		1 acute care hospital and 1 nursing home		85	18,804 buildings destroyed; 60,000 persons evacuated; 14 shelters opened, at least half unofficial, including a large, spontaneous encampment in a Walmart parking lot.
COVID-19	Ongoing					

ED, emergency department

the Hospital Preparedness Program (HPP) administered by the Office of the Assistant Secretary for Preparedness and Response (ASPR; CDC, n.d.-c; ASPR, 2020). Together, these grants provide federal funding to support readiness of the public health and medical systems to prepare and respond to all types of disasters.

Emergency Management Structure

5,21 Disaster response requires a highly coordinated effort, and no public health response can succeed without understanding concepts of emergency coordination and management. Emergency management overlays standard organizational management, but the interface is often poorly understood. A key principle of the **Incident Command System (ICS)** is the standardized management organizational chart that is flexible and scalable with personnel job descriptions (Figure 8.3). These well-defined standard roles can be filled by persons from various agencies or jurisdictions creating a smooth interface between agencies. Each agency's **Emergency Operations Center (EOC)** performs a regular planning cycle that integrates across levels of support.

Emergency response is based on the assumption that all disasters are local, meaning that the primary responsibility for the direct response on the ground is at the local level. Field incident command remains at the local level with other emergency operations in support of the response, often in a unified command. Additional resources are obtained through mutual aid provided by progressively larger jurisdictions at the county, regional, state, and federal levels upon request. Neighboring communities and organizations play a key role by

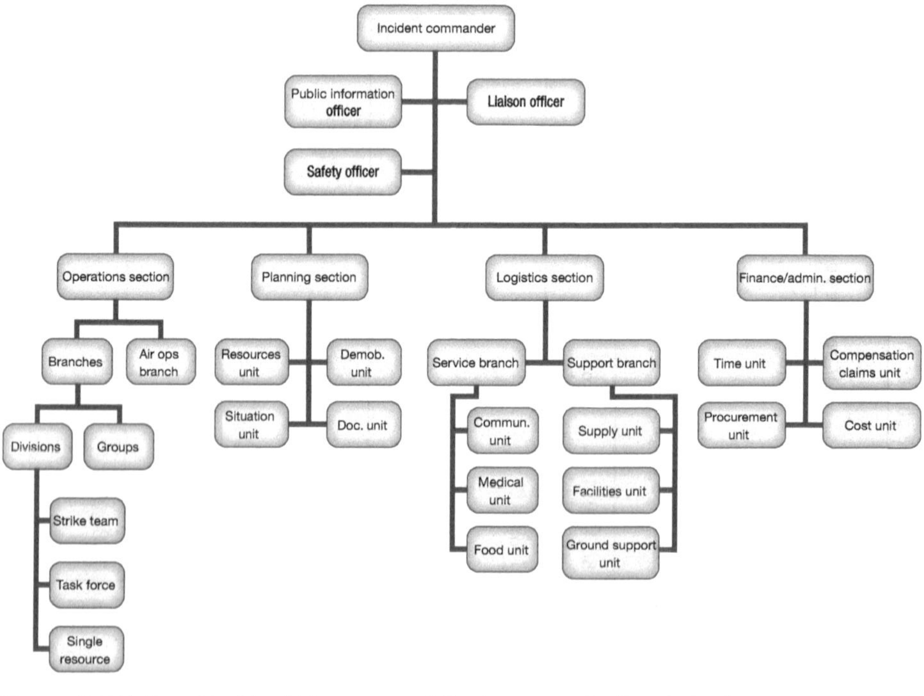

Figure 8.3 National Incident Management System organizational chart.

Source: FEMA ICS training.

providing support through a network of mutual aid and assistance agreements that identify the resources that communities may share during an incident (Figure 8.4).

Because large events may immediately overwhelm a local jurisdiction, emergency response agencies at the higher levels with greater resources may "lean forward" by engaging with the local jurisdiction and staging resources to more rapidly support resource needs. In large impact events, there is always an initial resource gap when the need far exceeds the resources in the affected area. During this initial period, accurate information is difficult to obtain, communications are often disrupted and inadequate, and the population is not receiving needed services. Public agencies are under extreme criticism and pressure during this period.

The ICS structure is not optional and following the **National Incident Management System (NIMS)** designed around ICS is required to receive federal reimbursement (Federal Emergency Management Agency [FEMA], n.d.-b).

The **National Response Framework (NRF)** provides emergency management policy and structure for how the United States responds to all types of incidents. It is built on scalable, flexible, and adaptable concepts identified in the NIMS to align key roles and responsibilities across the nation (U.S. Department of Homeland Security, 2019).

For optimal efficiency, emergency response services are divided into functional areas called **Emergency Support Functions (ESFs)**. There are 15 areas designated in the federal response plan. ESFs, now termed **essential community lifelines**, have proved to be an effective way to organize and manage resources to deliver core capabilities and maintain critical services. These are defined as services that enable the continuous operation of critical government and business functions: safety and security; food, water, and shelter; health and medical; energy (power and fuel); communications; transportation; and hazardous material. The Health and Medical Community Lifeline (ESF #8) is further described as medical care, public health, patient movement, fatality management, behavioral health, veterinary support, and health or medical supply chains.

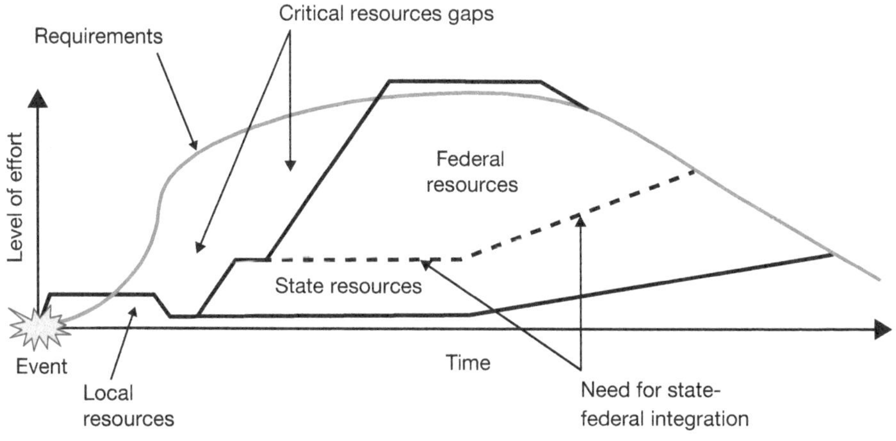

Figure 8.4 Time course of resource gaps and mutual aid.

Source: From FEMA.

In any disaster, the first overall objective is to save lives, the second is to minimize suffering, and the third is to protect property. This means public health and their healthcare partners have an immediate critical role to provide and support a broad range of services. The depth and breadth of public health responsibilities have generated robust discussion on the core competencies and functions for disaster response (Gibson et al., 2012; Khan et al., 2018).

Mitigation and Preparedness

As with any public health issue, prevention is paramount. Both **mitigation and preparedness** aim to put structure, process, policy, and laws in place to facilitate response and create agency and community resilience (U.S. Department of Housing and Urban Development [HUD], 1995). There is no agreement on any one method, and so there are many possible strategies for how to prepare communities. Reaching agreement for a particular community is the entire focus of the federal preparedness cooperative agreements and grants.

5

12,13, 21

Public health competencies needed to develop policies and plans that support individual and community health efforts

Operational plans must be developed for anticipated and potential disasters and for meeting health needs of the population. California and other earthquake-prone states have done extensive planning for large earthquakes as well as other high-risk disasters. It is better to plan for large events and scale down for a smaller event than to try to scale up from plans for smaller events. Planning must occur at all levels, from healthcare facilities and systems to local, state, and federal government. The U.S. Department of Homeland Security (DHS)/FEMA Region IX and the California Governor's Office of Emergency Services (OES) collaborated with public and private partners to create a base plan for catastrophic disasters (California OES, 2008), then these groups developed plans for specific events on the major earthquake faults (Northern California Bay Area, Southern California Los Angeles region, and northern rural California Cascadia Fault) that describe the joint state and federal response to a catastrophic earthquake. These plans are not static and are regularly reviewed and updated; in addition, exercises are designed to evaluate the plan and teach staff their roles. Planning is a complex function that engages multiple jurisdictional levels as well as all levels of public health staff.

Each of these plans has a section on public health and medical response. The public health response must consider all aspects of maintaining healthcare delivery as well as all risks to public health. They must also incorporate plans for the most vulnerable populations, including the aged, children, and those with functional and access needs.

The California Department of Public Health (CDPH) and **California Emergency Medical Services Authority (EMSA)** have developed the "Public Health and Medical Emergency Operations Manual," a medical and health operational guide for local response and the interface between local and state agencies (CDPH, 2011).

Prepared policy guidance serves several purposes: (a) it is a resource for local health officers and (b) it ensures consistency of messages among health jurisdictions that helps prevent public confusion and frustration. One example is guidance for wildfire smoke, originally developed in California (U.S. Environmental Protection Agency, 2016).

Public health competencies needed to assure a competent public and personal healthcare workforce 8

Each agency must train staff and develop the necessary structure to respond in accordance with federal, state, and local mandates and statutes. To assure a competent workforce, all public health personnel should understand basic emergency management and their potential role in a response structure, since they may be redirected to support a disaster response. ICS courses are available online through FEMA (n.d.-a). For most staff, including frontline staff, this should include the basic levels ICS 100, 200, and 700. Program management/supervisory–level personnel benefit from additional higher level courses, including ICS 300, 400, and 800; these courses should be required for those who will directly interface with the emergency response system at the local or state level. California EMSA has developed a course titled Medical Health Operations Center Support Activities (MHOCSA) that applies disaster management and ICS principles specifically to medical and health responses. It is designed to train the personnel who will staff the health and medical branch of their EOC.

Executive management, especially state and local health officers, must understand their authorities and responsibilities, which are substantial. They must also understand the authorities of the governor and other officials that are usually granted under an Emergency Services Act. The CDPH has detailed these powers and authorities in California in the *California Public Health and Medical Emergency Operations Manual* (CDPH, 2011).

Responding to an emergency is a routine and essential function of a public health department (Posid et al., 2013), yet evidence suggests that the healthcare workforce does not feel prepared to respond to disasters (Gowing et al., 2017).

4

Public health competencies needed to mobilize community partnerships to identify and solve health problems 8,9,13,14

Planning for emergencies and disasters requires engagement of partners that will be involved in response. Collaboration ensures that relationships are established prior to a response, and that roles, responsibilities, and agency interface are understood. The HPP grant requires jurisdictions to develop community healthcare coalitions to assure that all parts of the healthcare delivery system are engaged and integrated during a response. Healthcare systems and facilities have an obligation to plan and prepare that is supported by professional and quality organizations and may be required by law.

Hospital Preparedness

The Centers for Medicare and Medicaid Services (CMS) approved The Joint Commission's updated emergency management standards (implemented in 2017), which were created in response to the CMS final rule on emergency preparedness. The Joint Commission requires hospital preparedness efforts that include a vulnerability analysis, evacuation plans, internal response structure, preparedness and response plans, inventory of resources available, and engagement of leaders/executives. In addition to new requirements for hospitals, the most significant changes to the emergency performance standards were to home health settings and ambulatory healthcare.

Disasters in California and nationwide have shown that hospitals must be capable of continuing operations and sheltering patients in place for at least 3 to 5 days, since it could be several days before outside help and resources are able to reach the facility. Facilities with sufficient resources in-house for critical areas fare the best during disasters, and facilities that have corporate structures or associations with out-of-area organizations receive more timely help. California regulations require hospitals to be self-sufficient for 96 hours with subsistence needs for staff and patients, including food, water, and essential medical and pharmaceutical supplies; emergency and standby power systems to maintain temperature, lighting, and fire detection; and utilities, including sewage and sanitation. These are consistent with requirements from the CMS, The Joint Commission, and the National Fire Protection Association (NFPA). The California Hospital Association (CHA) coordinated a survey of acute care hospitals to determine their readiness to shelter in place and to create an inventory of emergency power equipment so that emergency response agencies could be prepared to replace generators or power connections during a response.

The California EMSA, in partnership with national organizations, has adapted principles of ICS to healthcare facilities. The Hospital Incident Command System is in the public domain and training courses are widely available (California EMSA, 2014). It has become a national standard and adopted by numerous other countries to help facilities rapidly organize to respond to internal and widespread emergencies.

Public health competencies needed to enforce laws and regulations that protect health and ensure safety

Public health agencies and public health officers are regulatory agencies with broad statutory powers to control infectious diseases and mitigate public health risks. This ranges from the power of isolation and quarantine to oversight and regulation of health facilities and providers. Many legal questions arise concerning public health authorities in an emergency (Public Health and Medical Emergency Powers, 2019). It is critical that agencies understand their emergency powers as well as those of the local and state emergency management agencies and the chief executive of the city/county/ state. In most states, the governor has the power to suspend, flex, or implement rules during a declared disaster. Some
3 authorities can be delegated to the state health officer. Health agencies can anticipate needs to flex regulatory requirements for facilities to support healthcare surge by pre-scripting emergency orders for the governor or health officer. (See more in the following section, Support for Healthcare Surge). The Association of State and Territorial Health Officers (ASTHO, n.d.-b) has developed legal preparedness and response resources that explain and support these authorities. California has catalogued public health powers and responsibilities for disaster response (Public Health and Medical Emergency Powers, 2019).

Other agencies are responsible for laws and regulations that will support public health and medical mitigation and response. For example, architectural standards are a critical earthquake mitigation strategy since structural collapse is one of the major causes of morbidity and mortality; healthcare facilities at all levels may be required to meet structural requirements. In California, the Office of Statewide Health Planning and Development (OSHPD, 2019) creates and enforces regulations for building standards designed to minimize damage from earthquakes. These have been strengthened over time as engineering solutions are developed and experience obtained from real events, but implementation and optimal standards are repeatedly delayed due to the cost of retrofitting or replacing a facility. Current standards address both the structural integrity of the building (Structural Performance Categories, SPC) and the bracing or anchoring of critical internal components (Nonstructural Performance Categories, NPC), such as restraining computers and cabinets to prevent them from injuring patients and staff. Maintaining structural safety and functional status is critical to avoid the need for immediate evacuation of numerous facilities at the same time. Although there is continual progress, there are still a significant number of hospital buildings at risk for structural failure (SPC 1 and 2) during a large earthquake in California (Table 8.2).

The Northridge earthquake in California was the impetus for stronger architectural standards, after four facilities were severely damaged and had to be demolished and four others evacuated due to nonstructural damage (Schultz et al., 2003; Figure 8.5). In Chile, although new hospitals were built to high standards, older hospitals constructed of unreinforced materials suffered extensive damage.

In addition to hospital construction standards, residential structural standards for both new construction and for retrofitting are critical to prevent death and injury from collapse, damage, and falling objects. Older residences should be reinforced and bolted to their foundation. Cabinets and bookshelves should be secured to the walls and cabinet doors fitted with special latches to decrease flying objects. Construction standards for offices and homes are updated according to experience and engineering advances. During the Loma Prieta earthquake, many older flats and apartments in San Francisco with insufficient support for upper levels due to open parking on the first level collapsed, leading to new requirements to retrofit the structures.

TABLE 8.2 SPC Ratings of Acute Care Hospital Buildings as of 1/23/20

SPC Category	Number (%) *N* = 3,043 as of 11/30/19	Definition
1	147 (4.8)	Significant risk of collapse and danger to the public
2	646 (21.6)	Does not significantly jeopardize life, but may not be repairable or functional following strong ground motion
3	379 (12.4)	May experience structural damage which does not significantly jeopardize life, but may not be repairable or functional following strong ground motion
4	795 (26.1)	May experience structural damage which may inhibit ability to provide services to the public following strong ground motion
5	1,140 (37.5)	Reasonably capable of providing services to the public following strong ground motion
N/A	69 (2.2)	

SPC, Structural Performance Categories

Source: From California Office of Statewide Planning and Development (OSHPD) {Development, #65}.

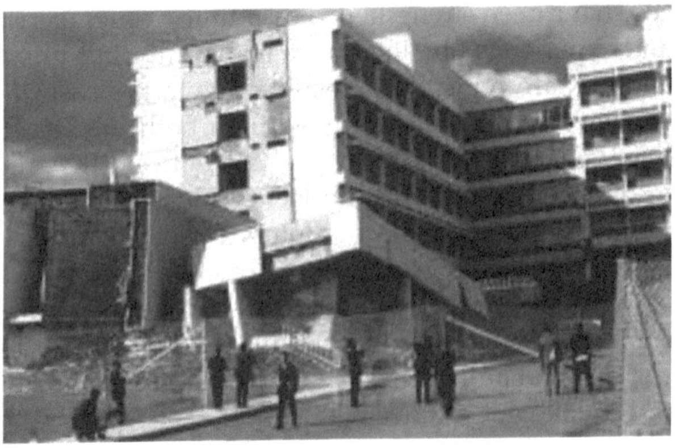

Figure 8.5 Hospital damage following Northridge Earthquake (1994).

Source: U.S. Geological Survey. USGS publication: https://pubs.usgs.gov/fs/old.2003/fs068-03

Public health competencies needed to inform, educate, and empower people about health issues

Disaster plans depend on individual and community preparedness. If this is lacking, the entire response will be magnified in difficulty and delayed in execution. No matter how prepared the healthcare system is for disasters like an earthquake, it must meet the entire community's needs in the aftermath of a large event. However, educating and motivating the public to take individual, household, business, and institutional preparedness measures to increase their resilience and decrease their total dependence on public services is very challenging. In a large earthquake, as in any large-scale disaster, relief services may not be adequate and widely available for up to 1 week, so residents are encouraged to have their own supply of food, water, lights and batteries, and first aid supplies. Despite regular disasters and persistent campaigns and public communication efforts, only a small percentage of people can be convinced to take action such as stockpiling 3 days of food and water, as recommended by federal and local emergency management agencies. Few have even developed family emergency plans for reuniting and communicating.

Research indicates that factors influencing preparedness attitudes and behaviors are complex and multifaceted, including demographic characteristics, trust in government efforts, previous exposure to a disaster, and number of dependents in a household (Greenberg et al., 2013; Kohn et al., 2012). While it seems completely rational, it is difficult to demonstrate that household preparedness is effective (Clay et al., 2019; Heagele et al., 2016; Levac et al., 2012). Given poor evidence for efficacy and the challenge of getting the public to address individual preparedness by stockpiling emergency supplies and creating an emergency plan, Los Angeles CDPH shifted its social media messaging for emergency preparedness to encourage social connectivity as a
19,20 central feature with an emphasis on community preparedness (Plough et al., 2013).

Business and industry have a self-interest in continuity plans following a disaster. Disruption of businesses that are part of a critical supply chain may have direct impact on public health response efforts as well as business revenue.

Physical damage at industrial sites may pose a risk to public safety from hazardous material spills or releases, which creates the need for public health engagement.

Response

Within the NRF, the term "response" includes actions to save lives, protect property and the environment, stabilize the incident, and meet basic human needs following an incident. All the components of NIMS—resource management, command and coordination, and communications and information management—support response. The **National Preparedness Goal** identifies 32 core capabilities that cover all areas of response. The Public Health, Healthcare, and Emergency Medical Services core capability is to provide lifesaving medical treatment and avoid additional disease and injury by providing targeted public health, medical and behavioral health support, and products to all affected populations.

Public health agencies usually open a **Department Operations Center (DOC)** to coordinate their internal activities and communications and send representatives to coordinate with the local emergency management agencies at the local and/or state level where their actions are requested and integrated into the overall response. A public health program will be tasked through the EOC of the emergency management agency that has statutory responsibility for managing the response to the disaster. Public health staff will continue to report to their usual manager unless assigned to work in an EOC within the ICS structure. In most local and state jurisdictions, under emergency law, all employees are to be designated as emergency responders during a disaster and may be assigned roles outside of their usual position but within their ability, skill, and safety level.

Initial Activation

Following a major emergency or disaster, the health and medical needs are overwhelming. The entire public health agency will be recruited to address myriad needs. As the extent of the damage becomes known, an emergency declaration may be declared by the local political leader. The local health officer may also declare a public health emergency. This may be rapidly followed by a declaration or proclamation at the state level and request for federal declaration. At each level, there may be a public health declaration as well. Emergency declarations or proclamations are not simply a formality; they are necessary to initiate statutory and regulatory emergency measures and funding. If required, initiation of mutual aid does not wait for an emergency declaration. (See the following Federal Support section.)

The first step is for the public health management/leadership to mobilize 2,3
their emergency management structure and personnel and then begin to reas-
sign other staff as disaster service workers. Representatives will respond to 1
the local, regional, or state EOC to represent ESF #8. These staff, following ICS
and NIMS principles, will serve as liaisons to synthesize situation status and
to field requests for mutual aid. 21

The high-level response goal for ESF #8 is to manage disaster-induced injuries and public health risks and maintain access to healthcare services. This requires evaluating and supporting the health needs of the population and the healthcare system.

Federal Support

The **Stafford Act (Robert T. Stafford Disaster Relief and Emergency Assistance Act**, Public Law 93–288, 42 U.S.C. 5121 et seq.) authorizes the president to provide financial and other assistance to local, state, tribal, territorial, and insular area governments; certain private nonprofit organizations; and individuals to support response, recovery, and mitigation efforts following a Stafford Act emergency or major disaster declaration. While federal assistance under the Stafford Act may only be delivered after a declaration, FEMA may predeploy federal assets when a declaration is likely and imminent. Most forms of Stafford Act assistance require a cost share.

The secretary of the HHS has the authority to take actions to protect the public health and welfare, declare a public health emergency, and prepare for and respond to public health emergencies. The Public Health Service Act (PHSA), as amended by the Pandemic and All-Hazards Preparedness Reauthorization Act, forms the foundation of the HHS's legal authority for responding to public health emergencies (PHSA, 42 U.S.C. §§ 201 et seq.). If the president declares an emergency or disaster and the secretary of the HHS declares a public health emergency, certain waivers to the provisions of the HIPAA Privacy Rule may be initiated. An interactive web-based decision tool is available to assist planners to determine how to access and use health information during a declared disaster (HHS, 2020a).

18,19, 20 Communications

Following a disaster or local emergency, risk communication is critical to inform the public and to direct them to helpful actions and services. The overall responsibility for public communication is through political leaders or their designees. The health agency director or public health officer will often be assigned to provide pertinent information on the status of health impact and services. The ICS structure includes a communications chief under the incident commander. The EOC sets up a **Joint Information Center (JIC)** to develop risk communications with a consistent message for both public and response partners. The local or state public health agency will hold situation status calls and regular situation status reports to update response partners, for example, local health officers and healthcare facilities, and to share critical resource status and needs. The challenge is to provide accurate and
3 timely information to various key stakeholders without compromising time to carry out other response activities. Typically, agency leadership will be
1 fully engaged in developing and delivering the message and program staff will provide updates and technical information. Information and messages should be reviewed with higher levels of emergency management to assure a coordinated message.

Public health competencies needed to monitor health status to identify and solve community health problems

Diagnose and investigate health problems and health hazards in the community

Epidemiology and Surveillance

Earthquakes have a specific epidemiological medical profile like any disease or public health event. The initial health impact is from traumatic injuries related to structural collapse, flying objects, and rubble. This creates critical injuries, blunt and penetrating trauma, and crush and orthopedic injuries. The most extreme example was in the 2010 Haiti earthquake when inadequately reinforced concrete structures collapsed, killing thousands and trapping many more, resulting in high burden of injuries with significant mortality and morbidity, including many amputations (Doocy et al., 2013). The same was found in the Northridge earthquake (Peek-Asa et al., 1998). Emergency department visits following the California Northridge earthquake experienced a major increase in lacerations and bruises with decreases in many minor ambulatory problems, including respiratory illness and general examinations. The stress will contribute to both cardiac and other acute events. Another source of early mortality in coastal areas is a tsunami that results from a large offshore earthquake as seen in the 2010 Chile earthquake and the 2004 Indonesian earthquake.

The terror and stress of an earthquake will have both physiological and
psychological impact. Evaluation of psychological impact is as important
as physical injury or illness but is not as well understood or addressed by
emergency response systems. Like other mass casualty situations, assessment
using screening tools can be accomplished that triage people for level of service needed (Schreiber et al. 2014; Sylwanowicz et al., 2018). The initial epide- 7
miological assessment focuses on exposure to traumatic events rather than a
psychological evaluation. Moreover, the assessment, as well as many initial
interventions, can be accomplished by people who are not licensed mental
health professionals. Behavioral health resources can then be applied in areas 1
and to persons with the greatest need. Without addressing the behavioral
health needs, scarce and overwhelmed healthcare resources will be diverted
to those exhibiting symptoms of psychological stress.

Epidemiological evaluation may be done in the community, within shelters,
or in healthcare facilities. One technique to obtain community level information is the **Community Assessment for Public Health Emergency Response
(CASPER)**. CASPER standardizes the assessment methodology by using a
modified cluster sampling methodology that involves selection of 30 clusters
selected proportional to size and seven households interviewed within each
cluster to provide estimates for the population. The CASPER Toolkit provides 1
a guidance document for public health practitioners and emergency management officials (CDC, n.d.-a). 2,3,4,7,11

Assessment needs to include availability of basic needs and services such as availability of shelter, food, water, and outbreaks of infectious diseases or toxic exposure. Following the 1994 Northridge earthquake in Los Angeles County, communication systems, water, food, shelter, sanitation means, power sources, and medical supplies were among the resources needed early in the disaster (Stratton et al., 1996).

As specific issues are identified, more focused epidemiological assessments will be required. Whenever there are large numbers of evacuated persons who are living in crowded shelters or tent communities, there is great concern for hygiene, food safety, and infectious disease outbreaks (Figure 8.6). For example, there were outbreaks of norovirus within shelters housing evacuees from the Camp Fire in California. Public health provided a clinical case

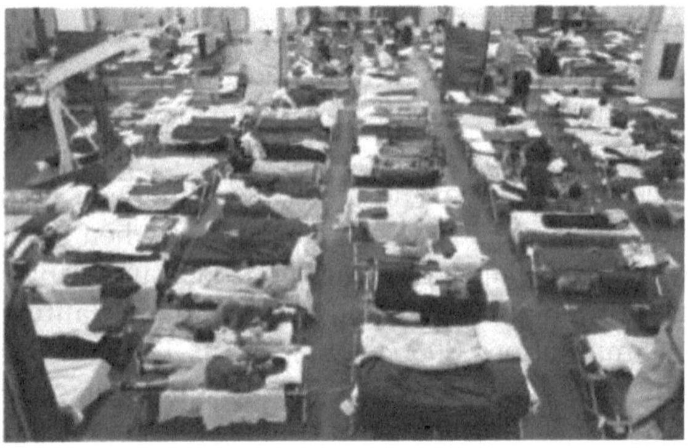

Figure 8.6 Disaster shelter (before COVID-19).

4 definition and protocols for management. Special isolation areas were established
1,2 (Figure 8.7). Infection control nurses visited each shelter daily and played a key
role in surveillance, health education of shelter staff, and monitoring infection control measures. Influenza was another threat that required monitoring and an immunization effort. Careful surveillance is also required to identify cases of measles and other highly infectious illness. Recent western-state fires during the COVID-19 pandemic required a redesign of congregate shelters to assure social distancing, such as housing individuals and families in tents rather than open shelters (Figures 8.8–8.9). Public health should not assume that the Red Cross can adequately monitor and manage health issues. Important sources of information are all health encounters within shelters and emergency department visits. Food safety and hygiene staff may be busy with impacted businesses but must also monitor food preparation and serving at shelters and other ad hoc community volunteer sites. Earthquakes may result in damage to industrial facilities, storage tanks, and pipelines, resulting in toxic spills or release.

One special area at the intersection of communications and epidemiology is mortality attributable to the event. This is always of high interest to the media and to the political leadership. Discrepancies in numbers elicit detailed questions and become a risk communication issue. Health agencies and emergency

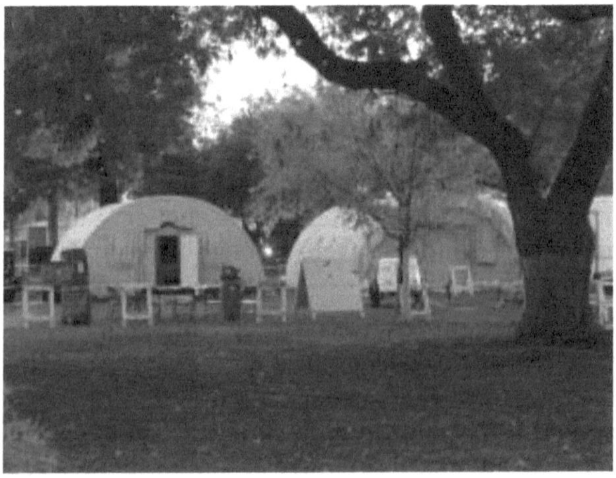

Figure 8.7 Isolation shelters for norovirus and respiratory infection patients.

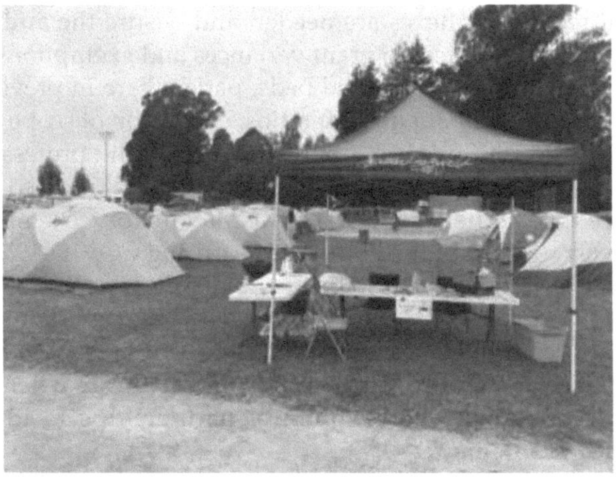

Figure 8.8 Outdoor sheltering during COVID-19.

management must agree to provide a single number at a specific time of day. This is analogous to the convention of counting shelter inhabitants at midnight.

Public health competencies needed to evaluate effectiveness, accessibility, and quality of personal and population-based health services

Assessment of healthcare resources and services is another critical area of evaluation. The Public Health Department and the Health and Human Services Agency must have a rapid initial assessment and current information on the status of all facilities and services. Health facility licensing and regulation are usually part of public health. The public health field licensing staff must determine whether facilities can safely continue operations and if the building is structurally sound. Public health executive leadership will need 3

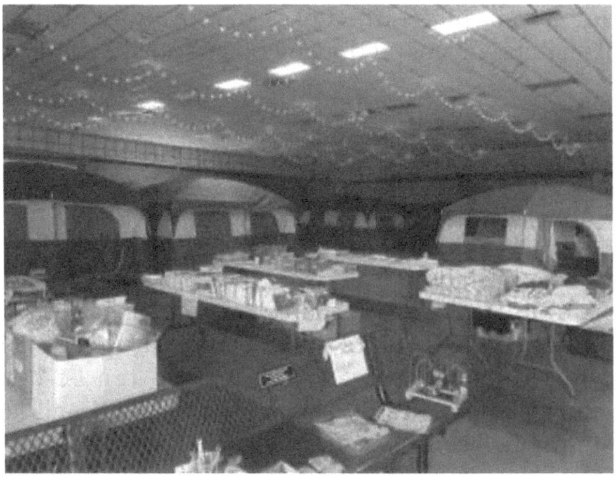

Figure 8.9 Indoor congregate general population shelter during COVID-19.

to determine what regulatory flexes are needed and ensure the authority from the governor or state health officer to grant variances and exemptions. This may include increasing the number of licensed beds, patient care in previously unlicensed areas, exemption from patient–staff ratios, expansion of scope of practice, emergency licensing and staff privileges of responding health professionals, and authorization of alternate care sites. Licensing staff approves the need for exemptions and monitors care. Emergency orders and regulatory exemptions have been used extensively to support healthcare surge during COVID-19. Healthcare surge measures are discussed further in the text that follows.

Public health competencies needed to link people to needed personal health services and assure the provision of healthcare when otherwise unavailable and mobilize community partnerships to identify and solve health problems

Healthcare Surge

In the aftermath of a large earthquake, response agencies will have to manage the increased need for services and resources in the face of damaged capacity and infrastructure. For the healthcare system, this translates to high demand at the same time capacity is diminished by damaged facilities, reduced staff, disrupted critical services such as power and transportation, interrupted patient services and access, and displaced community residents. Healthcare surge is the response to a sudden increase in demand for services that exceeds usual capacity. Surge is a complex multifaceted endeavor that involves inpatient care, outpatient care, and home health. Public health and their associated health agencies have a major role in supporting the healthcare system and assuring access to healthcare for all community residents. Preparing for surge caused by all types of emergencies is the primary objective of the HPP grant. California developed extensive surge guidelines that covers many aspects of the topic (CDPH, 2008a, 2008b, 2008c).

Maintaining healthcare services is also highly dependent on other services such as water, power, transportation, and supply lines. It also depends heavily on obtaining a wide range of resources. Plans can incorporate prescripted bundled resource requests to state or federal authorities designed to meet anticipated needs of large events. This avoids the need for individual requests with the risk of delays, omissions, and underestimates of need. California has bundled federal resource requests for catastrophic earthquakes that includes medical supplies,
10 emergency medical response teams, and many other anticipated shortages.

Assuring Healthcare

Following a major earthquake, the first priority is rescue and emergency care. The public is always the first responder and effects many rescues. Local fire personnel, followed by Urban Search and Rescue teams, locate, rescue, and initiate medical stabilization for persons trapped in collapsed structures. Federal teams from FEMA are available to supplement local personnel. The emergency medical services (EMS) system and emergency departments (EDs) are the first to feel impact from a disaster and can be quickly overwhelmed. EMS is part of public health in many states, but in all jurisdictions it works closely with public health to coordinate transportation and healthcare surge during disasters. Hospital evacuation in addition to a surge in 911 calls requires additional ambulance units that will first respond from neighboring jurisdictions. California has a system of ambulance strike teams that are routinely used in earthquakes, fires, and other multicasualty incidents. These consist of five ambulances of like type basic life support (BLS) or advanced life support (ALS) with a leader unit to provide resupply and communications. Initial ambulance strike teams are available within 2 hours with other teams arriving shortly. Up to 500 additional ground transport units are available through a national EMS contract with HHS-ASPR. EMS response may be compromised by rubble blocking transportation routes as well as gridlock from persons trying to evacuate the affected area, so air medical also plays an important role in patient transport during a major disaster (Figure 8.10).

There are several other means for EMS to address a large surge in demand (CDC, n.d.-b), but these are very difficult to initiate rapidly in a no-notice event:

1. Tiered dispatch: screen callers to determine acuity; prerecorded messages to selectively direct 911 calls with referral of non-life-threatening calls to advice lines.
2. Modify treatment and transport protocols to allow EMS personnel to assess, treat, release, and refer patients without transport.
3. Transport to facilities that do not traditionally receive 911 patients (e.g., clinics, urgent care, surgery centers, and alternate care sites).

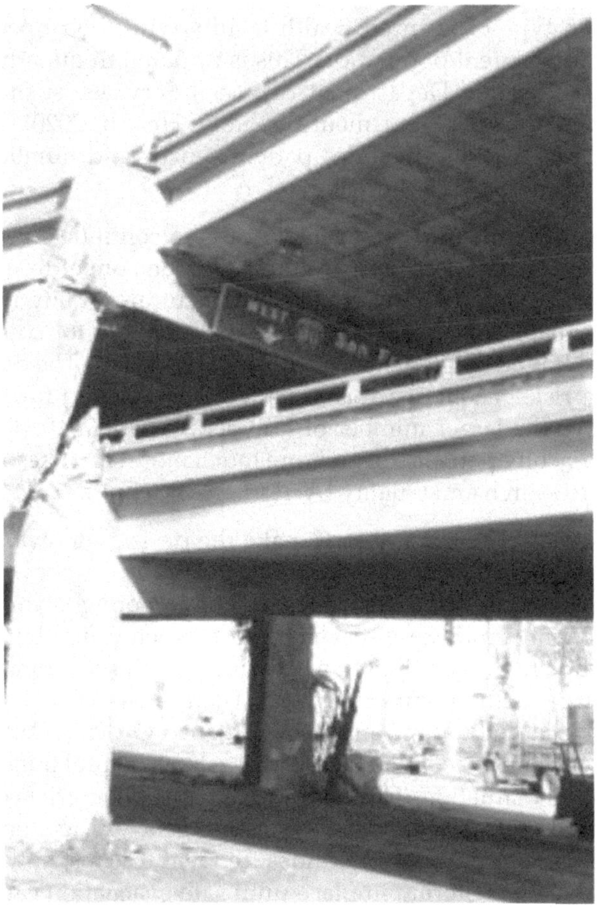

Figure 8.10 Freeway collapse, Oakland, California, Loma Prieta earthquake.

After the Northridge earthquake in Southern California, Urban Search and Rescue Teams and **Disaster Medical Assistance Teams (DMATs)** were important elements in the response. The acute phase of the emergency medical response ended within 48 to 72 hours and public health then became the predominant healthcare issue (Stratton et al., 1996).

Impacted acute care hospitals should immediately activate and staff their emergency operation center according to principles in the HICS.

Public health competencies needed to monitor health status to identify and solve community health problems and diagnose and investigate health problems and health hazards in the community

Healthcare Facility Support

Public health and the heath agency must rapidly assess facility status. This can be very challenging in the initial chaos after a large emergency, especially if communications are disrupted. One method is for facilities to report to the
1 public health and medical EOC or health branch. In California, facilities report to a local or regional medical and health coordinator in either the Public Health
13 or EMS Department that then reports the data to the State Medical and Health Coordination Center, California Health and Human Services. The Department
2 of Public Health generates a GIS map with the boundaries of the disaster and overlays of each type of licensed health facility with their operational status and status of their patient population. This is updated frequently and includes facilities licensed by the Department of Social Services, such as residential care facilities (California Department of Public Health, 2020). In addition to operational status, tracking includes patient census and numbers of patients evacuated.

An objective determination of hospital status to continue care requires engineers to evaluate structural safety and licensing personnel to evaluate ability to provide care safely within the structure. Structural stability may be specific to parts of the hospital and functional status may allow for continued care of current patients but no ability to admit additional patients. The decision to evacuate involves a risk–benefit analysis of patient safety and a further analysis of whether to move the larger number of low–acuity patients first or the smaller number of high-acuity patients that require much more scarce resources (Agency for Healthcare Research and Quality [AHRQ], n.d.; Schultz et al., 2003, 2007).

In extreme situations, hospital staff make the decision to evacuate based on
16 patient safety and begin moving patients outside of the facility without full consultation and without assuring transportation or accepting facilities. This is cer-
1 tainly true of not only rapidly approaching danger such as fires but also following an earthquake due to the certainty of numerous aftershocks, some of which may be nearly as large as the main movement. There have been several examples of this in California due to fires and the threatened Oroville Dam failure (Hick et al., 2017). Exercising evacuation before a disaster is helpful but does not reproduce an emergency situation (Haverkort et al., 2016). Experience in California and Israel emphasize that the decision of emergency evacuation is complex, with structural damage and loss of utilities frequent reasons; however, hospitals should be capable of sheltering in place until safe evacuation can be organized

(Adini et al., 2012; Schultz et al., 2003, 2007). Unless unsafe, hospitals and long-term care facilities should try to shelter in place initially.

Support for Healthcare Surge

Facilities continuing to care for patients and receiving additional patients from the disaster zone or from other facilities will require support for key elements of surge: staff, space, and supplies.

Emergency Orders and Regulatory Exemptions

Emergency orders and regulatory exemptions are a critical and effective means to support the emergency response in general and healthcare surge in particular. The first orders in a disaster expedite government operations by exempting procurement and personnel rules. Existing laws designate all state workers as emergency service workers who can be reassigned to the response efforts. Another broad area of emergency regulation to facilitate access to healthcare is to require health plans and systems to reimburse out of plan care, because patients may not be able to access their usual provider. Public health leadership requests and oversees regulatory exemptions while the facility licensing staff implements and monitors them.

Personnel

Healthcare personnel are highly dedicated and often will respond to their clinic or facility to assist, but many will be impacted themselves or unable to get to their place of employment. Hospital staff can be augmented through exemption of nurse–patient staff ratios, shifting personnel from less affected facilities within healthcare systems, or through volunteers. Hospitals may need to modify or exempt staff privileging requirements.

State regulatory exemptions may include expanding scope of practice for specific types of personnel such as paramedics and nurses, the use of nonconventional licensed personnel such as veterinarians and dentists, and exempting state licensing requirements to allow retired staff and out-of-state personnel to practice. Medical volunteers are provided liability protection.

Spontaneous volunteers are particularly problematic for healthcare, since professional license and skills must be validated. The **Emergency System for Advance Registration of Volunteer Health Professionals (ESAR-VHP)** is a federal program to support states and territories in establishing standardized volunteer registration programs for disasters and public health and medical emergencies (HHS, 2020b). The system is linked to the state licensing agencies to verify licensure and can be used to call up specific types of personnel or entire teams that are rostered within the database. Legal issues of using volunteers have been analyzed for public health officers by ASTHO (n.d.-a).

Emergency medical teams can be requested from local, state, or federal agencies. Disaster medical teams specialize in providing care in nontraditional settings such as shelters or alternate care sites. These teams may be organized locally **(Medical Reserve Corps)** or at the state or federal level. DMATs are federal teams coordinated by the HHS-ASPR as part of the **National Disaster Medical System (NDMS;** ASPR, n.d.-a). These teams come with sufficient equipment

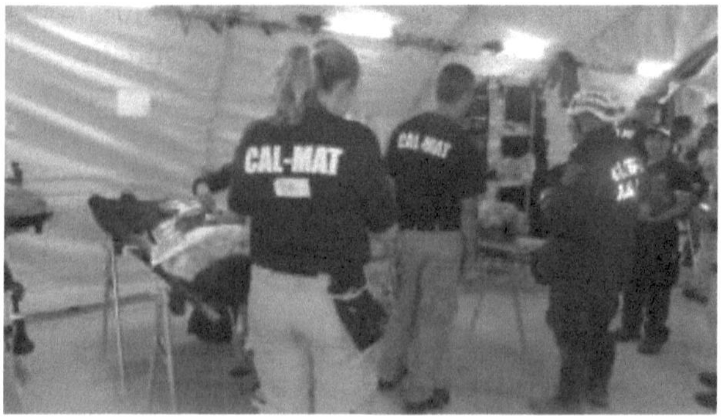

Figure 8.11 California Disaster Medical Assistance Team (CAL-MAT).

and supplies to rapidly set up and begin care that includes high-level emergency capabilities. They can also provide care within shelters or nearly any other structure. California has similar teams based on the DMAT model (CAL-MAT; Figure 8.11). The NDMS can also supply teams to support trauma and critical care, mortuary services, and even veterinary care in disaster areas. The U.S. Public Health Service Commissioned Corp also has teams that can be rapidly deployed into the field to support medical or mental healthcare. The Department of Defense can also supply teams of healthcare providers to supplement civilian healthcare.

Personal Health Information

One unique challenge to providing quality care outside of usual health facilities or within facilities that must treat patients who usually obtain their healthcare elsewhere is obtaining personal health information. One of the most common health needs for persons who had to evacuate their homes is replacement of medications, but few patients have an accurate record of their current medications. Fortunately, pharmacy chains now have electronic records for patients who obtain their prescriptions from that chain. But medical history can only be inferred from prescription medications. Integrated healthcare systems usually have electronic records integrated across their sites, but do not share their records with competitors. California EMSA has developed a solution from a federal grant that allows volunteer medical providers to use internet access to search patient records that are synthesized from the majority of major health systems within California. **Patient Unified Lookup System for Emergencies (PULSE)** is activated during an emergency and connects multiple local and national data sources (health information organizations and health systems), allowing disaster medical volunteers to check patient records for allergies, problem lists, and medications in order to allow the healthcare providers in Disaster Healthcare Volunteers (DHV) to make better clinical decisions (California EMSA, 2020).

Space and Beds

Bed capacity can be increased through licensing exemptions or regulatory interventions. The first step is to identify nontraditional and nonclinical spaces within the facility. Establishing alternate care sites in existing structures or shelters can provide additional treatment locations and decompress acute care hospital emergency departments and inpatient units. These have been widely established but

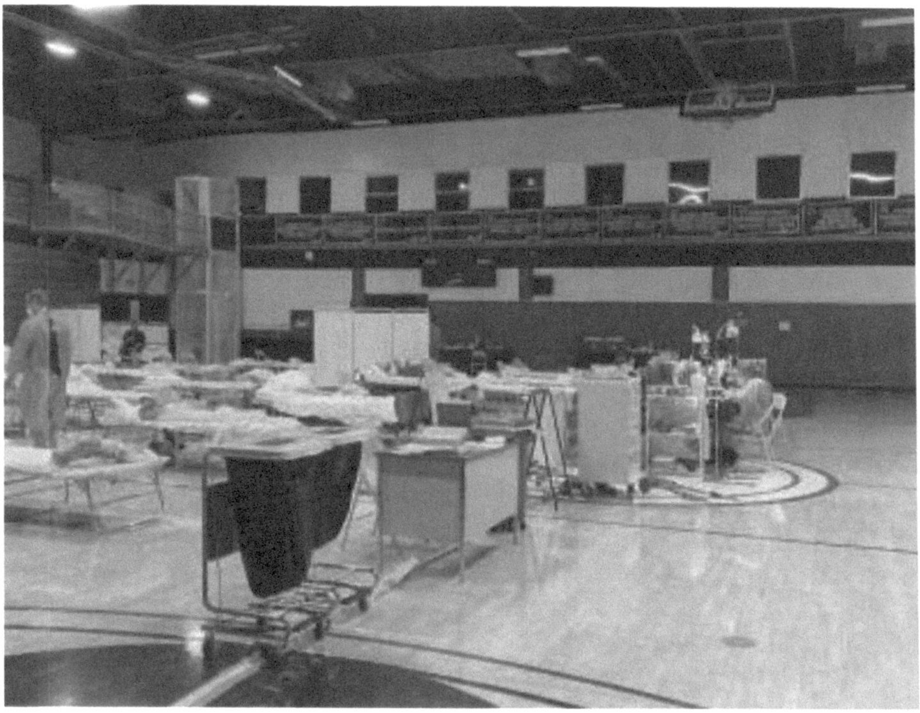

Figure 8.12 Alternate care site.

not highly utilized during COVID-19 (Figures 8.12–8.13). Mobile field hospitals are routinely used by the military and following disasters in other countries but are not commonly used in the United States due to the ability to move patients by ground or air to other nearby facilities. Following the Chilean earthquake, 14 field hospitals were set up on the site of damaged facilities until more permanent structures could be rebuilt (Gerdin et al., 2013). A field hospital was used in Joplin, Missouri, in 2011, following a tornado that destroyed the main community hospital. These facilities require licensing exemptions and approvals (Figure 8.14).

In addition to moving supplies and staff into the affected area, the other means of supporting patient care following a disaster is to decompress facilities by moving patients out of the area. Patient movement requires coordination of transportation and destination to assure that the appropriate level of care is maintained during and after transport. Bed availability and arrangements with receiving facilities are often the responsibility of the public health or health agency.

SUPPLIES

Supplies can usually be obtained through private supply chains, but in unusual situations with demand far exceeding supply (e.g., countermeasures for chemical, radiological, or biological attacks) local resources may be supplemented by federal stockpiles. The CDC manages the Strategic National Stockpile that can be mobilized within hours to supplement certain medical supplies (ASPR, n.d.-b).

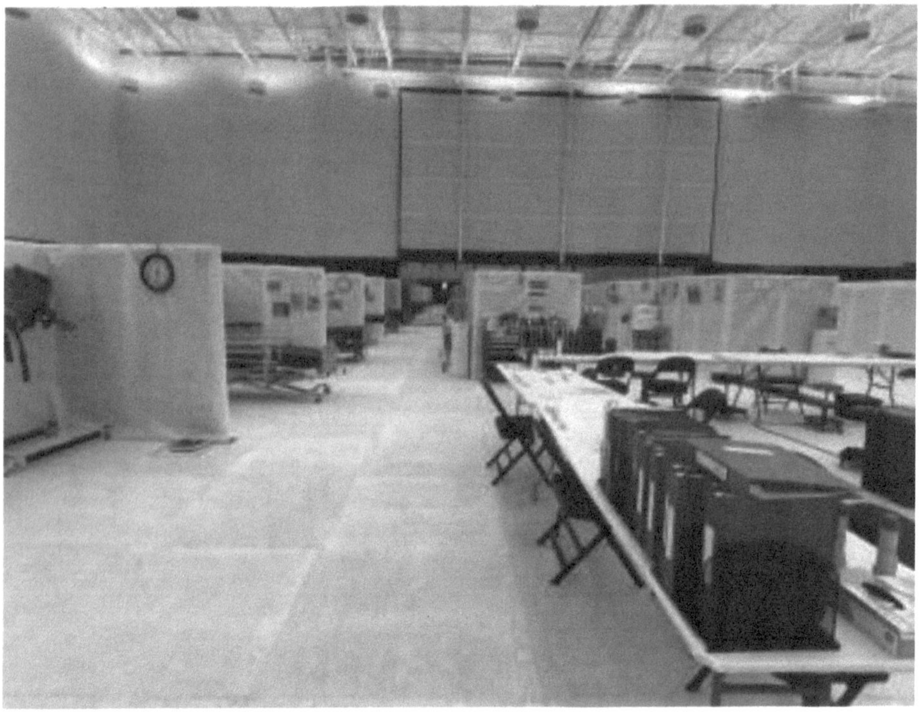

Figure 8.13 Alternate care site to support hospital surge during COVID-19.

Populations With Special Needs

One key responsibility is to assure supportive services and care for individuals with chronic conditions or with access and functional needs and those in medically underserved areas, which includes a large proportion of the population. For the population in shelters, this responsibility is shared by emergency support function for Mass Care and Shelter (ESF #6), usually the responsibility of the social services agency in partnership with the American Red Cross (ARC); however, ARC-managed shelters generally provide only first aid or very basic-level medical care, so the government health agency determines how to best provide care.

It is a difficult determination how to optimally provide care within shelters. Sometimes this can be done through a clinical area within a shelter, by cohorting shelter residents with medical needs, or establishing a separate medical shelter. National policy has shifted to providing care for those with access and functional needs as much as possible in general population shelters. California Department of Social Services has responsibility for coordination of Mass Care and Shelter

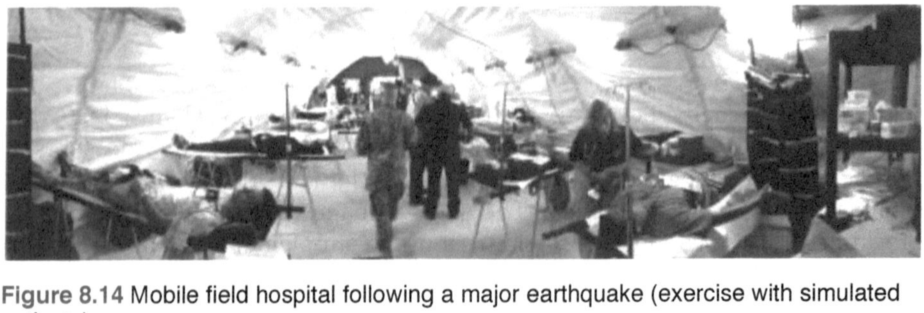

Figure 8.14 Mobile field hospital following a major earthquake (exercise with simulated patients).

(ESF #6) and deploys Functional Assessment Service Teams (FAST) to shelters to determine unmet functional and access needs (California Department of Social Services, n.d.). However, there is a spectrum of medical need that may require special medical shelters, including for patients in long-term care and convalescent facilities. In one recent event in California, a long-term care facility evacuated to the community shelter without prior notification or planning. This created an immediate need to set up a medical shelter to care for the patients until they could be repatriated or transferred to an appropriate facility. The HHS has federal medical stations that include caches of medical supplies that can be set up in nonmedical spaces to care for patients from these types of facilities. To avoid evacuation of skilled nursing and long-term care facilities that were experiencing widespread patient and staff COVID-19 outbreaks, California sent strike teams to support staffing gaps, establish effective infection control practices, and assure appropriate personal protective equipment for staff.

Outpatient and home care require attention to avoid additional load on hospitals and skilled nursing facilities. This emphasizes the need to mobilize community partnerships to mitigate disruption for patients. Dialysis is an example of a critical service that is highly specialized urgent or emergent care that is not easily shifted to other sites and must be continued through coordination of the community care network (Irvine et al., 2014).

Another large population that requires special consideration is children, who compose nearly 25% of the population. There are relatively few pediatric beds and specialty facilities for children in the community, so in a large-scale disaster, facilities that may not provide pediatric trauma care or intensive care may need to manage children until they can be safely transferred. This is currently an area of required planning for the HPP grant. Pediatric preparedness in emergency departments has been evaluated and shown to improve outcomes for pediatric patients (Remick et al., 2016). The ASPR is currently supporting development of regional networks for pediatric mutual aid to optimize sharing of expertise and other resoures (Western Regional Alliance for Pediatric Emergency Management, 2020).

Crisis Standards of Care

Management of scarce resources remains a complex and challenging problem for emergency management overall and especially in healthcare where it can make a difference in patient outcome and access to care. This has been termed "crisis care" or **"crisis standards of care" (CSC)**, which is defined as a substantial change in usual healthcare operations and level of care it is possible to deliver, which is made necessary by a pervasive or catastrophic disaster (Hanfling et al., 2013). In catastrophic disasters involving an overwhelming demand for medical care, CSC enables more effective use of the limited resources through fair, just, and equitable processes for making decisions across the region about who should receive treatments when there are not enough resources to provide patients with the level of care they would usually receive. Resources most often anticipated in shortage include EMS, intensive care, ventilators, or specific medications. However, immediately following an event, it could be any medical resource until additional support is available.

Implementation of CSC requires careful coordination and cooperation with all stakeholders through multiagency coordination groups (MACs; California Statewide Multi-Agency Coordination System Working Group, 2013). Prior

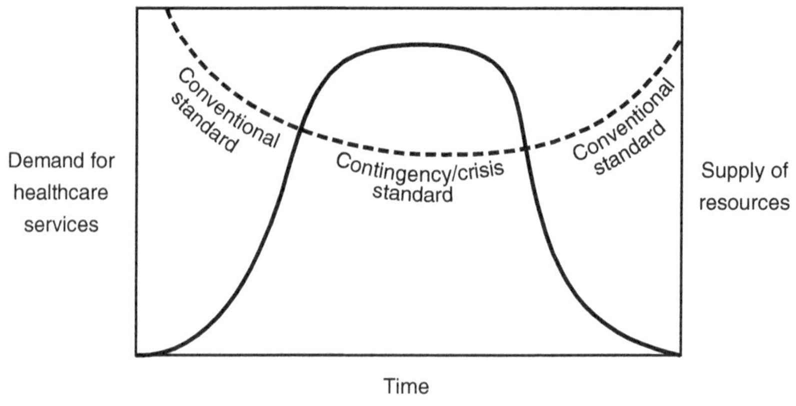

Figure 8.15 Relationship between supply, demand, and shift in standard of care in a sustained public health emergency.

Source: From Hanfling, D., Altevogt, B. M., Viswanathan, K., & Gostin, L. O. (Eds.). (2012). *Crisis standards of care: A systems framework for catastrophic disaster response.* National Academies Press. https://doi.org/10.17226/13351

planning and discussion for shifting to contingent or crisis care is critical, since it may be interpreted as rationing care. With guidance from the AHRQ, some state health agencies and healthcare systems have developed protocols or policies to address resource shortages (Institute of Medicine [U.S.] Committee on Guidance for Establishing Standards of Care for Use in Disaster Situations, 2012). Many more states developed or revised these during the waves of COVID-19 that overwhelmed hospital intensive care units. Ethical and legal concerns create intense scrutiny of CSC (Hodge et al., 2013).

Levels of care that can be provided in catastrophic scenarios have been defined (Hanfling et al., 2013; Figure 8.15):

Conventional care—Space, staff, and supplies are consistent with daily practice within the institution used during a multicasualty incident that triggers activation of the facility's emergency operations plan.

Contingency care—Space, staff, and supplies are not consistent with daily practice but have minimal impact on patient care practices and meet patient demand using local and regional resources.

Crisis care—Adaptive spaces, staff, and supplies are not consistent with the usual standards of care but provide the best possible care to patients given the circumstances and resources available. Local, regional, state, interstate, and national resources may be required to meet patient demand.

Behavioral Health

The most widespread and enduring impact will be the psychological stress and posttraumatic stress resulting from fear, anxiety over the loss of housing and services, and exposure to devastation and injuries of loved ones and community members (Dai et al., 2016; Farooqui et al., 2017). It is one of the most underestimated and persistent needs following a disaster and is often not addressed due to a lack of understanding the long-term impacts and a lack of sufficient resources at the local level (Alisha et al., 2019; Tanaka et al., 2019). Following the

2010 earthquake in Chile, government and health officials told a visiting Red Cross delegation that their greatest need for healthcare was behavioral health.

It is estimated that the majority of affected persons in a disaster area will have transitory distress symptoms, and 30% to 40% will develop a new incidence disorder such as posttraumatic stress disorder (PTSD) or depression. This includes 10% to 20% of responders. These disorders can be prevented in many people if addressed within the first month. California has developed response guides for local health departments that describe the resources and options for response (California EMSA, 2018; California Department of Public Health, California Emergency Medical Services Authority, 2018). The traditional one-on-one model of behavioral therapy is inadequate to address the overwhelming need (Abeldaño & Fernández, 2016; Macy et al., 2004; Shultz & Forbes, 2013).

The Substance Abuse and Mental Health Services Administration (n.d.) provides technical, financial, and personnel support for disaster planning and response. One underappreciated area is the needs of first responders who have very high rates of PTSD following disaster response. Posttraumatic stress is the most persistent health problem that should be addressed during recovery.

Other ESF #8 Areas of Responsibility: Veterinary Support and Mass Fatality

Veterinary support may be needed for animal care and rescue. It is difficult to convince people to evacuate unless arrangements are made for their pets or animals. Many human shelters now allow pets to accompany owners or colocate animal shelters with general population shelters. In either case, it requires additional levels of public health surveillance for hygiene and infectious disease. California rosters veterinary teams on their medical volunteer registry. They have rescued, sheltered, and treated domestic pets; large farm animals; exotic pets; and wildlife. During one large fire, they sheltered and delivered a pregnant giraffe from a wildlife sanctuary and even rescued fish from koi ponds.

Another little appreciated task that may be the responsibility of ESF #8 is mortuary services to identify and process bodies outside of the hospital. Special federal teams are available (DMORT).

Recovery

Public health competencies needed to evaluate effectiveness, accessibility, and quality of personal and population-based health services and research for new insights and innovative solutions to health problems

Recovery involves reestablishing services and infrastructure and begins during the response phase. Although the healthcare system may be most stressed by the initial demand for services following a large earthquake or other disaster, the system must continue to focus on providing care to the entire population and rapidly shift to recovery of usual services (Cartwright et al., 2017). Whereas some services and utilities may be restored within hours or days, others involving major destruction of infrastructure may take months or years. Severely damaged healthcare facilities may be demolished and rebuild to higher standards of earthquake resistance. Shelters may not close for months, especially if many homes have been destroyed and require extensive repair or rebuilding. Public health is responsible for continuously monitoring health status and approving reopening of healthcare facilities and repatriation of patients. Public health also has responsibility to monitor drinking water quality as utilities come back online, monitor the effects of environmental toxic spills, and monitor food safety as restaurants reopen.

One of the challenges for postdisaster assessment of healthcare is evaluating care provided in nontraditional settings. Care provided in shelters and alternate care sites by disaster medical teams or volunteer community providers often do not have electronic records or standardized clinical encounter forms. There are simple electronic records that can be loaded on portable electronic devices and uploaded into a central database; however, this requires considerable preparation. The ARC uses its own forms for medical screening, first aid, and treatment that are not readily aggregated and available for analysis.

Recovery is also a time to redouble efforts toward mitigation and preparedness. Immediately after a disaster, the issue of preparedness is prevalent and
18 urgent, creating a political window for additional funding and important program or resource gaps. Reimbursement from federal and state emergency funds
2,3 is predicated on prior declarations of emergency, adherence with emergency management principles, accurate financial record keeping, and specific eligible activities. Healthcare is generally not reimbursed from emergency funds but may be covered by health insurance. This may depend on prior emergency or executive orders and negotiations between regulatory agencies and health plans.

Evaluation of Response

Emergency management typically seeks immediate evaluation feedback from responders before they return to their usual jobs or move on to the next emergency. The initial discussion and evaluation of the response is known as the "hotwash." Each agency subsequently undertakes a more detailed after-action evaluation. These recommendations drive changes to the emergency plans and subsequent exercises to familiarize staff with new procedures.

Research

Research differs from after-action reports in that it may evaluate individuals in a community or quantitative analysis of relief efforts or healthcare interventions. Disaster science is relatively new, and most publications have been descriptive rather than analytical. Several publications have evaluated the disaster public health literature (Gowing et al., 2017; Khan et al., 2015; Savoia et al., 2017).

DISCUSSION QUESTIONS

1. Discuss how specific mitigation and preparedness measures can help reduce the number of deaths and injuries, as well as amount of property damage, due to earthquakes.
2. Give some examples for how enforcement of laws and regulations—both before and immediately after an earthquake—reduce impacts of earthquakes on populations.
3. Accessing healthcare for the wounded immediately after an earthquake is a high priority. Describe how public health, emergency medical services, and healthcare facilities respond to a sudden surge in healthcare needs.
4. The recovery phase after an earthquake may start within hours for some services; however, for some major destruction of infrastructure, it may take years to fully recover. Describe some of the aspects and elements of the recovery phase.

SUMMARY

TABLE 8.3 Select Essential Services of Public Health Demonstrated in Earthquake Response

Essential Service # and Definition	Context in Chapter Case	Competency # It Ties to	Importance for Emergency Preparedness, Response, or Recovery
1. Assess and monitor population health status, factors that influence health, and community needs and assets (Assessment)	Epidemiological evaluation conducted in the community, within shelters, or healthcare facilities	1, 2, 3	Assessment allows for determination of the magnitude of the problem as well as the impact of interventions.
2. Investigate, diagnose, and address health problems and hazards affecting the population (Assessment)	Evaluation of psychological and physical impact with assessment through screening tools	3, 4	Analyzing data and interpreting the results are critical in taking appropriate actions
3. Communicate effectively to inform and educate people about health, factors that influence it, and how to improve it (Policy Development)	Los Angeles County Department of Public Health shifted its social media messaging to encourage social connectivity with emphasis on community preparedness.	7, 8, 9, 18	Tailoring communication, taking into account language, cultural values, and the types of media used for receiving information, is important to reach all segments of the affected population.
4. Strengthen, support, and mobilize communities and partnerships to improve health (Policy Development)	HPP grant requires jurisdictions to develop community healthcare coalitions to assure that all parts of the healthcare delivery system are engaged and integrated.	8, 9, 13, 14	Effective public health actions require the trust and cooperation of the community which can only be achieved through outreach to create coalitions and partnerships.
5. Create, champion, and implement policies, plans, and laws that impact health (Policy Development)	California and other earthquake-prone states have done extensive planning for large earthquakes as well as other high-risk disasters.	12, 13, 21	Plans are not static and are regularly reviewed and updated; in addition, exercises are designed to evaluate the plan and teach staff their role.
6. Utilize legal and regulatory actions designed to improve and protect the public's health (Policy Development)	In most states, the governor has the power to suspend, flex, or implement rules during a declared disaster. Some authorities can be delegated to the state health officer.	16	Health agencies can anticipate needs to flex regulatory requirements for facilities to support healthcare surge by prescripting emergency orders for the governor or health officer.
7. Assure an effective system that enables equitable access to the individual services and care needed to be healthy (Assurance)	California has bundled federal resource requests for catastrophic earthquakes that include medical supplies, emergency medical response teams, and other anticipated shortages.	4, 7	Such bundling of federal resource requests helps avoid the need for individual requests with the risk of delays, omissions, and underestimates of need.
8. Build and support a diverse and skilled public health workforce (Assurance)	California EMSA developed a course, Medical Health Operations Center Support Activities (MHOC-SA), that applies disaster management and ICS principles to medical and health response.	21, 22	Such courses are important mechanisms to train the personnel who will staff the health and medical branch of their EOC.
9. Improve and innovate public health functions through ongoing evaluation, research, and continuous quality improvement (Assurance)	Public Health Department and the Health and Human Services Agency must have rapid initial assessment and current information on the status of all facilities and services.	2, 3, 4, 5	The public health field licensing staff [(Level 1)] must be able to determine whether facilities can safely continue operations and if the building is structurally sound.

(continued)

TABLE 8.3 Select Essential Services of Public Health Demonstrated in Earthquake Response (*continued*)

Essential Service # and Definition	Context in Chapter Case	Competency # It Ties to	Importance for Emergency Preparedness, Response, or Recovery
10. Build and maintain a strong organizational infrastructure for public health (Assurance)	Immediately after a disaster, the issue of preparedness is prevalent and creates a political window for funding an important program or resource gaps.	15	Importantly, reimbursement from federal and state emergency funds is predicated on prior declarations of emergency, adherence with emergency management principles, accurate financial record keeping, and specific eligible activities.

EOC, Emergency Operations Center; HPP, Hospital Preparedness Program; ICS, Incident Command System.

TABLE 8.4 Select CEPH Competencies Needed for Frontline Health Workers, Managers, and Leaders for Earthquake Emergency Preparedness, Response, and Recovery

Competency # and Definition	Context in Case/Chapter	Level	Importance for Emergency Preparedness, Response, or Recovery
4. Interpret results of data analysis for public health research, policy, or practice	Public health provided a clinical case definition and protocols for management after norovirus outbreaks.	Level 1	Such protocols can help to establish special isolation areas and ensure infection control nurses visit each shelter daily and play a key role in surveillance, health education of shelter staff, and monitoring infection control measures.
12. Discuss the policymaking process, including the roles of ethics and evidence.	Governor has the power to suspend, flex, or implement rules during a declared disaster. Some authorities can be delegated to the state health officer.	Level 3	As an illustration of the multiple dimensions of policy making, other agencies are responsible for laws and regulations that will support public health and medical mitigation and response. For example, architectural standards are a critical earthquake mitigation strategy since structural collapse is one of the major causes of morbidity and mortality.
13. Propose strategies to identify stakeholders and build coalitions and partnerships for influencing public health outcomes.	Facilities report to a local or regional medical and health coordinator in the Public Health or EMS Department that reports the data to the State Medical and Health Coordination Center.	Level 2	A Department of Public Health can generate a GIS map with the boundaries of the disaster and overlays of each type of licensed health facility with their operational status, status of their patient population, and track patient census and numbers of patients evacuated.
16. Apply leadership and/or management principles to address a relevant health issue.	Hospital staff make the decision to evacuate based on patient safety and will move patients outside of the facility.	Level 1	The decision for emergency evacuation is complex and may be due to structural damage and loss of utilities; however, hospitals should be capable of sheltering in place, at least initially, until safe evacuation can be organized.
18. Select communication strategies for different audiences and sectors.	Agency leadership will be fully engaged in developing and delivering the message.	Level 3	Information and messages should be reviewed with higher levels of emergency management to assure there is a clear, coordinated message.
21. Integrate perspectives from other sectors and/or professions to promote and advance population health.	Public health management/leadership mobilizes their emergency management structure and reassigns other staff as disaster service workers.	Level 2	The high-level response goal is to manage disaster-induced injuries and public health risks and maintain access to healthcare services. This requires evaluating and supporting the health needs of the population and the healthcare system.

Key: Essential services of public health; CEPH competencies; Leadership levels.

EMS, emergency medical services; GIS, geographic information system.

REFERENCES

Abeldaño, R. A., & Fernández, R. (2016). Community mental health in disaster situations. A review of community-based models of approach. *Ciência & Saúde Coletiva, 21*(2), 431–442. https://doi.org/10.1590/1413-81232015212.17502014

Adini, B., Laor, D., Cohen, R., & Israeli, A. (2012). Decision to evacuate a hospital during an emergency: The safe way or the leader's way? *Journal of Public Health Policy, 33*(2), 257–268. https://doi.org/10.1057/jphp.2012.2

Agency for Healthcare Research and Quality. (n.d.). *Hospital evacuation decision guide*. https://www.ahrq.gov/research/shuttered/hospevac4.html

Alisha, K. C., Gan, C. C. R., & Dwirahmadi, F. (2019). Breaking through barriers and building disaster mental resilience: A case study in the aftermath of the 2015 Nepal earthquakes. *International Journal of Environmental Research and Public Health, 16*(16), 2964. https://doi.org/10.3390/ijerph16162964

Assistant Secretary for Preparedness and Response. (n.d.-a). *Calling on NDMS*. https://www.phe.gov/Preparedness/responders/ndms/Pages/calling-ndms.aspx

Assistant Secretary for Preparedness and Response. (n.d.-b). *Strategic National Stockpile*. https://www.phe.gov/about/sns/Pages/default.aspx

Association of State and Territorial Health Officers. (n.d.-a). *Emergency Volunteer Toolkit*. https://www.astho.org/Programs/Preparedness/Public-Health-Emergency-Law/Emergency-Volunteer-Toolkit

Association of State and Territorial Health Officers. (n.d.-b). *Public health emergency law*. https://www.astho.org/Legal-Preparedness-Series/?terms=legal+authorities+in+disasters

California Department of Public Health. (2008a). *Standards and guidelines for healthcare surge during emergencies* (Vol. 1: Hospitals). https://www.calhospitalprepare.org/sites/main/files/file-attachments/volume1_hospital_final.pdf

California Department of Public Health. (2008b). *Standards and guidelines for healthcare surge during emergencies* (Vol. II: Government-authorized alternate care sites). https://www.cidrap.umn.edu/sites/default/files/public/php/258/258_acs.pdf

California Department of Public Health. (2008c). *Standards and guidelines for healthcare surge during emergencies* (Vol. III: Payers).

California Department of Public Health. (2011). *California public health and medical emergency operations manual*. https://www.calhospitalprepare.org/sites/main/files/file-attachments/finaleom712011.pdf

California Department of Public Health, California Emergency Medical Services Authority. (2018). *Resource typing guidance: Disaster mental/behavioral and spiritual care*. https://emsa.ca.gov/wp-content/uploads/sites/71/2018/11/EOM-Disaster-Behavioral-Health-Resource-Typing-Aides-10-25-2018.pdf

California Department of Public Health, California Emergency Medical Services Authority. (2020). *Real time mapping application for situational awareness*. https://www.cdph.ca.gov/Programs/EPO/Pages/real_time_mapping_application.aspx

California Department of Social Services. (n.d.). *Functional Assessment Service Team (FAST) program*. https://www.cdss.ca.gov/inforesources/mass-care-and-shelter/fast

California Emergency Medical Services Authority. (2014). *Hospital Incident Command System (HICS) guidebook* (5th ed.). Author. https://emsa.ca.gov/wp-content/uploads/sites/71/2017/09/HICS_Guidebook_2014_11.pdf

California Emergency Medical Services Authority. (2018). *California public health and medical emergency operations manual: Disaster behavioral health*. https://emsa.ca.gov/wp-content/uploads/sites/71/2018/11/EOM-Disaster-Behavioral-Health-10-26-2018.pdf

California Emergency Medical Services Authority. (2020). *Patient Unified Lookup System in Emergencies (PULSE)*. https://emsa.ca.gov/wp-content/uploads/sites/71/2020/03/EMSA-PULSE-Just-InTime-Training-4.1.20.pdf

California Office of Emergency Services. (2008). *California catastrophic incident base plan: Concept of operations*. https://www.caloes.ca.gov/individuals-families/catastrophic-planning

California Statewide Multi-Agency Coordination System Working Group. (2013). *California Statewide Multi-Agency Coordination System Guide*. https://www.caloes.ca.gov/PlanningPreparednessSite/Documents/10%20California%20Statewide%20Multi-Agency%20Coordination%20System(CSMACS)%20Guide%202-13-13.pdf

Cartwright, C., Hall, M., & Lee, A. C. K. (2017). The changing health priorities of earthquake response and implications for preparedness: A scoping review. *Public Health, 150*, 60–70. https://doi.org/10.1016/j.puhe.2017.04.024

Centers for Disease Control and Prevention. (n.d.-a). *Community Assessment for Public Health Emergency Response (CASPER)*. https://www.cdc.gov/nceh/hsb/disaster/casper/default.htm

Centers for Disease Control and Prevention. (n.d.-b). *Framework for expanding EMS system capacity during medical surge*. Department of Health and Human Services. https://www.cdc.gov/cpr/readiness/healthcare/Expanding-EMS-Systems.htm

Centers for Disease Control and Prevention. (n.d.-c). *Public Health Emergency Preparedness (PHEP) cooperative agreement*. https://www.cdc.gov/cpr/readiness/phep.htm

Clay, L. A., Goetschius, J. B., Papas, M. A., Trainor, J., Martins, N., & Kendra, J. M. (2019). Does preparedness matter? The influence of household preparedness on disaster outcomes during Superstorm Sandy. *Disaster Medicine and Public Health Preparedness, 14*, 71–79. https://doi.org/10.1017/dmp.2019.78

Dai, W., Chen, L., Lai, Z., Li, Y., Wang, J., & Liu, A. (2016). The incidence of post-traumatic stress disorder among survivors after earthquakes: A systematic review and meta-analysis. *BMC Psychiatry, 16*, 188. https://doi.org/10.1186/s12888-016-0891-9

Doocy, S., Jacquet, G., Cherewick, M., & Kirsch, T. D. (2013). The injury burden of the 2010 Haiti earthquake: A stratified cluster survey. *Injury, 44*(6), 842–847. https://doi.org/10.1016/j.injury.2013.01.035

Farooqui, M., Quadri, S. A., & Suriya, S. S. (2017). Posttraumatic stress disorder: A serious post-earthquake complication. *Trends in Psychiatry and Psychotherapy, 39*(2), 135–143. https://doi.org/10.1590/2237-6089-2016-0029

Federal Emergency Management Agency. (n.d.-a). *ICS resource training materials*. https://training.fema.gov/emiweb/is/icsresource/trainingmaterials

Federal Emergency Management Agency. (n.d.-b). *National Incident Management System (NIMS)*. https://training.fema.gov/nims

Gerdin, M., Wladis, A., & von Schreeb, J. (2013). Foreign field hospitals after the 2010 Haiti earthquake: How good were we? *Emergency Medicine Journal, 30*(1), e8. https://doi.org/10.1136/emermed-2011-200717

Gibson, P. J., Theadore, F., & Jellison, J. B. (2012). The common ground preparedness framework: A comprehensive description of Public Health Emergency Preparedness. *American Journal of Public Health, 102*(4), 633–642. https://doi.org/10.2105/AJPH.2011.300546

Gowing, J. R., Walker, K. N., Elmer, S. L., & Cummings, E. A. (2017). Disaster preparedness among health professionals and support staff: What is effective? An integrative literature review. *Prehospital and Disaster Medicine, 32*(3), 321–328. https://doi.org/10.1017/S1049023X1700019X

Greenberg, M. R., Dyen, S., & Elliott, S. (2013). The public's preparedness: Self-reliance, flashbulb memories, and conservative values. *American Journal of Public Health, 103*(6), e85–e91. https://doi.org/10.2105/AJPH.2012.301198

Hanfling, D., Hick, J. L., & Stroud, C. (2013). *Committee on Crisis Standards of Care: A toolkit for indicators and triggers*. National Academies Press. https://doi.org/10.17226/18338

Haverkort, J. J., Biesheuvel, T. H., & Bloemers, F. W. (2016). Hospital evacuation: Exercise versus reality. *Injury, 47*(9), 2012–2017. https://doi.org/10.1016/j.injury.2016.03.028

Heagele, T. N. (2016). Lack of evidence supporting the effectiveness of disaster supply kits. *American Journal of Public Health, 106*(6), 979–982. https://doi.org/10.2105/AJPH.2016.303148

Hick, J. L., Weil, J., Skivington, S., & Saruwatari, M. (2017). *The last stand: Evacuating a hospital in the middle of a wildfire*. ASPR Tracie. https://files.asprtracie.hhs.gov/documents/aspr-tracie-the-last-stand-evacuating-a-hospital-in-the-middle-of-a-wildfire.pdf

Hodge, J. G., Jr., Hanfling, D., & Powell, T. P. (2013). Practical, ethical, and legal challenges underlying crisis standards of care. *Journal of Law, Medicine & Ethics, 41*(Suppl. 1), 50–55. https://doi.org/10.1111/jlme.12039

Irvine, J., Buttimore, A., Eastwood, D., & Kendrick-Jones, J. (2014). The Christchurch earthquake: Dialysis experience and emergency planning. *Nephrology (Carlton), 19*(5), 296–303. https://doi.org/10.1111/nep.12222

Khan, Y., Fazli, G., & Henry, B. (2015). The evidence base of primary research in Public Health Emergency Preparedness: A scoping review and stakeholder consultation. *BMC Public Health, 15*, 432. https://doi.org/10.1186/s12889-015-1750-1

Khan, Y., O'Sullivan, T., & Brown, A. (2018). Public Health Emergency Preparedness: A framework to promote resilience. *BMC Public Health, 18*(1), 1344. https://doi.org/10.1186/s12889-018-6250-7

Kohn, S., Eaton, J. L., Feroz, S., Bainbridge, A. A., Hoolachan, J., & Barnett, D. J. (2012). Personal disaster preparedness: An integrative review of the literature. *Disaster Medicine and Public Health Preparedness, 6*(3), 217–231. https://doi.org/10.1001/dmp.2012.47

Levac, J., Toal-Sullivan, D., & O'Sullivan, T. L. (2012). Household emergency preparedness: A literature review. *Journal of Community Health, 37*(3), 725–733. https://doi.org/10.1007/s10900-011-9488-x

Macy, R. D., Behar, L., Paulson, R., Delman, J., Schmid, L., & Smith, S. F. (2004). Community-based, acute posttraumatic stress management: A description and evaluation of a psychosocial-intervention continuum. *Harvard Review of Psychiatry, 12*(4), 217–228. https://doi.org/10.1080/10673220490509589

Office of Statewide Planning and Development. (2019). *Seismic compliance program.* https://oshpd.ca.gov/construction-finance/seismic-compliance-and-safety

Office of the Assistant Secretary for Prepardness and Response, U.S. Department of Health and Human Services. (2020). *Hospital Preparedness Program (HPP).* https://www.phe.gov/Preparedness/planning/hpp/Pages/default.aspx

Peek-Asa, C., Kraus, J. F., Bourque, L. B., Vimalachandra, D., Yu, J., & Abrams, J. (1998). Fatal and hospitalized injuries resulting from the 1994 Northridge earthquake. *International Journal of Epidemiology, 27*(3), 459–465. https://doi.org/10.1093/ije/27.3.459

Plough, A., Fielding, J. E., & Chandra, A. (2013). Building community disaster resilience: Perspectives from a large urban county department of public health. *American Journal of Public Health, 103*(7), 1190–1197. https://doi.org/10.2105/AJPH.2013.301268

Posid, J. M., Bruce, S. M., Guarnizo, J. T., O'Connor, R. C., Jr., Papagiotas, S. S., & Taylor, M. L. (2013). Public health emergencies and responses: What are they, how long do they last, and how many staff does your agency need? *Biosecur Bioterror, 11*(4), 271–279. https://doi.org/10.1089/bsp.2013.0044

Public Health and Medical Emergency Powers. (2019). *California Department of Public Health, California Emergency Medical Services Authority, public health and medical emergency operations manual.* https://emsa.ca.gov/wp-content/uploads/sites/71/2019/03/New-EOM-Public-Health-and-Medical-Emergency-Powers-3-15-2019-002.pdf

Remick, K., Kaji, A. H., & Olson, L. (2016). Pediatric readiness and facility verification. *Annals of Emergency Medicine, 67*(3), 320–328.e321. https://doi.org/10.1016/j.annemergmed.2015.07.500

Savoia, E., Lin, L., Bernard, D., Klein, N., James, L. P., & Guicciardi, S. (2017). Public health system research in Public Health Emergency Preparedness in the United States (2009–2015): Actionable knowledge base. *American Journal of Public Health, 107*(Suppl. 2), e1–e6. https://doi.org/10.2105/AJPH.2017.304051

Schreiber, M., Shields, S., Formanski, S., Cohen, J. A., & Sims, L. V. (2014). Code triage: Integrating the National Children's Disaster Mental Health Concept of Operations across health care systems. *Clinical Pediatric Emergency Medicine, 15*(4), 323–333. https://doi.org/10.1016/j.cpem.2014.09.002

Schultz, C. H., Koenig, K. L., & Lewis, R. J. (2007). Decision making in hospital earthquake evacuation: Does distance from the epicenter matter? *Annals of Emergency Medicine, 50*(3), 320–326. https://doi.org/10.1016/j.annemergmed.2007.03.025

Schultz, C. H., Koenig, K. L., & Lewis, R. J. (2003). Implications of hospital evacuation after the Northridge, California, earthquake. *New England Journal of Medicine, 348*(14), 1349–1355. https://doi.org/10.1056/NEJMsa021807

Shultz, J. M., & Forbes, D. (2013). Psychological first aid: Rapid proliferation and the search for evidence. *Disaster Health, 2*(1), 3–12. https://doi.org/10.4161/dish.26006

Stratton, S. J., Hastings, V. P., & Isbell, D. (1996). The 1994 Northridge earthquake disaster response: The local emergency medical services agency experience. *Prehospital and Disaster Medicine, 11*(3), 172–179. https://doi.org/10.1017/s1049023x00042916

Substance Abuse and Mental Health Services Administration. (n.d.). *Disaster Technical Assistance Center.* https://www.samhsa.gov/dtac

Sylwanowicz, L., Schreiber, M., & Anderson, C. (2018). Rapid triage of mental health risk in emergency medical workers: Findings from Typhoon Haiyan. *Disaster Medicine and Public Health Preparedness, 12*(1), 19–22. https://doi.org/10.1017/dmp.2017.37

Tanaka, E., Tennichi, H., Kameoka, S., & Kato, H. (2019). Long-term psychological recovery process and its associated factors among survivors of the Great Hanshin-Awaji Earthquake in Japan: A qualitative study. *BMJ Open, 9*(8), e030250. https://doi.org/10.1136/bmjopen-2019-030250

U.S. Department of Health and Human Services. (2020a). *Disclosures for emergency preparedness—A decision tool.* https://www.hhs.gov/hipaa/for-professionals/special-topics/emergency-preparedness/decision-tool/index.html

U.S. Department of Health and Human Services. (2020b). *The emergency system for advance registration of volunteer health professionals (ESAR-VHP).* https://www.phe.gov/esarvhp/Pages/about.aspx

U.S. Department of Homeland Security. (2019). *National response framework* (4th ed.). Author. https://www.fema.gov/sites/default/files/2020-04/NRF_FINALApproved_2011028.pdf

U.S. Department of Housing and Urban Development. (1995). Office policy development and research. *Preparing for the "big one": Saving lives through earthquake mitigation in Los Angeles, California.* https://www.hsdl.org/?view&did=806248

U.S. Environmental Protection Agency, U.S. Forest Service, U.S. Centers for Disease Control and Prevention, California Air Resources Board, California Department of Public Health. (2016). *Wildfire smoke: A guide for public health officials.*

Western Regional Alliance for Pediatric Emergency Management. (2020). https://wrap-em.org/index.php

CHAPTER 9

WILDFIRES

EVALUATING THE CARDIORESPIRATORY HEALTH OF WILDLAND FIREFIGHTERS

DENISE M. GAUGHAN, MARK D. HOOVER, CHRISTOPHER A. KIRBY, AND STEPHEN S. LEONARD

KEY TERMS

Chronic Obstructive Pulmonary Disease
Cytokines
Enzyme-Linked Immunosorbent Assay (ELISA)
Free Radicals
In Vitro–In Vivo
Micro-Orifice Uniform Deposit Impactor (MOUDI)
National Multi-Agency Coordinating Group
Oxidized Low-Density Lipoprotein

INTRODUCTION

Wildland fires can pose grave occupational health risks to firefighters, as well as risks to wildlife, the environment, and communities. Cardiorespiratory health effects among firefighters are of special concern, along with risks of traumatic injury or death from firefighting-associated activities, such as entrapment in the fire, and from vehicle and air transport crashes. This case study chapter provides public health students and practitioners with an introduction and overview of the increasing risks from wildfires, health issues for firefighters, firefighting organization and practices, and vignettes of experiences and lessons learned from scientific field investigations and laboratory investigations of wildland firefighter (WLFF) health conducted by researchers

---

The following icons, located in the margins throughout the chapter and within the summary tables, denote essential services of public health, CEPH competencies, and leadership levels: Essential services of public health; CEPH competencies; Leadership levels.

at the National Institute for Occupational Safety and Health (NIOSH) and the Harvard School of Public Health.

THE INCREASING RISKS FROM WILDFIRES

According to wildland fire statistics collected by the U.S. government, the number and intensity of wildfires has grown over the past decades, with approximately 7.1 million acres being destroyed in an average North American wildland Fire season between 2010 and 2019 (National Interagency Fire Center [NIFC], 2020b). The year 2012 involved extremely arid conditions (i.e., the worst U.S. drought since 1934), and 9.3 million acres burned in wildfires. In 2018, the Camp Fire was the deadliest and most destructive wildfire in California history and the most expensive global natural disaster in 2018 in terms of insured losses (Reyes-Velarde, 2019). Similarly, Australia experienced one of its worst droughts in decades in 2019 and 2020, with 46.3 million acres ravaged by wildfires, killing 34 people, an estimated 1 billion animals, and destruction of over 5,900 buildings (Dickman, 2020). The growing annual extent and intensity of wildfires spurs increasing concern for the health of exposed individuals, especially the seasonal and permanent WLFFs employed each year by the U.S. federal government.

HEALTH ISSUES

Firefighters are known to have respiratory and cardiovascular problems (Adetona et al., 2016; Cascio et al., 2018; Yoo & Franke, 2009).[1] At the 1997 Consensus Conference on the Health Hazards of Smoke, WLFF health and safety experts reported that respiratory problems were common in WLFFs and accounted for 30% to 50% of visits to fire incident medical aid stations (Sharkey, 1997). Cardiovascular disease (CVD) events are the leading cause of on-duty and lifetime mortality among structural (career and volunteer) firefighters (Kales et al., 2003; Sardinas et al., 1986; Yoo & Franke, 2009). The deleterious effects of smoke exposure to structural firefighters have been extensively researched (Burgess et al., 2001; Centers for Disease Control and Prevention [CDC], 2006; Chia et al., 1990; Kales et al., 2003; Liu et al., 1992; Musk et al., 1979; Scannell & Balmes, 1995; Yoo & Franke, 2009). Exposure to particulates and other contaminants, heavy physical exertion, and cardiovascular strain have been found to be among the chief health hazards associated with structural firefighting (Delfino et al., 2009; Gaughan, Christiani, et al., 2014; Gledhill & Jamnik, 1992; Takeyama et al., 2005). Those findings, however, may not be generalizable to WLFFs for a number of reasons, including the difference in smoke composition, as well as the possible comparative younger age of WLFFs, the generally shorter career tenure of WLFFs, and the longer duration of respiratory exposures per incident (up to several weeks instead of just minutes or hours) for WLFFs as compared to structural firefighters. Additionally, structural firefighters routinely wear respiratory protection when responding to fires while WLFFs do not.

Studies examining respiratory symptoms and pulmonary function in WLFFs have found increases in symptoms, airways hyperresponsiveness, and declines

[1] Additional references of interest are Austin et al. (2001), Betchley et al. (1997), Burgess et al. (2001), Centers for Disease Control and Prevention (CDC) (2006), Chia et al. (1990), Gaughan et al. (2008), Guidotti & Clough (1992), Kales et al. (2003), Liu et al. (1992), Materna et al. (1992), Musk et al. (1979), Rothman et al. (1991), Sardinas et al. (1986), Scannel & Balmes (1995), Slaughter et al. (2004), and Takeyama et al. (2005).

in lung function cross-shift and cross-season (Betchley et al., 1997; Letts et al., 1991; Liu et al., 1992; Reh et al., 1994; Rothman et al., 1991; Sharkey, 1997; Slaughter et al., 2004). A longitudinal study conducted by NIOSH from May 2004 to May 2007 (Gaughan et al. 2008) observed significantly increased upper and lower respiratory symptoms, including cough, wheeze, sputum production, inflammatory indicators in sputum and nasal exudate, shortness of breath or chest tightness, shortness of breath while walking, and various eye, nose, and throat symptoms, postfire compared to preseason (i.e., health conditions of the firefighters after they conducted firefighting duties compared to their health conditions before they were deployed for firefighting duties in an annual firefighting season). This finding is consistent with observations made by Rothman et al. (1991), who observed a significant increase in eye irritation, nose irritation, cough, phlegm, and wheezing from preseason to late season among WLFFs, with strong associations noted for recent firefighting activity. In the longitudinal study by the NIOSH, the increased scores for lower respiratory symptoms observed postfire returned to near preseason levels during the postseason. Upper respiratory symptom scores remained significantly elevated at postseason compared to preseason, although scores were significantly lower at postseason compared to postfire. These observations suggest substantial recovery from respiratory tract effects of firefighting by the time of the authors' postseason assessment. Nevertheless, the finding in multifactor analyses that cumulative time spent fighting fires over a career was significantly associated with increased upper (but not lower) respiratory symptoms suggests that wildfire-associated exposure may produce a more sustained rhinitis/sinusitis (Gaughan et al., 2008). Conversely, Betchley et al. (1997) observed no significant increase in symptoms cross-season in their study of 53 WLFFs, but their postseason testing was done well over a month later in the season than the NIOSH study and may have allowed for more complete recovery. A practical limitation of longitudinal studies such as these is that not all crew members return to the same crew for multiple seasons. For example, in the NIOSH study, only half the members of one crew (10 out of 20) returned for the next season. The possibility that some crew members do not return because of health issues or health concerns raises the possibility that the actual magnitude of health effects may be underreported.

These previously observed increases in subjective symptoms and declines in objective measures of lung function suggest that wildland firefighting is associated with upper and lower airway inflammation and raise concern about potential risk of long-term respiratory effects, including asthma, **chronic obstructive pulmonary disease** (COPD), and upper airway conditions such as sinusitis.

Navarro et al. (2019) used a number of assumptions about smoke concentration levels, frequencies and durations of exposures per year, number of years in the career of a firefighter, and health effects of a given smoke exposure to estimate the relative risk of CVD mortality based on existing PM2.5 exposure–response relationships. An example of their assessment is that the lifetime risk of mortality from CVD for a firefighter who was exposed for 98 days per year for a career duration of 25 years would be 30% higher than the lifetime risk to someone who was not exposed in that manner.

Health risks to firefighters also include traumatic physical injury and even death. The fire with the greatest toll of deaths prior to 1950 was the Mann Gulch Fire in 1949, which occurred north of Helena, Montana, at the Gates of the Mountains area along the Missouri River. Thirteen firefighters died. This disaster directly led to the establishment of safety standards, some of which are still used today by all WLFFs. On July 6, 1994, nine members of a firefighting crew based in Prineville, Oregon, died after being overtaken by the fast-moving Storm King Fire west of Glenwood Springs, Colorado. Five other firefighters also died in the fire. On June 30, 2013, the 19 members of the Prescott Fire Department's wildfire fighting crew (known as the Granite Mountain Hotshots) perished in the Yarnell Hill Fire near Yarnell, Arizona, when their escape route was cut off by the approaching fire.

Health risks to firefighters also include exposures to infectious diseases. In 2020, in response to the COVID-19 pandemic, the **National Multi-Agency Coordinating Group** established three regional Area Command Teams that, along with partners at all levels of the fire community, developed protocols which were integrated into nine Wildland Fire Response Plans (WFRP; www.nifc.gov/fireInfo/covid-19.htm). Topics include: Fire Personnel Readiness; Modifying Strategies, Tactics, and Logistics; Drawdown Projections and Contingency Opportunities; and Leveraging Best Available Information Management and Technology. Tactical information is intended for local area fire managers, Incident Management Organizations, and the "boots on the ground" in the format of Best Management Practices. These region-specific WRFPs provide guidance and considerations for strategic and tactical information for maintaining continuity of wildland fire response in the presence of the COVID-19 virus for all levels of wildland fire response—from national level, regional level, and local level to module level.

WILDLAND FIREFIGHTING ORGANIZATION AND PRACTICES

The North American wildland fire season typically runs from May through November. The National Interagency Coordination Center (n.d.) mobilizes local, regional, and national firefighting resources. Firefighter assignments to specific fire incidents can be for up to 14 consecutive days, followed by two obligate days off. In some situations, assignments may be extended to 21 days; however, this is somewhat rare. While at a fire, the shift duration can vary, depending on the nature of the fire, the terrain and weather, and the available number of firefighters. Some shifts may extend to 12 hours or more. Thus, sleep deprivation may be reported as a pervasive concern among these workers. Moreover, resultant stress from sleep restriction may be an independent risk factor for cardiovascular morbidity (Austin et al., 2001).

The other demands of wildland firefighting can also be profound. Some crews may work from camps in remote areas, eating prepackaged food, with limited access to sanitation or shower facilities during their assignment. On larger fires, crews may be assigned to fire camps with hundreds if not thousands of other firefighters where hot meals, showers, and handwashing stations may be available under crowded conditions.

Additionally, a person's daily caloric consumption to maintain work performance and cognitive abilities at a wildland fire operation routinely can be quite high (e.g., 4,000 to 6,000 calories during arduous duty activities on the fireline; NWCC, 2020). The high level of duty activities is important to note because prolonged, intense exercise may amplify **oxidized low-density lipoprotein** generation, which is associated with atherosclerotic plaque (Ashley & Kannel, 1974), and because changes in body composition (defined as the ratio of fat to lean muscle) may hasten the development of CVD (Higgins et al., 1993; Lissner et al., 1991).

Examples of Firefighting Crew Types

As described in the following, firefighting crews are differentiated based on increasing levels of experience, leadership, and availability. Categories of federal WLFF crew types per the 2020 edition of the *Interagency Standards for Fire and Fire Aviation Operations* (commonly referred to as the Interagency Redbook) are Type 1, Type 2 IA (Initial Attack Capable), and Type 2 (NIFC, 2020a). Crews typically comprise 18 to 20 men and women, including a crew boss and squad bosses who supervise the crew's actual work. Duties may involve serving as "lead" workers, the individuals who oversee all crew operations; "line" workers, those who construct the fire line; "sawyers," the chain-saw operators who clear the way for fire line construction; and "swampers," who shadow the sawyers, removing the fallen debris. Fire line construction is defined as clearing vegetation and exposing bare soil by cutting, scraping, or digging to create a break in fuel availability. Mop-up operations involve extinguishing or removing burning material along or near a fire line after the fire has been controlled. When not on wildland fire assignments, crews are stationed at their home unit, and they perform project work such as collecting samples of vegetation, identifying plant species, documenting wildland fuel loading, and conducting prescribed burning and other fuel-reduction activities.

Smoke Jumpers

Smoke jumpers are specially trained Type 1 WLFFs who provide an initial attack response on remote wildland fires. They are transported by plane or helicopter and descend by parachute to the site of the fire. In addition to performing the initial attack on wildfires, and like other qualified WLFF professionals, they may also provide leadership for extended attacks on wildland fires. Shortly after smoke jumpers touch ground, they are supplied by parachute with food, water, and firefighting tools, making them self-sufficient for 48 hours. Today, nine smoke jumper crews operate in the United States. Seven are operated by the U.S. Forest Service (USFS), and two are operated by the Bureau of Land Management (BLM).

The minimum required physical fitness standards for smoke jumpers set by the National Wildfire Coordinating Group are carry a pack loaded with 110 lb for three miles within 90 minutes; run 1.5 miles in 11 or fewer minutes; and perform 25 push-ups in 60 seconds, 45 sit-ups in 60 seconds, and seven pull-ups.

Interagency Hotshot Crews

Type 1 Interagency Hotshot Crews (IHCs) are elite crews who often construct fire lines using hand tools during the most dangerous phases of wildland fire suppression. Type 1 crews often comprise 20 members. In the United States, hotshot crews are organized by agencies such as the USFS, the National Park Service, the Bureau of Indian Affairs, the BLM, and state/county agencies. The NIFC in Boise, Idaho, coordinates hotshot crews on the national level.

All IHC crew members are expected to strive to meet the fitness criteria developed by the National Wildfire Coordinating Group (Sharkey & Gaskill, 2009). These criteria include the ability to perform the following: 1.5 mile run in a time of 10:35 or less, 40 sit-ups in 60 seconds, 25 push-ups in 60 seconds, and chin-ups based on body weight as follows: four chin-ups for body weight more than 170 lb, five chin-ups for 135 to 170 lb, six chin-ups for 110 to 135 lb, and seven chin-ups for less than 110 lb.

Engine, Helitack, and Air Tanker Crews

Engine crews are generally made up of 3 to 5 WLFFs. A typical wildland fire engine is an off-road vehicle able to carry water for use in firefighting. Many wildland fire engines also carry foam to use on wildland fuels to help extend the use of the limited water supply they have. Engine crews are used in initial response to a fire, sometimes providing structure protection, holding burnout operations, patrolling, providing structure protection, and conducting mop-up activities.

Helitack crews are specially trained in the tactical and logistical use of helicopters for fire suppression. These crews can be rapidly deployed and are often the first to respond to a wildland fire. Some helitack crews are also trained to "rappel" from a hovering helicopter in areas where the terrain or vegetation does not allow the helicopter to land. Others are trained in operations for rescue missions on fires. Other helitack duties may be loading and unloading thousands of pounds of equipment and supplies needed for firefighting, commonly called "cargo," and manifesting and loading and unloading firefighters headed to the fireline (USFS, 2017). Air tanker crews use fixed-wing aircraft to apply water or other fire suppressants to the fire area.

The Incident Command System

The Incident Command System (ICS) is part of the National Incident Management System and was created in response to a series of destructive wildfires in southern California in 1970 (FEMA, 2020). National, state, and local emergency responders required a tool to effectively provide command and control functions while coordinating the efforts of many individual agencies and departments working together to stabilize a disaster while protecting life, property, and the environment. The ICS is used by emergency responders across the nation as well as by local governments and agencies. ICS is successful because it uses a common organizational structure with standardized management principles. The ICS is a management system designed to enable effective and efficient domestic incident management by integrating a combination of facilities, equipment, personnel, procedures, and communications operating within a common organizational structure. ICS is normally structured to facilitate activities in five major functional areas: command, operations, planning, logistics, and finance/administration. The incident commander typically is supported by a public information officer, a liaison officer, and a safety officer. The ICS is a scalable structure, and it may also include intelligence and investigations, as well as epidemiology. It is a fundamental form of management, with the purpose of enabling incident managers to identify the key concerns associated with the incident—often under urgent conditions—without sacrificing attention to any component of the command system.

Emergency Responder Health Monitoring and Surveillance

A plan for monitoring emergency responder health and conducting surveillance for diseases and health conditions associated with emergency responders is essential to ensure the health and safety of the responders. The NIOSH has worked with the U.S. National Response Team (NRT, www.nrt.org), and a number of federal agencies, state health departments, labor unions, and volunteer emergency responder groups to develop the Emergency Responder Health Monitoring and Surveillance™ (ERHMS™) framework (NIOSH, 2020a). The ERHMS™ framework provides recommendations for protecting emergency responders during small and large emergencies in any setting. It may be used by all who are involved in the deployment and protection of emergency responders, including incident command staff; response organization leadership; health, safety, and medical personnel; and emergency responders. ERHMS™ training is available online (CDC, 2020). The application of ERHMS™ in wildland firefighting situations could be a useful augmentation to the ICS.

VIGNETTES ON EVALUATING THE CARDIOVASCULAR HEALTH OF WILDLAND FIREFIGHTERS

Within the many areas of knowledge, skills, and abilities that public health practitioners require to understand, communicate, and manage the health risks associated with wildland fires, an area of special expertise involves the harnessing of the multiple disciplines of exposure assessment, field and laboratory methodologies, medicine, and epidemiology and biostatistics. The following sections present examples of how the integration of these disciplines was carried out for the field portion and for the laboratory portion of longitudinally designed NIOSH and the Harvard School of Public Health studies of the cardiorespiratory effects of particulate exposures in two IHCs (Gaughan et al., 2008; Gaughan, Piacitelli, et al., 2014; Gaughan, Siegel, et al., 2014; Leonard et al., 2007).

Field Issues for Evaluating the Cardiorespiratory Health of Wildland Firefighters

To successfully design and implement an epidemiological study in the organizationally and logistically complex wildfire environment, a number of field issues had to be anticipated, communicated, and managed. From 2004 through 2006, NIOSH public health practitioners applied epidemiological methods to monitor the respiratory health status of affected firefighters by collecting medical and exposure data preseason, during a wildfire or prescribed fire setting, and postseason (in October, a minimum of 2 weeks' postfire exposure) consisting of all members of two Type 1 IHCs employed by the National Park Service. The Alpine IHC of Rocky Mountain National Park was studied preseason; for 7 days while fighting the Boundary Fire (Fox, AK, July 2004), which was a very large and intense wildfire; for 7 days while working the Tuolumne Grove Fire (Yosemite National Park, CA, October 2005), a less intense prescribed burn; and for 6 days while fighting the Red Eagle Fire (Glacier National Park, MT, August 2006), a large wildfire.

In addition, the Arrowhead IHC of Sequoia and Kings Canyon National Parks was studied preseason and for 3 days while fighting the South Sundance Fire Complex (Sundance, WY, July 2005), a smaller wildfire that was nearly completely contained during the period of testing. Preseason participation was 100% for both crews in all years. In May 2011, a follow-up study of the Alpine IHC was conducted by the Harvard School of Public Health and NIOSH. This cross-sectional survey expanded the medical data collection to include measures of arterial stiffness and oxidative stress.

Consistent with the essential public health service of communicating effectively and the essential public health service of strengthening, supporting, and mobilizing communities and partnerships to improve health, members of the wildfire research team made formal presentations and question-and-answer sessions to each crew at the beginning of each fire season detailing the proposed health study methods. Written informed consent was obtained from each crew member. End-of-season presentations about the study results to date were made to each crew at the conclusion of each fire season. Similar presentations were made as well to the NIFC, the DOI, and the USFS stakeholders at various times during the study. In addition, a daylong workshop of stakeholder experts was held in March 2005 at the NIOSH to discuss the first-year results and future study plans in detail.

In addition, consistent with the essential public health service to build and support a diverse and skilled public health workforce, the NIOSH trained the occupational health technicians who conducted lung function testing on federal WLFFs. This was part of the larger medical standards program to ensure safety that has been established by the DOI (see www.nifc.gov/medical_standards/Program/index.html). The technicians received the 16-hour NIOSH spirometry certification at no cost. Following training, the technicians were provided with the spirometry equipment and supplies. The technicians submitted spirometry test results (tracings) for quality review by the NIOSH for 1 year. Feedback from trained NIOSH experts was then provided back to technicians.

As public health practitioners who were external partners to the formal wildland fire ICS, the NIOSH investigators undertook a number of steps to become familiar with, and to become qualified to participate in, the details and procedures of wildland firefighting. These actions are consistent with the essential public health service to build and support a diverse and skilled public health workforce and can serve as an example to other public health practitioners who may want or need to become directly involved in emergency response involving specialized situations. NIOSH technicians began by becoming certified in Basic Firefighter Training and Wildland Fire Behavior (S130/190) and Introduction to the Incident Command System (ICS-100) at the Arizona Wildfire Academy, Prescott, Arizona; the Colorado Wildfire Fire and Incident Management Academy, Alamosa, Colorado; the Utah Fire and Rescue Academy, Orem, Utah; and the local USFS, Morgantown, West Virginia. The National Fire Academy S130/190 and the ICS-100 courses are also now available online (U.S. Fire Administration, n.d.). Field technicians were also fitness-rated at the moderate level in what is known as the Work Capacity Field Test (WCFT; Figure 9.1). This test involves walking two miles in 30 minutes wearing a 25-lb weight vest and is an annual requirement of the National Wildfire Coordinating Group (2021). The WCFT was administered in the spring by the local USFS preceding preseason data collection.

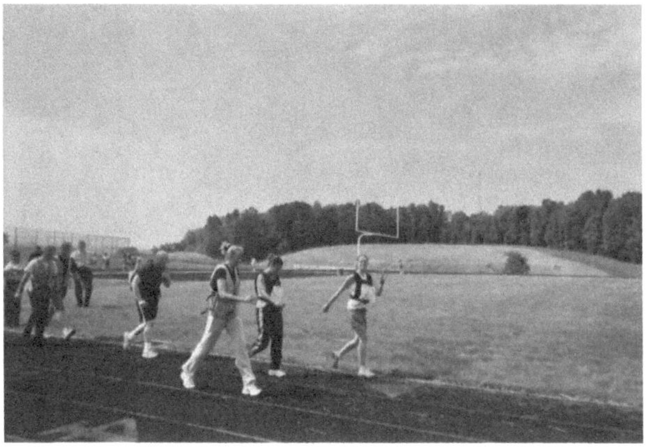

Figure 9.1 NIOSH wildland fire research team members preparing for participation in wildfire field activities by taking the U.S. Forest Service's annual Work Capacity Field Test, Morgantown, West Virginia.

Medical Data of Interest

Medical field technicians on the wildland fire research team collected questionnaire data, blood pressure, spirometry, bronchial hyperresponsiveness, exhaled breath carbon monoxide (CO), blood, urine, pulse wave velocity for arterial stiffness assessment, and sputum and nasal lavage for markers of inflammation (Figure 9.2).

Additionally, to diagnose and investigate public health problems associated with affected firefighters, spirometry and exhaled breath CO were collected pre- and post-shift (Figure 9.3). Samples were placed on dry ice and shipped overnight to the NIOSH in Morgantown, West Virginia, for processing. Technicians collecting spirometry had completed the NIOSH 16-hour spirometry certification training course (NIOSH, 2020b), and all were trained in their designated procedures following standard manual of procedures (MOPs).

Environmental Data of Interest

To understand the concentrations and composition of smoke to which the firefighters were exposed, personal and area sampling devices were provided to

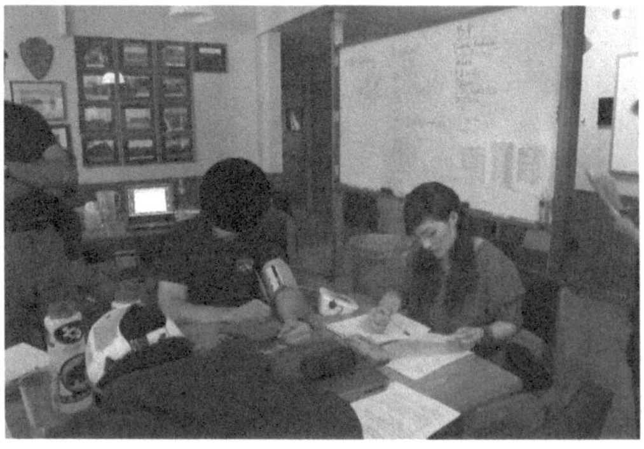

Figure 9.2 A wildland fire research team member applies epidemiology skills by collecting preseason medical data from an IHC crewmember at the Alpine IHC home base, Rocky Mountain National Park, Estes Park, Colorado.

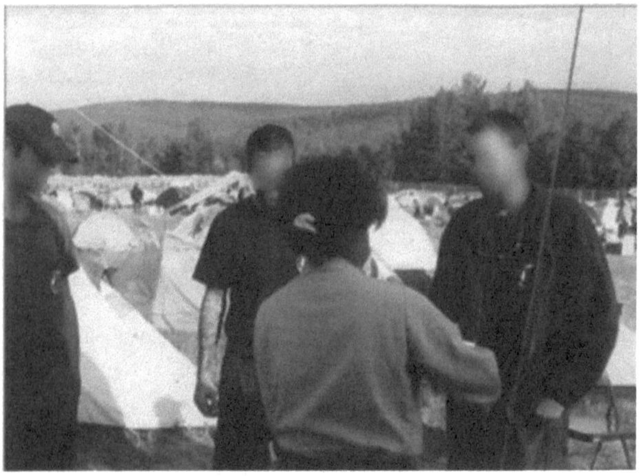

Figure 9.3 A wildfire research team member meets with IHC crewmembers to conduct pre-shift exhaled breath CO testing at the Boundary Fire, Fox, Alaska.

the crews by the NIOSH investigators. Figure 9.4 shows research team members packing field equipment into the fire area.

Environmental field technicians collected sets of aerodynamically size-selected aerosol samples using the **Micro-Orifice Uniform Deposit Impactor (MOUDI)** model 110 with rotator (MSP, Inc., Minneapolis, MN) for area samples. Each Hotshot agreed to wear a personal real-time (RT) personal breathing zone CO monitor (Industrial Scientific Corporation, Oakdale, PA); and one of the following: a filter cassette with a 10-mm nylon respirable cyclone to measure respirable particulate concentration and either a respirable levoglucosan (LG, an indicator of burning biomass) concentration or a respirable crystalline silica concentration; a personal cascade impactor to measure particle size distribution, total concentrations of particulates and LG, and respirable concentrations of particulates and LG; or a personal DataRAM monitor (Thermo Scientific Corporation, Franklin, MA) to measure RT particulate in the size range of 0.1 to 10 μm. NIOSH environmental field technicians shadowed the crews, periodically checking the personal and area samplers for the duration of the shift. At the conclusion of the work shift, the samplers would be returned to a technician

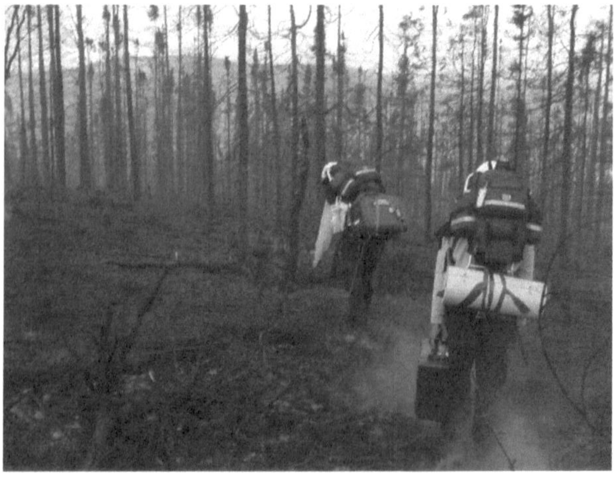

Figure 9.4. Wildfire research team members packing field equipment into the fire area at the Boundary Fire, Fox, Alaska.

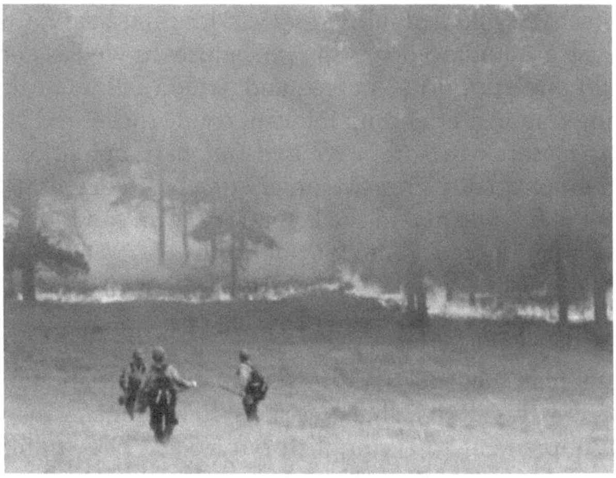

Figure 9.5 View of the Alpine IHC approaching the fire line at the Tuolumne Grove Fire, Yosemite National Park, California.

staying at a local hotel who would charge the pumps and place the filters on nitrogen or dry ice for shipment back to the NIOSH in Morgantown, West Virginia, for processing. Figure 9.5 shows sampler-equipped firefighter crew members approaching a fire line.

Laboratory Issues for Evaluating the Cardiorespiratory Health of Wildland Firefighters

To successfully design and implement an epidemiological study in the organizationally and logistically complex wildfire environment, a number of laboratory issues had to be anticipated, communicated, and managed. The following sections describe both general and specific thought processes and actions that were taken in the NIOSH respiratory studies. These can serve as an example for public health practitioners who may be faced with the coordination of laboratory issues in their own areas of emergency response practice. Planning and cooperation between the principal investigators, the team leaders of the laboratory, and the skilled technicians who carry out the research are crucial for the success of the project. As part of the laboratory team's goals they must keep in mind the 10 essential public health services. Assessment and monitoring of the health status of WLFF populations are performed by the field team. Investigation, diagnosing, and identifying hazards affecting the WLFF population are performed through literature searches and epidemiology studies. Communicating effectively to inform and educate people about the hazards will come through the publication of findings in scientific journals and presentations of data at conferences. Strengthening, supporting, and mobilizing communities and partnerships to improve health will be a result of information and data the laboratory investigation provides. While the laboratory cannot create and implement policies and laws, the data and findings are used to establish these through recommended exposure limits and hazard identification. The laboratory findings and publications will provide a basis for legal and regulatory actions designed to improve and protect the public's health. The identification of specific hazards and biological pathways involved can help assure an effective system of individual services and healthcare. Up-to-date training and the use of standard operating procedures as well as good laboratory practice will build and support a diverse and skilled public health workforce. Providing ongoing training, attending relevant conferences, and staying abreast of other scientific research will improve and innovate public health functions resulting in continuous quality improvement. Effective interactions and communication between the field team and the laboratory team can build and maintain a strong organizational infrastructure for public health.

Project Planning for Sample Collection and Analysis

The first questions that need to be addressed in any occupational health study are, why are we doing this study, what questions do we hope to answer, and what strategy will we implement to accomplish our goals? The strategy to answer these questions will help determine the biological and toxicological endpoints to be measured and must be developed by the principal investigator or team leader. The laboratory must also look at the assets they have; personnel, equipment, instruments, and laboratory skill sets will all be used in assessing possible endpoints. Once the goals, strategy, and endpoints have been determined it is important for the laboratory team and field team to meet. Encouraging all personnel involved to see not just their individual responsibilities but also the "big picture" is essential for idea exchange, independent thinking and maximizing individual contributions to the project.

Communication is the most important aspect in any situation where field teams and laboratory teams are working together. It is vital that both groups work together and prepare for the study as thoroughly as possible prior to its start. The field team must understand what sample types the laboratory will need and how they will be treated, handled, and shipped back to the laboratory. The laboratory must recognize that the field team will be working in difficult, even dangerous, conditions, and once on-site they may have very limited access to electrical power, refrigeration, or any supplies or materials that they may run short of. Communication starts with both teams, or team representatives, meeting and discussing the sampling strategy and requirements. The laboratory team should present a prioritized "wish list" of analysis endpoints, and together both teams can access what they can realistically collect. Items to be considered include samplers, collection materials, sample volume, sample storage, and sample shipment back to the laboratory. Samplers can be heavy and may require batteries or generators to take collections. The field team may also only be able to deploy a limited number of these samplers. Personal samplers are smaller but also require batteries, time, and a trained individual to place them on the firefighters (Figure 9.6).

All samplers require some sort of filter and replacement filters, which require proper storage and handling to prevent contamination before use, as well as proper installation into the sampler. The laboratory and field teams need to agree on the volumes to be collected based on the time on-site and materials present. This will allow the laboratory team to determine number and types of endpoints they can measure and prioritize them. Handling and storage of samples will be a challenge in the field environment. Will the samples need to be refrigerated, frozen, or stored under a special head gas? These needs may necessitate coolers, blue ice, dry ice, and special gas tanks. The research team must ask the field team if these needs can be met. Shipping of the samples must also be considered. What kind of access to shipping points does the field team have,

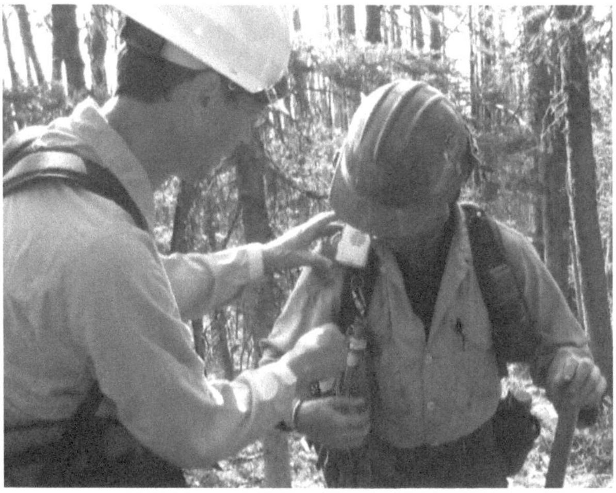

Figure 9.6 Wildfire research team member installing a personal air sampler on a wildland firefighter at the Red Eagle Fire, Glacier National Park, Montana.

or will they directly carry the collected samples back to the laboratory when they return from the site? Labeling is paramount for effective communication between field and laboratory teams. Both teams must agree on a simple, clear method for labeling the samples in order to avoid any confusion and assist in a smooth transition from field to laboratory. Filters, tubes, bottles, or any other collection vessels should be pre-labeled before going into the field to avoid mistakes. Sitting on a mountainside in 90-degree heat with your eyes watering from smoke exposure may make a simple task in the laboratory difficult in the field.

Skills needed for this area of the project are leadership, strategic planning, interpersonal communication, and organizational management.

Goals of the Laboratory Research Team

Determining the research strategy generates a selection of productive endpoints. The chosen endpoints then dictate sample types and sample volumes to possibly be collected by the research team. Beyond the physical dangers, WLFFs are exposed to a variety of inhaled hazards (Broyles, 2013). These inhaled hazards can vary depending on location, material of burn, temperature of burn, and weather conditions (EPA, 2021). Wildfire smoke particle toxicity depends on volume, size of particles, and chemical makeup. Important characteristics of inhaled particle toxicity are particle size and aerodynamic diameter, which together determine how far into the respiratory tract a particle can penetrate and be deposited. Different locations in the respiratory tract have different methods of dealing with and clearing particles as well as various sensitivities to their effects. The chemical characteristics of a particle are also important in determining its toxicity once it is deposited in the respiratory tract (Cheng et al., 1999). Is it soluble, insoluble, or persistent? Soluble particles may transmit their components into the bloodstream or other areas of the respiratory tract, while persistent particles may cause chronic conditions (Tarlo, 2012). As shown in Figure 9.7, there are three basic regions in the respiratory tract: nasopharyngeal (nose, sinuses, pharynx), tracheobronchial (trachea, upper bronchus), and pulmonary (bronchioles, alveoli).

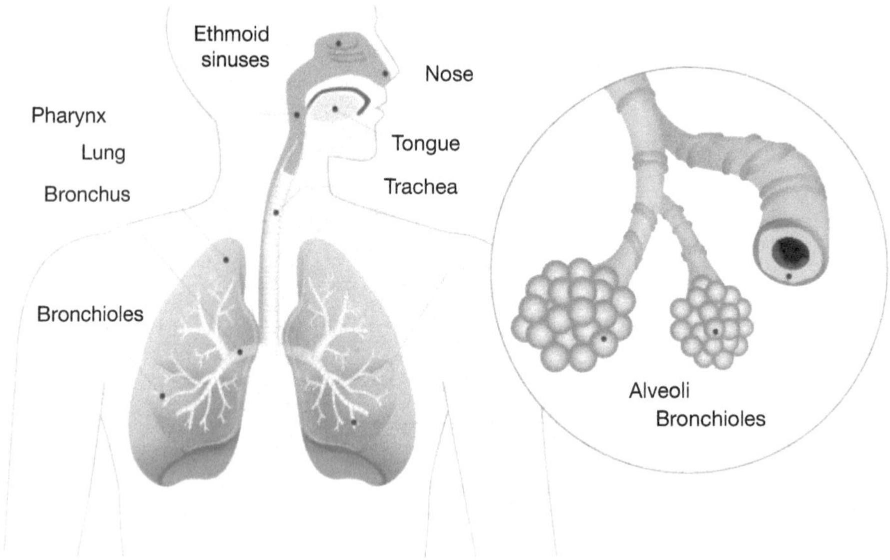

Figure 9.7 Respiratory tract showing major areas of possible exposure.

Clearing particles from these areas takes different forms. The mucociliary escalator covers most of the bronchi and bronchioles. It is composed of mucus-producing goblet cells and ciliated epithelium particles that are trapped in the mucus; cilia movement directs the particles into the pharynx, where they are swallowed and cleared (Stuart, 1984). If a particle is inhaled and deposited in the pulmonary region, which is composed of the lung's small bronchioles and alveolar sacs, the particle encounters a sensitive, high surface area environment specifically designed to absorb. The alveolar sacs are made up of a thin layer of cells and therefore it is relatively easy for toxins to cross into the bloodstream. This area is defended by macrophages that engulf and destroy most particles and bacteria; however, persistent particles can remain in the alveolar sacs and may cause chronic toxic conditions (Oberdörster et al., 1994). These physical and chemical characteristics of the particles are factors that the laboratory must consider when planning their analysis.

Skills needed for this part of the study are a comprehension of physics and a grasp of how surface area influences particle behavior in the respiratory tract, of the chemistry of particles and how this can impact their toxicity, and of basic human physiology and structure of the bronchopulmonary zone.

Type of Exposure Model

An important part of the particle analysis and testing is deciding whether to use either **in vitro or in vivo** testing. In vitro assays include those performed or taking place in a test tube, culture dish, or elsewhere outside a living organism. These can include chemical, enzymatic, cellular, and ex vivo organ systems. In vitro systems can provide good models of reaction systems if properly used. They provide testing for determination of initial toxicity and dosages without using animals. In vitro assays can also provide valuable mechanistic information of biological pathways involved in reactions. When using in vitro cellular systems there are many choices available. Cell lines provide relatively durable cells which can be grown in media and used in exposure assessments (D. D. Allen et al., 2005).

One disadvantage of cell lines is that they are transformed cells and may not provide an accurate model of cells in living systems. Primary cells are cells that are taken directly from living tissue and established for growth in vitro (Roggen, 2011). This increases their relevance as a model of living systems, but they are more challenging to culture. Both cell lines and primary cells have advantages and drawbacks, so the selection of an in vitro cellular system is dependent on experimental conditions. In addition to different cellular systems, cells themselves can be grown and maintained in a variety of ways. Cells can be grown in a suspension of media, on the surface of culture plates while immersed in liquid media, or even in an air–liquid interface, where the top surface of the cell is exposed to the atmosphere while the base of the cell is bathed in media (Lacroix et al., 2018). Air–liquid interface cell culture allows direct access to the cells for vapor, gas, and small particle exposures.

In vivo animal models can provide a "whole system" approach to test exposures, and the interaction of multiple biological pathways can be measured at once (Nemmar, 2013). Crosstalk between various biological systems through signaling can influence modulation of an organism's response. In vivo systems can also provide information for short-term, long-term, and repeated exposures as well as chronic outcomes, none of which may be an option with in vitro systems. Exposures can be accomplished through inhaled material, intratracheal instillation, dermal exposures, injection, and ingestion. The use of animals in research carries tremendous ethical responsibility for their proper care, handling, and use. When animal exposures are used, the researcher must try to maximize the number of useful endpoints that can be obtained from each animal. Before any animals are ordered, the researcher must also provide a protocol to their Institutional Animal Care and Use Committee (IACUC), which will review the plan. In addition, the researcher must establish the reasoning behind the study, need for the study, novelty of the study, and statistical justification for the number of animals requested. This is usually a multi-step procedure with the IACUC adding refinements and clarifications throughout the process. Only once the researcher has shown animal use justification and proper animal handling techniques are they permitted to use animals in the project. The in vitro or in vivo system that the laboratory uses depends on the skills and instrumentation laboratory members possess, as well as the experimental model and specific aims of the study.

Skills needed include cell culture techniques, sterile method, dilution calculations, IACUC-certified courses on specific animals used, and animal anatomy knowledge.

Sample Characterization

Particles and fumes that penetrate into the respiratory system may have multiple effects and potentially cause varied types of toxicity and damage. The following is an example of the sample analysis plan we developed for wildfire smoke; however, this is not meant to be an all-encompassing strategy. Each situation will need to have a unique sampling and analysis plan developed by the research team.

For our wildfire study, airborne particles were collected and separated into discrete sizes using an MOUDI, including using a specialized nano-MOUDI device to collect particles in the ultrafine (smaller than 100 nm) size range

(Leonard et al., 2010; Figure 9.8). The MOUDI separates particles based on their size, which allows the researchers to understand which particles may penetrate to different depths in the respiratory system.

The MOUDI impactors are used for collecting size-fractionated particle samples in the 0.056 to 10 μm aerodynamic diameter range, which can be used for the collection of particles for gravimetric and/or chemical analyses. The different MOUDI models can hold different numbers of size stages, and the classic MOUDIs hold various impaction stages and cut sizes. Particle deposits are collected on standard 47-mm substrates that can be analyzed to determine mass or examined via chemical analysis or microscopy. Nano-MOUDIs increase the size range and number of fractions that can be captured. Personal cascade impactors are smaller devices that can be worn on an individual. Figure 9.9 illustrates the value of using particle size–selective sampling to characterize the wildfire aerosols.

An additional important aspect of the sample collection is the type of filter used in the aerosol impactors. Filter types should be compatible with both the collected material and the endpoint analysis to ensure there is no chemical interference from the filters themselves.

Wildfire smoke contains many different elements and characteristics. Because no two smoke samples are identical, we wanted to develop a broad analysis plan to investigate wildfire smoke's possible effects. Potential methods in particle characterization include mass spectrometry, x-ray diffraction, the

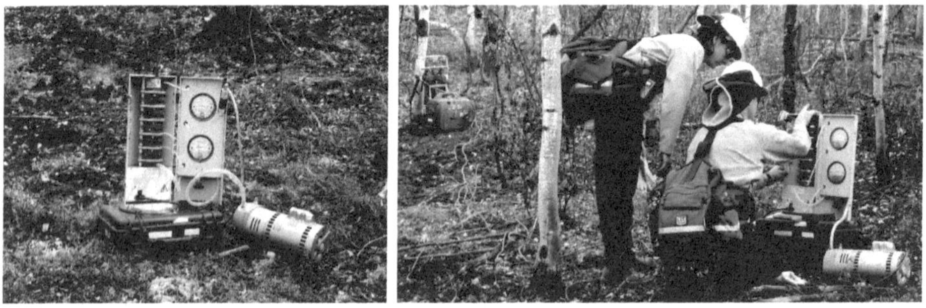

Figure 9.8 MOUDI particle collector (left) and MOUDI being set up by wildfire research team members in the field (right).

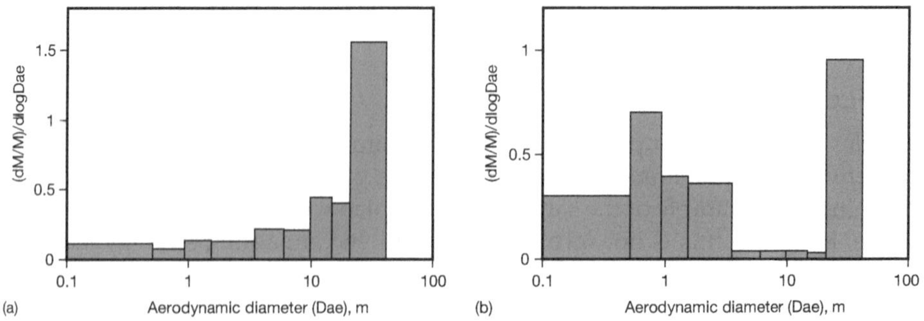

Figure 9.9 Normalized personal cascade impactor particle size distributions for (A) airborne particle mass and (B) airborne levoglucosan. Note that airborne particle mass is mostly associated with larger particles, while airborne levoglucosan is bimodally distributed.

Brunauer–Emmett–Teller (BET) method, and dynamic light scattering (DLS). Mass spectrometry separates isotopes, molecules, and molecular fragments according to mass (El-Aneed et al., 2009). The sample is vaporized and ionized, and the ions are accelerated in an electric field, deflected by a magnetic field, and launched into a curved trajectory yielding a distinctive mass spectrum. This can be matched to known samples, and the elemental profile of the sample can be determined. X-ray diffraction scatters x-rays through the regularly spaced atoms of a crystal, which obtains data about the structure of the crystal (Ameh, 2019). The BET method uses the physical adsorption of gas molecules on a solid surface for the measurement of materials, specific surface area (Gelb & Gubbins, 1998). DLS can be used to measure particle size down to the nanometer (Stetefeld et al., 2016).

In our wildfire study we first investigated the smoke's basic reactivity. When a smoke particle interacts with the lung, how could it react? Many particles were found to contain Fe2+ or other transition metals that can generate **free radicals** upon exposure to cells (Leonard et al., 2007). The high heat and freshly generated nature of wildfire smoke potentially make it likely to contain reactive materials. Therefore, a free radical analysis on the samples was performed using several methods: electron paramagnetic resonance (EPR; Davies, 2016), measurement of intracellular reactive oxygen species (ROS; Halliwell & Gutteridge, 2015), and the comet assay (Glei et al., 2016). A free radical is an uncharged molecule, typically highly reactive and short-lived, having an unpaired valence electron. In biology, a primary interest is the hydroxyl and superoxide radicals. It is important to note that radicals play an important role in a healthy biological system and are not always damaging. Hydroxyl radicals are an important part of the cellular defense system and superoxide radicals are integral to the mitochondrial electron transport chain, which is essential for generating cellular energy (Cogliati et al., 2018). Balancing these radicals in cellular systems is important. If the redox state is out of balance then the cells can accrue damage (Figure 9.10).

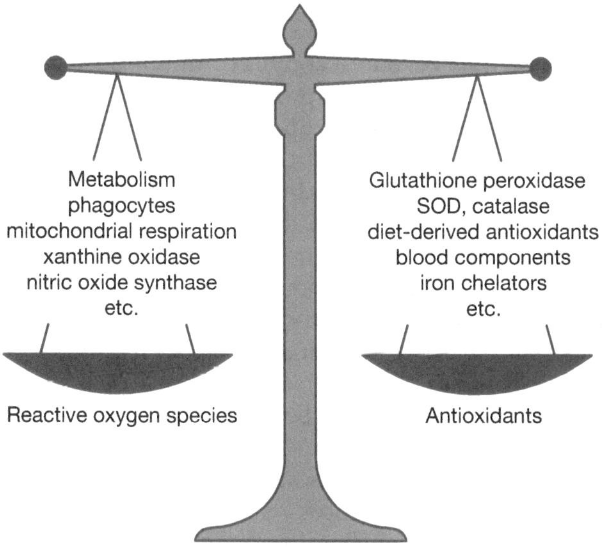

Figure 9.10 Illustration of how the ability of the body to balance radical generators and radical scavengers is important to overall health.

SOD, superoxide dismutase.

Free radicals can be detected by EPR in chemical, enzymatic, cellular, organ, and whole-body systems. As part of our wildfire study we used EPR in chemical and cellular systems. We first reacted wildfire smoke with hydrogen peroxide and macrophage cells to measure the basic reactivity of the smoke (Leonard et al., 2007). The wildfire smoke may react with the hydrogen peroxide to generate hydroxyl radicals. With the addition of a "spin trap," in this case 5,5-dimethyl-1-pyrroline N-oxide (DMPO), we can trap and measure the radicals. If the smoke does generate hydroxyl radicals, then we can determine its relative reactivity and ability to produce damaging radicals. Other assays and spin traps can measure superoxide radicals and nitroxide radicals. Superoxide radicals can be measured using EPR with the spin trap 5-(diethoxyphosphoryl)-5-methyl-1-pyrroline-N-oxide (Halliwell & Gutteridge, 2015) or by using various cell-staining methods. Nitroxide radicals can be measured using EPR and using light emissions such as luminescence and fluorescence. Depending on the study goals and laboratory capabilities, these assays may be used in your study.

Skills needed include a background in chemistry and physics and knowledge of chemical analysis, particle-sizing techniques, and materials testing.

Exposure Endpoints of Interest

As part of your initial proposal, it is critical to determine the endpoints that you wish to measure as part of your specific aims. These depend on the lab's abilities and the scope of the project. How many personnel do you have available for the study? How much sample do you have to work with? Are you looking at acute, chronic, or both types of endpoints? Are you using an in vitro or in vivo model? What is the timeline for obtaining finished results? All these questions will help you devise your endpoints and the data you will gather to address your specific aims.

The effects of inhaled material may be acute, eliciting a quick response, or chronic, either persistent for a long time or constantly recurring. Acute effects may exist only for a short duration, and recovery time may be brief, whereas chronic effects may last for years and present significant health problems (Tarlo, 2012). Inhalation of material may cause short-term coughing, congestion, and shortness of breath, or it may become a chronic condition such as asthma, COPD, pulmonary fibrosis, asbestosis, silicosis, pneumonitis, and other lung conditions. The study design should consider the scope of these responses. Some endpoints we used in our wildfire study included cell viability, cell membrane damage, redox reactions, DNA damage, and cytokine activation and release. Cell viability is useful to determine basic toxicity and dosage parameters (Stoddart, 2011). If your intended dose kills all or most of the cells, then your other measurements will be irrelevant due to a lack of cell responses. A dosage profile should be determined to document a range of cell injury. An LD50 (lethal dose) is a valuable measure to establish since it is the amount of substance required to kill 50% of the test population. This provides a useful basis for comparison to other exposure substances. Cell membrane damage can be used to measure cell trauma that did not result in death. Lactate dehydrogenase (LDH) can be measured in exposed cells as a gauge on how "leaky" the cells have become after treatment (M. Allen et al., 1994). LDH is found in cell cytosol, and as cell membranes are damaged, they allow LDH to pass through. Therefore, elevated LDH levels indicate cell membrane damage. Redox reactions and measurement of a cell's redox state can give information of the health of a cell as well as what it may be responding to and signaling to other cells. As mentioned earlier, EPR is one method we used in our study for measuring free radicals in cells; however, others included hydrogen peroxide and intracellular ROS determination. Hydrogen peroxide, while not a radical, is considered an ROS and provides a precursor for the hydroxyl radical. Elevated levels of hydrogen peroxide can indicate the activation of cellular defenses and an increased redox potential. Measurement of intracellular ROS utilizes the stain dichlorofluorescein (DCFH). This stain is a probe that can penetrate cell membranes and is easily oxidized to fluorescent dichlorofluorescein (DCF)(Aranda et al., 2013). Measurement of this fluorescence can be used to determine the redox state of the exposed cells. The ability of wildfire smoke to cause cellular DNA damage was measured utilizing the comet assay (Glei et al., 2016). The comet assay uses a layer of gel which the cellular DNA is drawn through by applying an electric charge. The electric charge causes material to migrate through the gel, and the smaller a component is, the less resistance present, and the faster it will move through the gel layer. Undamaged DNA will remain in one continuous ribbon and move as one mass. Damaged DNA will be broken up into sections of various sizes that will be viewed as a smearing of broken DNA as it is drawn through the gel at various rates. As shown in Figure 9.11, this results in undamaged DNA appearing as a ball while damaged DNA looks like a comet possessing a tail of DNA pieces smearing behind the central mass.

Our wildfire study also included measurement of cytokines. **Cytokines** are any number of substances, such as interferons, interleukins, and growth factors, which are secreted by cells and influence other cells (Dinarello, 2000). There are many types of cytokines with various functions. Cytokines can be induced by oxidative stress and subsequently trigger the release of other cytokines. This may lead to increased oxidative stress and gives them an important role in chronic inflammation, as well as other immunoresponses. In contrast, cytokines can also play a role in anti-inflammatory pathways and are possible therapeutic treatments for pathological inflammation or peripheral nerve injury. There are both pro-inflammatory and anti-inflammatory cytokines which regulate these pathways, and an imbalance in these cytokines can lead to cell and tissue injury. Cytokines are usually measured using an **enzyme-linked immunosorbant assay (ELISA)**. ELISAs use a capture antibody on a solid support, generally one well of a 96-well plate (Figure 9.12), that pulls cytokines out of a biological fluid and permits the measurement using a colorimetric, chemiluminescent, or fluorescent signal. When examining oxidative stress, useful cytokines to measure are IL-1β, IL-6, IL-8, and TNF-α. IL-1β is an important mediator of inflammatory response, and it is involved in a variety of cellular activities, including cell proliferation, differentiation, and apoptosis. IL-6 can act as both a pro-inflammatory cytokine and an anti-inflammatory myokine. IL-8 has two primary functions. First, it

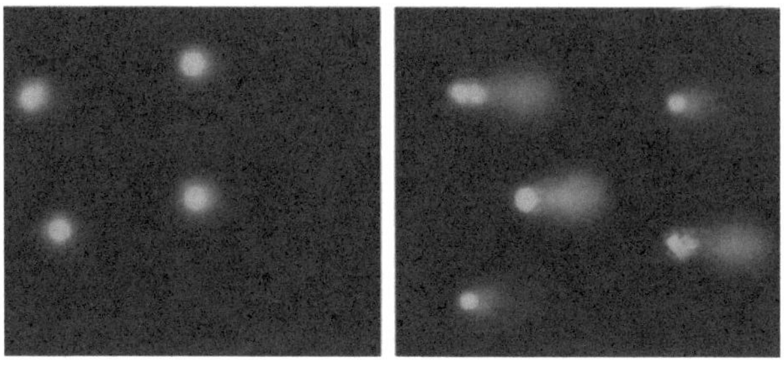

Figure 9.11 Comet assay control DNA (left) and wildfire smoke-exposed DNA (right).

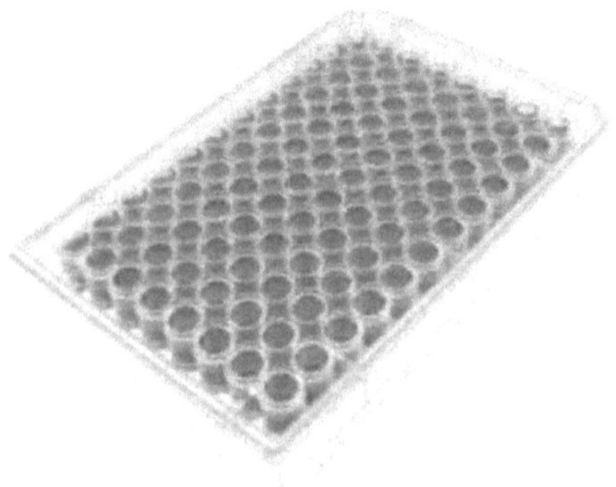

Figure 9.12 An example of a 96-well plate.

induces chemotaxis in cells, causing them to migrate, and second, it stimulates phagocytosis. TNF-α is involved in systemic inflammation and is one of the cytokines that make up the acute phase reaction. Our wildfire study plan is just an example of how different assays can be assembled to form research goals. In addition to what was mentioned, there are many other assays and methods that can be used for sample analysis and toxic response determination.

Skills needed include biology, chemistry, biochemistry, cell physiology, physiology, specific instrumentation knowledge, and specific assay protocols.

Data Analysis and Presentation of Finding

As part of your initial study plan, the statistician will help you determine the proper number and layout of samples you will need in order to provide statistical power to your results. Data analysis will include statistical models that allow you to determine the significance of differences in your results. Observing a difference in raw data isn't adequate to produce a statement about the research, so the data must be statistically analyzed to determine significance.

At the end of your study you will need to communicate your findings to other scientists, academic institutions, government agencies, occupational organizations, and the people directly involved with the exposures. Communication methods for your findings include presenting a poster at a meeting, giving an oral presentation, or publishing a paper. Posters and oral presentations permit for interaction between the presenter and audience, allowing follow-up issues to be addressed. Published papers undergo a peer-review process before release and allow a wide audience to view your results.

Skills needed include math, statistics, sampling power calculation, scientific writing, graphical presentation, oral presentation, and communication.

DISCUSSION QUESTIONS

1. Are wildfires related to climate change? Defend your position.
2. Discuss other ways to protect firefighter health.
3. Laboratory professionals provide vital services in public health. Discuss some of the ways laboratory professionals work behind the scenes.
4. Explore and research laboratories in your geographic area as a class project. Where are they located? What services do they provide? How do they communicate with public health departments? What disease is most frequently reported at labs in your area?

SUMMARY

TABLE 9.1 Select Essential Services of Public Health Demonstrated in the Wildfire Response

Essential Service # and Definition	Context in Chapter Case	Competency # It Ties to	Importance for Emergency Preparedness, Response, or Recovery
1. Assess and monitor population health status, factors that influence health, and community needs and assets (Assessment)	Assessment and monitoring the health status of wildland firefighter (WLFF) populations.	2, 3, 4	The health and well-being of firefighters must be considered in any community's preparedness and response plans. Firefighters provide direct services in emergencies. Jurisdictions should have comprehensive plans to assess fire exposure hazards and complications in its firefighter workforce.
2. Investigate, diagnose, and address health problems and hazards affecting the population (Assessment)	Investigating, diagnosing, and identifying hazards affecting the WLFF population via literature searches and epidemiology studies	1, 2, 3, 4	Based on previous studies and evaluation data, communities must anticipate and plan for treating firefighters on the front line of an event. In addition, epidemiologists and health scientists can report findings in presentations and publications to inform public health policies.
3. Communicate effectively to inform and educate people about health, factors that influence it, and how to improve it (Policy Development)	Communicating effectively to inform and educate people about the hazards	18, 19	Advance warning of the imminent threat of an advancing wild fire is essential for protecting communities in its path. Public health officials must also provide education to their constituents on how to protect themselves in the event of wildfires. Appropriate messages must be developed in advance and be ready to disseminate.
5. Create, champion, and implement policies, plans, and laws that impact health (Policy Development)	Data and findings are used to establish policies through recommended exposure limits and hazard identification.	4, 5	Policies, plans, and laws in place before a wildfire event can aid in a rapid response, reducing bureaucratic delays in decision-making. Knowledge of who is in charge of specific activities and required approvals can eliminate time wasted when boots on the ground are necessary.
8. Build and support a diverse and skilled public health workforce (Assurance)	Up-to-date training and use of standard operating procedures as well as good laboratory practice	21, 22	Laboratory technicians are in demand in public health. Jurisdictions are often short of the laboratory professionals they require for rapid processing of samples to detect disease outbreaks and identify trends. In addition, many schools of public health have eliminated or reduced training programs. Building laboratory capacity should be a priority for public health.
9. Improve and innovate public health functions through ongoing evaluation, research, and continuous quality improvement (Assurance)	Providing ongoing training, attendance at relevant conferences, and staying abreast of other scientific research	1, 2, 3, 4	Public health professionals interested in wildfire response can contribute by conducting evaluations of events using data from responses to inform program and policy improvement. Long-term research could be conducted on related issues, such as erosion and mudslide, in appropriate areas. Causes of wildfires is another area of inquiry that could be undertaken by health scientists.
10. Build and maintain a strong organizational infrastructure for public health (Assurance)	Effective interactions and communication between the field team and the laboratory team	21	Building laboratory capacity should be a high priority in all jurisdictions. Laboratory technology is changing rapidly with computer applications and diagnostic tests based on DNA analysis. Constant review and upgrades to laboratory processes are essential efforts to maintain quality.

TABLE 9.2 Select CEPH Competencies Needed for Frontline Health Workers, Managers, and Leaders for Wildfire Emergency Preparedness, Response, and Recovery

Competency # and Definition	Context in Case/Chapter	Level	Importance for Emergency preparedness, response, or recovery
2. Select quantitative and qualitative data collection methods appropriate for a given public health context.	Medical field technicians collect questionnaire data, blood pressure, spirometry, bronchial hyperresponsiveness, exhaled breath carbon monoxide (CO), blood, urine, pulse wave velocity, and sputum and nasal lavage.	Level 1	Frontline data and specimen collectors provide the basic units of analysis for all biological tests. These public health professionals are indispensable for all scientific inquiries. They are skilled in medical procedures. Frontline scientists, who collect data through surveys, are equally important for gathering information for surveillance and decision-making.
4. Interpret results of data analysis for public health research, policy, or practice.	Local U.S. Forest Service administered Work Capacity Field Test to field technicians for fitness rating.	Level 2	Midlevel managers and supervisors partner with staff at Level 1 to ensure quality of methodologies is maintained, offer day-to-day guidance and oversight to teams, and use collected and analyzed data for decision-making.
7. Assess population needs, assets, and capacities that affect communities' health.	Occupational health technicians trained by the NIOSH to conduct lung function testing on Federal WLFF	Level 1	Skilled professionals at this level interact with affected populations to administer vital assessments to address public health problems.
13. Propose strategies to identify stakeholders and build coalitions and partnerships for influencing public health outcomes.	A day-long workshop of stakeholder experts was held in March 2005 at the NIOSH to discuss the first-year results and future study plans in detail.	Level 2	Managers and supervisors plan strategies to collaborate with stakeholders and create opportunities for communities and public health professionals to meet and share knowledge and concerns.
16. Apply leadership and/or management principles to address a relevant health issue.	NIOSH worked with the U.S. National Response Team and federal agencies, state health departments, labor unions, and volunteer emergency responder groups to develop the Emergency Responder Health Monitoring and Surveillance™ framework.	Level 3	Public health agency leaders collaborate with other agency level leaders and make the decisions and policies, based on the ground work and data results provided by Levels 1 and 2, to advocate for policies and practices to benefit the public's health.
19. Communicate audience-appropriate (i.e., non-academic, non-peer audience) public health content, both in writing and through oral presentation.	Members of the wildfire research team made formal presentations and question-and-answer sessions to each crew at the beginning of each fire season detailing proposed study methods.	Levels 1, 2, 3	All levels communicate in their respective audiences and have important roles for conveying health security information to the public, to community collaborators, to the media, to agency partners, and to others. Each level crafts messages appropriate for the recipient audience.

Key: Essential services of public health; CEPH competencies; Leadership levels.

WLFF, wildland firefighters

ACKNOWLEDGMENTS

The creation of this chapter would not have been possible without the extensive wildfire health studies that the authors and their many colleagues and collaborators were able to conduct over many years. The authors especially thank the Alpine and Arrowhead IHCs for their participation in the study. We thank the U.S. Department of the Interior, the National Park Service, and the NIFC for arranging for the crews' participation. The authors also thank all the incident management teams that assisted with the collection of data at the fires. In addition, the authors thank their many research colleagues for assistance with various aspects of protocol development, data collection at the fires, and other field and laboratory studies, data analysis, and manuscript preparation and review, especially those from the Field Studies Branch in the NIOSH Respiratory Health Division, the Pathology and Physiology Research Branch in the NIOSH Health Effects Laboratory Division, the NIOSH Western States Office, Colorado State University, and the Harvard School of Public Health. Special recognition for their significant support of these studies goes to Gregory Wagner, MD; to David Weissman, MD; and to David Christiani, MD, MPH. Significant appreciation also goes to Christopher Piacitelli, MS; Jean Cox-Ganser, PhD; Paul Siegel, PhD; and Lester Kobzik, MD. DMG currently serves as an epidemiologist at the National Institutes of Health, Intramural Research Program, Baltimore, Maryland. MDH was a research physical scientist in the NIOSH Respiratory Health Division, Field Studies Branch prior to his retirement from the NIOSH at the end of 2018.

We dedicate this chapter to the memory of all WLFF who have been injured or lost their lives in the line of duty.

DISCLAIMER

The findings and conclusions in this report are those of the authors and do not necessarily represent the views of the National Institute for Occupational Safety and Health, Centers for Disease Control and Prevention, the NIH, or the USDA. Mention of any company or product does not constitute endorsement.

REFERENCES

Adetona, O., Reinhardt, T. E., Domitrovich, J., Broyles, G., Adetona, A. M., Kleinman, M. T., Ottmar, R. D., & Naeher, L. P. (2016). Review of the health effects of wildland fire smoke on wildland firefighters and the public. *Inhalation Toxicology, 28*(3), 95–139. https://doi.org/10.3109/08958378.2016.1145771

Allen, D. D., Caviedes, R., Cárdenas, A. M., Shimahara, T., Segura-Aguilar, J., & Caviedes, P. A. (2005). Cell lines as in vitro models for drug screening and toxicity studies. *Drug Development and Industrial Pharmacy, 31*(8), 757–768. https://doi.org/10.1080/03639040500216246

Allen, M., Millett, P., Dawes, E., & Rushton, N. (1994). Lactate dehydrogenase activity as a rapid and sensitive test for the quantification of cell numbers in vitro. *Clinical Materials, 16*(4), 189–194. https://doi.org/10.1016/0267-6605(94)90116-3

Ameh, E. S. (2019). A review of basic crystallography and x-ray diffraction applications. *The International Journal of Advanced Manufacturing Technology, 105*(7), 3289–3302. https://doi.org/10.1007/s00170-019-04508-1

Aranda, A., Sequedo, L., Tolosa, L., Quintas, G., Burello, E., Castell, J. V., & Gombau, L. (2013). Dichloro-dihydro-fluorescein diacetate (DCFH-DA) assay: A quantitative method for oxidative stress assessment of nanoparticle-treated cells. *Toxicology In Vitro, 27*, 954–963. https://doi.org/10.1016/j.tiv.2013.01.016

Ashley, F. W., & Kannel, W. B. (1974). Relation of weight change to changes in atherogenic traits: The Framingham Study. *Journal of Chronic Diseases, 27*(3), 103–114. https://doi.org/10.1016/0021-9681(74)90079-4

Austin, C. C., Wang, D., Ecobichon, D. J., & Dussault, G. (2001). Characterization of volatile organic compounds in smoke at municipal structural fires. *Journal of Toxicology and Environmental Health, Part A, 63*(6), 437–458. https://doi.org/10.1080/152873901300343470

Betchley, C., Koenig, J. Q., van Belle, G., Checkoway, H., & Reinhardt, T. (1997). Pulmonary function and respiratory symptoms in forest firefighters. *American Journal of Industrial Medicine, 31*(5), 503–509. https://doi.org/10.1002/(sici)1097-0274(199705)31:5<503::aid-ajim3>3.0.co;2-u

Broyles, G. (2013). *Wildland firefighter smoke exposure*. U.S. Department of Agriculture, U.S. Forest Service.

Burgess, J. L., Nanson, C. J., Bolstad-Johnson, D. M., Gerkin, R., Hysong, T. A., Lantz, R. C., Sherrill, D. L., Crutchfield, C. D., Quan, S. F., Bernard, A. M., & Witten, M. L. (2001). Adverse respiratory effects following overhaul in firefighters. *Journal of Occupational and Environmental Medicine, 43*(5), 467–473. https://doi.org/10.1097/00043764-200105000-00007

Cascio, W. E. (2018). Wildland fire smoke and human health. *Science of the Total Environment, 624*, 586–595. https://doi.org/10.1016/j.scitotenv.2017.12.086

Centers for Disease Control and Prevention. (2006). Fatalities among volunteer and career firefighters—United States, 1994-2004. *Morbidity and Mortality Weekly Report, 55*(16), 453–455. https://www.cdc.gov/mmwr/preview/mmwrhtml/mm5516a3.htm

Centers for Disease Control and Prevention. (2020). *Emergency Responder Health Monitoring and Surveillance (ERHMS) online training course (WB2873)*. https://emergency.cdc.gov/training/erhmscourse

Cheng, Y.-S., Zhou, Y., & Chen, B. T. (1999). Particle deposition in a cast of human oral airways. *Aerosol Science and Technology, 31*, 286–300. https://doi.org/10.1080/027868299304165

Chia, K., Jeyaratnam, J., Chan, T., & Lim, T. (1990). Airway responsiveness of firefighters after smoke exposure. *British Journal of Industrial Medicine, 47*(8), 524–527. https://doi.org/10.1136/oem.47.8.524

Cogliati, S., Lorenzi, I., Rigoni, G., Caicci, F., & Soriano, M. E. (2018). Regulation of mitochondrial electron transport chain assembly. *Journal of Molecular Biology, 430*(24), 4849–4873. https://doi.org/10.1016/j.jmb.2018.09.016

Davies, M. (2016). Detection and characterization of radicals using electron paramagnetic resonance (EPR) spin trapping and related methods. *Methods, 109*, 21–30. https://doi.org/10.1016/j.ymeth.2016.05.013

Delfino, R. J., Brummel, S., Wu, J., Stern, H., Ostro, B., Lipsett, M., Winer, A., Street, D. H., Zhang, L., Tjoa, T., & Gillen, D. L. (2009). The relationship of respiratory and cardiovascular hospital admissions to the Southern California wildfires of 2003. *Occupational and Environmental Medicine, 66*(3), 189–197. https://doi.org/10.1136/oem.2008.041376

Dickman, C. (2020). More than one billion animals killed in Australian bushfires. *University of Sydney News*. https://www.sydney.edu.au/news-opinion/news/2020/01/08/australian-bushfires-more-than-one-billion-animals-impacted.html

Dinarello, C. A. (2000). Proinflammatory cytokines. *Chest, 118*(2), 503–508. https://doi.org/10.1378/chest.118.2.503

El-Aneed, A., Cohen, A., & Banoub, J. (2009). Mass spectrometry, review of the basics: Electrospray, MALDI, and commonly used mass analyzers. *Applied Spectrometry Reviews, 44*(3), 210–230. https://doi.org/10.1080/05704920902717872

Environmental Protection Agency. (2021). *Wildfire smoke: A guide for public health officials*. U.S. Environmental Protection Agency. https://www.airnow.gov/sites/default/files/2021-09/wildfire-smoke-guide_0.pdf

Federal Emergency Management Agency. (2020). *National Incident Management System*. https://www.fema.gov/national-incident-management-system

Gaughan, D. M., Christiani, D. C., Hughes, M. D., Baur, D. M., Kobzik, L., Wagner, G. R., & Kales, S. N. (2014). High hsCRP is associated with reduced lung function in structural firefighters. *American Journal of Industrial Medicine, 57*, 31–37. https://doi.org/10.1002/ajim.22260

Gaughan, D. M., Cox-Ganser, J. M., Enright, P. L., Castellan, R. M., Wagner, G. R., Hobbs, G. R., Bledsoe, T. A., Siegel, P. D., Kreiss, K., & Weissman, D. N. (2008). Acute upper and lower respiratory effects in wildland firefighters. *Journal of Occupational and Environmental Medicine, 50*(9), 1019–1028. https://doi.org/10.1097/JOM.0b013e3181754161

Gaughan, D. M., Piacitelli, C. A., Chen, B. T., Law, B. F., Virji, M. A., Edwards, N. T., Enright, P. L., Schwegler-Berry, D. E., Leonard, S. S., Wagner, G. R., Kobzik, L., Kales, S. N., Hughes, M. D., Christiani, D. C., Siegel, P. D., Cox-Ganser, J. M., & Hoover, M. D. (2014). Exposures and cross-shift lung function declines in wildland firefighters. *Journal of Occupational and Environmental Hygiene, 11*(9), 591–603. https://doi.org/10.1080/15459624.2014.895372

Gaughan, D. M., Siegel, P. D., Hughes, M. D., Chang, C. Y., Law, B. F., Campbell, C. R., Richards, J. C., Kales, S. F., Chertok, M., Kobzik, L., Nguyen, P. S., O'Donnell, C. R., Kiefer, M.,

Wagner, G. R., & Christiani, D. C. (2014). Arterial stiffness, oxidative stress, and smoke exposure in wildland firefighters. *American Journal of Industrial Medicine, 57*(7), 748–756. https://doi.org/10.1002/ajim.22331

Gelb, L., & Gubbins, K. (1998). Characterization of porous glasses: Simulation models, adsorption isotherms, and the Brunauer–Emmett–Teller analysis method. *Langmuir, 14*(8), 2097–2111. https://doi.org/10.1021/la9710379

Gledhill, N., & Jamnik, V. K. (1992). Characterization of the physical demands of firefighting. *Canadian Journal of Sports Science, 17*(3), 207–213.

Glei, M., Schneider, T., & Schlormann, W. (2016). Comet assay: An essential tool in toxicology research. *Archives of Toxicology, 90*, 2315–2336. https://doi.org/10.1007/s00204-016-1767-y

Guidotti, T. L., & Clough, V. M. (1992). Occupational health concerns of firefighting. *Annual Review Public Health, 13*, 151–171. https://doi.org/10.1146/annurev.pu.13.050192.001055

Halliwell, B., & Gutteridge, J. M. C. (2015). *Free radicals in biology and medicine*. Oxford University Press.

Higgins, M., D'Agostino, R., Kannel, W., Cobb, J., & Pinsky, J. (1993). Benefits and adverse effects of weight loss. Observations from the Framingham Study. *Annals of Internal Medicine, 119*(7 Pt. 2), 758–763. https://doi.org/10.7326/0003-4819-119-7_part_2-199310011-00025

Kales, S. N., Soteriades, E. S., Christoudias, S. G., & Christiani, D. C. (2003). Firefighters and on-duty deaths from coronary heart disease: A case control study. *Environmental Health, 2*(1), Article 14. https://doi.org/10.1186/1476-069X-2-14

Lacroix, G., Koch, W., Ritter, D., Gutleb, A. C., Søren, T. L., Loret, T., Zanetti, F., Constant, S., Chortarea, S., Rothen-Rutishauser, B., Hiemstra, P. S., Frejafon, E., Hubert, P., Gribaldo, L., Kearns, P., Aublant, J.-M., Diabaté, S., Weiss, C., de Groot, A., & Kooter, I. (2018). Air–liquid interface *in vitro* models for respiratory toxicology research: Consensus workshop and recommendations. *Applied In Vitro Toxicology, 4*(2), 91–106. https://doi.org/10.1089/aivt.2017.0034

Leonard, S. S., Castranova, V., Chen, B. T., Schwegler-Berry, D., Hoover, M., Piacitelli, C., & Gaughan, D. M. (2007). Particle size-dependent radical generation from wildland fire smoke. *Toxicology, 236*(1–2), 103–113. https://doi.org/10.1016/j.tox.2007.04.008

Leonard, S. S., Chen, B. T., Stone, S. G., Schwegler-Berry, D., Kenyon, A. J., Frazer, D., & Antonini, J. M. (2010). Comparison of stainless and mild steel welding fumes in generation of reactive oxygen species. *Particle and Fibre Toxicology, 7*, 32. https://doi.org/10.1186/1743-8977-7-32

Letts, D., Fidler, A. T., Deitchman, S., & Reh, C. M. (1991). *Health hazard evaluation report: U.S. Department of the Interior, National Park Service, Southern California* (NIOSH HETA Report No. 91-152-2140, NTIS No. PB92-133347). U.S. Department of Health and Human Services. https://www.cdc.gov/niosh/hhe/reports/pdfs/1991-0152-2140.pdf

Lissner, L., Odell, P. M., D'Agostino, R. B., Stokes, J., Kreger, B. E., Belanger, A. J., & Brownell, K. D. (1991). Variability of body weight and health outcomes in the Framingham population. *New England Journal of Medicine, 324*(26), 1839–1844. https://doi.org/10.1056/NEJM199106273242602

Liu, D., Tager, I., Balmes, J., & Harrison, R. (1992). The effect of smoke inhalation on lung function and airway responsiveness in wildland fire fighters. *American Review of Respiratory Disease, 146*, 1469–1473. https: doi.org/10.1164/ajrccm/146.6.1469

Materna, B. L., Jones, J. R., Sutton, P. M., Rothman, N., & Harrison, R. J. (1992). Occupational exposures in California wildland fire fighting. *American Industrial Hygiene Association Journal, 53*, 69–76. https://doi.org/10.1080/15298669291359311

Musk, A. W., Smith, T. J., Peters, J. M., & McLaughlin, E. (1979). Pulmonary function in firefighters: Acute changes in ventilatory capacity and their correlates. *British Journal of Industrial Medicine, 36*, 29–34. https://doi.org/10.1136/oem.36.1.29

Navarro, K. M., Kleinman, M. T., Mackay, C. E., Reinhardt, T. E., Balmes, J. R., Broyles, G. A., Ottmar, R. D., Naher, L. P., & Domitrovich, J. W. (2019). Wildland firefighter smoke exposure and risk of lung cancer and cardiovascular disease mortality. *Environmental Research, 173*, 462–468. https://doi.org/10.1016/j.envres.2019.03.060

National Institute for Occupational Safety and Health. (2020a). *Emergency Responder Health Monitoring and Surveillance (ERHMS)™*. https://www.cdc.gov/niosh/erhms

National Institute for Occupational Safety and Health. (2020b). *NIOSH Spirometry Training Program*. https://www.cdc.gov/niosh/topics/spirometry/training.html

National Interagency Coordination Center (n.d.). *About us*. https://www.nifc.gov/nicc/about/about.htm

National Interagency Fire Center. (2020a). *Interagency Standards for Fire and Fire Aviation Operations Standards for fire and fire aviation operations (2020 Redbook)* (NFES 2724). Interagency Standards for Fire and Fire Aviation Operations Group, National Interagency Fire Center.

National Interagency Fire Center. (2020b). *Total wildland fires and acres (1926–2019)*. https://www.nifc.gov/fireInfo/fireInfo_stats_totalFires.html

National Wildfire Coordinating Committee. (2020, November). *Firefighter nutrition*. https//www.nwcg.gov/committee/6mfs/firefighter-nutrition

National Wildfire Coordinating Group. (2021). *Work Capacity Test (WCT)*. https://www.nwcg.gov/term/glossary/work-capacity-test-wct

Nemmar, A. (2013). Recent advances in particulate matter and nanoparticle toxicology: A review of the in vivo and in vitro studies. *BioMed Research International, 2013*, 279371. https://doi.org/10.1155/2013/279371

Oberdörster, G., Ferin, J., & Lehnert, B. (1994). Correlation between particle size, in vivo particle persistence, and lung injury. *Environmental Health Perspectives, 102* (Suppl. 5), 73–179. https://doi.org/10.1289/ehp.102-1567252

Reh, C. M., Letts, D., & Deitchman, S. (1994). *Health hazard evaluation report: U.S. Department of the Interior, National Park Service, Yosemite National Park, California* (NIOSH HETA Report No. 90-0365-2415, NTIS No. PB95-242541). U.S. Department of Health and Human Services, Public Health Service. https://www.cdc.gov/niosh/hhe/reports/pdfs/1990-0365-2415.pdf

Reyes-Velarde, A. (2019, January 11). California's Camp Fire was the costliest global disaster last year, insurance report shows. *Los Angeles Times*. https://www.latimes.com/local/lanow/la-me-ln-camp-fire-insured-losses-20190111-story.html

Roggen, E. L. (2011, February 7). *In vitro* toxicity testing in the twenty-first century. *Frontiers in Pharmacology, 2*. https://doi.org/10.3389/fphar.2011.00003

Rothman, N., Ford, D. P., Baser, M. E., Hansen, J. A., O'Toole, T., Tockman, M. S., & Strickland, P. T. (1991). Pulmonary function and respiratory symptoms in wildland firefighters. *Journal of Occupational and Environmental Medicine, 33*(11), 1163–1167. https://doi.org/10.1097/00043764-199111000-00013

Sardinas, A., Miller, J. W., & Hansen, H. (1986). Ischemic heart disease mortality of firemen and policemen. *American Journal of Public Health, 76*(9), 1140–1141. https://doi.org/10.2105/ajph.76.9.1140

Scannell, C. H., & Balmes, J. R. (1995). Pulmonary effects of firefighting. *Occupational Medicine, 10*(4), 789–801.

Sharkey, B. J. (Ed.). (1997). *Health hazards of smoke: Recommendations of the consensus conference, April 1997*. U.S. Department of Agriculture, U.S. Forest Service.

Sharkey, B. J., & Gaskill, S. E. (2009). *Fitness and work capacity: 2009 Edition* (NWCG PMS 304-2, NFES 1596). National Wildfire Coordinating Group.

Slaughter, J. C., Koenig, J. Q., & Reinhardt, T. E. (2004). Association between lung function and exposure to smoke among firefighters at prescribed burns. *Journal of Occupational and Environmental Hygiene, 1*(1), 45–49. https://doi.org/10.1080/15459620490264490

Stetefeld, J., McKenna, S. A., & Patel, T. R. (2016). Dynamic light scattering: A practical guide and applications on biomedical sciences. *Biophysical Reviews, 8(4)*, 409–427. https://doi.org/10.1007/s12551-016-0218-6

Stoddart, M. J. (2011). Cell viability assays: Introduction. In M. J. Stoddart (Ed.), *Methods in molecular biology (methods and protocols): Mammalian cell viability* (Vol. 740, pp. 1–6). Humana Press.

Stuart, B. O. (1984, April). Deposition and clearance of inhaled particles. *Environmental Health Perspectives, 55*, 369–390. https://doi.org/10.1289/ehp.8455369

Takeyama, H., Itani, T., Tachi, N., Sakamura, O., Murata, K., Inoue, T., Takanishi, T., Suzumura, H., & Niwa, S. (2005). Effects of shift schedules on fatigue and physiological functions among firefighters during night duty. *Ergonomics, 48*(1), 1–11. https://doi.org/10.1080/00140130412331303920

Tarlo, S. (2012). Occupational lung disease. In L. Goldman & A. I. Schafer (Eds.), *Goldman's Cecil medicine* (24th ed., Vol. 1, pp. 567–574). Elsevier.

U.S. Fire Administration. (n.d.). *National Fire Academy online courses*. https://www.usfa.fema.gov/training/nfa/courses/online.html

U.S. Forest Service. (2017). *Wildland Fire Learning in Depth Series: Wildland fire management personnel*. https://www.nps.gov/articles/wildland-fire-management-personnel.htm

Yoo, H. L., & Franke, W. D. (2009). Prevalence of cardiovascular disease risk factors in volunteer firefighters. *Journal of Occupational & Environmental Medicine, 51*(8), 958–962. https://doi.org/10.1097/JOM.0b013e3181af3a58

CHAPTER 10

EXTREME HEAT EVENTS AND PUBLIC HEALTH

MARYAM KARIMI, ROUZBEH NAZARI, AND SAMAIN SABRIN

KEY TERMS

Anthropogenic Sources
Cluster Analysis
Cumulative Health Vulnerability Index (CHVI)
Global Warming
Greenhouse Gas
Machine Learning
Paris Climate Agreement
Permafrost

INTRODUCTION

Climate change is a complex global phenomenon that poses serious risk to all aspects of human society along with increasing dangers to human health and life (World Health Organization [WHO], 2018a). Extreme heat events are among the major impacts caused by climate change that we have been experiencing for the last 2 decades. The National Aeronautics and Space Administration (NASA) has reported that, since 2001, the United States has recorded 17 of the 18 hottest years on record. During the summer and fall of 2017, the excessive heat events broke every past state record, and the annual average temperature was warmer than usual (National Oceanic and Atmospheric Administration [NOAA], 2017). According to the NOAA, the highest temperatures on record statewide were observed in the states of Arizona, Georgia, New Mexico, North Carolina, and South Carolina, resulting in an increased number of heat-related mortalities. Heat events are now considered one of the major concerns to public health. This chapter discusses 10 essential public health services and core competencies aiming to understand extreme heat events and tackle potential heat-attributable health burdens.

The following icons, located in the margins throughout the chapter and within the summary tables, denote essential services of public health, CEPH competencies, and leadership levels: Essential services of public health; CEPH competencies; Leadership levels.

GLOBAL WARMING AND ANTHROPOGENIC EMISSION

Future **global warming** highly depends on both past and future human-induced emissions of greenhouse gases. The sources of **greenhouse gas** emission from daily human activities are referred to as **anthropogenic sources**, which include fossil fuel combustion in the transportation sectors and electric utility, land-use modification, agriculture, waste management, treatment, and industrial processes. Also, there are many natural sources of greenhouse gases such as volcanos, thawing **permafrost**, wetlands, and so on. However, the anthropogenic sources play a significant role in emitting *greenhouse gases* such as methane, carbon dioxide, nitrous oxide, many synthetic halocarbons, and chemicals. Climate models predict the level of human-induced climate change based on a combination of past change with historical emission data and future change with expected ongoing emissions of heat-trapping gases. The extent of global temperature surges by the end of this century will be largely governed by the magnitude of present and future emissions from the anthropogenic sources. However, there are significant variances between scenarios with lower emissions compared to the fossil-fuel-intensive high-emission scenarios compared to scenarios in which emissions are reduced (Fahad et al., 2017). The most recent climate model (CMIP5) projects human-induced climate change by considering a wide range of human activities including lower emission scenarios as previously considered in RCP 2.6, which resulted in less warming with the assumption of 70% emission reduction from current levels by 2100. On the contrary, the RCP 8.5 model, assuming a continuous increase in emissions, projects extensive warming by the end of the century compared to the intermediate-emissions scenarios (RCP 4.5, RCP 6.0).

HEAT WAVES IN THE UNITED STATES

Heat waves are becoming more common with different intensity levels over the contiguous United States. The National Climate Assessment projects 20 to 30 more days with heat over 90 °F in most areas by 2050. Dahl et al. (2019) recently predicted that the number of days with a heat index above 100 °F will double nationwide and that days with a heat index above 105 °F will triple by 2100. Scientists are projecting average temperature to rise by 3 to 5 °F by the mid-2030s and 2.8 to 10.8 °F by the end of the 21st century under lower emissions scenarios (B1 or RCP 4.5; Wuebbles et al., 2017). Predicted warming by the mid- and late century shown in Figure 10.1 is statistically significant from the near present (1976–2005). Climate Science Special Report from the 4th National Climate Assessment (NCA4) has estimated a 1.2 °F rise in the annual average temperature of the 1986–2016 period relative to the 1901–1960 period. They observed the highest average warming temperatures in the Great Plain North followed by Alaska, the Southwest, the Northwest, and the Northeast national climate assessment regions (Figure 10.2, top panel). Also, the annual average temperatures have been projected to rise up to 4.21 °F, 5.29 °F (RCP 4.5, RCP 8.5) by the mid-century and 5.57 °F, 9.49 °F (RCP 4.5, RCP 8.5) by the late century in the Midwest region (Figure 10.2, bottom panel). The NCA4 report also predicted 2.5 °F average nationwide warming for the mid-century (2021–2050) relative to the 1976–2005 period using all RCP scenarios, and much greater rises for the late century (2071–2100) by 2.8 °F to 7.3 °F (1.6 °C to 4.1 °C) in a lower scenario (RCP 4.5) and 5.8 °F to 11.9 °F (3.2 °C to 6.6 °C) in the higher scenario (RCP 8.5). All these observations and projections imply record-breaking temperatures and continuous extreme heat events (EHEs) that may be common phenomena in the coming decades.

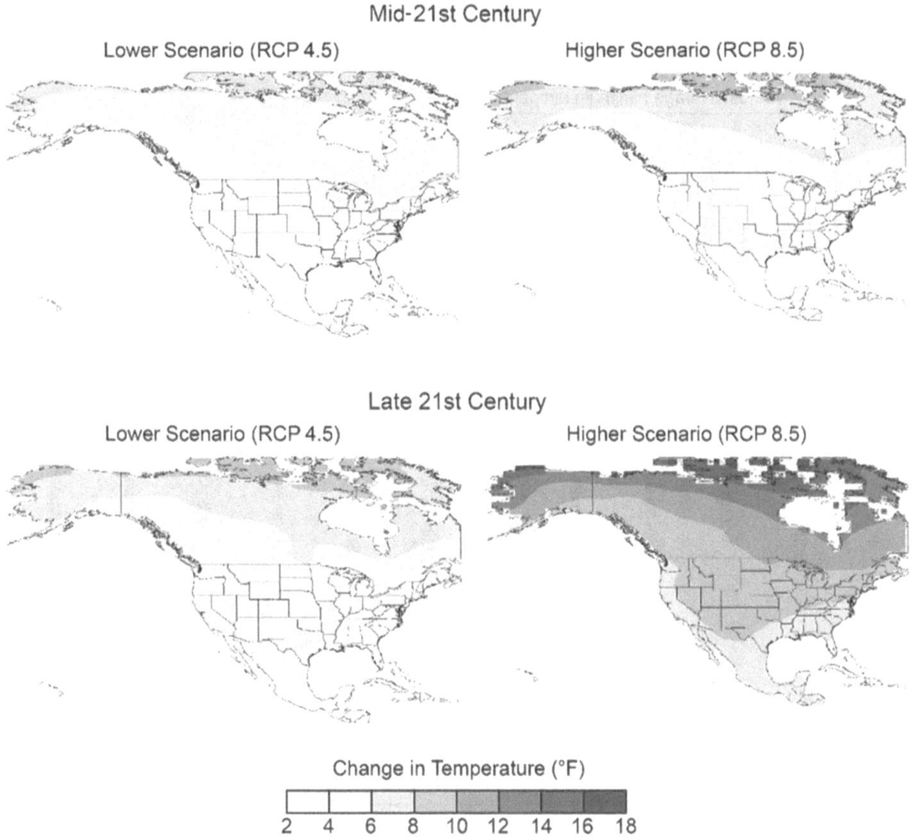

Figure 10.1 Projected changes in annual average temperatures (°F) between mid-century (2036–2065, top) or late century (2070–2099, bottom) and the average for near present (1976–2005).

Source: CICS-NC and NOAA NCEI. Public domain.

DEFINITION OF AN EXTREME HEAT EVENT

The term "extreme heat" is defined as "summertime temperatures that are substantially hotter and/or more humid than average for that location at that time of year" by the Centers for Disease Control and Prevention (CDC; 2017). However, the interpretation of feeling heat depends on several meteorological variables including temperature, humidity, solar radiation, and cloud cover that varies with time of year and location. Places around the globe have different extreme heat criteria corresponding with local standards to deal with the warmest summer weather. These criteria may also change for a geographic area over the course of summer months, which is unreliable to specify a fixed absolute criterion of a maximum temperature of at least 90 °F. Nevertheless, heat events are identified in many ways. Some compare current weather to the historical meteorological baselines, while some assess present and forecasted weather using site-specific weather-based mortality algorithms to identify EHEs. An example of identifying criteria could be an actual or forecasted daily high temperature exceeding the 95th percentile of historical distribution for a certain period. Likewise comparing with historical 20th-century data, the U.S.

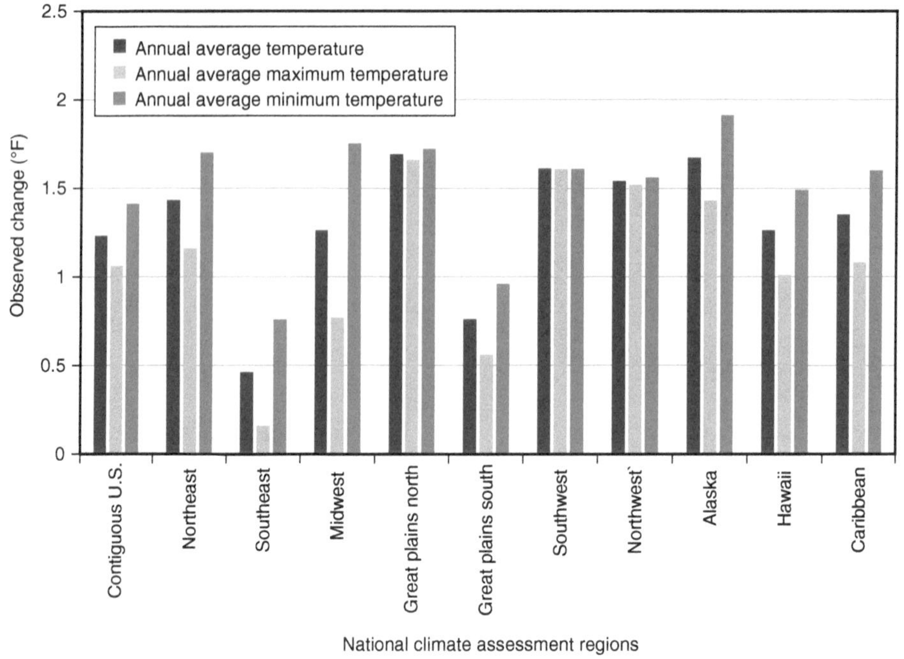

(A)

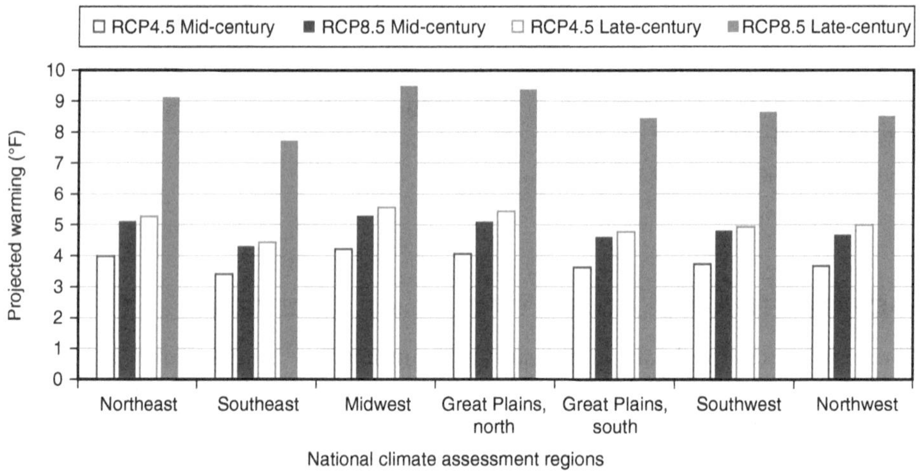

(B)

Figure 10.2 (A) Observed changes in (1986–2016) annual average temperatures (°F) from the first half of the last century (1901–1960) for the contiguous United States (1925–1960), Alaska, Hawaii, and the Caribbean. (B) Projected changes in the mid and late century average temperature from the near present (1976–2005) in the United States.

Source: Data from Vose, R., Easterling, D. R., Kunkel, K., & Wehner, M. (2017). Temperature changes in the United States. In D. J. Wuebbles, D. W. Fahey, K. A. Hibbard, D. J. Dokken, B. C. Stewart, & T. K. Maycock (Eds.)., *Climate science special report: Fourth National Climate Assessment, volume I* (pp. 185–206). U.S. Global Change Research Program. https://doi.org/10.7930/J0N29V45

NOAA reported a 1.7 °F rise in the global average temperature during the summer of 2019.

HEAT-RELATED HAZARDS AND MORTALITY AND MORBIDITY

Environmental, ecological processes and social vulnerability in a community govern any climate-related health impacts varying in scale, duration, and intensity (Crowley, 2016). Extreme heat can similarly impose direct health effects and indirectly affect human life by changing or stressing components of the environment. The frequency, intensity, and duration of the heat events are expected to increase, so the effects of EHEs on public health have become an exigent issue. EHEs have already caused more mortalities than any natural disaster (CDC, 2017). Different heat-stress conditions such as heat stroke, cramps, and exhaustion can be initiated by extreme heat (Karimi et al., 2017); when the internal body cannot maintain a consistent temperature around 98.6°F to sustain normal physiological activities, body temperature and sweating rate increase. Emergency treatment becomes necessary to avoid permanent damage or even death in cases of EHEs (Davis & Novicoff, 2018). Increased hospital admissions due to diabetes; cardiovascular, kidney, and respiratory disorders; and mental illnesses are associated with heat waves. Also, chronic dehydration and occupational heat stress may lead to chronic kidney disease (Isaksen et al., 2015).

Around 125 million people were exposed to the EHEs globally during 2000 to 2016, while 70,000 heat-related deaths in Europe were recorded due to the June to August EHEs in 2003 with 56,000 additional deaths during a 44-day long EHE in 2010 in the Russian Federation (WHO, 2018b). Table 10.1 lists average daily heat-related mortalities observed in nine European cities for different study periods (Scortichini et al., 2018). The table also projects mortalities with the EHEs expected to occur once every 30 years (on average) in 15 U.S. cities (Atlanta, Boston, Chicago, Dallas, Detroit, Houston, Los Angeles, Miami, New York, Philadelphia, Phoenix, San Francisco, Seattle, St. Louis, and Washington, D.C.). The mortalities have been projected in three warming scenarios (3 °C, 2 °C, 1.5 °C) by the end of the 20th century. Major cities like New York, Los Angeles, Miami, Chicago, and Philadelphia are expected to see between 1,484 and 5,798 deaths per city for each 1-in-30-year event at 3 °C warming and between 984 and 3,818 deaths if the cities can meet the **Paris Climate Agreement's** goal of limiting global warming by 2 °C (Lo et al., 2019). Studies are also linking harmful air pollutants with the elevated temperature in urban areas. Hence, respiratory problems can be indirectly linked with the EHEs.

Besides many direct effects on individual and community health, heat may also cause indirect impacts such as altered behavior; high-crime rates; increased demand on health services; higher risks of gastrointestinal diseases; marine algae blooms; and potential disruption in the power, water, and transportation infrastructure.

URBAN HEAT ISLANDS

A common term related to extreme heat phenomena in the city areas is "urban heat islands" (UHIs). Urban areas that replace previous areas with hard paves experience overheating and higher ambient temperature than

TABLE 10.1 Observed Mortalities in Nine European Cities and Projected Mortalities in 15 U.S. Cities

Observed Heat-Related Mortalities in Nine European Cities			
City	**Observed Period**	**Total Mean Daily Deaths**	
Helsinki	1990–2010	17	
Stockholm	1990–2010	29	
London	1990–2010	144	
Paris	1991–2009	108	
Budapest	1992–2010	65	
Rome	1992–2010	53	
Barcelona	1991–2009	36	
Valencia	1994–2010	15	
Athens	1992–2010	73	
Projected Heat-Related Mortalities per 1-in-30-Year EHE in 15 U.S. Cities			
City	**3 °C increase**	**2 °C increase**	**1.5 °C increase**
New York	5,798	3,818	3,082
Los Angeles	2,561	1,802	1,476
Miami	2,359	1,465	1,124
Chicago	1,781	1,145	906
Philadelphia	1,484	984	800
Detroit	1,372	910	732
Dallas	901	595	446
Houston	792	538	440
Seattle	725	446	341
Phoenix	526	310	226
Washington, DC	486	312	251
Atlanta	446	346	312
St. Louis	351	269	234
Boston	330	215	172
San Francisco	328	253	214

EHE, extreme heat event.

the surrounding suburban and rural areas, which is defined as UHI phenomena. According to the United Nations (UN), more population has started living in cities than rural areas since 2007 (Department of Economic and Social Affairs [DESA], 2018), and 55% of the global population were reported to live in urban areas by 2018. Following that trend of the urban population growth, two-thirds of the world population is expected to shift toward urban regions by 2050, with significant increases (90%) in Asia and Africa. Since the numbers and scale of urban areas are globally rising along with population growth, UHI effects may pose higher risk of heat waves for the people living in cities.

HEALTH INEQUITIES AND HEAT EVENTS

Many factors determine people's level of vulnerability toward EHEs. For example, city dwellers, people working outdoors, vulnerable age groups (children, older adults), and people with a history of chronic diseases are at highest risk for heat-related mortality and morbidity. The capacity to adapt with mitigation strategies to reduce heat exposure is often determined by the societal vulnerabilities. The socially vulnerable populations such as low-income groups, socially isolated, people without access to education or health insurance, and people lacking adaptive capacity mostly suffer from the heat events. In many metropolitan cities, minorities and low-income individuals are more likely to live in neighborhoods devoid of green spaces with more paved and impervious surfaces and with limited access to air conditioning. These neighborhoods can exhibit 22 °F higher nighttime temperature than surrounding areas (Rudolph et al., 2018). Since 2013, 52% of African Americans, 32% of Asian Americans, and 21% of Hispanics are residing in the heat-stress areas across the United States (Rudolph et al., 2018). Moreover, mortality rate in the rural areas is about 3% higher than the urban areas due to limited access to healthcare services, transportation, and useful information; higher numbers of outdoor workers; and a large older adult population. Heat-related mortality rates in crop workers were 20 times higher than the usual U.S. rate during 1992 to 2006, illustrating greater risks for people in outdoor occupations (Rudolph et al., 2018). Some risk factors during the EHEs could be social isolation, age, and cognitive or physical impairment. High mortality in older adults living alone was observed in the 2003 European heat wave (Gamble et al., 2016). Limited mobility and cognitive impairment also constrain the ability to move to safer cool places and the ability to understand the severity of EHE risks. Limited regulation in core body temperature makes the process of coping with outdoor temperature more difficult for the vulnerable age groups of children and older adults. Moreover, people with underlying diseases including chronic ones such as diabetes, cardiovascular and respiratory problems, and obesity fall under the group of high-heat morbidity risks.

DETERMINANTS OF HEAT-RELATED HEALTH RISKS

The nature and scale of heat-related impacts vary as a function of individual acclimatization capacity and adaptive capacity of a community, institutions, and infrastructure to the changing climate preparedness for the heat events, in addition to location, duration, and intensity of EHEs. Factors that can dominate health risks can be categorized as environmental and nonenvironmental risk factors, and are listed in Figure 10.3.

Environmental Risk Factors

The factors or conditions in the environment that can pose potential heat-related hazards are defined as environmental risk factors. The built environment of a location and its weather conditions such as air temperature, humidity, wind speed, and solar radiation have direct effects on the human thermal comfort level. When the temperature gets warmer than the limit people are usually accustomed to, the vulnerability of losing control of inner temperature increases. One of the commonly used indices to understand multiple meteorological parameters is Heat Index, which combines relative humidity with the

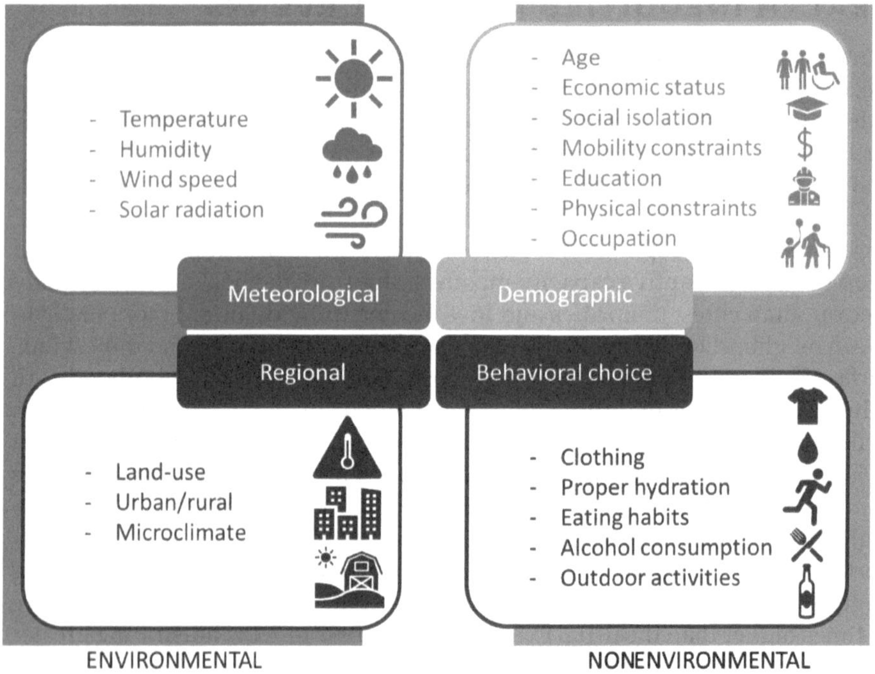

Figure 10.3 Factors affecting health risks attributable to extreme heat events.

air temperature to understand human-perceived temperature. However, the index is not properly designed to capture dry wind scenarios and often assumes shaded condition with light wind velocity. There is also increased risk associated with the hot, dry wind condition that may lead to rapid dehydration. Since regions with comparatively cooler climate do not mandate buildings to be equipped with air conditioning, persistent heat waves for several days over 90 °F can pose increased risk for inhabitants along with the limited access to emergency care, transportation, and cooling centers. Regional characteristics such as extent of urbanizations, local urban design, urban microclimate, and the geographic location can play a significant function in determining an individual's health risks. An example of environmental factors within an urban setting can be buildings with dark roofs and ground urban areas mostly paved with dark and hard materials that absorb 60% to 95% of solar energy instead of reflecting to atmosphere. Cities usually have a significantly warmer microclimate (defined as a set of local atmospheric conditions varying from the surrounding areas) than the surrounding areas even without the EHEs due to UHIs' effects. Hence, vulnerability in urban areas can become multifold difficult in terms of providing efficient public health services.

Nonenvironmental Risk Factors

Demographics, individual health conditions, and behavioral preferences are nonenvironmental risk factors. These sociodemographic parameters include people within vulnerable age groups (children and older adults), people with limited access to education, people who are socially isolated, and low-income marginalized populations. Those who have preexisting health conditions such as diabetes, heart disease, and obesity lack the adaptive capacity to tolerate the EHEs. Individual behavioral choices or habits can also profoundly affect one's health risk during an

EHE. These choices might include wearing dark clothes that restrict the cooling process via evaporation of perspiration; exposing skin to the sun; failing to consume enough water, which is critical to regulate core body temperature; consuming alcohol, which impairs judgment and limits perspiration; participating in outdoor activities that increase sun exposure, and eating high-protein and hot food that increases core body heat with high metabolic rate.

PUBLIC HEALTH ACTIONS TO ADDRESS EXTREME HEAT EVENTS

It is crucial for proper public health services to predict, control, and improve the health burdens that increasing numbers of EHEs may impose. The American Public Health Association (APHA) and a group of federal, state, and local agencies and stakeholders developed a standard framework for public health action in 1994, which includes 10 essential public health services. Public health professionals should confront practicality in developing and implementing EHE response plans via essential public health services (addressed in the following subsection) because the severity, intensity, and occurrence of extreme heat vary regionally. The effects of EHEs also vary by population groups due to unequal susceptibility within different population criteria. The response planning and policy implementation must be multidisciplinary to address overall complexity in meteorological systems. Understanding regional variation, health inequalities, and complex climatic scenarios are required to consider public health actions to address EHE effects based on the 10 essential public health services.

10 Essential Services of Public Health and Core Competencies

Case studies of heat-related events in the following section will be used to demonstrate the 10 essential services of public health and related competencies (Table 10.2). Additionally, Table 10.3 lists the CEPH competencies required for frontline health workers, managers, and leaders for heat-related emergency preparedness, response, and recovery. Examples were drawn from Philadelphia, Phoenix, and Toronto. Philadelphia first experienced EHEs in the summer of 1991, which caused 20 mortalities. In 1993, the city experienced similar conditions from July 4 to July 14 that resulted in 105 heat-related deaths, with minimum daily temperatures of at least 90 °F. In response to these two recurrent events, Philadelphia launched an EHE forecasting system in advance of 2 days and built a Heat Task Force that identified relevant agencies and departments to develop an integrated communication system. Phoenix is one of the hottest cities in the United States, where 100 °F to 110 °F is usual and some days are above 120 °F; residents are mostly acclimatized to high temperature. In mid-July 2005, several heat mortalities were reported in Phoenix from consecutive days (2-weeks duration) of record-breaking high temperatures. In response to that event, Phoenix prioritized using homeless shelters and air-conditioning facilities to limit severe heat exposure. Toronto, on the other hand, evolved its own program from perceived local health risks as a proactive and precautionary response instead of originating as an immediate response from a specific heat event. The city started its program with a temperature threshold to initiate health alerts in 1998 as an effort to address health issues of the homeless people. A full-fledged plan was in action starting in the summer of 2001 and is an example of an effective program learned from relevant case studies prior to local-level implementation.

Service 1: Monitoring Extreme Heat Event-Attributable Mortality and Morbidity Toward Exploring Solutions

Competencies applied in this essential service include tracking the trends in EHE-attributable illnesses and mortalities. This requires data from a variety of sources, including public health tracking or surveillance systems, that can determine the extent and trends of heat-related mortality and morbidity rates over time; forecast EHE conditions in advance; identify clusters of health burdens, affected regions, and vulnerable populations; and assess the availability of cooling centers. Different types of data including environmental, social, and health risks are critical to design policies, assess, and execute public health interventions. Environmental data consist of meteorological factors and physical parameters of a region such as built environment, existing or lost vegetation, waterbodies, and land elevation, while social parameters address the aspects of health inequalities including social status.

These data can be directly collected from the community or can be simulated using other independent variables over time through different statistical or quantitative methods. For example, land surface temperature (LST) can be

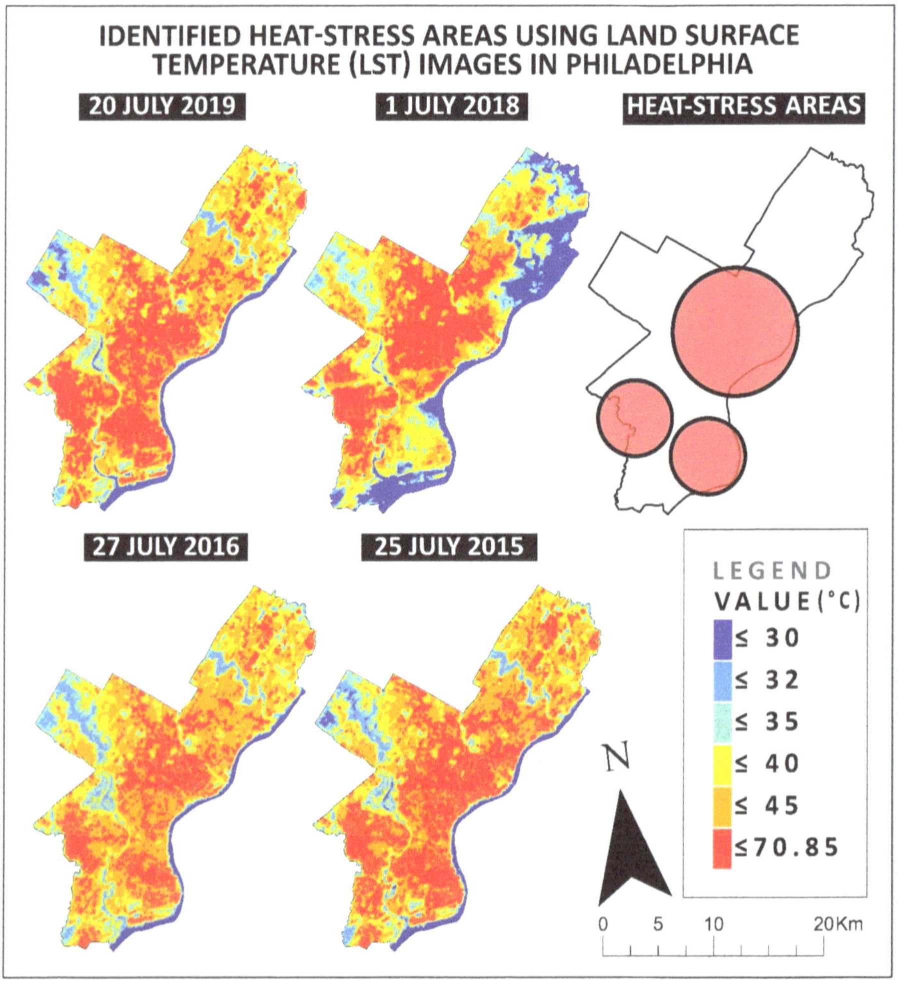

Figure 10.4 Identified heat-stress areas using LST images in Philadelphia, Pennsylvania.

LST, land surface temperature.

derived from the satellite images and used as an indicator of heat stress within a study area. Observing LST over a course of time can be a useful way to identify regions most vulnerable to extreme heat. As case studies, LST maps have been derived using the satellite images from Landsat 8 via remote-sensing techniques for Philadelphia, Pennsylvania, and Birmingham, Alabama. Figure 10.4 shows the heat-stress areas in Philadelphia at 30-m resolution, which have been identified from derived LST images over the summer and winter months. Similarly, Figure 10.5 locates heat-stress regions in the city of Birmingham. By incorporating LST data with other environmental and

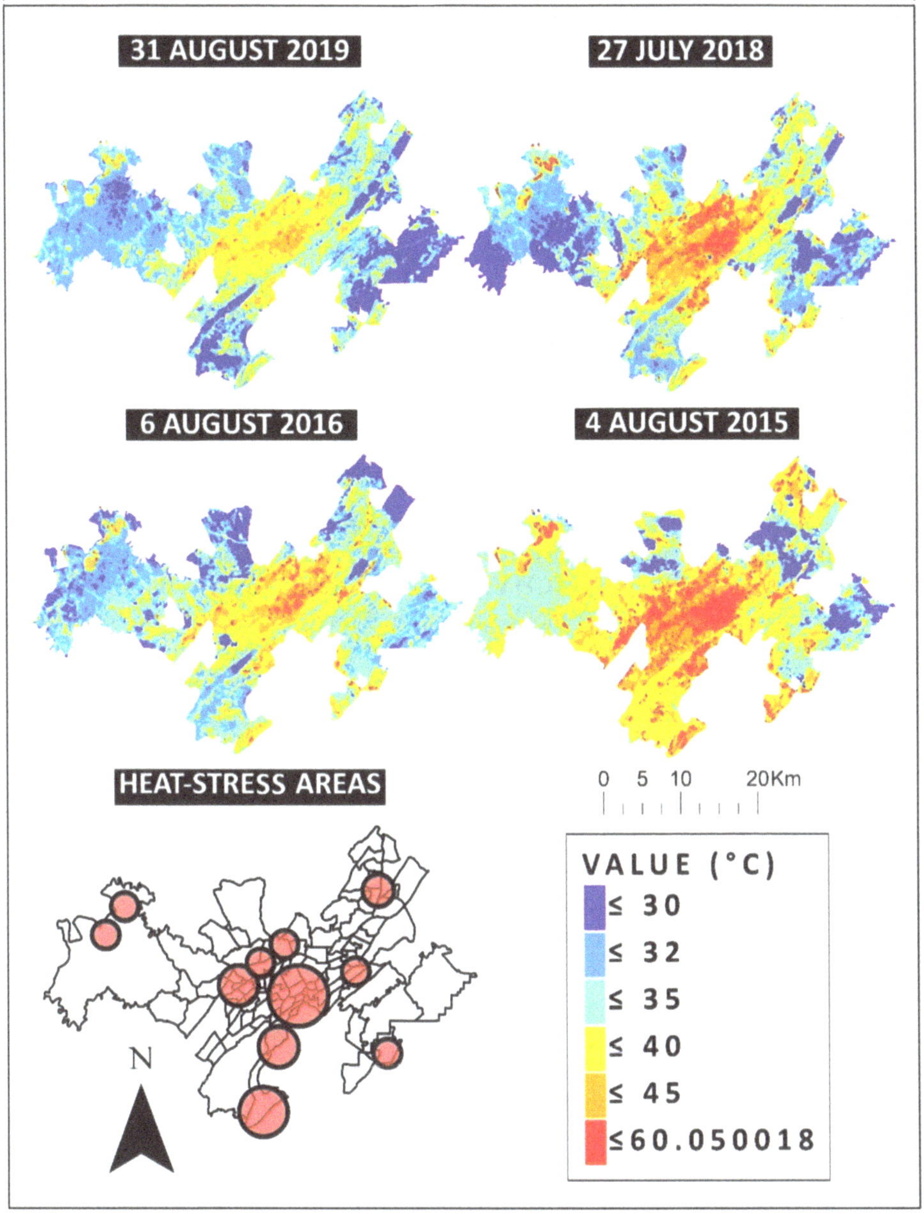

Figure 10.5 Identified heat-stress areas using land surface temperature images in Birmingham, Alabama.

socioeconomic factors, useful public health tools can be developed for public health research that can lead to formulating policy and implementation of an early EHE warning system. In addition, clinical data such as heat-illness syndromic surveillance data, patients' laboratory data, pharmaceutical use, and emergency hotline call tracking data from local healthcare services can be combined with the warning system. All these data are useful for performing a heat vulnerability assessment and can demonstrate the need for potential neighborhood greening and mitigative measures to address the UHIs with a high number of people who have social risk factors.

Service 2: Investigating Extreme Heat Event-Attributable Health Problems at the Community Level

Competencies applied for this essential public health service include identifying, diagnosing, and understanding heat-related health problems and hazards at the community level. Data on the availability of healthcare, health insurance, and accessibility of medical treatment can be utilized to model health vulnerability during EHEs. However, to track health effects attributed to EHEs specifically, a comprehensive structure is required in the health system with enhanced capacity in diagnosis and investigation since EHEs can initiate many health issues including emerging vector-borne diseases that need to be monitored at regional scale. The existing system is highly limited by the lack of geo-located high-resolution health data, which limits the researchers to access data at the local level. The data can also be constrained by temporal and spatial consistency.

Understanding the extent to which EHEs can cause health hazards is the main concern of this competency, which helps develop effective strategies for proper health system responses. Several methods have been proposed to quantify EHE-attributable health impacts via risk assessment techniques. For example, a **cumulative heat vulnerability index (CHVI)** was developed to map EHEs and related vulnerability for 2,081 census block groups in Maricopa County of Arizona; a similar susceptibility index has been mapped using the spatiotemporal dimensions of environmental and demographic parameters for the Milwaukee metropolitan area of Wisconsin (Christenson et al., 2017), census tracts of San Juan City in Puerto Rico (Méndez-Lázaro et al., 2018), New York State (Nayak et al., 2018), New York City (Karimi et al., 2018), and census grids of Camden in New Jersey (Sabrin, Karimi, Fahad, et al., 2020; Sabrin, Karimi, & Nazari, 2020). There are few examples of mapping methods to track vulnerability. Participatory vulnerability assessment integrates qualitative detailed survey data with available data. The map overlay method utilizes available knowledge about related health outcomes. **Cluster analysis** defines areas of similar degrees of susceptibility. Hazard mapping locates the areas of extreme heat exposure (one relatable example could be FEMA flood maps). Time activity patterns can be useful to map health outcome data in the spatial and temporal dimensions. **Machine learning** technique uses available explanatory variables and health outcomes data to train a forecast model using machine learning algorithms.

Service 3: Disseminate Public Health Information About Extreme Heat Event Health Issues

The aim of this competency is to establish effective health communication among the research scientists, public health professionals, and policy makers to inform potential EHE-attributable health issues. There are significant gaps in people's knowledge about the occurrence and importance of EHEs along with climate change effects. This indirectly reflects the individual views of health aspects and hinders adaptive capacity, which makes this competency more critical. Different groups accounting for ethnic and cultural differences, varying levels of health vulnerabilities, and EHE understanding should be targeted to empower them with access to necessary health resources during the extreme events. Information on heat vulnerability assessment should be shared with partners including community-based organizations, social services agencies, residents, schools, healthcare providers and institutions, and emergency management agencies to promote awareness of heat-illness prevention and to prompt mitigative suggestions for the local and community agencies to address EHE vulnerability. For example, both Toronto and Philadelphia organize public announcements about the timing, duration, and severity of forecasted EHEs and information on the availability of cooling centers, heat exposure symptoms, and tips on cooling techniques during EHEs, as well as phone lines to be used to report EHE-related health issues. They also established direct contact with areas and individuals at higher risk, enhanced outreach measures to cooling center provisions for the homeless, designated specific infrastructures with air conditioning as cooling centers, and aided public transportation. Philadelphia media recommends practice of the buddy system where friends, families, neighbors, or block captains check on the residents at risk during the events. Government agencies like the U.S. Environmental Protection Agency (EPA) also share useful tips via websites to establish communication with people from all sectors. Identifying vulnerable areas and people is the primary step in the mitigation processes. Many researchers have proposed spatial frameworks to assess the EHE-related vulnerability using high-resolution data sets (Karimi et al., 2018; Sabrin, Karimi, Fahad, et al., 2020; Sabrin, Karimi, & Nazari, 2020), so they can be utilized as a prediction tool in locating high-risk areas at greater details. NOAA recently released publicly accessible tools developed from similar frameworks to precisely target vulnerable populations to protect and prepare for the EHEs (Leslie & Bateman, 2017).

Service 4: Organizing Community Partnerships Toward Implementing Adaptive Measures

Organizing community partnerships among academia, private institutions, and federal, state, and local government agencies is critical to build integrated multisector and interdisciplinary responses to health problems. Such partnership usually develops from the local or state level starting with identifying health problems, locating vulnerable areas and populations, proposing policies, and implementing adaptive measures. New partnerships must be developed in addition to maintaining existing relationships with public health collaborators such as city planners, architects, and transportation planners who are driven by energy-efficient, climate-resilient city-building designs and low-emission environment-friendly transportation systems. In addition, the religious communities can share governance in disseminating public health information.

The multisector partnership will promote expansion in the green infrastructure and spaces, which enhances community access to cooler spaces like parks, waterfronts, tree canopy, and urban streams and addresses UHI effects. Public awareness campaigns can be useful to share information about heat-related illnesses with community residents at the neighborhood level. Local clinicians can be trained to protect patients from heat-related illnesses.

Communities should be informed about resources for financial support to deal with heat, such as the Low-Income Home Energy Assistance Program (LIHEAP). Philadelphia uses block captains elected by block residents who represent a critical point of communication between health departments and the public during EHEs and help in coordinating neighborhood improvement projects. Block captains and their neighbors, community groups, and units are currently working together to identify high-risk and isolated individuals during EHEs.

Service 5: Designing Policies That Safeguard Community and Individual Health

Public health professionals and healthcare providers in collaboration with scientists can effectively spread information on the EHE-attributable health impacts, provide evidence on the mortality–morbidity assessment data in terms of different EHE scenarios, and play significant roles in developing plans and policies by addressing EHE risks. Identified regions within county or municipality levels can be targeted for vigilant policies to implement proper rescue plans and health surveillance at the local level, as well as involve the healthcare providers, educate residents, and designate cooling centers. Other plans can be beneficial to mitigate EHEs: cool and green roof programs, broadcasting helpful tips during EHEs, establishing a website, maintaining a phone line in multiple languages with information on cooling centers and heat illness prevention, issuing media publicity of EHE-relevant information, and providing an emergency warning system in collaboration with local weather forecasters to use a standard terminology for heat.

After experiencing severe extreme heat waves in 1993, Philadelphia has developed an organized field team consisting of city health department staffs who follow up with the high-risk individuals identified from a developed phone system (Heatline calls). The Maricopa County Department of Public Health (MCDPH) engaged with a diverse array of stakeholders from 45 participating organizations to bridge climate change and public health, elevating the health and equity impacts of extreme heat in November 2016. The MCDPH developed a formal strategic plan for Maricopa County in a second summit in May 2017. Community partners identified five strategic directions in a series of three meetings (MCDPH, 2017):

- Celebrate incremental success and climate and health champions.
- Encourage community awareness and public education about climate and health.
- Promote environmental and climate action for a better community.
- Coordinate research and collaborative efforts to catalyze change.
- Develop a strategic and targeted communication plan.

Service 6: Implementing Regulatory Measures Toward Supporting Public Health and Safety

Public health professionals can offer scientific knowledge before enacting law and regulations to address EHEs. After policies are legislated, state and government agencies can enforce regulations to protect city dwellers during EHEs. For example, agencies can establish associations with employers and local Occupational Safety and Health Administration (OSHA) officials to ensure that outdoor workers and others vulnerable to heat are informed and that employers are mindful of their responsibilities to prevent occupational heat-related illness, especially providing shaded cool areas, plenty of drinking water, extended breaks for workers, and adjusted work schedules to reduce physical demands during the hottest times of day. Emergency services and law enforcement should train police and first responders to recognize heat-related illness in vulnerable populations and ensure the heat response plan includes strategies to reach homebound individuals. Utilities and other agencies must inform residents about and ensure enforcement of "disconnection rules" that prohibit electricity cutoffs.

Service 7: Connecting People With Appropriate In-Person Healthcare and Ensuring Services When Necessary

A health response program to address EHE issues must include an integrated infrastructure to provide healthcare during a disaster. Preparing for heat waves requires planning in local, regional, and national emergency medical systems, including specialized services, and expanding capacity in disaster response. Such requirements have been incorporated in the National Response Plan under Emergency Support Function #8, which is called Public Health and Medical Services. Medical planning during a disaster must address the issue of interrupting normal medical services during extreme events and planning accordingly. Also, local codes require facilities such as assisted-living establishments to monitor and automate air cooling systems to remain within comfortable temperatures in all living and communal areas. Housing conditions and susceptibility of household members can be monitored to provide EHE health information and refer to social programs and services providing financial support (for rebates, subsidies, air conditioning, tree planting) that can save lives from heat-related illnesses.

Service 8: Securing a Competent and Well-Prepared Personal–Public Healthcare Workforce

A successful health system relies on a professional, competent workforce. The workforce should be well prepared to deal with potential health impacts, including additional challenges in future years that require collected endeavors from all sectors. The health system should be updated with a set of competencies including specialized professionals with multidisciplinary backgrounds. Systematic training programs should be designated for the public health professionals that will address state and local health officials' recommended essential services. It is also beneficial to train health professionals about emerging knowledge in nontraditional disciplines such as urban health, ecology, vulnerability modeling, and economic impacts in developing a wider range of expertise.

Service 9: Assessing Efficiency, Convenience, and Quality of Public Health Services

Besides planning and implementing mitigative measures, it is also the responsibility of the health professionals to determine accountability for the effectiveness, accessibility, and quality of the interventions. This evaluation process helps to improve public health endeavors in EHE response plans and communication strategies between stakeholders. This requires a reliable system with a properly trained public health workforce and vigorous inspection capacity. Intermittent evaluation of available service and the degree to which the mitigative measure is reducing the UHI phenomena is necessary for this public health competency. For example, Phoenix provides cooling centers as a critical heat adaptation service for the people who cannot afford air conditioning and developed a regional heat relief network in Maricopa County consisting of seven dozen facilities. These facilities provide free access during the summer months and additional services including food supply, water distribution, overnight shelter, and a counseling program. The MCDPH conducted a large-scale survey and used these findings to better understand the community need during EHEs, which can be an example of an evidence-based interactive approach toward evaluating adaptive programs. This approach can be used as important guidance to promote climate justice by establishing an evidence-based platform about the pros and cons of adaptive or mitigative programs.

Service 10: Exploring New and Innovative Insights for Health Impact Solutions

The final essential service of public health is to encourage researchers about innovations and techniques on adaptive strategies. These activities also include scientific research on emerging health impacts related to EHEs and best practice standards in public health and linking academicians and professionals to conduct health policy analysis, epidemiological studies, and research on health systems. Examples include promoting the sharing of data resources and protocols to enhance climate-based research, synchronizing funding applications to public and private organizations, and relating EHE-attributable health adaptation strategies among universities.

CONCLUSION

Severe heat waves are now a rising public health concern as we are expected to see a spike in extreme heat events by the end of the 21st century. Greenhouse gas emissions from our present and future activities will directly dictate the intensity of coming heat waves. Since the beginning of the 21st century, we have already experienced many record-breaking heat waves of varying intensity, making EHEs one of the major causes of global mortalities. Our bodies struggle to cope with high temperatures to which we are not normally acclimatized. Moreover, additional social, environmental, and biological susceptibilities render any adaptation measure more difficult. EHEs can affect a large group of vulnerable populations within short periods, which demands a rapid emergency response to minimize grave damages in public health. Also, there is insufficient public awareness toward health risks resulting from extended exposure to EHEs. Hence, climate change along with EHEs calls for effective mitigative measures to protect and prepare vulnerable populations so public health professionals can serve people regardless of health inequalities and without disrupting existing healthcare capacity and resources such as electricity, water, and transportation infrastructure. The 10 essential public health services and core competencies developed by the APHA provide a systematic and coordinated framework to understand complex climatic conditions and tackle potential health burdens posed by EHEs. Hands-on multidisciplinary and feasible public health services at the community, local, and state levels can save millions of lives during the extreme events.

DISCUSSION QUESTIONS

1. Discuss how public health professionals can partner with urban planners to mitigate heat-stress areas.
2. Discuss the paradox of freon use in air-conditioning units for cooling, while the substance is actually a greenhouse gas and a contributor to global warming.
3. Discuss the social determinants of heat-related injuries. Who is likely to be affected, and why?
4. Why do people lock children and pets in cars with tragic results? Discuss.

SUMMARY

TABLE 10.2 Select Essential Services of Public Health Demonstrated in Heat-Related Emergencies and Events

Essential Service # and Definition	Context in Chapter Case	Competency # It Ties to	Importance for Emergency Preparedness, Response, or Recovery
1. Assess and monitor population health status, factors that influence health, and community needs and assets (Assessment)	Land surface temperature (LST) maps using satellite images from Landsat 8 via remote sensing techniques for Philadelphia, Pennsylvania, and Birmingham, Alabama	1, 2, 3, 4	Monitoring the health status of populations affected by the impact of climate change is increasingly becoming urgent. Public health scientists should collect data among people and places experiencing extreme heat events (EHEs) and monitor trends over time.
2. Investigate, diagnose, and address health problems and hazards affecting the population (Assessment)	Cumulative heat vulnerability index developed to map EHEs and related vulnerability for 2,081 census block groups in Maricopa County of Arizona	3, 4	Knowledge of places experiencing increasing EHEs and why these areas are vulnerable will aid in preparing populations living there, aid in strategies to reduce harm caused by EHEs, and aid in revitalizing environments for resilience.
3. Communicate effectively to inform and educate people about health, factors that influence it, and how to improve it (Policy Development)	Toronto and Philadelphia organize public announcements about EHEs and information on cooling centers, heat exposure symptoms, and tips on cooling techniques.	18, 19	Populations living in hot zones must receive comprehendible information for protection of self and family members in advance of seasonal heat waves. Public health professionals are critical to conveying this important information to save lives.
4. Strengthen, support, and mobilize communities and partnerships to improve health (Policy Development)	Philadelphia uses elected block captains who are a critical point of communication between health departments and the public while coordinating neighborhood improvement projects.	13, 14	Going forward, in anticipation of climate change-related EHE, public health professionals must partner with communities and organizations to ensure that populations are prepared for EHE in advance and understand what to do.
5. Create, champion, and implement policies, plans, and laws that impact health (Policy Development)	After heat waves in 1993, Philadelphia developed an organized field team of city health department staff, who follow up with the high-risk individuals.	12, 13	Policies and plans in place for addressing EHE in advance help communities reduce associated morbidity and mortality, ensuring that roles and responsibilities of responders, leaders, and others are clear on concrete activities and expectations.
6. Utilize legal and regulatory actions designed to improve and protect the public's health (Policy Development)	Agencies can establish associations with employers and local Occupational Safety and Health Administration officials to ensure outdoor workers and others vulnerable to heat are informed.	13, 14	Regulations to protect people who must work outside during heat seasons ensure that employers know what to do to protect the workforce. Employers must ensure that workers are not overexposed to heat and provide hydration for vulnerable workers.
7. Assure an effective system that enables equitable access to the individual services and care needed to be healthy (Assurance)	Local codes require facilities (assisted-living establishments) to monitor and automate air cooling systems to remain within comfortable temperatures in living and communal areas.	5, 21	Public health professionals should work in communities to inspect vulnerable or marginal congregate living spaces, nursing homes, schools and day-care centers, and other places with large numbers of people to ensure air conditioning apparatuses are adequate to cool the volume of inhabitants.

(continued)

TABLE 10.2 Select Essential Services of Public Health Demonstrated in Heat-Related Emergencies and Events (*continued*)

Essential Service # and Definition	Context in Chapter Case	Competency # It Ties to	Importance for Emergency Preparedness, Response, or Recovery
8. Build and support a diverse and skilled public health workforce (Assurance)	Training health professionals about knowledge in nontraditional disciplines–urban health, ecology, vulnerability modeling, and economic impacts	21, 22	A skilled public health workforce is essential for understanding climate change and related issues. Persons considering careers in public health that address extreme heat should have a broad knowledge of climate change, health disparities, health equity, and vulnerable populations, as well as geographic trends in EHE.

TABLE 10.3 Select CEPH Competencies Needed for Frontline Health Workers, Managers, and Leaders for Heat-Related Emergency Preparedness, Response, and Recovery

Competency # and Definition	Context in Case/Chapter	Level	Importance for Emergency Preparedness, Response, or Recovery
3. Analyze quantitative and qualitative data using biostatistics, informatics, computer-based programming, and software, as appropriate.	Clinical data, patients' laboratory data, pharmaceutical use, and emergency hotline call tracking data from local healthcare services can be combined with the warning system.	Level 1	Mastery of computer-based qualitative and quantitative data analytical software is essential for Level 1 professionals. Rapidly analyzing both kinds of data is important for informing preparedness and response activities.
7. Assess population needs, assets, and capacities that affect communities' health.	Local codes require facilities such as assisted-living establishments to monitor and automate air cooling systems in all living and communal areas.	Level 2	At Level 2, deeper understanding of population characteristics and needs, economic diversity, populations with special needs, children, and others at risk is required. Knowledge of a community's assets, to include infrastructure, funds, and other resources, is important for middle-level managers also.
13. Propose strategies to identify stakeholders and build coalitions and partnerships for influencing public health outcomes.	Agencies can establish associations with employers and local *Occupational Safety and Health Administration* officials to ensure that outdoor workers and others vulnerable to heat are informed.	Level 2	Workplace hazards can be avoided or mitigated through communicating public health recommendations to employers and other stakeholders.
15. Evaluate policies for their impact on public health and health equity.	Maricopa County Department of Public Health conducted a large-scale survey and used these findings to better understand the community need during extreme heat events (EHEs).	Level 3	At Level 3, policy makers and other decision-makers use data generated on previous events to evaluate responses. Identification of what worked and gaps can be determined by reviewing after-action reports. At Level 3, policies can be introduced to ensure health disparities are addressed and processes to include health equity are undertaken. What can be done to improve services to the underserved, for example?
18. Select communication strategies for different audiences and sectors.	Philadelphia uses block captains elected by block residents who are a critical point of communication between health departments and the public.	Levels 1, 2, 3	At all levels appropriate messages should be crafted based on the target audiences.
20. Describe the importance of cultural competence in communicating public health content.	National Oceanic and Atmospheric Administration released publicly accessible tools developed to target vulnerable populations to protect and prepare for the EHEs.	Level 3	Understanding diversity in a community should be a priority for decision-makers at this level. Without this critical knowledge, responses may miss vulnerable populations or may not serve them in appropriate ways.

Key: Essential services of public health; CEPH competencies; Leadership levels.

REFERENCES

Centers for Disease Control and Prevention. (2017). *Climate change and extreme heat events*. https://www.cdc.gov/climateandhealth/pubs/extreme-heat-guidebook.pdf

Christenson, M., Geiger, S. D., Phillips, J., Anderson, B., Losurdo, G., & Anderson, H. A. (2017). Heat vulnerability index mapping for Milwaukee and Wisconsin. *Journal of Public Health Management and Practice, 23*(4), 396–403. https://doi.org/10.1097/PHH.0000000000000352

Crowley, R. A. (2016). Climate change and health: A position paper of the American College of Physicians. *Annals of Internal Medicine, 164*(9), 608–610. https://doi.org/10.7326/M15-2766

Dahl, K., Licker, R., Abatzoglou, J. T., & Declet-Barreto, J. (2019). Increased frequency of and population exposure to extreme heat index days in the United States during the 21st century. *Environmental Research Communications, 1*(7), 075002. https://doi.org/10.1088/2515-7620/ab27cf

Davis, R. E., & Novicoff, W. M. (2018). The impact of heat waves on emergency department admissions in Charlottesville, Virginia, U.S.A. *International Journal of Environmental Research and Public Health, 15*(7), 1436. https://doi.org/10.3390/ijerph15071436

Department of Economic and Social Affairs. (2018). *Revision of world urbanization prospects*. Population Division of the UN Department of Economic and Social Affairs. https://population.un.org/wup

Fahad, G. R., Nazari, R., Daraio, J., & Lundberg, D. J. (2017). Regional study of future temperature and precipitation changes using bias corrected multi-model ensemble projections considering high emission pathways. *Journal of Earth Science and Climatic Change, 8*(9). https://doi.org/10.4172/2157-7617.1000409

Gamble, J. L., Balbus, J., Berger, M., Bouye, K., Campbell, V., Chief, K., Conlon, K., Crimmins, A., Flanagan, B., Gonzalez-Maddux, C., Hallisey, E., Hutchins, S., Jantarasami, L., Khoury, S., Kiefer, M., Kolling, J., Lynn, K., Manangan, A., McDonald, M., . . . Hallisey, E. (2016). Populations of concern. In A. Crimmins, J. Balbus, J. L. Gamble, C. B. Beard, J. E. Bell, D. Dodgen, R. J. Eisen, N. Fann, M. D. Hawkins, S. C. Herring, L. Jantarasami, D. M. Mills, S. Saha, M. C. Sarofim, J. Trtanj, & L. Ziska (Eds.), *The impacts of climate change on human health in the United States: A scientific assessment* (pp. 247–286). U.S. Global Research Program. http://dx.doi.org/10.7930/J0R49NQX

Isaksen, T. B., Yost, M. G., Hom, E. K., Ren, Y., Lyons, H., & Fenske, R. A. (2015). Increased hospital admissions associated with extreme-heat exposure in King County, Washington, 1990–2010. *Reviews on Environmental Health, 30*(1), 51–64. https://doi.org/10.1515/reveh-2014-0050

Karimi, M., Nazari, R., Dutova, D., Khanbilvardi, R., & Ghandehari, M. (2018). A conceptual framework for environmental risk and social vulnerability assessment in complex urban settings. *Urban Climate, 26*, 161–173. https://doi.org/10.1016/j.uclim.2018.08.005

Karimi, M., Vant-Hull, B., Nazari, R., Mittenzwei, M., & Khanbilvardi, R. (2017). Predicting surface temperature variation in urban settings using real-time weather forecasts. *Urban Climate, 20*, 192–201. https://doi.org/10.1016/j.uclim.2017.04.008

Leslie, J., & Bateman, J. (2017). *NOAA releases new tool to help prepare and protect vulnerable populations from extreme heat*. https://www.nesdis.noaa.gov/content/noaa-releases-new-tool-help-prepare-and-protect-vulnerable-populations-extreme-heat

Lo, Y. E., Mitchell, D. M., Gasparrini, A., Vicedo-Cabrera, A. M., Ebi, K. L., Frumhoff, P. C., Millar, R. J., Roberts, W., Sera, F., Sparrow, S., Uhe, P., & Williams, G. (2019). Increasing mitigation ambition to meet the Paris Agreement's temperature goal avoids substantial heat-related mortality in US cities. *Science Advances, 5*(6), eaau4373. https://doi.org/10.1126/sciadv.aau4373

Maricopa County Department of Public Health. (2017). *Climate and health strategic plan for Maricopa County 2016–2021*. https://www.maricopa.gov/DocumentCenter/View/38688/Climate-and-Health-Strategic-Plan-2016-2021-PDF

Méndez-Lázaro, P., Muller-Karger, F. E., Otis, D., McCarthy, M. J., & Rodríguez, E. (2018). A heat vulnerability index to improve urban public health management in San Juan, Puerto Rico. *International Journal of Biometeorology, 62*(5), 709–722. https://doi.org/10.1007/s00484-017-1319-z

National Oceanic and Atmospheric Administration. (2017). *National climate report - Annual 2017*. https://www.ncdc.noaa.gov/sotc/national/201713

Nayak, S. G., Shrestha, S., Kinney, P. L., Ross, Z., Sheridan, S. C., Pantea, C. I., Hsu, W. H., Muscatiello, N., & Hwang, S. A. (2018). Development of a heat vulnerability index for New York State. *Public Health, 161*, 127–137. https://doi.org/10.1016/j.puhe.2017.09.006

Rudolph, L., Harrison, C., Buckley, L., & North, S. (2018). *Climate change, health, and equity: A guide for local health departments*. Public Health Institute and American Public Health Association. http://climatehealthconnect.org/wp-content/uploads/2018/10/APHA_ClimateGuide18_pp10web_FINAL.pdf

Sabrin, S., Karimi, M., Fahad, M. G. R., & Nazari, R. (2020). Quantifying environmental and social vulnerability: Role of urban heat island and air quality, a case study of Camden, NJ. *Urban Climate, 34*, 100699. https://doi.org/10.1016/j.uclim.2020.100699

Sabrin, S., Karimi, M., & Nazari, R. (2020). Developing vulnerability index to quantify urban heat islands effects coupled with air pollution: A case study of Camden, NJ. *ISPRS International Journal of Geo-Information, 9*(6), 349. https://doi.org/10.3390/ijgi9060349

Scortichini, M., de'Donato, F., De Sario, M., Leone, M., Åström, C., Ballester, F., Basagaña, X., Bobvos, J., Gasparrini, A., Katsouyanni, K., Lanki, T., Menne, B., Pascal, M., & Michelozzi, P. (2018). The inter-annual variability of heat-related mortality in nine European cities (1990–2010). *Environmental Health, 17*(1), 1–10. https://doi.org/10.1186/s12940-018-0411-0

World Health Organization. (2018a). *COP24 special report: Health and climate change*. https://apps.who.int/iris/handle/10665/276405

World Health Organization. (2018b). *Heat and health*. https://www.who.int/news-room/fact-sheets/detail/climate-change-heat-and-health

Wuebbles, D. J., Fahey, D. W., Hibbard, K. A., Dokken, D. J., Stewart, B. C., & Maycock, T. K. (Eds.). (2017). *Climate science special report: Fourth national climate assessment (NCA4)* (Vol. I). U.S. Global Change Research Program. https://doi.org/10.7930/J0J964J6

CHAPTER 11

PUBLIC HEALTH RESPONSE TO BIOTERRORISM

LESSONS FROM THE 2001 ANTHRAX ATTACKS AS A FOUNDATION

ALLISON P. CHEN, ALEXANDER H. CHANG, AND EDBERT B. HSU

KEY TERMS

Ciprofloxacin
Dispersant
Doxycycline
Prophylaxis

INTRODUCTION

To maintain a healthy society, public health personnel at all levels must remain vigilant in protecting the nation from all forms of biological threats. Biological threats may be either naturally occurring or man-made. Naturally occurring biological threats include outbreaks of an identified virus, such as Ebola, or the COVID-19 pandemic resulting from a novel virus such as SARS-CoV-2. Other biological threats include bacterial exotoxins affecting our food, such as Shiga toxin from *E. coli* O157:H7, or climate change affecting our agricultural supply chain. Man-made biological threats include the accidental or intentional contamination from laboratory agents or biological weapons, which exploit the properties of microbes or their toxins to intentionally produce harm in humans, animals, or plants. This chapter focuses on an important historical

---

The following icons, located in the margins throughout the chapter and within the summary tables, denote essential services of public health, CEPH competencies, and leadership levels: Essential services of public health; CEPH competencies; Leadership levels.

case of bioterrorism on U.S. soil involving a deliberate attempt to cause harm using biological agents.

The 2001 anthrax attacks, sometimes referred to as Amerithrax after the code name of the ensuing investigation, were biological attack events in the United States involving the mailing of anthrax-laced letters to news media offices and congressmen. Two sets of letters, the first set postmarked September 18, 2001, and the second set postmarked October 9, 2001, were sent to the *New York Post* and Tom Brokaw at NBC News in New York City and Senators Patrick Leahy and Thomas Daschle in Washington, DC. Evidence suggests that an additional letter was likely sent to American Media, Inc. (AMI) in Boca Raton, Florida, although no physical letter was ever found. In total, there were 22 cases of anthrax as a result of the letters, with five deaths (Federal Bureau of Investigation [FBI], 2010).

The anthrax attacks began less than a month after the September 11 World Trade Center attacks, and thus occurred in an existing climate of national security concern. They severely tested public health resources and response capabilities at the local, state, and federal levels and remain an event from which lessons are drawn regarding responses to bioterrorism and other major emergencies.

BACKGROUND OF THE ANTHRAX ATTACKS

Bioterrorism Concerns Prior to 2001

During the 1970s and 1980s, concern over nuclear weapons largely overshadowed concern over biological weapon threats. It was not until the 1990s that the possibility of a major biological attack on the United States began to become a political issue of some note, with this new attention the result of several factors (Cohen & Cook, 2006). These included growing alarm about the threat posed by newly emerging or reemerging infectious diseases, bolstered by the recent HIV/AIDS pandemic, as well as the rise of drug-resistant microbes (Lederberg et al., 1992). In addition to naturally occurring pathogens, there was the emergence of evidence regarding the biological weapons programs of countries such as Russia and Iraq (Davis, 1999). High-profile terrorism incidents, including a sarin gas attack in Tokyo perpetrated by a group that had also attempted to develop biological agents, drew attention to threats from nonstate actors as well (Cohen & Cook, 2006). An outbreak of West Nile virus in New York City in 1999, marking the first appearance of the virus in the Western Hemisphere, was at one point suspected to have been a bioterrorist attack, although it was determined that this was not the case and the appearance was natural, not deliberate (U.S. General Accounting Office [GAO], 2000).

In 2000, the U.S. National Intelligence Council issued a report examining the potential national and international impact of diseases of concern, as well as scenarios regarding them and existing capabilities to address them. The focus was on naturally occurring diseases, although it was acknowledged that the risk of a bioterrorist attack was growing as well. The report anticipated disease to "complicate US and global security over the next 20 years" (National Intelligence Estimate, 2000).

There was a recognition that the U.S. public health system was underprepared to handle growing biological threats. Studies conducted in the late 1990s indicated that the system suffered from outdated laboratories, a lack of trained staff, a lack of biological attack response plans in almost 80% of hospitals, and insufficient infrastructure for communication, such as no access to email in almost 20% of local health departments (Frist, 2002).

Legislation arose in the United States in response, although implementation and investment of actual resources was lackluster. The landmark Public Health Threats and Emergencies Act was passed in late 2000, but it received little attention from lawmakers at the time, and it seemed unlikely that its initiatives would be fully funded. It did indicate an understanding that public health capability to respond to disease and bioterrorism threats needed to be improved, and laid the foundation for measures taken after the 2001 anthrax attacks (Frist, 2002).

Background of Anthrax Disease

Anthrax is an infectious disease caused by the spore-forming *Bacillus anthracis* bacteria. Symptoms vary based on the route of infection, with the most common routes being cutaneous, gastrointestinal, inhalation, and injection. The disease is rare in humans, and typically transmitted from infected animals through either direct or indirect contact. Person-to-person transmission has not been observed but is thought to be possible through contact with an infected individual's skin lesions (Centers for Disease Control and Prevention [CDC], n.d.-a, n.d.-b, n.d.-c, n.d.-d; Mayo Clinic, 2020).

Victims of the 2001 attacks contracted either cutaneous or inhalation anthrax. Cutaneous anthrax enters through the skin through an open wound and results in a generally mild infection, with a localized sore and swelling. In contrast, inhalation anthrax is the most severe form. Resulting from inhalation of spores, it can initially result in flu-like symptoms, developing into difficulty breathing and shock. The disease is 85% to 90% fatal without treatment, and approximately 45% fatal with intervention (CDC, n.d.-a, n.d.-b, n.d.-c, n.d.-d). Eleven victims of the 2001 attacks contracted cutaneous anthrax, and 11 contracted inhalation anthrax. All the deaths were from cases of inhalation anthrax.

Bacillus anthracis has been classified as a Tier 1 agent by the U.S. government, designating it as a pathogen with the highest risk of "deliberate misuse" and the potential to "pose a severe threat to public health." Anthrax is considered a likely candidate for a biological agent for several reasons, including that spores can be readily found or produced, are hardy and long lived in the environment, can be released discreetly, and have a history of use as a bioweapon (CDC, n.d.-a, n.d.-b, n.d.-c, n.d.-d).

The 2001 Anthrax Attacks

The first of two sets of anthrax-laced letters were postmarked September 18, 2001, from Trenton, New Jersey, and were sent to the *New York Post* and NBC News. Individuals infected by these letters began noticing symptoms in late September but were not formally diagnosed until mid-October (ABC News, 2001; Begley & Isikoff, 2001).

The first victim to be formally diagnosed, and the first victim to die from the attack, was Robert Stevens, a photo editor for American Media, Inc., in Florida. His case formed the basis for the consideration that a contaminated letter had been mailed to AMI, despite one never being found. He was admitted to the hospital on October 2, 2001; diagnosed with inhalation anthrax on October 4, 2001; and expired the following day (ABC News, 2001). Another hospitalized AMI employee, who worked in the mailroom, was subsequently diagnosed with anthrax. An examination of the AMI building found traces of anthrax, and the building was closed.

On October 12, the New York City Department of Health confirmed the first case of cutaneous anthrax, broadening the known scope of the attacks (Holtz et al., 2003). The victim was an employee at NBC who had been infected by the letters sent on September 18 (GAO, 2003).

The second set of letters were also postmarked from Trenton, on October 9, 2001, and were sent to the Washington, DC, offices of Senators Patrick Leahy and Thomas Daschle. After the contaminated letter to Senator Daschle was found on October 15, congressional mail was quarantined and kept unopened until it could be checked for hazards; through this, the letter to Senator Leahy was discovered (Associated Press, 2001; *New York Times*, 2001).

In addition to individuals at the letters' targeted sites, victims of the attacks included postal workers and unconnected civilians who received cross-contaminated mail. Of the four other victims, in addition to Robert Stevens, who died as a result of the attacks, two were postal workers in Washington, DC—Thomas Morris and Joseph Curseen, Jr. The remaining two—Kathy Nguyen of New York City and Ottilie Lundgren of Connecticut—were infected as a result of receiving mail that had come into contact with contaminated letters or equipment (Nakashima & Russakoff, 2001). Lundgren was the last fatality, dying on November 21, 2001. Seventeen other individuals contracted anthrax as a result of the contaminated letters but recovered.

There were six epicenters of the attack where cases were concentrated: Florida; New York; New Jersey; the Capitol area in Washington, DC; the Washington, DC, regional area (including places in Maryland and Virginia), and Connecticut (GAO, 2003). The presence of anthrax was detected in over 50 locations, including three outside of the epicenters: postal-related facilities in Indiana, Missouri, and North Carolina (National Response Team, 2004). In total, 35 mail facilities were contaminated, with two facilities so severely affected that they were closed for over 2 years (U.S. Department of Justice, 2010).

Contaminated letters contained two different preparations of anthrax, one that was coarse and brownish and another that was a fine powder. The former was responsible for most cases of cutaneous anthrax; the latter was responsible for most cases of the more dangerous inhalation anthrax. Furthermore, silicon was found with the anthrax, raising the question of whether it had been deliberately weaponized by adding a silica **dispersant**. Ultimately it was determined, due in part to the location in the spores of the silicon, that there was no evidence for this type of weaponization (U.S. Department of Justice, 2010).

Investigation of the Attacks

The U.S. government undertook a 7-year-long investigation led by the FBI that was unprecedented in its size to identify the individual or individuals responsible for the anthrax attacks. The "Amerithrax Task Force" consisted of 25 to 30 investigators from the FBI and U.S. Postal Inspection Service at most times, in addition to federal prosecutors. More than 10,000 witness interviews were conducted, while about 6,000 pieces of potential evidence and 5,700 environmental samples were collected. Over 1,000 people, from the United States, as well as other nations, were investigated as suspects.

Suspects were identified based on factors including access to the pathogen used, their connection to the area in New Jersey where the letters were postmarked, potential motive, and tips. At the same time, efforts were made to genetically characterize the anthrax found in the letters as well as to determine the source of the contaminated letters and envelopes.

The strain of anthrax used was determined to be the Ames strain, originally isolated in Texas in the 1980s and distributed to laboratories worldwide, including the U.S. Army Medical Research Institute of Infectious Diseases (USAMRIID) in Maryland. Investigators also concluded that the anthrax used had not been genetically engineered.

The investigation identified Dr. Bruce E. Ivins of USAMRIID as the most likely perpetrator of the attacks, based initially on his access to the Ames strain, as well as suspicious behavior around the time of the attacks. Later, evidence recovered from his property and office further lent credence to Dr. Ivins as the individual responsible. Although he committed suicide before he could be indicted, continued investigation after his death reinforced the likelihood that he acted alone in mailing the contaminated letters (U.S. Department of Justice, 2010).

ROLES OF THE 10 ESSENTIAL SERVICES OF PUBLIC HEALTH

Assess and Monitor Population Health Status, Factors That Influence Health, and Community Needs and Assets

The response to the anthrax attacks was complicated by unique features of the event. One such feature was the fact that several geographical regions were affected at the same time. Naturally occurring disease outbreaks usually begin in one limited area and are handled at least initially by local and state public health departments, with federal agencies such as the CDC becoming involved when more resources or specialized knowledge are needed or the disease spreads beyond a state's borders. Consistent with this, at the time of the attacks the prevailing model was that data would be collected and monitored initially by local and state health departments. These data were expected to come mostly from frontline clinical staff noting outbreaks unusual in pattern or causative agent (GAO, 2003).

Monitoring of anthrax cases during the attacks began when on October 2, 2001, Robert Stevens was suspected to have anthrax when he was admitted to the hospital in Palm Beach County, Florida. The local Palm Beach County Health Department (PBCHD) and the Florida Department of Health (FDOH) were notified that day. An epidemiological investigation was launched by the PBCHD and the FDOH, and on October 4, after anthrax was confirmed by the state laboratory and the CDC, employees from the FDOH and the CDC began to assist the investigation in Palm Beach County (CDC, 2001c). Another employee from the AMI location where Stevens worked was diagnosed with anthrax on October 5, although he had been originally hospitalized before Stevens.

Epidemiologists used enhanced case findings, established retrospective and prospective surveillance, conducted environmental sampling, and distributed surveys at the AMI location where Stevens worked. Environmental sampling showed that the AMI location was contaminated with anthrax, although Stevens' home and other locations he had visited had no contamination. Nasal swabs of employees in the AMI building identified one additional individual infected with anthrax (CDC, 2001c).

On October 9, the CDC was notified by the New York City Department of Health of a suspected cutaneous anthrax case. Employees were subsequently dispatched from the CDC to New York City to assist local efforts. The case was confirmed on October 12. As of October 19, when the CDC issued an update on the anthrax cases in its *Morbidity and Mortality Weekly Report* (*MMWR*), four total cases had been confirmed, two in Florida and two in New York City. The report asserted at this time that the four cases were considered the result of intentional exposure (CDC, 2001b).

Throughout the course of the anthrax attacks, local, state, and federal public health agencies surveilled for anthrax cases in every state in the United States (Jernigan et al., 2002). The CDC was responsible for overall coordination, acting on behalf of the U.S. Department of Health and Human Services, and its teams supported other health departments' efforts especially in the six epicenters. Teams from the CDC relied on traditional epidemiological investigation approaches, a "two-pronged" strategy that involved investigating a case or confirmed exposure in conjunction with surveillance to find additional cases (GAO, 2003). Over 100 officers from the CDC's Epidemic Intelligence Service were deployed to respond to the anthrax attacks, including some 50 in Washington, DC, and almost 40 in New York City, some of whom were already there responding to the September 11 World Trade Center attacks. Officers were involved in collecting epidemiological data, contact tracing, and collecting clinical samples, among other monitoring roles (Hamilton, 2006).

In regions of concern, surveillance was also conducted in healthcare facilities through provider reporting and review of patient medical records. Any individual, not only healthcare workers and law enforcement, but the public as well, could report potential cases, and these were investigated with individuals who were potentially infected or exposed being interviewed. If a report met the surveillance case definition, which outlined criteria for determining confirmed and suspected cases (CDC, 2001d), it was forwarded to the CDC. Locations suspected to be contaminated were environmentally sampled (Jernigan et al., 2002).

These procedures indicate a reliance on frontline clinical staff to monitor health conditions in their area in conjunction with epidemiological investigators to preempt the emergence and contain the spread of health problems. Investigators must apply epidemiological methods and will most likely be responsible for analysis and interpretation of collected data, while clinical staff, with guidance from investigators, select and utilize appropriate quantitative and qualitative data collection methods.

Investigate, Diagnose, and Address Health Problems and Hazards Affecting the Population

Naturally occurring cases of anthrax in humans are rare in the United States, and mostly associated with contact with infected animals or animal products.

Between 1955 and 2000, there were 235 reported cases of human anthrax infection in the United States, of which only 11 were of inhalational anthrax (Brachman, 2002).

As a result, most clinicians and public health officials had not encountered a case of anthrax before and lacked experience in identifying cases. Healthcare facilities sought guidance from the CDC on differentiating anthrax, especially inhalational anthrax, from other diseases such as influenza with similar initial presentation (GAO, 2003). They expected specific instructions on identifying and treating cases, received in a timely manner due to the speed at which the outbreak was progressing and the improved outcomes of patients whose inhalational anthrax was detected early. Because the infections were deliberately introduced, even clinicians in areas unconnected to the known epicenters were warned to be on the lookout for cases, and needed guidance.

However, the CDC itself lacked experience addressing anthrax. At the time of the attacks, it did not have adequate background information on the disease, including a roster of experts around the United States who could be contacted, or a comprehensive review of the existing scientific literature. A need to assemble this information before developing and issuing guidance led to delays in the process, and information was often slow to reach clinicians (GAO, 2003). For example, there was once a 6-day delay between when physicians were told the CDC would be releasing guidelines on October 20 to when the guidelines were actually published in the agency's October 26 *MMWR*, a notable gap when the outbreak was accelerating. As a result, in the meantime frontline practitioners often created, and sometimes even disseminated, their own procedures and guidance. One physician later stated in an interview for a study on responses to the 2001 attacks: "We created what we needed to create" (Gursky et al., 2003).

On November 2, 2001, in the *MMWR*, the CDC published flowcharts to assist clinical evaluation of patients with suspected inhalational or cutaneous anthrax. These included a list of potential symptoms, diagnostic tests that should be run, therapies, and when to notify public health authorities. The CDC also regularly described in the *MMWR* cases of anthrax that had been identified to date, including the age and occupation of the patient, symptoms, results of tests performed, treatments given, and outcome if known (CDC, 2001c). However, the fact that updates only occurred weekly hampered its usefulness, as did its comparatively limited regular readership at the time (Gursky et al., 2003). While the broader perspective of the CDC, including receipt of information from locations across the United States, as well as greater research resources in comparison to frontline staff, meant that they were expected to provide diagnostic and evaluative guidance, and ultimately did provide guidance, when there were delays or problems with distribution, frontline staff also developed their own diagnostic and evaluative strategies from experience.

Communicate Effectively to Inform and Educate People About Health, Factors That Influence It, and How to Improve It

Communication needed to occur between the multitude of individuals, organizations, and agencies involved in the response to the attacks in order to coordinate an effective response; at the same time, information needed to be provided to the media and to the public.

The effectiveness of communication between different actors in the public health response was very variable. Communication among local and state response organizations, such as public health agencies, hazardous materials units, and police and fire departments, was largely productive since channels already existed, and additional conference calls instituted during the attacks were helpful in conveying information and opening dialogues (GAO, 2003). However, coordination suffered in areas with complicated jurisdictional designations, such as the Washington, DC, regional area, where the response involved the Maryland, Virginia, and DC health departments (Gursky et al., 2003).

Communication between public health agencies and local hospitals was relatively effective, though methods differed from place to place. Faxes, emails, CD-ROMs, website updates, and hotlines were among the methods used by public health officials to get information to clinicians (GAO, 2003). In Washington, DC, regular conference calls organized by the DC Hospital Association allowed physicians in the area to share information about their patients' clinical symptoms and discuss treatment and diagnostic options (Gursky et al., 2003). However, contacting physicians with private practices was more difficult. Many did not have an email or reliable access to the web, and rosters of telephone numbers held by public health agencies were not always current. Instead, institutions, associations, and their affiliated physicians who could access regularly updated information were depended upon to relay what they had received; it was generally agreed that relying on physicians to spread public health information was inconsistent and did not ensure good coverage (GAO, 2003).

The CDC struggled with synthesizing the enormous amount of information it was receiving and with disseminating its own guidance. It began by relying mostly on the Health Alert Network (HAN) and the *MMWR*, as well as the Epidemic Information Exchange (Epi-X), to communicate (M'ikanatha et al., 2003). Later, when these proved to be insufficient for the rapidly evolving situation, and when more regular communication with the media became needed, the CDC also adopted twice-daily press releases and daily telebriefings (GAO, 2003).

The criminal investigation that was ongoing during the outbreak hampered communication. Information collected in association with the investigation was not always provided to public health officials, and restrictions were placed on what could be shared to clinicians (GAO, 2003).

A significant dimension of communication during the attacks was dissemination of information to the media and public. The American population was still shaken by the September 11, 2001, attacks when the anthrax events began, and declarations of Islamic faith on the contaminated letters raised concern about whether the attacks were linked (U.S. Department of Justice, 2010). Uncertainty about who was responsible for the letters, how many of them there might be, and where they might appear fueled nationwide alarm. An October 13 CNN/Time Magazine poll indicated that almost half of Americans feared they or someone close would be exposed to anthrax (CNN, 2001a, 2001b, 2001c).

Every major news organization covered the events as they unfolded, providing information not only about the ongoing cases but also the history of anthrax, its usual prevalence and distribution, its clinical features, and its treatment. An October 20, 2001, article in the *British Medical Journal* observed, more seriously than not: "Any doctor could learn as much about anthrax through reading a newspaper as they could through reading a medical text" (Charatan, 2001).

There were some sources, especially on the internet, that capitalized on the uncertainty, in some cases to sell the prophylactic ciprofloxacin (Belongia et al., 2005). Major news organizations, however, tried to avoid contributing to panic by reiterating the small number of cases, that anthrax is not contagious from person to person, and that exposure did not necessarily mean a person would develop the disease (Associated Press, 2001; Charatan, 2001; CNN, 2001a, 2001b, 2001c; *New York Times*, 2001). They published recommendations on how to handle suspicious packages, and some media organizations included numbers for hotlines or ways to contact authorities. When possible, they provided distilled information from public health agencies, such as CNN's "Ten Things You Need to Know About Anthrax," with information from the CDC (CNN, 2001a, 2001b, 2001c).

Getting information from public health authorities to the news media was often challenging. An important communication-related competency is to choose the right communication strategy for each audience, which in public health may range from subject-matter experts to an unfamiliar member of the population. The news media can be an essential partner in a communication strategy; however, during the anthrax attacks different officials and agencies placed varying degrees of importance on communicating with the media, which had trouble reaching officials, especially at the CDC, in the early weeks of the outbreak (Gursky et al., 2003). The ongoing criminal investigation meant that there were further restrictions on information that could be distributed.

Particularly problematic was inconsistency in information and messaging. The rapidly changing situation and differences in developments and responses in different areas of the country meant that reporting was sometimes outdated or contradictory. For example, there was confusion regarding the use of **ciprofloxacin** versus **doxycycline** as a prophylactic. Ciprofloxacin was initially recommended. However, after the effectiveness of doxycycline was demonstrated, it began to be the drug of choice due to fewer side effects, among other considerations. This change was not clearly communicated in all areas where **prophylaxis** was being administered; especially in places where prophylaxis programs began after the change, individuals questioned why they were not being given what had previously been broadcast as the recommended drug. In Washington, DC, the miscommunication led to accusations of racial bias in how individuals were being treated, also highlighting the importance of cultural competence and sensitivity in public health communication (Gursky et al., 2003).

The impact of consistency in messaging and clarification of uncertainty can also be seen in the 2019–2020 COVID-19 pandemic, notably with information about mask wearing in the United States. At the beginning of the outbreak in March 2020, citizens were discouraged from wearing masks, likely to prevent shortages that would affect healthcare workers. However, in the early summer, masks began to be recommended as states lifted restrictions on public activities, but the given rationale was not that they would protect the wearer, but they could prevent the wearer, who might be an asymptomatic carrier, from transmitting the disease to others (University of California San Francisco, 2020). Then, in an update in November 2020, the CDC asserted that masks also protect the wearer (NPR, 2020). While these changes reflect an evolving situation and evolving knowledge about the disease, the contradictory messaging has also led to confusion that has, in some cases, fueled resistance to mask wearing.

As seen from these examples, during a disease outbreak, including one that results from bioterrorism, public health officials have roles and responsibilities not only regarding communicating with clinicians, organizations, and agencies involved in response but also communicating with the media and public. Especially with the current environment in which information is available from a staggeringly varied number of sources on a constant basis, it is important for public health officials to provide timely, ongoing, straightforward, honest, empathetic, and useful information, as it becomes available, to outlets that are able to disseminate this information effectively (Tumpey et al., 2018). This is needed to preempt or minimize the potentially dangerous influence of false, misleading, or inflammatory messaging that can undermine other public health responses, such as by prompting refusal to participate in public health efforts.

Strengthen, Support, and Mobilize Communities and Partnerships to Improve Health

During the anthrax attacks, local law enforcement, emergency medical services, fire departments, and other emergency response organizations were involved in surveillance, investigation, and environmental sampling activities. The local police or fire department would often be the one initially reached by a concerned resident encountering a suspicious package. In collaboration with the local health department, collected samples were evaluated for credibility before they were sent for laboratory analysis to determine the presence of anthrax to avoid swamping an already severely overstretched laboratory system (Trust for America's Health, 2011). This demonstrates the critical nature of establishing partnerships and collaborations both in advance of and during a public health crisis.

The nonprofessional civilian population has traditionally not been expected to play a significant role in response to bioterrorism incidents. After the attacks, there were calls to provide the public with more information in the event of a future bioterrorist attack, and it was suggested that nonprofessional community members and organizations could be mobilized, since often the populace is a good source of surveillance, and community members can be used to spread information effectively (Glass & Schoch-Spana, 2002). Furthermore, the increase of community involvement may help to identify or bring attention to issues of structural inequity.

In 2020, the COVID-19 pandemic has seen civilian employees and volunteers in the more formal roles of contact tracers nationwide.

Create, Champion, and Implement Policies, Plans, and Laws That Impact Health

As the response to the attacks progressed, frontline policies and plans, including communication protocols, what type of information was relevant for which involved party, the use of protective equipment, who should receive prophylaxis, and clinical and environmental testing standard practices, needed to be developed and followed locally. This involved coordination and agreement between public health officials and agencies, postal officials, federal investigators, and local first responders (GAO, 2003).

Existing plans from before 2001 primarily involved partnerships between local and state public health officials and law enforcement and emergency responders. Incorporation of other organizations such as the postal service, environmental agencies, and the military, all of whom were involved in the anthrax attacks response, had not been as widely expected. As a result, necessary communication, safety, and testing policies were created throughout the event. This also highlights the importance of being able to efficiently identify stakeholders and response partners during a specific bioterrorism or outbreak incident, as they may not be the same as in prior events.

Interaction with hospitals for the purpose of setting up screening and prophylaxis clinics was also a consideration that lacked existing frameworks in many local areas. The timeline for establishing these clinics was often very tight, with some clinics set up within 24 hours. Plans were developed for selecting appropriate locations, ensuring sufficient staff, and stocking supplies and medications. There were some areas that had existing procedures in place regarding these issues, and their response time was improved as a result (GAO, 2003).

At the overall federal level, the CDC used working groups of between six to eight subject matter experts in order to develop plans and guidance for clinical and environmental activities. These working groups had to review and incorporate information that was coming in on a constant basis. As a result of the evolving situation, some CDC policies and guidelines changed throughout the event. For example, since the first anthrax cases were linked to contact with opened contaminated letters, the CDC initially considered individuals who would have only come into contact with sealed contaminated letters to be at low risk (CDC, 2001d; GAO, 2003). However, after five individuals from Washington, DC–area mail facilities developed inhalation anthrax without contact with opened letters, guidance was revised, including guidance on who should receive prophylaxis (Dewan et al., 2002).

Utilize Legal and Regulatory Actions Designed to Improve and Protect the Public's Health

Bioterrorism events may be overt or covert; in the former case, the event is clearly identifiable as an attack, while in the latter case the event may initially appear to be naturally occurring. The overt or covert nature of an event can influence the balance of public health and law enforcement response. While the first anthrax case was best classified as covert, by the time additional victims were identified it became evident that these were deliberate infections (Butler et al., 2002).

The response to the attacks required coordination between public health and law enforcement in order for the activities and investigation conducted by one not to interfere with the other. For instance, the processing of samples during the attacks, in addition to being necessary for public health purposes, also needed to adhere to standards, be consistent between laboratories with regard to protocols and reagents, and maintain a chain of custody, such that the results would stand during legal proceedings. Additionally, interviews with potentially infected and exposed individuals needed to be conducted for both public health and law enforcement reasons; however, multiple interviews of the same individual ran the risk of inconsistent statements, which could be challenged in court. To address this, in some cases law enforcement officers and epidemiologists conducted interviews together. Security clearance was another point of consideration. At the time public health workers largely did not have national security clearances and in some cases were denied access to certain information by the FBI as a result, to the detriment of the response (Butler et al., 2002).

After the anthrax attacks, there was a recognition that public health and law enforcement officers would likely be working closely together in the future, and policies have been developed to address this specific relationship. This provides an example of the necessity of building coalitions and partnerships with groups that may not have traditionally worked extensively with public health officials. It also indicates a role for both public health officials and policy makers in evaluating, on a specific and individual basis, whether regulations surrounding information sharing should be adjusted during a bioterrorist attack if it would significantly improve the public health response.

Assure an Effective System That Enables Equitable Access to the Individual Services and Care Needed to Be Healthy

The majority of individuals who sought medical attention during the anthrax attacks were "concerned and potentially exposed" but ultimately not infected. These individuals predominantly visited their usual healthcare locations or emergency rooms (Barbera & Macintyre, 2002).

The significant group of individuals receiving medical intervention were those receiving postexposure prophylaxis. Over 32,000 individuals started antimicrobial prophylaxis after potential exposure, while about 10,000, concentrated in the six epicenters, were recommended to continue with a full 60-day regimen as a result of confirmed exposure risk (Army Medical Logistics Command, 2013; Jernigan et al., 2002). Ciprofloxacin and doxycycline were the main agents used, while amoxicillin was an option for vulnerable populations such as children and pregnant women due to concern over side effects of the prior two compounds (CDC, 2001a).

Prophylaxis was ultimately recommended for individuals who had been in the same location as an individual with inhalation anthrax, a location where environmental samples had shown presence of anthrax and there was a risk of aerosolization, or a location where a contaminated letter had been opened (Jernigan et al., 2002). Centralized distribution and refill clinics were established to provide prophylaxis, with the antimicrobials coming from the National Pharmaceutical Stockpile (Perkins et al., 2002).

A survey of approximately 6,000 individuals intended to receive the 60-day regimen found that 97% were able to get an initial supply of antimicrobials without problems, and about 80% of the remaining respondents ultimately received prophylaxis. However, adherence was low, with only 44% of respondents completing the 60-day course (Shepard et al., 2002). In a study of Washington, DC, postal workers receiving prophylaxis, a similarly low percentage, 40%, fully adhered to the regimen. The study found that intervention by public health workers, such as group sessions and actively distributing informational materials to individuals, improved adherence. Common reasons for nonadherence included adverse effects from the antimicrobials, concerns about potential long-term effects, belief they were at low risk, and a lack of information about anthrax, the prophylactics, and environmental results from their workplace (Jefferds et al., 2002).

The data about adherence indicate the importance of continued contact, or at least the availability of frontline public health staff to answer questions and address concerns of individuals involved in long-term interventions.

Build and Support a Diverse and Skilled Public Health Workforce

The scope of the response to the anthrax attacks strained public health workforce capacity. Individuals were needed to follow up on tips and investigate suspected cases, conduct surveillance and tracing, staff hotlines, test tens of thousands of specimens for anthrax including clinical and environmental samples, administer prophylactics, communicate between agencies and with healthcare workers and the media, and, in addition, carry on a portion of their normal duties.

Laboratory Response Network (LRN) laboratories across the country played a significant role in processing samples, processing over 120,000 between October and December 2001. Even Level A laboratories, which were not official members of the LRN and were only supposed to handle clinical samples, were receiving anthrax-associated environmental specimens (Snyder, 2005). The New York City Public Health Laboratory received 3,000 times its usual number of samples, and went from two personnel to deal with suspected bioterrorism-related samples to 75 personnel per shift (Heller et al., 2002).

The CDC sent over 350 of its employees to the epicenters of the attacks, including over 90% of its active Epidemic Intelligence Service officers, but state and local capacity remained strained. Departments pulled staff from other projects and jobs, but training was required before they could work effectively, requiring the investment of time, personnel, and resources. In some cases, such as with staffing hotlines, limited training led to poorer performance (GAO, 2003). The redeployment of staff also meant that regular public health duties could not be performed while the event was ongoing.

While the situation was managed, numerous officials reported later that their facilities and personnel may not have been able to cope had the attacks gone on longer, been larger in scope, or if another public health emergency had occurred simultaneously. The anthrax attacks sharply illustrated the necessity of surge capacity and flexibility in deployment. Since many of the roles involved in the frontline response to a bioterrorist attack require training, staffing needs cannot be effectively met without preexisting planning and structures. This requires leadership from managers and higher level public health officials, who are in the position to think in a systems manner, remain aware of how changes in personnel and personnel needs in a particular location or for a particular task affect other parts of the public health system, and hire or create procedures accordingly.

IMPROVE AND INNOVATE PUBLIC HEALTH FUNCTIONS THROUGH ONGOING EVALUATION, RESEARCH, AND CONTINUOUS QUALITY IMPROVEMENT

The anthrax attacks and responses to them provided numerous public health lessons. In the immediate aftermath, however, there was an apparent lack of available official analyses addressing the public health response to the attacks. This was observed by an article providing its own summary of the response, published in June 2003 in the journal *Biosecurity and Bioterrorism* (Gursky et al., 2003). The article noted that one report that had the potential to be comprehensive was not publicly released due to concerns of the Department of Defense about "sensitive information" contained within (Gursky et al., 2003). Later in October 2003, a fairly extensive report was issued by the GAO to William Frist, Senate Majority Leader and himself a trained physician. It outlined the strengths and weaknesses of local/state and federal actions taken during the events. The benefits provided by existing plans, and reasonably effective communication between emergency response agencies at the state and local level, as well as the CDC's support of local and state responses, were noted as strengths. On the other hand, problems getting information to clinicians, the CDC's struggles with incorporating incoming information and issuing guidelines in a timely manner, a lack of coordinated and effective communication with the media and public, inconsistency in messaging, and the unsustainable strain put on public health workers and resources were noted as weaknesses (GAO, 2003). These judgments are fairly consistent across analyses and reports about the anthrax attacks, which were subsequently released and continue to be. Summarizing the events and response and evaluating them in this manner can create invaluable resources that serve as guidance for public health leaders, officials, and policy makers when managing future outbreaks.

The attacks prompted increased federal investment in the public health system, including an unprecedented $3 billion allocated in December 2002 to combat bioterrorism, of which one-third was intended to strengthen state and local capacity. Additional resources were provided by the 2002 Public Health Security and Bioterrorism Preparedness and Response Act. Improvements made to public health infrastructure over the next decade included increases in available laboratory personnel at the state level, establishment of electronic communication systems with healthcare providers, and improvements to surge capacity. All 50 states developed CDC-approved plans to address a bioterrorist attack (Trust for America's Health, 2003, 2011).

Research into anthrax was also conducted in the aftermath of the attacks, and recommendations regarding diagnosis, prophylaxis, decontamination, and treatment were reviewed. Respectively, 2001 and 2002 saw about 340 and 550 new publications regarding anthrax on the PubMed database, whereas the topic had previously averaged fewer than 100 publications per year.

CONCLUSION

The 2001 anthrax attacks tested a U.S. public health system and a nation that was growing more aware of the threat of bioterrorism but had not fully prepared to meet it. It proved to be an unprecedented public health crisis, involving a disease few public health officials or clinicians had experience with, emerging in different geographical areas almost simultaneously, and occurring during an already fraught time. It indicated some gaps in existing public health responses, especially with regard to communication and capacity, and some ways to improve, including by holding regular briefings or meetings, preemptively training staff members and considering the flexibility of surge capacity, and maintaining protocols for coordination among various agencies. These observations can also be extended to other public health crises, and lessons from the 2001 attacks will ideally serve to help strengthen public health responses at large.

DISCUSSION QUESTIONS

1. Research the Epidemic Intelligence Service program online. Discuss the training program and how it aided in the anthrax response.
2. Discuss the anthrax events in 2001 as acts of bioterrorism. Who were the targets? Speculate, on why.
3. Boots on the ground epidemiology is fundamental to investigate outbreaks and emergency medical events. How has this approach changed over time, with advances in technology?
4. In 2001, social media did not play a role in communication during the anthrax response. How might the response have been different had social media been involved? Better, worse? Defend your position.

SUMMARY

TABLE 11.1 Select Essential Services of Public Health Demonstrated in the 2001 Anthrax Attacks

Essential Service # and Definition	Context in Chapter Case	Competency # It Ties to	Importance for Emergency Preparedness, Response, or Recovery
1. Assess and monitor population health status, factors that influence health, and community needs and assets (Assessment)	Epidemiological investigation launched by the PBCHD and FDOH on October 4th	1, 2, 3, 21	Epidemiologists were deployed to investigate the anthrax exposure event, to identify the source of exposure and its mechanism, and to collect data among postal workers given antibiotics for postexposure prophylaxis to ascertain adverse events.
3. Communicate effectively to inform and educate people about health, factors that influence it, and how to improve it (Policy Development)	In Washington, DC, regular conference calls organized by the DC Hospital Association allowed physicians to share information about their patients' symptoms and treatment options.	18, 19	Public health epidemiologists, doctors, and scientists communicated regularly with other government agencies to provide consistent messages to the public via the media.
4. Strengthen, support, and mobilize communities and partnerships to improve health (Policy Development)	CDC used working groups of subject matter experts to develop plans and guidance for clinical and environmental activities.	2, 3	Lessons learned in the anthrax response were used to guide the development of medical counter-measure strategies and strengthen community capacity to respond to mass medical emergencies requiring dispensation of medicines.
6. Utilize legal and regulatory actions designed to improve and protect the public's health (Policy Development)	Recognition that public health and law enforcement officers would need to work together in the future, and policies have been developed to address this specific relationship.	13, 14, 21	Lessons learned from the anthrax response revealed gaps in communication among response actors and influenced subsequent congressional mandates for improved emergency preparedness activities.
7. Assure an effective system that enables equitable access to the individual services and care needed to be healthy (Assurance)	Centralized distribution and refill clinics established to provide prophylaxis, with antimicrobials coming from the Strategic National Pharmaceutical Stockpile.	7	Enhancements to the Strategic National Stockpile containing medical equipment for emergencies and plans for deploying the supplies were strengthened in jurisdictions.
9. Improve and innovate public health functions through ongoing evaluation, research, and continuous quality improvement (Assurance)	Research into anthrax was also conducted in the aftermath of the attacks; 2001 and 2002 saw about 340 and 550 new publications, respectively, regarding anthrax.	2, 3, 4, 12, 13, 14	The anthrax events were foundational to our understanding of emergency preparedness through lessons learned.

CDC, Centers for Disease Control and Prevention; FDOH, Florida Department of Health; PBCHD, Palm Beach County Health Department.

TABLE 11.2 Select CEPH Competencies Needed for Frontline Health Workers, Managers, and Leaders for Biochemical Emergency Preparedness, Response, and Recovery

Competency # and Definition	Context in Case/Chapter	Level	Importance for Emergency Preparedness, Response, or Recovery
1. Apply epidemiological methods to settings and situations in public health practice.	Data was expected to come mostly from frontline clinical staff noting outbreaks unusual in pattern or causative agent.	Level 1	At Level 1, boots on the ground—for example, the Epidemic Intelligence Service Officers of CDC—were deployed to serve in multiple activities including conducting interviews with government officials, hospital workers, and others. Officers collected clinical samples. Some were deployed to the hospital where one of the victims worked. Others participated in interviewing postal workers to document adverse events associated with antibiotics prescribed for post exposure prophylaxis.
2. Select quantitative and qualitative data collection methods appropriate for a given public health context.	Surveillance was also conducted in healthcare facilities through provider reporting and review of patient medical records.	Level 1	At Level 1, EIS officers were assigned to assist with syndromic surveillance and provided support to hospitals for review of medical records.
9. Design a population-based policy, program, project, or intervention.	The CDC was responsible for overall coordination, acting on behalf of the U.S. Department of Health and Human Services, and its teams supported other health departments' efforts.	Level 3	At Level 3, CDC leaders met with other agencies in the Department of Health and Human Services and other federal agencies to ensure an efficient coordination of the response and used scientific principles for guiding the investigation.
18. Select communication strategies for different audiences and sectors.	Faxes, emails, CD-ROMs, website updates, and hotlines were among the methods used by public health officials to get information to clinicians.	Level 2	At Level 2, managers developed mechanisms to inform the public of response activities and to provide recommendations for self-protection, using accurate and clear language.
22. Apply a systems thinking tool to visually represent a public health issue in a format other than standard narrative.	Leadership from managers and higher level public health officials are required to think in a systems manner to meet staffing needs.	Level 3	At Level 3, leaders applied knowledge of the public health systems, agency functions, regulatory concerns, partnerships, and resources to rapidly respond.

Key: Essential services of public health; CEPH competencies; Leadership levels.

CDC, Centers for Disease Control and Prevention.

REFERENCES

ABC News. (2001, January 6). Fla. man hospitalized with anthrax. *ABC News*. https://abcnews.go.com/Health/story?id=117206&page=1

Army Medical Logistics Command. (2013). *Information paper: Anthrax infections and anthrax vaccine*. https://www.amlc.army.mil/Portals/73/Documents/USAMMA%20Anthrax%20Info%20Paper.pdf?ver=2020-03-04-140130-947

Associated Press. (2001, December 6). Anthrax letters sent to Leahy and Daschle called identical. *New York Times*. https://www.nytimes.com/2001/12/06/national/anthrax-letters-sent-to-leahy-and-daschle-called-identical.html

Barbera, J., & Macintyre, A. (2002). The reality of the modern bioterrorism response. *The Lancet, 360*, S33–S34. https://doi.org/10.1016/S0140-6736(02)11812-5

Begley, S., & Isikoff, M. (2001 October 22). Anxious about anthrax. *Newsweek*. http://www.ph.ucla.edu/epi/bioter/anxiousanthraxerinoconnor.html

Belongia, E., Kieke, B., Lynfield, R., Davis, J. P., & Besser, R. E. (2005). Demand for prophylaxis after bioterrorism-related anthrax cases, 2001. *Emerging Infectious Diseases, 11*(1), 42–48. https://doi.org/10.3201/eid1101.040272

Brachman, P. (2002). Bioterrorism: An update with a focus on anthrax. *American Journal of Epidemiology*, 155(11), 981–987. https://doi.org/10.1093/aje/155.11.981

Butler, J., Cohen, M., Friedman, C., Scripp, R. M., & Watz, C. G. (2002). Collaboration between public health and law enforcement: New paradigms and partnerships for bioterrorism planning and response. *Emerging Infectious Diseases, 8*(10), 1152–1156. https://doi.org/10.3201/eid0810.020400

Centers for Disease Control and Prevention. (n.d.-a). *Federal Select Agent Program*. https://www.selectagents.gov/compliance/guidance/biosafety/definitions.htm

Centers for Disease Control and Prevention. (n.d.-b). *The threat of an anthrax attack*. https://www.cdc.gov/anthrax/bioterrorism/threat.html

Centers for Disease Control and Prevention. (n.d.-c). *Types of anthrax: Inhalation anthrax*. https://www.cdc.gov/anthrax/basics/types/inhalation.html

Centers for Disease Control and Prevention. (n.d.-d). *What is anthrax?*. https://www.cdc.gov/anthrax/basics/index.html

Centers for Disease Control and Prevention. (2001a). Notice to readers: Update: Interim recommendations for antimicrobial prophylaxis for children and breastfeeding mothers and treatment of children with anthrax. *Morbidity and Mortality Weekly Report, 50*(45), 1014–1016. https://www.cdc.gov/mmwr/preview/mmwrhtml/mm5045a5.htm

Centers for Disease Control and Prevention. (2001b). Update: Investigation of anthrax associated with intentional exposure and interim public health guidelines, October 2001. *Morbidity and Mortality Weekly Report, 50*(41), 889–893. https://www.cdc.gov/mmwr/preview/mmwrhtml/mm5041a1.htm

Centers for Disease Control and Prevention. (2001c). Update: Investigation of bioterrorism-related anthrax and interim guidelines for clinical evaluation of persons with possible anthrax. *Morbidity and Mortality Weekly Report, 50*(43), 941–948. https://www.cdc.gov/mmwr/preview/mmwrhtml/mm5043a1.htm

Centers for Disease Control and Prevention. (2001d). Update: Investigation of bioterrorism-related anthrax and interim guidelines for exposure management and antimicrobial therapy, October 2001. *Morbidity and Mortality Weekly Report, 50*(42), 909–919. https://www.cdc.gov/mmwr/preview/mmwrhtml/mm5042a1.htm

Charatan, F. (2001). Anthrax and the US media. *BMJ, 323*(7318), 942. https://doi.org/10.1136/bmj.323.7318.942

CNN. (2001a, October 21). *Anthrax letter found at* New York Post. https://www.cnn.com/2001/HEALTH/conditions/10/20/anthrax/

CNN. (2001b, October 14). *New anthrax exposures in New York*. https://www.cnn.com/2001/HEALTH/conditions/10/14/anthrax/index.html

CNN. (2001c, October 24). *Ten things you need to know about anthrax*. https://www.cnn.com/2001/HEALTH/conditions/10/12/inv.anthraxqanda/index.html

Cohen, D., & Cook, A. H. (2006). At the intersection of public health and national security: The evolution of smallpox policy in the Clinton and G. W. Bush administrations. *Politics & Policy, 23*(1), 156–194. https://doi.org/10.1111/j.1747-1346.2006.00008.x

Davis, C. (1999). Nuclear blindness: An overview of the biological weapons programs of the former Soviet Union and Iraq. *Emerging Infectious Diseases, 5*(4), 509–512. https://doi.org/10.3201/eid0504.990408

Dewan, P., Fry, A., Laserson, K., Tierney, B. C., Quinn, C. P., Hayslett, J. A., Broyles, L. N., Shane, A. L., Winthrop, K. L., Walks, I., Siegel, L., Hales, T., Semenova, V. A., Romero-Steiner, S., Elie, C.,

Khabbaz, R., Khan, A. S., Hajjeh, R. A., & Schuchat, A. (2002). Inhalational anthrax outbreak among postal workers, Washington, D.C., 2001. *Emerging Infectious Diseases, 8*(10), 1066–1072. https://doi.org/10.3201/eid0810.020330

Frist, B. (2002). Public health and national security: The critical role of increased federal support. *Health Affairs, 21*(6), 117–130. https://doi.org/10.1377/hlthaff.21.6.117

Glass, T., & Schoch-Spana, M. (2002). Bioterrorism and the people: How to vaccinate a city against panic. *Clinical Infectious Diseases, 34*(2), 217–223. https://doi.org/10.1086/338711

Gursky, E., Inglesby, T. V., & O'Toole, T. (2003). Anthrax 2001: Observations on the medical and public health response. *Biosecurity and Bioterrorism, 1*(2), 97–110. https://doi.org/10.1089/153871303766275763

Hamilton, D. H. (2006). The epidemic intelligence service: The Centers for Disease Control and Prevention's disease detectives. *AMA Journal of Ethics, 8*(4), 261–264. https://doi.org/10.1001/virtualmentor.2006.8.4.mhst2-0604

Heller, M. B., Bunning, M. L., France, M. E. B., Niemeyer, D. M., Peruski, L., Naimi, T., Talboy, P. M., Murray, P. H., Pietz, H. W., Kornblum, J., Oleszko, W., Beatrice, S. T., Joint Microbiological Rapid Response Team, & New York City Anthrax Investigation Working Group. (2002). Laboratory response to anthrax bioterrorism, New York City, 2001. *Emerging Infectious Diseases, 8*(10), 1096–1102. https://doi.org/10.3201/eid0810.020376

Holtz, T. H., Ackelsberg, J., Kool, J. L., Rosselli, R., Marfin, A., Matte, T., Beatrice, S. T., Heller, M. B., Hewett, D., Moskin, L., Bunning, M. L., Layton, M., & New York City Anthrax Investigation Working Group. (2003). Isolated case of bioterrorism-related inhalational anthrax, New York City, 2001. *Emerging Infectious Diseases, 9*(6), 689–696. https://doi.org/10.3201/eid0906.020668

Jefferds, M. D., Laserson, K., Fry, A. M., Roy, S. L., Hayslett, J., Grummer-Strawn, L., Kettel-Khan, L., & Schuchat, A. (2002). Adherence to antimicrobial inhalational anthrax prophylaxis among postal workers, Washington, D.C., 2001. *Emerging Infectious Diseases, 8*(10), 1138–1144. https://doi.org/10.3201/eid0810.020331

Jernigan, D. B., Raghunathan, P. L., Bell, B. P., Brechner, R., Bresnitz, E. A., Butler, J. C., Cetron, M., Cohen, M., Doyle, T., Fischer, M., Greene, C. M., Griffith, K. S., Guarner, J., Hadler, J. L., Hayslett, J. A., Meyer, R., Petersen, L. R., Phillips, M., Pinner, R. W., . . . National Anthrax Epidemiologic Investigation Team. (2002). Investigation of bioterrorism-related anthrax, United States, 2001: Epidemiologic findings. *Emerging Infectious Diseases, 8*(10), 1019–1028. https://doi.org/10.3201/eid0810.020353

Lederberg, J., Shope, R. E., & Oaks, S. C., Jr. (Eds.). (1992). *Emerging infections: Microbial threats to health in the United States.* National Academies Press. https://doi.org/10.17226/2008

Mayo Clinic. (2020). *Anthrax.* https://www.mayoclinic.org/diseases-conditions/anthrax/symptoms-causes/syc-20356203

M'ikanatha, N., Lautenbach, E., Kunselman, A., Julian, K. G., Southwell, B. G., Allswede, M., Rankin, J. T., & Aber, R. C. (2003). Sources of bioterrorism information among emergency physicians during the 2001 anthrax outbreak. *Biosecurity and Bioterrorism, 1*(4), 259–265. https://doi.org/10.1089/153871303771861469

Nakashima, E., & Russakoff, D. (2001, December 3). Link made in anthrax deaths of 2 women. *Chicago Tribune.* https://www.chicagotribune.com/news/ct-xpm-2001-12-03-0112030138-story.html

National Intelligence Estimate. (2000). *The global infectious disease threat and its implications for the United States.* https://www.dni.gov/files/documents/infectiousdiseases_2000.pdf

National Response Team. (2004). *Observations and lessons learned from anthrax responses.* https://nrt.org/sites/2/files/ANTHRAX_Observations%20LL%20Report_02_14_06.pdf

New York Times. (2001, October 16). *Responding to anthrax attacks.* https://www.nytimes.com/2001/10/16/opinion/responding-to-anthrax-attacks.html

NPR. (2020). *Wear masks to protect yourself from the coronavirus, not only others, CDC stresses.* https://www.npr.org/sections/health-shots/2020/11/11/933903848/wear-masks-to-protect-yourself-from-the-coronavirus-not-only-others-cdc-stresses

Perkins, B. A., Popovic, T., & Yeskey, K. (2002). Public health in the time of bioterrorism. *Emerging Infectious Diseases, 8*(10), 1015–1018. https://doi.org/10.3201/eid0810.020444

Shepard, C., Soriano-Gabarro, M., Zell, E., Hayslett, J., Lukacs, S., Goldstein, S., Factor, S., Jones, J., Ridzon, R., Williams, I., Rosenstein, N., & CDC Adverse Events Working Group. (2002). Antimicrobial postexposure prophylaxis for anthrax: Adverse events and adherence. *Emerging Infectious Diseases, 8*(10), 1124–1132. https://doi.org/10.3201/eid0810.020349

Snyder, J. (2005). The laboratory response network: Before, during, and after the 2001 anthrax incident. *Clinical Microbiology Newsletter, 27*(22), 171–175. https://doi.org/10.1016/j.clinmicnews.2005.10.003

Trust for America's Health. (2003). *Ready or not? Protecting the public's health in the age of bioterrorism.* https://www.tfah.org/wp-content/uploads/archive/reports/bioterror03/Bioterror.pdf

Trust for America's Health. (2011). *Remembering 9/11 and anthrax: Public health's vital role in national defense.* https://nasemso.org/wp-content/uploads/TFAH911Anthrax10YrAnnvFINAL.pdf

Tumpey, A., Daigle, D., & Nowak, G. (2018). Communicating during an outbreak or public health investigation. In S. A. Rasmussen & R. A. Goodman (Eds.), *The CDC field epidemiology manual.* https://www.cdc.gov/eis/field-epi-manual/chapters/Communicating-Investigation.html

U.S. Department of Justice. (2010). *Amerithrax investigative summary.* https://www.justice.gov/archive/amerithrax/docs/amx-investigative-summary2.pdf

U.S. General Accounting Office. (2000). *West Nile virus outbreak: Lessons for public health preparedness.* https://www.gao.gov/products/hehs-00-180

U.S. General Accounting Office. (2003). *Public health response to anthrax incidents of 2001.* https://www.gao.gov/assets/250/240162.pdf

University of California San Francisco. (2020). *Still confused about masks?* https://www.ucsf.edu/news/2020/06/417906/still-confused-about-masks-heres-science-behind-how-face-masks-prevent

CHAPTER 12

CHEMICAL DISASTERS AND PUBLIC HEALTH EFFECTS

THE BHOPAL CHEMICAL INDUSTRIAL DISASTER

ALEXANDER H. CHANG, ALLISON P. CHEN, AND EDBERT B. HSU

KEY TERMS

Aldicarb Oxime
Methyl Isocyanate Gas
Mustard Gas
Nongovernmental Organizations (NGOs)
Sarin Gas

INTRODUCTION

There are several types of chemical disasters necessary for public health personnel to consider. The first is the deliberate use of chemical agents, such as **mustard gas** or **sarin gas**. While the Geneva Protocol has banned the use of chemical and biological weapons, the use of chemical weapons has reared its ugly head in terrorist attacks and in armed conflicts that violate the rules of war. The second type of chemical disaster is the unintentional release of hazardous compound(s), typically from factories or plants. In this chapter, the focus is on the latter: chemical industry disasters.

The modern world has brought with it large-scale industries—all dependent on raw materials and chemicals; massive plants synthesize and produce these chemicals that are crucial to our everyday life. Much of what goes into producing foods and goods is taken for granted; however, a large global infrastructure exists to sustain a myriad of chemical reactions, virtually around the

---

The following icons, located in the margins throughout the chapter and within the summary tables, denote essential services of public health, CEPH competencies, and leadership levels: Essential services of public health; CEPH competencies; Leadership levels.

clock. These large industries bring with them disasters— inherently man-made— involving the unintentional release of hazardous substance(s). Such disasters can have a devastating impact on a population; not only can there be casualties, but there can also be long-term effects on human health and the environment. From an historical case study, public health professionals can garner insight into the inherent risks found in the chemical industry and the services designed to protect the public, and a real-world response.

On the night of December 2, 1984, 45 tons of **methyl isocyanate gas** was released from the Union Carbide pesticide plant in Bhopal, Madhya Pradesh State, India, in one of the world's worst chemical disasters. The methyl isocyanate gas drifted to the surrounding densely populated town, where 500,000 people were exposed with over half a million injuries and a resultant death toll of 2,259. This case illustrates the importance of public health competencies pertaining to the hazards of chemical plants and the application of competencies post disaster. The case of Bhopal is indelibly etched into the annals of disasters and leaves a legacy of positive changes in the chemical industry and public health.

BACKGROUND OF THE CHEMICAL INDUSTRY

Bhopal is not an isolated incident—far from it. Since the Industrial Revolution, factories have been deeply embedded into modern infrastructure, and with larger scales of production comes increasing potential for environmental impacts and disasters. Over the last century there have been several notable public health catastrophes including mercury pollution in Minamata, Japan (1932–1969); the Seves, Italy, dioxin release in 1976; and the Love Canal disaster in 1978 (Lucchini et al., 2017). The nature of the large-scale chemical industry is one of the most problematic challenges public health needs to acknowledge.

Chemical plants should not be situated solely within local public health issues; rather, they are best framed from a global perspective. Chemical industries are transnational, and the manufacturing processes of toxic chemicals are typically trade secrets cloaked in matters of a technical nature. With the larger scale comes the burdening of larger populations, often in developing countries. Historically, transnational corporations have exhibited a "lack of care regarding worker and public health" (Broughton, 2005). Examples include toxic waste disposal, asbestos, tobacco, and a plethora of other industrial unpleasantries. Thus, the goal of public health comes to an impasse; the prioritization of profit over public health concerns by transnational corporations and even governments is often at odds with the welfare and well-being of producer populations.

The history of Bhopal's disaster can also be contextualized against a backdrop of the history of technology and environmentalism. The synthesis of the chemical carbaryl (marketed as Sevin) was deemed to be safer and better than chlorinated pesticides. Carbaryl pesticides became commonly used in the United States and were heavily marketed as a boon to crops ravaged by pests in developing countries such as in Latin America and India. The exigent need for pesticides globally with the willingness of some countries to bear the burden of producing toxic compounds fueled an environment that led to Bhopal.

LINKING PEOPLE TO NEEDED HEALTH SERVICES

Several years after the disaster, Union Carbide Corporation (UCC) financed a 500-bed hospital for the long-term medical care of survivors in 1991. UCC set up the

Bhopal Hospital Trust in 1992, and the Bhopal Memorial Hospital & Research Centre (n.d.) was opened in 1998, with the first outreach health center beginning that year in April. The hospital currently has 17 departments. Its motto is "Caring is a way of life" and states its objectives as: (a) to provide state-of-the-art super-specialty medical facilities to all registered gas victims and their entitled dependents; (b) to carry out basic, clinical, and epidemiological disciplines in all disciplines in the hospital; and (c) to utilize the existing infrastructure to train doctors, nurses, and paramedical personnel (Bhopal Memorial Hospital & Research Centre, n.d.).

In 1985, UCC gave $5 million as part of the relief package, which was used to set up four community clinics in gas-affected areas. While the last clinic closed in 1995, the remaining funds were transferred to the Bhopal Hospital Trust.

ASSESS AND MONITOR POPULATION HEALTH

After the incident, the Ministry of Gas Relief set up a research institute in Bhopal. During a 10-year period, the Indian Council of Medical Research (ICMR) conducted many studies and started publishing articles in 1995. The ICMR performed longitudinal cohort studies studying the various effects of methylisocyanate. Roughly 520,000 persons were exposed, and "20.3% or 80,021" were selected for the study (Eckerman, 2005). The ICMR has subsequently published studies on the health effects of the gas as well as several manuals for health problems associated with the Bhopal tragedy (Bhopal Disaster, 1987). These studies provide invaluable data on the short-term and long-term effects of methylisocyanate on the human body. The effect on the eyes, respiratory tract, and the central and peripheral nervous system were well-documented (Dhara et al., 2002). High-impact cytology research investigated the chromosomal aberrations caused by methylisocyanate exposure (Goswami et al., 1990). Not only was posttraumatic stress disorder (PTSD) studied, but the intent to treat PTSD in disaster victims is also evidenced by the neurology and psychiatry departments in the Bhopal Memorial Hospital and Research Centre and their outreach programs (Eckerman, 2005).

The First Essential Public Health Service is to "assess and monitor population health status, factors that influence health, and community needs and assets" (Centers for Disease Control and Prevention [CDC], n.d.). Studying the effects of methylisocyanate and the specific needs of the affected population embodies the First Essential Public Health Service. Fundamental to providing care to the public is "maintaining an ongoing understanding of health" (CDC, n.d.). Conducting longitudinal studies using various methods and technologies is crucial to developing a data set that identifies key issues to be addressed. In addition to acquiring data, monitoring the health status of a population engages the community and establishes rapport between community members, experts, and key partners.

COMMUNICATE EFFECTIVELY TO INFORM AND EDUCATE

One of the core tenets of public health is the duty to inform, educate, and empower, the Third Essential Public Health Service (CDC, n.d.). The Bhopal disaster has led to a renewed commitment to the community and a "never again" mentality toward disasters. A significant part of having a meaningful emergency plan is to have well-informed citizens as well as educated responders.

Working in the Bhopal plant required a degree in chemical or mechanical engineering; however, due to industry conditions, training was abridged, and security measures resulted in truncated education. Prioritization of public health in large-scale industrial projects is the bedrock of good design. One critic of modern engineering processes points out that "safety engineers are brought in at the end and wind up adding safety devices to control rather than to eliminate the hazards" (Johnson, 2005). This leads to a compliance-oriented mitigation of risk, resulting in a bare minimum of safety precautions, if that. In short, there is absolutely no commitment to systemic elimination of threats. Even in the education and training of engineers, process-safety is not prioritized. Without properly training both corporate leadership and engineering personnel in safety, it is impossible to achieve any meaningful mitigation of risk. Post-Bhopal, India has witnessed an increased commitment to understanding risk, educating employees as well as responders and government officials.

UTILIZE LEGAL AND REGULATORY ACTIONS

After the disaster, not only was the Ministry for Environment and Forests established in 1985, but several acts and regulations were also put into place. The Factories Act, containing a provision for "Hazardous Processes," was amended in 1987, and the Environment Act was passed in 1986. Several rules were also passed such as the "Model Rules" and the "Manufacture, Storage, and Import of Hazard Chemicals Rules" in 1989. The Public Liability Insurance Rules were amended in 1992, designed to protect the public.

The Emergency Planning, Preparedness, and Response to Chemical Accident Rules, which list hazardous chemicals including methyl isocyanate, were passed in 1996, representing a triumph of public health and disaster medicine (Bare Acts Live, 2016). These rules mandate the necessity of having an emergency preparedness plan both by district authorities and the operators of factories. Additionally, the Environment Protect Agency (in India) was established, leading to a legislative infrastructure to prevent future Bhopal-like disasters from being repeated. Thus, public health competencies are propagated on multiple levels on a legislative and infrastructure level.

Much progress has been made in advocating for human rights and victims of disasters as well as offering guidelines for transnational companies. One seminal document, "The UN Human Rights Norms for Business: Towards Legal Accountability," states categorically that "[t]ransnational corporations and other business enterprises bear responsibility for the occupational health and safety of their workers." Not only does this champion the dignity of workers, but it also sets a standard on which public health competencies can be built.

The Fifth Essential Public Health Service is to "create, champion, and implement policies, plans, and laws that impact health." Creating policies, laws, and plans not only sets a ceiling of legitimate actions for companies and organizations but also establishes precedents that establish public health-oriented thinking among stakeholders and community members alike.

RISK ASSESSMENTS FOR INDUSTRY

Concerns of safety, risk, and operational standards need to be addressed with a public health-oriented ethos on all levels. At the entry level, interactions with the community are important; however, there are policy and strategy decisions that need to be made as well. Critics have argued that perhaps communities that cannot respond to large-scale incidents, much less understand the inherent risk, should not be selected for installations. Advocating for public health and mitigating risk while regulating large corporations and industrial development is a challenge for the modern world.

Much like pandemics, chemical disasters "are no respecters of state borders." A year after the Bhopal disaster, on August 11, 1985, a UCC plant in West Virginia had a similar valve malfunction and a large cloud of **aldicarb oxime** (a compound mixed with methyl isocyanate) was released (Franklin, 1985). Although there were no casualties, there were at least one hundred cases of people sickened by the gas. After the Bhopal incident, this revelation made it evident that American plants were no safer. Congress acted and subsequently passed the 1986 Emergency Planning and Community Right to Know Act, which "help[ed] increase the public's knowledge and access to information on chemicals at individual facilities, their uses, and releases into the environment" (Environmental Protection Agency, n.d.).

The Disaster Management Institute was established in 1987 by the Government of Madhya Pradesh (Eckerman, 2005). The fruits of this public health success include "Refresher Course for Top Executives: Management of Chemical Accidents" as well as documents on emergency preparedness and response. This epitomizes the implementation of public health competencies.

A meaningful assessment of risk must be conducted for any large-scale industrial complex. Inherent in any structure and process is risk; the consequences of structural or procedural failure must be well established and understood. Different stakeholders need to ask fundamental yet critical questions such as (a) What are the consequences if an accident were to happen? (b) How will such an accident affect the community? (c) How could such effects be mitigated? Indispensable to the welfare of the public is understanding what is at stake and for whom.

The Second Essential Public Health Service is to "investigate, diagnose, and address health problems and hazards affecting the population" (CDC, n.d.). Post-incident investigations of Bhopal revealed that operating standards in the facility were subpar; fundamentally, this revealed a mismatch of risk understanding and operational execution. However, the lessons learned from the disaster have led to a public health ethos found in the Disaster Management Institute, a beacon of public health and disaster medicine, born from the tragedy of the Bhopal gas disaster (http://dmibhopal.mp.gov.in). Many lessons emerged from Bhopal, and the consequences of "hazards affecting the population" will always be at the forefront of future planning and development projects.

BUILD A DIVERSE AND SKILLED WORKFORCE

Disaster experts point out that crises are by definition "low probability, high impact" events. It is imperative to understand that the risk of high-impact needs to shift operating standards for the better. The higher the risk, the broader reaching the public health actions should be, including but not limited to (a) creating a larger buffer zone, (b) instilling higher safety standards, and (c) educating the community. Every industrial complex necessitates an operational mindset that puts a priority on public health and the well-being of the community, requiring public health-competent personnel in all stakeholder positions at various levels in the community leadership, governmental organizations, and corporate structures.

After the Bhopal incident, the state of shock and the magnitude of the tragedy catalyzed a transformation in the labor environment. Advocacy for working conditions, employment safety standards, and benefits increased dramatically. Working synergistically with the rules and regulations and new departments, nascent labor organizations have initiated the burgeoning public health movement in India.

The Eighth Essential Public Health Service is to "build and support a diverse and skilled public health workforce" (CDC, n.d.). Imperative to a public health–oriented society is the influential presence of a diverse workforce well-versed in public health. Advocacy for equitable working conditions is a cornerstone of health-oriented labor environments and, consequently, public health.

STRENGTHEN, SUPPORT, AND MOBILIZE COMMUNITIES AND PARTNERSHIPS

The aftermath of Bhopal witnessed numerous community partnerships, both local and on a global scale. Many small **nongovernmental organizations (NGOs)** rushed to the aid of the disasters, and long-term efforts of organizations such as the WHO sending representatives demonstrate the level of concern the global community felt. The European Economic Consortium (EEC) sent hundreds of tons of milk powder for children.

Local NGOs worked with survivors and mobilized healthcare and clinical support while international organizations formed networks to address broader issues such as environmental issues, human rights, education, trade, and transnational companies (Eckerman, 2005). The Fourth Essential Public Health Service is "strengthen, support, and mobilize communities and partnerships to improve health" (CDC, n.d.). Due to the transnational nature of the Bhopal disaster, public health-conscious organizations stepped in to aid the victims and advocate for change.

PUBLIC HEALTH IMPROVEMENTS

Though a Bhopal-scale event has not occurred in recent years, in the chemical factories themselves, it is hard to ascertain how much progress has been made. Methyl isocyanate is still used in industrial processes, and carbaryl is still widely used as a pesticide. The lack of Bhopal-scale incidents perhaps is indicative of progress achieved through integration of public health competencies into industrial infrastructures and communities alike. Community residents and leaders as well as public health officials need to establish open dialogue regarding chemicals and the processes to manufacture them, as well as any factors that could affect the health of a community. A well-informed public leads to a better outcome; various mechanisms of disseminating information need to be implemented such that residents living in proximity to industrial plants (and any other industrial complexes) are aware of the geographic hazards. Leaders of communities, public health officials, and socially active individuals (e.g., neighborhood watch), as well as transnational corporations, need to make a concerted effort to embrace, integrate, and apply the public health competencies on all tiers of the chemical industry.

Indeed, the tragedy of Bhopal has catalyzed a global movement toward public health competencies. The 10th Essential Public Health Service is to "build and maintain a strong organizational infrastructure for public health" (CDC, n.d.). Tragedies and catastrophes necessitate societies to create infrastructures that put public health values at its core. The case of Bhopal serves as an exemplar for the needs of the 10 Essential Public Health Services.

DISCUSSION QUESTIONS

1. Research and locate chemical plants in your state. If the plants have websites, review at least one and discuss the information presented there. Discuss safety information.
2. Review media reports on the catastrophic event in Bhopal. Discuss varying interpretations of the events. Also, review published public health literature on the event. Compare and contrast styles of reporting.
3. Should the government regulate use of toxic chemicals? Why or why not?
4. Discuss other toxic exposure events of which you are aware. What were lessons learned or outcomes?

SUMMARY

TABLE 12.1 Select Essential Services of Public Health Demonstrated in the Bhopal Chemical Disaster

Essential Service # and Definition	Context in Chapter Case	Competency # It Ties to	Importance for Emergency Preparedness, Response, or Recovery
1. Assess and monitor population health status, factors that influence health, and community needs and assets (Assessment)	Studying the effects of methylisocyanate and the specific needs of the affected population	2, 3, 4	Public health professionals involved in preparedness activities have an obligation to monitor the health of people who work in chemical plants and their working conditions to prevent adverse events.
2. Investigate, diagnose, and address health problems and hazards affecting the population (Assessment)	Post-incident investigations of Bhopal revealed that operating standards in the facility were subpar.	3, 4	After an event such as the Bhopal disaster, epidemiologists and health scientists must investigate exposures to document immediate and long-term results of toxic exposures. In addition, learning from the disaster can inform public health practices for inspection of chemical plants and making recommendations for enhancing safety precautions.
4. Strengthen, support, and mobilize communities and partnerships to improve health (Policy Development)	Many small nongovernmental organizations rushed to the aid of the disasters, and long-term efforts organizations sent representatives.	13, 14, 16, 21	Communities near chemical plants should be aware of potential hazards through communication strategies. Members of the community and organizations within the communities should be included in preparedness planning.
5. Create, champion, and implement policies, plans, and laws that impact health (Policy Development)	Ministry for Environment and Forests established in 1985 with several acts and regulations put into place	7, 12, 13, 14	Environmental policies and plans should be in place for geographic areas with chemical and other hazardous material plants. The plans for protection should be practiced with drills and include all relevant stakeholders, in advance of an emergency. Local communities should be aware of planning activities and be involved.
7. Assure an effective system that enables equitable access to the individual services and care needed to be healthy (Assurance)	Union Carbide Corporation financed a hospital for long-term medical care of survivors.	7, 9	Any populations identified as underserved or vulnerable living near a chemical or other hazardous material plan should be taken into account in preparedness planning activities. Members of these communities should serve as advisors on preparedness committees. Plans to provide medical services to vulnerable populations in an emergency should be devised in advance.
8. Build and support a diverse and skilled public health workforce (Assurance)	Advocacy for working conditions, employment safety standards, and benefits increased dramatically after Bhopal.	21	To function as a public health professional in chemical disaster preparedness, one must have a comprehensive knowledge of chemical and other toxic hazards, the use of these materials, and their transporting mechanism; potential harm to people and animals; potential food and water contamination; and best practices for children, pregnant women, and vulnerable populations. This comprehensive knowledge is essential.

TABLE 12.2 Select CEPH Competencies Needed for Frontline Health Workers, Managers, and Leaders for Chemical Disaster Emergency Preparedness, Response, and Recovery

Competency # and Definition	Context in Case/Chapter	Level	Importance for Emergency Preparedness, Response, or Recovery
2. Select quantitative and qualitative data collection methods appropriate for a given public health context.	Studying the effects of methylisocyanate and the specific needs of the affected population.	Level 1	At Level 1, epidemiologists and health scientists collect and analyze the data on the toxic exposures and negative effects on people in or around the chemical plant from hospital records or other sources. They can use the data to shed light on the conditions contributing to the worst outcomes or best outcomes. This information can inform improvement of plant working conditions.
7. Assess population needs, assets, and capacities that affect communities' health.	Local nongovernmental organizations worked with survivors and mobilized healthcare and clinical support.	Level 2	At Level 2, managers and supervisors can design a data gathering or evaluation strategy to answer specific questions about the event, and work with data collectors and analysts to implement the strategy. In addition, managers and supervisors can identify resources and strategies to assist survivors, families, and other affected persons to ensure broad coverage in the response activities.
14. Advocate for political, social, or economic policies and programs that will improve health in diverse populations.	Advocacy for working conditions, employment safety standards, and benefits increased dramatically.	Level 2	At Level 2, managers and supervisors can advocate for improved working conditions in chemical plants by creating data reports with findings suggesting specific actions.
15. Evaluate policies for their impact on public health and health equity.	In 1987, the Factories Act, containing a provision for "Hazardous Processes," was amended and the Environment Act was passed in 1986.	Level 3	At Level 3, public health leaders review data reports, after-action reports, evaluation studies, and other sources of information to design public policy for changing practice in chemical plants toward a greater awareness of hazards to people and specific action for better protection of workers.
16. Apply leadership and/or management principles to address a relevant health issue.	The Disaster Management Institute established by government with a course for top executives on management of chemical accidents.	Level 3	At Level 3, public health professionals can work with governmental agencies and organizations to share information on hazards in chemical plants, creating awareness of concerns for worker safety, obtaining buy-in for collaboration, and identifying resources for prevention and mitigation.

Key: Essential services of public health; CEPH competencies; Leadership levels.

REFERENCES

Bare Acts Live. (2016). *The chemical accidents (emergency planning, preparedness and response) rules, 1996.* http://www.bareactslive.com/ACA/ACT533.HTM

Bhopal Disaster. (1987). *Manual of mental health care for medical officers.* ICMR Centre for Advanced Research on Community Mental Health.

Bhopal Memorial Hospital & Research Centre. (n.d.). *About us.* http://bmhrc.ac.in/content/3_1_AboutUs.aspx

Broughton, E. (2005). The Bhopal disaster and its aftermath: A review. *Environmental Health, 4*(1), Article 6. https://doi.org/10.1186/1476-069X-4-6

Centers for Disease Control and Prevention. (n.d.). *10 Essential Public Health Services.* https://www.cdc.gov/publichealthgateway/publichealthservices/essentialhealthservices.html

Dhara, V. R., Dhara, R., Acquilla, S. D., & Cullinan, P. (2002). Personal exposure and long-term health effects in survivors of the Union Carbide Disaster at Bhopal. *Environmental Health Perspective Expansion, 110*(5), 487–500. https://doi.org/10.1289/ehp.02110487

Eckerman, I. (2005). *The Bhopal saga* (pp. 105–224). Universities Press.

Environmental Protection Agency. (n.d.). *What is EPCRA?* https://www.epa.gov/epcra/what-epcra

Franklin, B. (1985, August 12). Toxic cloud leaks at carbide plant in West Virginia. *The New York Times.* https://www.nytimes.com/1985/08/12/us/toxic-cloud-leaks-at-carbide-plant-in-west-virginia.html

Goswami, H. K., Chandorkar, M., Bhattacharya, K., Vaidyanath, G., Parmar, D., Sengupta, S., Patidar, S. L., Sengupta, L. K., Goswami, R., & Sharma, P. N. (1990). Search for chromosomal variations among gas-exposed persons in Bhopal. *Human Genetics, 84*(2), 172–176. https://doi.org/10.1007/bf00208935

Johnson, J. (2005). Process safety since Bhopal. *Chemical and Engineering News, 83*(4), 32–34. https://doi.org/10.1021/cen-v083n004.p032

Lucchini, R. G., Hashim, D., Acquilla, S., Basanets, A., Bertazzi, P. A., Bushmanov, A., Crane, M., Harrison, D. J., Holden, W., Landrigan, P. J., Luft, B. J., Mocarelli, P., Mazitova, N., Melius, J., Moline, J. M., Mori, K., Prezant, D., Reibman, J., Reissman, D. B., . . . Todd, A. C. (2017). A comparative assessment of major international disasters: The need for exposure assessment, systematic emergency preparedness, and lifetime health care. *BMC Public Health, 17*(1), Article 46. https://doi.org/10.1186/s12889-016-3939-3

CHAPTER 13

NUCLEAR DETONATION AS A PUBLIC HEALTH THREAT

A CASE APPROACH FOR PREPAREDNESS

ROBERT M. LEVIN

KEY TERMS

Acute Radiation Syndrome (ARS)
Disaster Medical Assistance Teams (DMATs)
Disaster Mortuary Operational Response Team (DMORT)
Electromagnetic Pulse
Emergency Alert System (EAS)
Emergency Operations Center (EOC)
Federal Radiological Monitoring and Assessment Center (FRMAC)
Interagency Modeling and Atmospheric Assessment Center (IMAAC)
Joint Information Center (JIC)
National Disaster Medical System (NDMS)
Office of Emergency Services (OES)
Personal Protective Equipment
Plume Mappers Group
Principal Federal Official (PFO)
Prophylactic Potassium Iodide (KI)
Radiological Assistance Program (RAP)
Stochastic Effects

The following icons, located in the margins throughout the chapter and within the summary tables, denote essential services of public health, CEPH competencies, and leadership levels: Essential services of public health; CEPH competencies; Leadership levels.

INTRODUCTION

Concern about a nuclear event occurring on American soil is not new. It began with fears that the Soviet Union, having developed nuclear weapons a short time after the United States did, would use those weapons against America. This, of course, set in motion an emotionally and financially draining arms race that lasted for decades and likely is still going on. Diplomacy was aimed at preventing a nuclear war from happening as this would devastate one or both countries and its destructive reach in terms of fallout would extend well beyond the borders of both those countries. With the dissolution of the Soviet Union, these fears momentarily subsided but then rumors and worries about the illicit sale of radioactive nuclear materials became more prevalent. As international terrorism established itself, a different, more limited but nevertheless terrifying scenario was now feared; this was the threat of a terrorist group developing an improvised nuclear device and detonating it on American soil. To this day, this remains a possibility. This chapter imagines the story of just such an event and postulates its impact as well as our nation's likely response.

TYPE OF EVENT: NUCLEAR DETONATION

Description of the Event[1]

On May 2, 2019, at 9:30 a.m., a large explosion and flash were heard and seen emanating from the Port of Los Angeles. There are some reports that the flash was seen at a distance of 100 miles. Subject matter experts were quick to recognize that the date coincided with the execution by American forces of Osama bin Laden 8 years earlier.

According to an aerial evaluation 24 hours later, there was nearly complete destruction of all structures at the port to within half a mile from what was presumed to be the epicenter of the blast. Larger structures like cranes and storage facilities were twisted and partially disintegrated and smaller objects like the transport containers that were offloaded from ships were either pulverized or blown and crumpled. Dozens of cargo transport ships were sunken or laying on their sides in the water. Damage decreasing in severity can be seen out to a mile from the center of the blast. Residents report shattered glass in structures 2.8 miles from the port.

There are numerous reports of shrapnel injuries to people as far as 2 miles away. There appears to be at first approximation a 95% fatality rate among those within four blocks, falling to a 1% death rate at six blocks. People experienced ruptured ear drums as far as seven to eight blocks away. Fatalities were due to the extreme heat from the explosion, rapid acceleration and deceleration from the blast force, and from objects large and small that became shot-like projectiles.

[1] [NOTE: It is confirmed that this is the warning used on official documents from the Joint Regional Intelligence Center and is for information only in this chapter to acquaint students with what an official communication would look like] May 3, 2019 Joint Regional Intelligence Center (JRIC) Ventura:

Warning: This document is Unclassified//For Official Use Only (U//FOUO). It contains sensitive information that cannot be released to the public or outside of the public safety community.

An irregularly shaped mushroom cloud rose above the blast site that could be seen for miles around. It is estimated to have reached 5 miles in height. Physicists and law enforcement sources feel that this was a nuclear detonation. This was confirmed by area emergency department physicians who have been seeing numerous patients presenting with a range of injuries that are consistent with a nuclear event. Patients have reported to emergency departments with burns; headache, nausea, diarrhea, and vomiting, which are consistent with radiation poisoning; acceleration/deceleration injuries; shrapnel wounds; ruptured ear drums; and blindness or other retinal injuries that doctors say is attributable to looking at the flash from the nuclear detonation. While a number of structural fires were started by the blast, emergency department physicians say that the vast majority of burns they are seeing are from the heat of the blast itself, so-called flash burns, and not from these fires. Medical authorities say further health impacts that should be anticipated from those exposed to the blast itself include more severe manifestations of radiation sickness that will materialize over the next few days and weeks. Fatal prompt radiation doses can be expected to be experienced by individuals who had direct line-of-sight exposure up to 1 mile from the blast. Potentially the greatest source of impending human casualty is radiation sickness from exposure to fallout. It is hoped that the latter will be minimized by the public information campaign promoted over the last few years in Southern California urging the public to "Get Inside. Stay Inside. Stay Tuned," should there ever be a nuclear detonation.

Communications in the area have been compromised. Some of this can be attributed to disabling or destruction of power stations and communications hubs directly impacted by the blast and some by the **electromagnetic pulse** generated by the blast, a sharp, high-voltage spike that disrupts electronic devices including automobiles, cell phones, and appliances within a 3-mile perimeter from the site of the explosion.

A fallout plume is being tracked via satellite by the National Weather Service, by radar images from towers in Ojai and Santa Ana and by the **Interagency Modeling and Atmospheric Assessment Center**[2] **(IMAAC)**. With westerly winds at 3 to 5 miles per hour for the last 26 hours, the fallout plume has moved about 100 miles inland with diminishing impact (Figure 13.1).

Most of the potential damage to human health from the fallout can be expected to be found within the first 9 miles of the plume. This is because of the greater concentration of heavier fallout particles raining down earlier within this range and the relatively rapid decay in the intensity of the radiation over the first few hours. The number of fallout casualties will be reduced by taking action such as sheltering in place or by successful evacuation. The jet stream winds of 150 miles per hour present at 5 miles above the earth will carry the finer particles in the fallout for great distances across the United States but will be less immediately injurious; the impact on health in these distant sites may not be known for decades.

Unprecedented traffic congestion is being experienced on all major highways out of Los Angeles—in some places, traffic has completely stopped, resulting in traffic congealment. On many highways, vehicles haven't moved

[2] The IMAAC collects and disseminates atmospheric dispersion models and hazard prediction information. Through plume modeling, the IMAAC provides emergency responders with predictions associated with hazardous material releases to aid in the decision-making process for public and environmental protection.

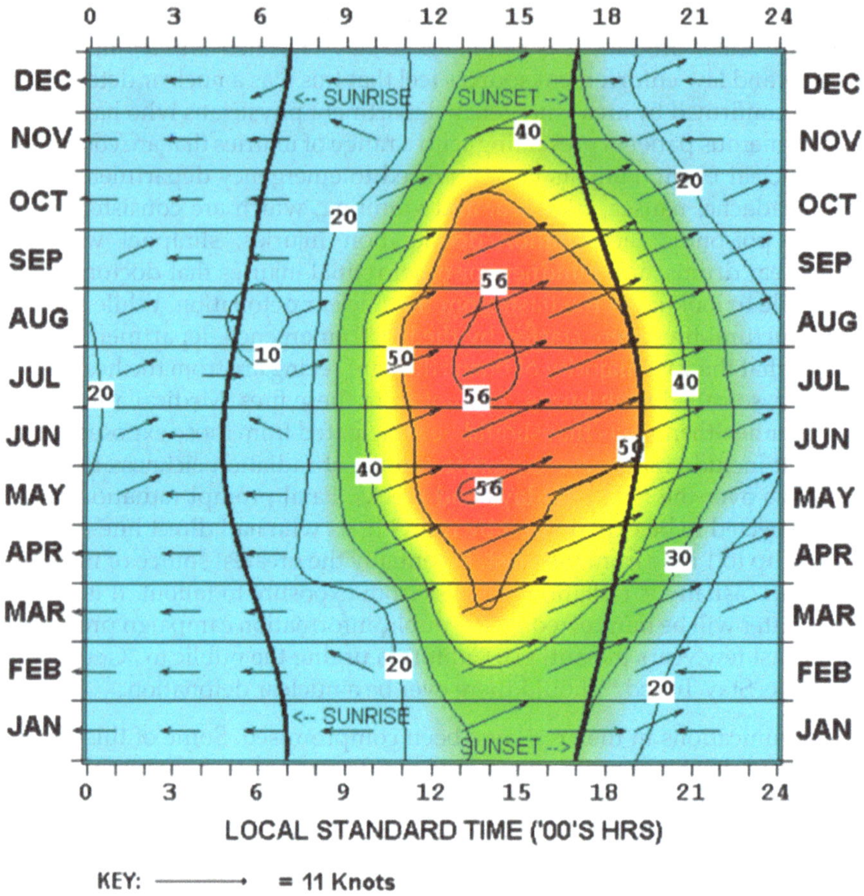

Figure 13.1 Prevailing wind direction and speed for Los Angeles International Airport.

Source: Reproduced with permission from Fisk, C. J. *Diurnal and seasonal wind variability for selected stations in Southern California climate regions*, P2.19.

in hours. Cars have been immobilized due to breakdowns, collisions, and running out of gas. The roads off highway exits are similarly affected for blocks with long lines at gas stations, with most gas stations rationing or out of gas entirely. Ambulances, law enforcement vehicles, and fire trucks have been impeded in responding to emergency calls due to the congestion. Resupply of grocery stores, gas stations, and pharmacies is also paralyzed. Law enforcement is utilizing motorcycles, bicycles, mopeds, Segways, foot, and horseback where available to respond to calls. Looting is breaking out in several surrounding communities, with some grocery store owners simply opening their doors and trying to control people from taking excessive amounts of products. There are reports that other major cities in the United States are experiencing similar traffic congestion as residents fear that their city may be the next target.

Subject matter experts from the Lawrence Livermore Lab estimate the detonation to be due to a 10-kiloton (kT) device. This is the approximate size of the nuclear bomb detonated over Hiroshima. Based on the size, it is believed that the bomb was likely of terrorist origin and not a state-sponsored device. State-sponsored bombs would be expected to be at least 100 kT.

Response Activities

Analysts feel that the Port of Los Angeles was selected because of the significant and long-lasting impact that its destruction would have on America's economy (Davis et al., 2014; National Council on Radiation Protection and Measurements, 2011). Increased scrutiny is being paid to other major ports in the United States on the chance that additional such attacks are planned. Particular attention is being focused on other ports on the West Coast of the United States. Over 50% of all American trade with the rest of the world is conducted through West Coast ports.

Direct concussive effects from the blast on Ventura County were not seen. Nevertheless, this incident in Los Angeles County is having a major impact on Ventura County. An uncontrolled mass evacuation from Los Angeles into Ventura County is being seen along with a degree of hysteria, gridlock on roadways, and the arrival of additional and overwhelming numbers of injured. Many of those who are fleeing are experiencing confusion, anxiety, fear, and psychological trauma.

Reassuring public information is being sent out on both traditional and social media. The County Behavioral Health Department is responding by setting up kiosks at Reception Centers and staffing them with counselors. The department is understaffed under normal circumstances and has never had to respond to a disaster of this magnitude. Behavioral Health has called for mutual aid to bring more providers into the county.

To contact loved ones, the public is being told to use the Red Cross Safe & Well website: disastersafe.redcross.org. Safe & Well provides a central location for people *in disasters* to register their current status, and for their *loved ones* to access that information. Additionally, messaging is being sent out as to how to assist others. Residents are being told that fleeing Los Angeles residents may show up at their door looking for shelter and they are encouraged to welcome them. If there is a concern about fallout contamination, residents should have their visitors go to the back of their dwelling, take off their outer layer of clothing, double bag it, leave it at the rear property line, and come into the house to shower and wash their hair. These procedures remove over 99% of the fallout from someone's body. As a part of this message, residents are being reminded that welcoming visitors during such times is a test of their compassion and 2
humanity. The planning section chief has asked the public information officer to get information about external decontamination to the **Emergency Alert** 21
System (EAS) stations for broadcast to the public. 2

The fallout plume from a nuclear detonation presents a radiation-related danger. Assessing the fallout plume is an essential part of planning for public 3
health actions and communication with the public. In the early phase immediately following the blast, members of the public who are near and some who 18,19,20
are distant from the hypocenter ("ground zero" of the detonation) are looking for guidance as to whether to shelter in place or evacuate. The initial instruction for everyone is to shelter in place and listen to a radio for specific information regarding shelter in place and evacuation through the EAS. Elected officials, emergency medical services, the Office of Emergency Services per- 3
sonnel, and public health leadership will need to discuss the multiple dimen- 16
sions of a nuclear incident and the ethics in what and when to communicate with the public. During the planning phases for this disaster scenario, it had 2,3
been determined that the plume map should be shared with the public. The

public in Ventura County is being told to "Get Inside. Stay Inside. Stay Tuned," until it becomes clarified that the fallout is not going to be a threat to them. If credible direction to "Get Inside. Stay Inside. Stay Tuned" reaches the public in a timely manner (within minutes after the explosion), it has the potential to keep tens of thousands of people from fleeing their homes and turning what might otherwise be a chaotic and risky situation on Los Angeles and Ventura County highways into a more manageable one. This message is reinforced by early placement of plume maps on the internet and television. In this way, those who are not in the path of fallout should feel comfortable with their decision to stay at home and those who are in the path of fallout are being told that it is safer to shelter in place than to flee. It appears after the first 24 hours that the fallout will not be an immediate threat to Ventura County residents. Nevertheless, a proportion of the population is fleeing.

If planning a response to a nuclear explosion is to have a single major benefit, it is to diminish or prevent altogether the number of people exposed to fallout. This has the potential to save tens of thousands of lives and prevent radiation-related illness in many more. Sheltering in place will keep some vehicles off the roadways and improve the chances for the orderly evacuation of many Los Angeles residents (and the movement of emergency response vehicles). The chaos that is being seen from massive self-evacuation is leading to unprecedented highway and surface street traffic congealment and preventing the timely exodus of those who would most benefit from evacuation. People who might have stayed safely and comfortably in their homes may find themselves stuck for hours or even days in their cars exposed to the groundshine (radiation) of fallout. If highway and surface street movement is at a standstill, then encouraging the evacuation of individuals who are threatened by fallout puts them in the position of going from bad to worse. They leave the greater protection and comfort afforded them from being in a building to the lesser protection and comfort of an automobile.

5 To provide the most reliable information about the fallout plume to both decision-makers and the public, Ventura County has brought together a team
16,21 of subject matter experts to form a **Plume Mappers Group** (Federal Emergency Management Agency [FEMA], 2011). Its purpose is to create redundancy so that
2 if the most reliable plume maps are not available, a backup plume map will be. Representatives from a number of disciplines within the county (National Weather Service, HazMat, Air Pollution Control District, Public Health, **Office of Emergency Services [OES]**, Information Technology) have developed a hierarchy of plume map quality and how and when these maps will be acquired. Individuals from within this group have been charged, trained, and exercised to rapidly locate the relevant information and to draw plume models over GPS street maps of Ventura County. Upon hearing that a nuclear explosion had occurred, these plume mappers initiated their work on their own.

Evacuation announcements broadcast to the public are suggesting that individuals who feel they must evacuate should bring with them enough food, water, medication, cash, and clean clothes to last them a week as well as items of personal value (photos, etc.), pillows, blankets, and emergency go-bags they may have created.

The Lawrence Livermore Laboratory has advised that no one should evacuate in the first 5 hours after a nuclear explosion. Their work shows that the amount of radiation someone would experience in the first hours while evacuating exceeds the amount that is experienced by someone who is sheltering in place. At various times after the first 5 hours, taking into consideration the decay in radioactivity of the fallout, there may be some slight advantage to evacuation into another area with little or no fallout. It would be of the utmost importance to know that traffic conditions were favorable for possible evacuation.

The Department of Energy's (DOE) **Radiological Assistance Program (RAP)** and their Remote Sensing Laboratories (which have planes and helicopters that measure radiation contamination) are assigned to respond to a nuclear emergency from a terrorist attack. The RAP team is to arrive at the site of an emergency within 4 to 6 hours and conduct a radiological assessment of the area. In responding to an emergency, they use radiation detectors and air-sampling equipment to measure contamination (Figure 13.2).

These teams coordinate environmental monitoring with specialized equipment, and collect and analyze data on the type, amount, and extent of the release. This information is being used to determine what further areas may be evacuated.

1,2

1,2,3,4

2

Two million people in 1 million cars are estimated to have arrived or be heading in the direction of Ventura County. Ventura County's infrastructure currently supports 850,000 people. Many of these evacuees say they are

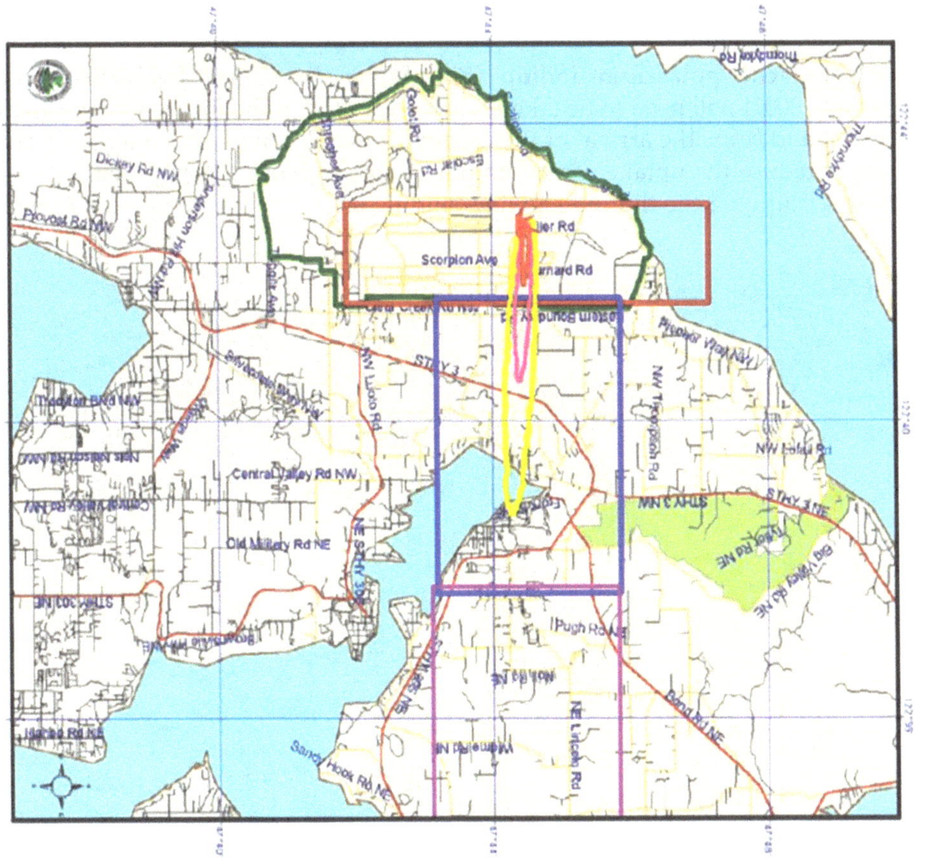

Figure 13.2 Ground deposition contour levels (ovals) for AM-241 (a radionuclide) measured with the helicopter system. The rectangles indicate the area covered during each helicopter flight

Source: From Bowman, D. R., & Daigler, D. M. (2002, October 1). *NNSA/NV consequence management capabilities for radiological emergency response.* U.S. Department of Energy. https://www.osti.gov/servlets/purl/804083

traveling through the county to get to locations further north. Some Ventura County residents are also fleeing because they fear nuclear fallout. Millions more are leaving Los Angeles and heading north, east, and south into other counties. There are four highways that head north through the county from Los Angeles. These contain a total of eight northbound lanes that can carry 250,000 cars a day in each direction. With contraflow, 13 lanes could be enlisted for northbound traffic to carry 400,000 cars per day, but this has not been instituted. The California Highway Patrol (CHP) is resisting this for reasons of emergency and resupply vehicles' access to Los Angeles. At the northern end of Ventura County, there is only one highway with two lanes. Flow has slowed to a two-lane rate all the way back to the San Fernando Valley in northern Los Angeles County. Given current conditions, it will likely take as much as 2½ days for these vehicles to get through Ventura County (Figure 13.3).

The three major water districts have been called and asked to check with their individual vendors as to the integrity of their water systems. They have been requested to increase monitoring of their wells and distribution systems.

Public service announcements (PSAs) are being released to the public at regular intervals on decontamination, avoidance of internal and external contamination, health implications of radiation exposure, plume information, and sheltering techniques.

Prophylactic potassium iodide (KI; Center For Drug Evaluation and Research, 2001) will need to be taken where indicated in the first few hours after the blast and *before* the arrival of the fallout plume. When used correctly, KI can block or reduce the uptake of radioiodine (a cancer-causing component of fallout) by occupying the thyroid's iodine-binding sites. The risk of thyroid cancer

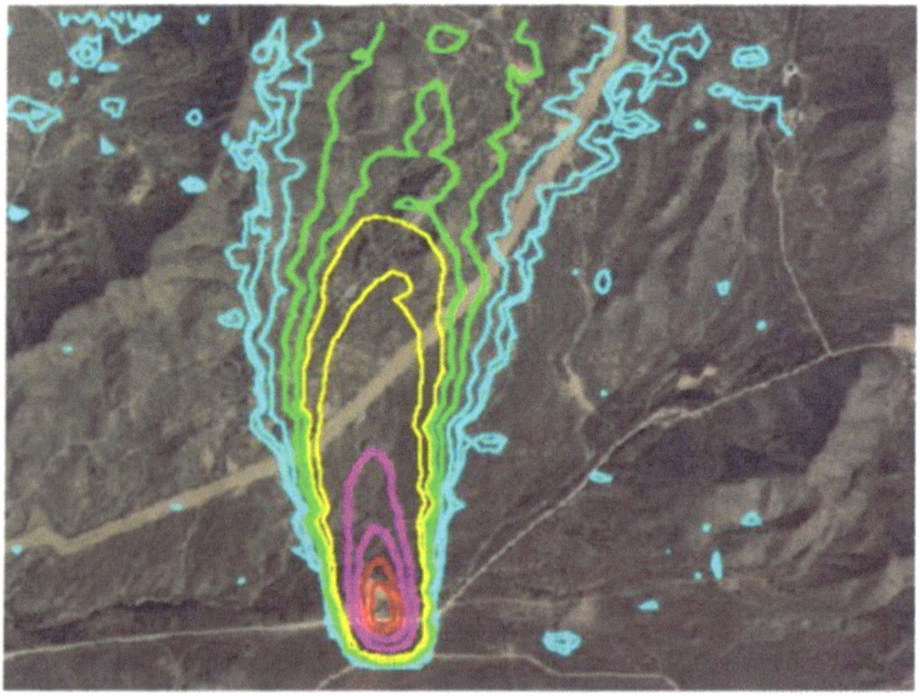

Figure 13.3 Graphical information system data fusion product. Radiation contours measured with the helicopter system are overlaid on a digital photo.

is inversely related to age since cancer takes time to develop. Fetuses, infants, and young children are at greatest risk and may be harmed by small amounts of radioiodine. Although caution should be taken when administering KI to pregnant women and to newborns in the first month of life, the benefits of short-term administration of KI as a thyroid- blocking agent far exceed the risks of administration to any age group. Among 7 million adults who took stable iodine in Poland following Chernobyl, only two severe adverse reactions were reported, both in persons with a known allergy to iodine. Public Health can mobilize its community partners to arrange for the prepositioning of KI in persons' homes in the community. Although the planning and resource mobilization would be done at leadership levels, the actual implementation of providing KI to homes would be done by front-line personnel who are operating under supervision.

Reception Centers (refugee shelters) have been, and more are being, set up by the Red Cross. Not only is this an example of mobilizing community partners (such as the Red Cross) and developing appropriate policies (such as where to establish Reception Centers and how to staff them), but it also is
an example of systems thinking in looking at the totality of resources needed 4,5
to meet the many needs of the population. A liaison has been identified with
that organization who will work with the **Emergency Operations Center** 7,9,22
(EOC). For some, displacement is likely to last several months and perhaps longer. Reestablishing routines, providing hope, allowing for opportunities to be productive, giving people a chance to control some of their destiny, stress reduction activities (including exercise), and making mental health services available will all contribute to a sense of well-being among the displaced (Becker, 2009). Unified Command has been established and is working with partners from the **Joint Information Center (JIC)**. This partnership allows for consistency and increased efficiency so that the Ventura County Public Information Officer (PIO) can share information regarding Reception Centers, EAS radio stations, and the like with the Los Angeles County PIO for broadcast to Los Angeles County residents.

The planning section chief in Ventura County has contacted his Los Angeles counterpart with information for Los Angeles County residents about Ventura County Reception Centers, Ventura County radio station phone numbers for the EAS stations, and the importance of self-decontamination, if needed, *before* beginning their journey out of Los Angeles County. The planning section chief for Los Angeles County has been asked to put this information out to Los Angeles County residents who are evacuating toward Ventura County and points north. Los Angeles County has been urged to broadcast this information over its EAS stations at a minimum, as well as any other functioning mechanisms of communication available.

Red Cross Reception Centers contain radiation detection systems to screen those seeking shelter and to decontaminate evacuees as needed. These are being set up in conjunction with HazMat. Once an evacuee has been cleared of any contamination or successfully decontaminated, they are given a wristband. Evacuees who pass through the decontamination process present no risk to the Reception Center staff.

The Red Cross is constantly evaluating its sheltering capacity against the volume of evacuees and creating more capacity as needed. This is an example of applying the essential service of evaluation utilizing the competencies of

9 assessing the population's needs and evaluating the impact of policies on public health nurses or skilled volunteer nurses who are on-site at each Reception
7,15 Center. Certain conditions, like second-degree burns, are being managed at the
Reception Center. Patients are referred for management of more serious con-
2,3 cerns such as vomiting within 12 hours of exposure to radiation. The demand for
medical care and the acuity of need is high. Since there are not enough Ventura County physicians who are knowledgeable about treatment of radiation-exposed patients to meet the need, the Medical Emergency Radiological Response Teams (MERRTs) have been requested in accordance with Emergency Support Function (ESF) #8.[3] This is an example of why, in a nuclear incident, it is important that there be a means for linking people to needed personal health services.

Red Cross Reception Centers will not house pets for reasons of sanitation and safety. The head of Animal Services activated its disaster plan. Animal Services has colocated animal shelters next to Red Cross shelters as needed to care for the evacuees' pets. Stray animals are being picked up and housed at the animal shelter. All animals are being provided essential medical care regardless of cost. Medications will not be made available to treat animals that are showing signs of acute radiation syndrome.

Included in ESF #8 is triage, treatment, and transportation of victims of the
7 disaster and evacuation of victims out of the disaster area. The EOC Medical Branch has deployed the **National Disaster Medical System (NDMS)**, a nationwide mutual aid network that includes medical response, patient evacuation, and definitive medical care consisting of precommitted acute care hospital beds. NDMS provides **Disaster Medical Assistance Teams (DMATs),** which can assist in the care of victims at the location of a disaster. Other resources mentioned by the ESF #8 include sending an assessment team into the county that assists in determining specific health needs and priorities and an assessment of the health system infrastructure; specialty DMATs that address mass burn injuries and contamination; casualty clearing and staging; individual clinical care specialists to work alongside of local doctors; restocking of health and medical facilities with pharmaceuticals, supplies, and equipment; monitoring of injury and disease patterns; monitoring the health and well-being of emergency workers; and extensive assistance related to radiological exposures, including collection of relevant samples, advice on protective actions and provision of technical assistance, and consultation on medical treatment and decontamination of victims. The ESF #8 delineates resources that ensure the safety of regulated foods, drugs, biological products, and medical devices following a nuclear disaster. These resources will arrange for the seizure, removal, and/or destruction of contaminated products. This is an important environmental health status monitoring function for public health undertaken by front line workers with supervision, utilizing appropriate data collection methods and analysis that must continue in a disaster setting.

Medical facilities are being set up at Oxnard Airport to stabilize and decontaminate the sickest patients for airlift transport to other cities for treatment. Non-hospital facilities (school gymnasia, mobile medical units, warehouses, arenas, and so on) are being recruited to shelter and treat mass casualties. There are an exceptionally large number of burn victims. Given transport problems

[3] Emergency Support Function #8—The Public Health and Medical Services Annex provides federal assistance to supplement local resources in response to a disaster, emergency, or incident that may lead to a public health, medical, behavioral, or human service emergency.

(congestion on the roads, limited ambulances, limited hospital beds available within driving distance) it will be impossible to move patients in significant numbers for probably 2 days or more. The average physician's knowledge of severe burn management is limited. Skilled physicians and nurses are coming in from all over the country. Hospitals are being asked to provide expedited emergency credentialing for these doctors and nurses.

The Planning Section within the Health Care Agency (HCA) Departmental Operations Center (DOC) is sending medical information to the clinics, hospitals, offices, and outposts where doctors and nurses are providing medical treatment. An emphasis is being placed on medical information about radiation-related illness, injuries related to a nuclear detonation, and steps that
health professionals can take to avoid radiation contamination. This is an 8
example of working interprofessionally (at frontline, supervisory, and leadership levels) to provide "just in time" training to assure a competent and 18,19,21
knowledgeable personal healthcare workforce in a disaster setting.

The 211 system[4] is answering calls on health concerns from Ventura County 1,2,3
residents. A public health nurse and representatives from the Red Cross and HazMat have been sent to the 211 system to provide expertise to the operators in answering questions from the public.

Hospitals have been directed to activate their emergency plan—Hospital Emergency Incident Command System (ICS). The EOC has asked hospitals to immediately "lock down," providing only two entrances: one for triage and patients and another for personnel, staff, and officials. Each hospital has established an Assessment Center on its grounds, separate and away from the emergency department. An Assessment Center is a collaborative effort between each hospital and HazMat. The HazMat installation (a decontamination center) is a part of the overall Assessment Center. HazMat has set up the radiation monitoring and decontamination component whereas the overall Assessment Center, which involves triage, referral, patient monitoring, and limited treatment, has been established by the hospital.

At the hospital-based Assessment Centers, those who have various levels of radiation exposure are being triaged into distinct groups. These are weighty and often sobering decisions. Patients can be categorized as those unlikely to survive due to high exposure to heat or radiation (palliative care only), those with acute radiation syndrome who are sick and require hospitalization, those receiving radiation doses of more than 30 or 40 rem but who do not require medical care, those with skin contamination, those with internal contamination, and those who have had no significant exposure. Persons who require treatment but are not sick enough for hospital admission are sent to nearby physicians' offices. Under unusual circumstances (grave injury, heart attack, etc.), patients are sent to the emergency department without radiation monitoring clearance. Evacuees who feel they might have been exposed to radiation are being told to contact the Centers for Disease Control and Prevention (CDC) at 1 800 CDC-INFO (232-4636) or on its website for long-term tracking, as well as for health-related information and available services and resources.

Rapid radiological triage is accomplished by documenting the symptoms of nausea, vomiting, and diarrhea. Vomiting is the most useful indicator of

[4] 211 is a 24-hour hotline that provides individuals and families health information, social services, and referrals.

TABLE 13.1 External Radiation by Onset of Vomiting

Vomiting Post Incident	Estimated Dose	Degree of Acute Radiation Syndrome
Less than 10 minutes	>800 rads	Lethal
10-30 minutes	600-800 rads	Very Severe
Less than 1 hour	400-600 rads	Severe
1-2 hours	200-400 rads	Moderate
More than 2 hours after	<200 rads	Mild

Source: Adapted from Kaufman, J. C. *LA County's response in a radiological event* [PowerPoint presentation]. County of Los Angeles Public Health.

significant exposure (Table 13.1). As time from exposure to vomiting increases from within 1 hour to between 1 and 4 hours and then greater than 4 hours, prognosis will vary from fatal outcome to needing some follow-up but not requiring hospitalization, respectively.

It should be noted that stress reactions can induce nausea and vomiting. However, any person exhibiting these symptoms in the time frames listed earlier is being assumed to have been exposed until this is excluded by further medical evaluation and the history of how far the person was from the hypocenter of the blast. Studies of peripheral blood cell counts, especially of lymphocytes during the following days, can confirm the prognoses described earlier.

Other steps being taken are the discharge of hospitalized patients deemed sufficiently stable to be managed at home; the cancelation of elective admissions and surgeries; calling in off-duty staff, and extending existing staff hours; and identifying additional space within the hospital for patient care, anticipating the management of unprecedented numbers of burn patients, patients with blunt trauma and shrapnel wounds, and patients with acute radiation syndrome.

The medical examiner has full authority and responsibility for the management of dead bodies. There is no basis for the fear that dead bodies cause epidemics. At the time of death, victims are not likely to be sick with "epidemic causing infections" (plague, cholera, typhoid). A **Disaster Mortuary Operational Response Team (DMORT)** will be requested if a significant increase in dead bodies comes to Ventura County. DMORT brings a complete morgue with workstations for autopsies together with equipment and supplies. Specifically, the Weapons of Mass Destruction (WMD) DMORT Team will be requested, which, in addition to performing autopsies, has the capacity to decontaminate between 5 to 50 deceased persons per hour.

Contaminated dead bodies are not being brought to hospitals. Contaminated pieces of shrapnel or other highly contaminated objects that find their way into the hospital are being handled with tongs, set far aside, and turned over to the hospital radiation safety officer for immediate shielding and sequestration. Contaminated water is being allowed to enter the usual drainage system. Contaminated human waste is being treated by the routine protocol for ordinary human waste.

6 A declaration of emergency from the county and a request from the county to
16,21 the governor to do likewise is an important step in a disaster. Such declarations
are a way of using the essential service of legal authority and tools for public
3 health benefit by applying the competencies of leadership and governance by
elected officials and/or public health officers.

First responders have been asked to remember that the cause of this mass casualty incident is a crime. Clothing removal and medical treatment must be performed, but healthcare workers at all levels have been told to stay alert to the potential evidentiary value of all items. It is possible that the perpetrator(s) may be among those treated, and evidence may be found in their possessions or on their clothing.

Trained counselors are on-site in the emergency departments, the hospitals, 4,7
and the Assessment Centers. They have been briefed on radiological issues 21
so they can use this knowledge in their counseling sessions. The National Institutes of Mental Health (NIMH) has developed trauma intervention strategies for the public. 1

Hospital employees have expressed concern about radiation contamination. Training about potential health effects and **personal protective equipment** coming from leadership on the ground is allowing them to respond effectively during this incident. Numerous one-page educational materials in hard copy and on the internet have been made available to healthcare workers throughout the county. Special precautions are being taken to protect pregnant employees. Employees are being instructed in the principles of TIME, DISTANCE, and SHIELDING for minimizing personal exposure to radiation contamination.

The agriculture commissioner has been notified about possible impending radiation risks to Ventura County agriculture and has disseminated this information to county farmers. The agriculture commissioner has the authority to prohibit the harvest of any lot of produce or seize and hold a crop. He is instructing farmers to provide dairy animals and poultry with shelter, stored feed, and protected water supplies.

The late phase of response involves reconstruction and long-term recovery. This begins when Los Angeles and Ventura Counties have demarcated those areas that will be uninhabitable for a prolonged period and have designated the areas where cleanup efforts may prove to be achievable. This process involves convening stakeholders and technical subject matter experts who will identify and evaluate the restoration of affected sites.

This stage is oriented toward the reordering and reopening of activities, communications, utilities, roads, and the general physical environment. It includes recovery and cleanup actions to reduce radiation levels in the environment to acceptable levels. Public Health decisions and goals will include addressing long-term chronic health issues and concerns, and the protection of children and other sensitive populations. Economic and social objectives will be to minimize disruption to businesses and communities and maintain property values. The return and normalization of airports and the seaport to pre-event function is important for convenience and business. The military base must be returned to normal function for national security purposes. Hospital
capacity, water, and sewage must be restored, and the recovery of private 4,9
property and adequate food, fuel, and power assured. Long-term needs for
federal and state resources must be determined. An after-action report on the 3,21
event will be conducted with input from various partners and stakeholders. 1,2,3

The CDC is the lead agency for population monitoring and is responsible for assisting the county and the state in the long-term monitoring of people for external and internal contamination. Through dose reconstruction, the

amount of radiation to which individuals have been exposed will be determined.
1,2 The CDC will help the county and state create a registry of people who may have
1,2,3, been exposed to radiation and monitor these people to see if they are having
4,21 health effects due to either radiation exposure or stress. Hospitals must ensure
that their Assessment Centers keep sufficient records of the radiologically con-
1,2 taminated to achieve follow-up.

Health Hazards and Risks

Forty thousand injured (Benjamin et al., 2009) people will be entering Ventura County in need of some kind of medical attention, from cuts and bruises to heart attacks, as well as burns, broken bones, and embedded objects (shrapnel-type injuries). Humans will be killed and injured by rapid acceleration and deceleration. Many people will be exposed to radiation, and some are concerned that they have been "injured" from fallout.

The treatment of injuries takes precedence over radio-contamination concerns. Removal of all clothing will generally eliminate about 90% of external contamination. It is highly unlikely that residual radiation levels from the patient will constitute a hazard to medical personnel. The only exception to this would be if a piece of radioactive metal from the blast penetrated the patient (radioactive shrapnel). Such a seriously injured patient would probably have been triaged past the peripheral Assessment Center without decontamination. Patients in the emergency department with penetrating injuries should therefore be monitored quickly with a handheld monitor to make sure that they are not a hazard to others.

Most burns will be due to the heat of the blast and not from fires. The instinctive reflex to cover one's eyes will limit the number of people with blindness. Numerous people will have ruptured ear drums. There will be delayed medical attention due to crowding of healthcare facilities.

Aside from the destructive effects of the blast itself, nothing is more problematic and fearsome than the accompanying radiation. Radioactivity will manifest itself in two major ways. The first will be the initial pulse known as "prompt radiation," defined as the radiation within 1 minute of the blast. Fatal doses of prompt radiation following a 10-kT blast may be seen out to a mile or more. The second will be the radiation emanating from "fallout." Fallout is produced when the fission from the blast ionizes dirt, concrete, metal, and the like, which then condenses to produce a radioactive mushroom cloud. A ground detonation produces more fallout than an air detonation because of its greater proximity to ionizable solid material.

Prompt radiation has four submicroscopic components: alpha and beta particles, gamma rays, and neutrons. Neutrons are heavy particles released from the nuclei of atoms. These pieces of atomic shrapnel penetrate solid objects. They can damage human organs immediately by wiping out bone marrow or damage genetic material in cells resulting in mutations for long-term damage, leading to cancer or to genetic defects in future offspring.

Gamma rays are essentially the same as x-rays and penetrate the body with much the same effect as neutrons. The beta and alpha particles can only penetrate the body as far as the skin and so are much less dangerous. They are more likely to cause serious effects in humans when they contaminate someone internally after being swallowed or inhaled.

The long-term or delayed effects of radiation, like cancer and genetic abnormalities, are called **stochastic effects**. These effects are "late" and add incremental risks to those that individuals already naturally have. Everyone has some risk of getting cancer or passing on a birth defect. The stochastic effect is the additional risk that occurs after exposure to a specific radiological exposure. Because the impact of radiation-related risks can only be measured in populations, not in individuals, it is their frequency, not their severity, that is dose-dependent.

The short-term or early health effects of radiation, like the vomiting seen in early acute radiation syndrome, are called deterministic effects. High doses of radiation damage too many cells for the body to repair. Too many damaged cells in the same location may lead to impaired organ function. Low doses of radiation have the potential to cause stochastic effects. Large doses cause acute illness and death. Survivors of large doses are subject to stochastic effects as well.

The unit for measuring the amount of radiation someone has been exposed to is the millisievert (mSv). This is the international term. The older American term is still in common usage and is referred to as rem. Ten mSv equal 1 rem.

In the average year, most humans throughout the world receive about 0.35 rem (3.5 mSv) from natural background radiation. Most humans can tolerate up to 50 rem (500 mSv) per year without any severe effects. Acute doses of radiation up to about 200 rem (2,000 mSv) are tolerated by most people with minimal deterministic effects. Four hundred rem (4,000 mSv) over a short period, as with the prompt radiation exposure from a nuclear blast, would be about 50% fatal within 4 to 8 weeks without medical intervention. For children, older adults, and the chronically ill, 200 rem would be 50% fatal. At 800 rem (8,000 mSv) there would be 100% fatality within 1 to 2 weeks without medical intervention. Medical treatment at these levels of exposure carries no guarantee of success.

Fallout radiation includes alpha and beta particles and gamma rays but not neutrons. The most significant damage to cells is done to the cellular DNA. Most DNA damage is repaired by the cellular systems. If correctly repaired, there will be no consequences. An unrepaired or incorrectly repaired cell will either die, be unable to reproduce, or remain genetically modified. If many cells in an organ are injured, that organ will either function poorly or not at all. If the organ is the intestinal tract, the individual may have diarrhea, vomiting, or bloody stool. If the organ is the brain, there may be confusion or coma. If the organ is the bone marrow, there may be uncontrolled bleeding or infection.

The stochastic effects of cancer and hereditary disease result from individual cells that have survived but resisted repair after radiation exposure. The increased risk of cancer is small. The same can be said for fetal deformities. Most abortions performed following the Chernobyl incident were unnecessary. Abortion is not recommended for exposures of less than 10 rem (100 mSv), and, above this, counseling based on the individual circumstance (such as age of the fetus) is advised. Real risks of cancer and deformity do exist, but they tend to be incremental and highly overblown in the public's imagination.

Health officials can work backward from the patient's symptoms and how long they began after exposure to radiation to estimate what dose of radiation they received (dose reconstruction). Another technique that may be used to estimate radiation dose takes advantage of how sensitive the lymphocytes in the bone marrow are to radiation.

Assessments of radiation measurements result in protective actions: These actions must be taken to prevent deterministic effects and minimize stochastic effects in both first responders and local residents. Taking actions that avoid exposure is much more effective than medical treatment after exposure has occurred. Medical actions taken after exposure will reduce health consequences by a factor of perhaps two or three, while *limiting* exposure will reduce these same consequences by multiples of tens to thousands.

Other actions driven by radiation assessments will inform decisions about evacuation, land use, and crop harvest and treatment. Credible estimates of radiation exposure by locale and population group will even affect psychological morbidity. Accurate and complete monitoring and its intelligent interpretation are the basis upon which a restoration of normality rests.

An assessment of dose that an individual has been exposed to will usually be reconstructed rather than directly measured at the time of the exposure. Those exposed by prompt radiation will have their dose estimated by the symptoms they develop and the period over which the symptoms develop. Those exposed to radiation from fallout will be exposed both to external radiation from radioactive materials transported by the cloud and deposited on the ground, as well as to internal radiation due to the inhalation or swallowing of radioactive materials. Some experts believe that internal contamination from fallout will be minimal. Accurate estimates of an individual's exposure can be made based on the isotopes identified in the area, the known decay rate of those isotopes, the time of the arrival of the fallout cloud, the time of evacuation of the individual, the time of measuring the quantity of radioactivity, and such unique information as the amount of body covered by clothing, when clothing was discarded, and if steps were taken to avoid inhalation of the dust (e.g., a wet handkerchief over the mouth).

The absorbed dose of radiation is thought to be approximately 20 times more harmful to the rest of the body, in terms of late (or stochastic) health effects, than it is to the thyroid. This is due in part to the fact that many Americans already have partial "blocking" of their thyroids, much as they would strive to achieve by taking potassium iodide tablets, because of the ubiquitous iodination of table salt and the high levels of iodine in seafood, milk-based products, and egg yolks.

An attack involving the release of radiation will create uncertainty, fear, and terror. Following the intentional detonation of a nuclear bomb, the management of acute psychological and behavioral responses is likely to be second in importance only to the direct effects of the nuclear explosion itself.

Radiation, an invisible, odorless, and poorly understood threat, has been a cause of extreme public anxiety in the past, as demonstrated by the public's response to the Three Mile Island, Chernobyl, and Goiania, Brazil, accidents. In the aftermath of the event, the public must rely on healthcare providers and scientists to determine who has been contaminated. Those who have been exposed or fear they may have been exposed may experience feelings of vulnerability, anxiety, and a lack of control.

Affected individuals fall into one of three groups: those who are distressed, those who manifest behavioral changes, and those who may develop psychiatric illness. General healthcare providers should manage most of these patients. Some individuals may exhibit behavior changes such as decreasing travel, staying home, refusing to send children to school, and increasing substance use and abuse. Fortunately, for most people, distress and psychological and behavioral symptoms related to the exposure will diminish over time.

Following the Chernobyl accident there has been a continual decline in the health and psychological well-being of the local people that is not radiation-related. Noncancer health effects seem to be related to the physical and psychological stresses that remain from the accident. Many unrelated major and minor health problems can be anticipated to be blamed on radiation effects following a nuclear event.

The significance of nonradiation effects cannot be overstated. In a study about the psychological development of Belorussian children exposed in utero to radiation in the Chernobyl accident compared to children from noncontaminated areas, no differences could be related to the radiation itself, but a significant correlation was found linking emotional stress in children to anxiety among parents.

Prior technological disasters, terrorist attacks, and use of novel weapons in the context of war suggest that healthcare providers' offices, medical clinics, and hospitals will be deluged with symptomatic and asymptomatic patients seeking evaluation and care for possible contamination following a radiation event.

Following a radiological event, people will turn to their own healthcare providers for information and guidance. Healthcare providers will play a key role in determining how patients and the public respond to a radiological event. A well-organized, effective medical response will instill hope and confidence, reduce fear and anxiety, and support the continuity of basic community functions.

There are three major problems that might occur to the drinking water in Ventura County following a nuclear detonation: radioactive contamination, a physical disruption of the water conduits, and an interruption in electrical power. Actual radioactive contamination is not likely to occur in large part due to the dilutional effect. Should this occur, water purveyors will shut down the supply. A physical disruption in water supply might occur to those areas of Ventura County serviced by the Los Angeles–based Metropolitan Water District. If one of these two types of supply interference were to occur, the status of restoration of flow and the potability of the water would be reported frequently on EAS radio stations and other news outlets. Suffice it to say that following a nuclear disaster, if a home faucet is running, the water is almost certainly safe to drink. The third form of problem is an interruption of electricity. Without electricity, water pumps and wastewater treatment plants cannot function. A lack of drinking water, poor sanitation, and the close quarters offered in an affected emergency shelter could create the conditions for spreading communicable diseases, such as *Salmonella*, *Shigella*, *Escherichia coli (E. coli)*, and noroviruses.

There may be disruptions in the normal food distribution channels that could result in rationing. If grocery stores run out of food, basic food items will need to be distributed by the county at designated locations and to shelters. Hoarding should be anticipated. Law enforcement personnel should be involved in monitoring grocery stores to prevent hoarding, rioting, and looting.

A refrigerator will keep foods cool for about 4 hours without power if it is unopened. Thawed food from a freezer can usually be eaten if it is still "re-frigerator cold," or refrozen if it still contains ice crystals. Food that has been at temperatures greater than 40 °F for 4 hours or more, and any food that has an unusual odor, color, or texture, should be discarded. A full freezer that has not been opened will hold food safely for 48 hours.

Water is needed to flush toilets. A toilet can be flushed with a bucket of water when there is no water pressure. Additional water sources in the home include water in the water heater tank, pool, and spa.

Morbidity and Mortality

Estimates are 99,000 will be dead of all causes by 8 weeks (National Security Council Led Domestic Readiness Group, 2016). The majority of deaths following a nuclear detonation are due to radiation, not direct blast effects. It can be assumed that 45,000 people will die from the blast in the first day;[5] 9,000 will die instantly; within four blocks of the hypocenter of the blast there will be a 95% fatality rate, 28% at five blocks and 1% at six blocks; 138,000 will suffer some form of injury; 131,000 of these will be injured by fallout and the remainder from the concussive effects from the blast, from burns or from shrapnel. Some of these will die.

A 10-kT nuclear detonation in a large urban area can be expected to produce 1,100 trauma cases, 1,700 burns, 700 cases of acute radiation syndrome, 3,200 multiple traumatic injuries, and 3,600 people who are blinded by the blast, 2,500 of whom will have had flash blindness and 1,100 with retinal burns. Numerous people will have ruptured ear drums from the blast pressure.

Traumatic injuries may be sorted into two categories: severe and mild. The severe injuries call for major or minor surgery to repair deep penetrating injuries, severe blunt force trauma resulting in internal organ damage or some other crush-related injury, and open fractures. Mild injuries are defined as nonoperative. These include such things as concussions, simple lacerations, closed fractures, ligamentous injuries, and others. This category includes shrapnel injuries from glass.

Most burns by far are due to the flash and heat from the immediate explosion. Roughly 95% of burn injuries are associated with the flash. Only 2% to 4% are attributable to flame burns alone (Table 13.2).

TABLE 13.2 Relative Distribution of Flash and Flame Burns at Hiroshima and Nagasaki

Flash Burn (%)	Flame Burn (%)	Both (%)
82.9	1.9	14.9
90.9	3.4	5.7

Source: Adapted from Oughterson, A. W., & Warren, S. (Eds.). (1956). *Medical effects of the atomic bomb in Japan* (Table 5.1). McGraw-Hill.

[5] Even in Hiroshima and Nagasaki there were occasional survivors within five city blocks of the nuclear detonation. These individuals were likely to find themselves in one of the few, modern concrete structures within the blast radius. In Hiroshima, almost 100% of people died within a five-block radius (approximately 0.8 square mile), and 80% died between six and ten blocks (an additional 2.3 square miles). Due to the more substantial buildings in modern Los Angeles and their associated protective effect, it is assumed that fewer people will die from the blast's immediate effects.

Whether from prompt radiation or from fallout, increasing amounts of radiation will cause predictable disease syndromes in the exposed. This group of illnesses is generally referred to as **Acute Radiation Syndrome (ARS)**. This spectrum of acute illness is caused by radiation to the entire body at a high dose for a short time. Depending on how high the dose and how resistant to radiation the different organs of the body are, different disease syndromes may be seen.

There are three classic ARS syndromes. At the lower range of dangerous doses of radiation is the bone marrow syndrome, also called hematopoietic syndrome. This syndrome is seen beginning at doses of 70 rem (700 mSv). The higher the dose above this, the more likely it is to be fatal. Symptoms begin with decreased appetite (anorexia), nausea, and vomiting. These symptoms may last from a few minutes to days. The radiation kills the stem cells in the bone marrow. These die off over a period of 1 to 6 weeks. During this period, the effected person may appear perfectly well. Then the patient experiences anorexia, fever, and malaise. All the different blood cell lines are diminished. The absent blood cells lead to infection and hemorrhage. Most deaths occur within a few months. Sometimes the radiation fails to kill all the marrow cells, and so they repopulate the bone marrow. Patients whose radiation exposure was limited to only causing the bone marrow syndrome will often completely recover. People who receive 120 rem (1,200 mSv) may die. At a dose of 250 to 500 rem, 50% will die.

The second ARS syndrome is the gastrointestinal syndrome. This is seen at about 1,000 rem (10,000 mSv) of exposure. Not only are the bone marrow cells killed, but the cells lining the gastrointestinal tract are as well. The initial symptoms are anorexia, nausea, vomiting, cramps and diarrhea. These symptoms are seen within a few hours after exposure and last for about 2 days. The patient may feel well thereafter for a period that lasts less than a week. Then the patient experiences malaise, anorexia, severe diarrhea, fever, dehydration, and electrolyte imbalance. The patient dies of infection, dehydration, and electrolyte imbalance within 2 weeks of their initial radiation exposure. At an exposure of 1,000 rem or above, 100% of people are expected to die.

The third and worst ARS syndrome is the cardiovascular/central nervous system syndrome. This is seen at an exposure of 5,000 rem (50,000 mSv). Sometimes this is seen at an exposure as low as 2,000 rem. Symptoms include extreme nervousness and confusion, severe nausea, vomiting, watery diarrhea, loss of consciousness, and burning sensations of the skin. Symptoms develop within minutes of exposure and last for minutes to hours. Occasionally the patient has a partial improvement but then returns to having watery diarrhea, convulsions, and coma. This occurs 5 to 6 hours after the initial radiation exposure. Within 3 days the patient is dead. No one survives.

Skin damage should be expected in many patients and will vary depending on the thermal exposure or radiation dose. Skin lesions that appear to be burns of various depths may appear immediately or in hours, days, or weeks. Lesions that appear early, remain, and resolve at the accustomed rate of thermal burns are probably just that. At radiation doses beginning around 300 rads, erythema may develop in a few hours but can disappear a few hours later and reappear later. Skin lesions that appear *late* are likely to be related to radiation as opposed to thermal causes.

Roles and Responsibilities of Key Players

Many actions will require coordination between agencies (U.S. Department of Homeland Security [DHS], 2016). Management and coordination of these groups is provided by an ICS, which describes a standardized structure for disaster response. This will be established early during the incident to coordinate response activities from multiple disciplines and stakeholders.

Coordination of the response effort must be established early on. Coordination promotes professionalism and accuracy; inspires confidence in government response by the local population; provides assets to the county; establishes which, if any, of the county's resources will be sent to other jurisdictions; and identifies and creates the available and functioning communication needed to efficiently respond to a disaster (e.g., satellite phones, the Auxiliary Communications Services,[6] placement of liaison personnel). Volunteers and donations should be screened and assigned for effective use by the Red Cross. The disaster response must be documented to provide maximum reimbursement.

Coordination will be needed between the Ventura County Operational Area and the Los Angeles Operational Area (LA County EOC) for the purpose of sharing situation status and receiving LA County's plume models. The CHP will monitor traffic flow along Highways 101, 118, 126, and 1 and coordinate traffic in affected areas. Caltrans will work with this effort.

The Ventura County Sheriff's Department and city police departments will coordinate with CHP to manage traffic problems and general backup. The sheriff will be the lead for crisis management at the local level that includes crowd control, rioting, and looting. The CHP may be needed to assist with intelligence, evacuation, and emergency notifications and provide information on radiation to the first responders.

The California Office of Emergency Services will provide information systems[7] as well as staff to assist in the county EOC. OES staff will administer the structure of mutual aid and response coordination for the State. They can provide additional expertise in overall coordination with federal agencies as well as requesting appropriate agencies to provide expertise in radiation, environmental health, utilities, water supply, and legal and political issues. The Federal Bureau of Investigation (FBI) will be the lead agency in the response. The Department of Energy will play a role in providing support and technical advice during any radiological event.

During most disasters, aside from the National Guard, the military cannot be expected to participate in the response. Therefore, local civil authorities are unacquainted with military assets. A nuclear detonation by a terrorist organization may allow for such a response. To facilitate and legalize the military's involvement, a state of war will likely be declared, authorizing the military to assume broad powers. The naval base in Ventura has extensive resources including an airport; construction equipment; medical capacity, mostly in the manner

---

[6] Licensed radio amateurs used during emergencies who are used to overcoming the barriers to radio communications. They may also use a wide range of communication modes like TV, data, voice, or Morse code to exchange messages.

[7] The Organization for the Advancement of Structured Information Standards, which is a consortium that seeks agreement on intelligent ways to exchange information over the internet, works on cybersecurity, and the Response Information Management System is an internet-based system used to coordinate and manage the state's response to disasters.

of personnel; berthing and staging areas; and policing capability. Numerous agencies, departments, and offices within the federal government are mandated to perform specific duties during disasters. These resources will support but not displace the Ventura County response in areas such as the handling of dead bodies and the stabilization of sick and wounded at an airport staging site for transport to distant medical facilities.

County responders will run the early phase of the response by necessity. State and federal assets may not be available to Ventura County for hours or days due to the realities of mobilization and the prioritization of needed expertise and resources to the most affected areas. As federal assets (DHS, 2006) arrive on scene, they will be included in the unified command structure.

The responsibilities of the various participants in this response will change as the incident progresses. When the detonation of a nuclear device is first detected, the Ventura County OES will be notified and will notify other response partners that will make up the members of the Unified Command (including, but not limited to, the Sheriff's Office, FBI, Ventura County Public Health [VCPH], and Fire Department/HazMat) and the Plume Mappers and open the EOC. The DHS Homeland Security Operations Center will be notified to provide support until a Joint Field Office (JFO) is operational. Protective actions will be ordered by VCPH (shelter in place, KI recommendations). Many federal assets will be expected to self-deploy under their own authority.[8] The county will request a disaster emergency declaration from the state, which is a necessary step to request personnel and financial reimbursements under California laws and regulations.

Fire departments, including city and county, will be the lead agencies for the decontamination operation. HazMat (a unit of the fire department) will monitor and decontaminate people in three settings: at five Red Cross Reception Centers; at Assessment Centers located at the county's eight hospitals; and at three independent sites in the county. The fire department will place portal radiation monitors at Reception Centers, make perimeter and access control decisions in conjunction with federal resources,[9] evaluate public safety concerns in conjunction with public health and environmental health, make recommendations to law enforcement regarding evacuations, and give notifications to neighborhoods that need to be evacuated. The Environmental Health Division has its own HazMat unit that declares clear those sites that require hazardous material or radiological agent cleanup and decontamination.

County Public Works serve as the lead for structural and infrastructural needs assessment for property and roadways and will refer calls to the appropriate agency for other problems they encounter (e.g., Southern California Edison for downed power lines). Public Works has several hundred barricades. These would be useful at sites in the county that are set up for decontamination of the public. They may also be useful with patient flow at Assessment Centers.

Public Health will activate its DOC and together with Emergency Medical Services (EMS) provide medical response operations; communication with

[8] Health and Human Services, FBI, Occupational Safety and Health Administration (OSHA), Environmental Protection Agency (EPA), and DOE.
[9] The Federal Radiological Monitoring and Assessment Center (FRMAC).

hospitals, ambulance companies, and healthcare providers; and coordination of medical and health resources during emergency response and recovery.[10] Emergency contract agreements and the mutual aid system will be utilized as will a request to evaluate the status of the healthcare system in Ventura County. Medical and health resource requests will be made.[11] Additional staffing will be requested.[12] Health staff may also be sought from the Naval Base Ventura.

A number of federal agencies will be expected to be represented in the Unified Command for an improvised nuclear device incident to support the response in accordance with the National Response Plan[13] (NRP). Ventura County will place a liaison at that EOC (which houses the Unified Command). It is also possible that Ventura County will be named the site of the event's EOC due to the possibility of significant degradation of Los Angeles County's capability. Thus, the County of Ventura would have two different EOCs, that of Los Angeles and its own. Every effected county will likely open their own EOC. The DHS will designate a **Principal Federal Official (PFO),** who will be responsible for coordinating federal assets.[14]

Field measurements for radiation in Ventura County will be utilized, if the **Federal Radiological Monitoring and Assessment Center (FRMAC)** is available, to provide data collection, analysis, and interpretation to Ventura's EOC. If FRMAC is not available, local HazMat field personnel will perform radiological monitoring and assessment.

It is hoped that between 12 and 24 hours the JFO will become operational and additional federal teams will be made available.[15] Protective Action Guides[16] (PAG; U.S. Environmental Protection Agency, 2017) will be provided by the JFO to state and local decision-makers. The state will request, and be granted, a major disaster or emergency declaration from the federal government. The DHS will declare an Incident of National Significance. A Robert T. Stafford Disaster Relief and Emergency Assistance Act declaration will facilitate funding for public and individual assistance and recovery operations.

As data become available, federal, state, and local officials will have better information with which to make protective action decisions, assist emergency workers, and inform the public. Federal protective action recommendations will be provided to state and local governments on public dose limits, restrictions regarding consumption of food and water, and dose reduction actions. Actions may include relocation, control of public access, decontamination of radiological "hot spots," response worker dose monitoring, population monitoring, food and water controls, and clearance of private property for return to habitation.

[10] The Standardized Emergency Management System (SEMS) is the cornerstone of California's emergency response system and the fundamental structure for the response phase of emergency management and the Regional Disaster Medical Health Coordinator (RDMHC), Region 1. SEMS is utilized in the DOC.
[11] Through the RDMHC.
[12] From the Disaster Medical Assistance Teams (DMATs); the Commissioned Corps Readiness Force (CCRF) for the U.S. Public Health Service; the Visiting Nurses Association; students from schools of medicine, pharmacy, nursing, and public health; retired and other volunteer healthcare workers; and the Medical Reserve Corps.
[13] DHS, FBI, DOE, the EPA, the Nuclear Regulatory Commission (NRC), OSHA, U.S. Army Corps of Engineers, and the Department of Defense (DoD).
[14] A Nuclear Incident Response Team (NIRT) will be stood up by DHS, incorporating the RAP, the Aerial Measuring System, FRMAC, Radiation Emergency Assistance Center/Training Site, and the Radiological Emergency Response Team.
[15] The NIRT, Domestic Emergency Support Team, and the Advisory Team for Food and Health may become available.
[16] PAGs are radiation dose guidelines that trigger public safety measures, such as evacuation or staying inside, to protect public health after a radiation emergency has occurred.

The Red Cross will accept donations, direct and register volunteers, and send representatives to the EOC for liaison. The PIO will disseminate information about these activities to the public.

MITIGATION

Mitigation efforts are those actions that can be taken to lessen the impacts of a disaster. Some of these can be accomplished in advance and some are taken as part of the response.

The United States is less prepared for a nuclear detonation on our soil than any other imaginable disaster other than an alien invasion from outer space. A major nuclear detonation is the only potential disaster we might face for which we are, compared to all other disasters, relatively unprepared (Burkle et al., 2017). The cause of this lack of preparation is that our elected officials fear the public's reaction to an open discussion of how to protect ourselves from a nuclear detonation and, perhaps, wrongly believe there is nothing we can do to lessen the consequences of such an attack.

The first step in this preparedness process is a public information campaign.[17] That campaign would leave our populace with an understanding and immediate recall of a simple slogan, "Get Inside. Stay Inside. Stay Tuned" (Kisken, 2017). In addition to concern about how the public might react to such a campaign, there is the challenge of making a low-incidence, high-consequence event important and relevant to the public.

We cannot possibly ready our response if we are afraid of public opinion. This will be particularly tragic when what evidence we have says the public is thirsting for this kind of knowledge. If we are afraid of public opinion, we will be unable to openly train our first responders. Numerous, very public event-specific responses would need to be exercised; unique challenges presented by the significant road congestion seen with a massive exodus of people from a nuclear bomb–affected area would require special training for law enforcement (road clearance, response to looting, disruptions at gas stations, alternate ways to move around our county when roads are not open) and the fire department (responding to healthcare calls, fires, setting up and running decontamination units outside hospital emergency departments and reception centers; Levin, 2011). The entire healthcare apparatus would need to train on dealing with victims of radiation exposure and fears about their own contact with contaminated patients. These activities would inevitably come to the public's attention. Furthermore, procuring government funds to create needed response infrastructure would be noticed by the public as well as the education of both parents and children about how students could best be made safe should a nuclear attack occur during school hours.

As far as the belief that there is nothing that can be done to lessen the consequences of a nuclear attack, this is based on old Cold War notions about an all-out nuclear assault. It is estimated that 100,000 lives could be saved upon the detonation of an improvised nuclear device with an educated public and prepared local first responders (Johns Hopkins Center for Health Security, n.d.).

---

[17] Ventura County is the only county of 3,142 counties and county equivalents in the United States that has launched a public information campaign preparing its populace to respond to a nuclear detonation. The public response to this campaign was greeted without panic and with significant gratitude and relief that local government was addressing this issue.

Given the fact that memory and information about the last nuclear detonation is scant, complete preparation for a nuclear event is an approachable but unachievable goal.

Public communication about immediate protective actions that the public should take ("Get Inside. Stay Inside. Stay Tuned."), how those receiving others who are fleeing a detonation should be welcomed ("This is a test of our humanity."), and education about the risks and myths of radiation exposure are indicated. The challenge is to craft messages that the public will perceive as relevant and memorable without causing undue alarm. Advance messaging must anticipate and resolve the questions, "What do you know that we don't know? Why are you telling us this now?" Participation and consensus from community leaders and other stakeholders in the community must be sought early in the development of a public education program. Elected officials and business and religious leaders may play an important role in soothing anxieties should these arise.

An education program must be based on each county's unique populations (including languages and typical methods of information acquisition) and communications assets available in the county (television, radio, internet, social networking, reverse 911, 211, health educators, reaching parents through their school-aged children). Public Health information via public service announcements, press releases, interviews, press conferences, and town hall meetings should be utilized. Messages should be developed collaboratively with stakeholders, such as the American Medical Association, the American Hospital Association, and others, that should also participate in their dissemination. Ideally, people will find enough interest in the campaign that they will want to learn more and education that goes into further depth should be made available on the county's website. Education about nuclear explosion preparedness must become a part of the canon of disaster topics that are taught in our country, especially in our schools of public health, in an ongoing manner.

Additional educational efforts should expand the knowledge of journalists and promote their partnering with first responders in covering the consequences of a nuclear detonation, so they promote helpful messaging. This will include effective ways to communicate clinical information to lay audiences. Social media will be sending erroneous and harmful information that professional journalists can counteract.

Public Health, nationally and locally, must develop materials that are brief and relevant to patients who have been exposed to radiation or have some other trauma-related medical problem. Other written materials must deal with the risks of radiation exposure to medical staff. Health departments must establish traditional and alternate ways of transmitting these documents to medical providers and be ready to do so in the event of a nuclear detonation. The Public Health Department should bring together all hospitals in the county to address and plan for a major surge in healthcare needs.

Providers must be trained in disaster response, including altered standards of care and how these may affect triage and treatment decisions, the legal and ethical basis for allocating scarce resources in a mass casualty event, how to note the signs and symptoms of radiation exposure and poisoning, and how to recognize and manage the effects of stress on themselves and their patients. Stress management measures should be planned for providers and their families. If laboratory or radiology testing are overwhelmed, treatment based on physical examination, history, and clinical judgment will occur. Good Samaritan laws will be in effect to reassure practitioners.

Protocols will need to be developed and practiced before the event, and usual and routine standards and practices will need to be modified at the time of an event based on public health and disaster law. Each hospital should exercise its capability to manage surge, the acquisition or training of personnel who know how to use radiation detection equipment, appropriate and adequate **personal protective equipment (PPE)** for Emergency Department (ED) staff, an exercised plan for a patient Assessment Center outside of the ED with associated decontamination capability, and a radioactive debris management plan.

Triage would be practiced and focus on identifying and reserving treatment for individuals who have a critical need for treatment and are likely to survive. The goal would be to allocate resources to maximize the number of lives saved. Complicating conditions, such as underlying chronic disease, may have an impact on an individual's ability to survive. Guidance documents should address the triage of patients based upon their likelihood of survival. Emergency department access may be reserved for immediate-need patients; ambulatory patients may be diverted to clinics and physicians' offices, or alternate care sites where "lower level" hospital ward care can be provided. Intensive or critical care units may become surgical suites and regular medical care wards may become isolation or other specialized response units. Tabletop exercises for medical leaders will address these potential scenarios.

The usual scope of practice standards will not apply (Sokol, 2006). Nurses may assume some of the functions of physicians, and physicians may perform outside their specialties. Credentialing of providers may be granted on an emergency or temporary basis. Equipment and supplies will be rationed and used in ways consistent with achieving the ultimate goal of saving the most lives. Disposable supplies may be reused. Documentation standards will not be maintained. Providers will not have time to obtain informed consent or be able to fully document the care provided. HIPAA laws will not be complied with in the usual way.

Hospitals should expect to not have enough trained staff. Some staff will be afraid to leave home or may be unable to travel to work. Stress and long hours will occur. Out-of-county volunteers and/or mutual aid may need to be utilized. Critical equipment, such as ventilators, may not be used without staff who are trained to operate them. Delays in hospital care due to backlogs of patients should be anticipated. Patients will be waiting for scarce resources, such as operating rooms, radiological suites, and laboratories. Patients may need to be transported out of county to receive care.

Plans for the delivery of healthcare following a nuclear event must address the special needs of several groups within the general population. These include children, people with physical or cognitive disabilities, persons with preexisting mental health or substance abuse problems, frail or immunocompromised adults and children, non-English speakers, the homeless, and people without vehicles.

The responsibilities of the medical examiner's office will include evidence collection since victims of terrorism are part of a crime scene and the perpetrators themselves may have become victims of the crime. Medical examiners will want to address in advance what protective equipment will be needed to ensure the safety of personnel, how to ensure radiation safety in the mortuary, the performance of abbreviated examinations due to an overwhelming workload, tests that are needed and available to make an accurate diagnosis, what federal resources can be called on to assist the medical examiner, and how to accommodate the cultural sensitivities and attitudes toward death and the handling of dead bodies. The number of fatalities will make it difficult to notify next of kin. Burial and cremation capacity may be overwhelmed, and the standards for timeliness of death certificates may not be met.

The challenge of transporting patients will be unprecedented. If the roads are in gridlock, patients may need to be transported between hospitals that are very near one another by gurney on sidewalks. Helicopters landing on the roofs or in the parking lots of hospitals will be utilized to transport patients out of the county. Oxnard Airport will need to plan on the arrival of large transport planes to move patients to distant sites.

The three major water purveyors in Ventura County will exercise their call tree (which is composed of approximately 150 individual water vendors) to initiate their reporting of systems integrity to their area captains as soon as they hear of any possible detonation of a nuclear device within 100 miles. These captains call into their respective purveyor (Calleguas, United, and Casitas Water Districts) who will report to their representative at the EOC.

Grocery store or grocery chain managers should work with experienced disaster planners to have a plan ready to ration their stock as soon as a nearby nuclear detonation is reported. Grocery stores should develop memoranda of understanding with their distributors to dispatch food supply trucks early, frequently, and preferentially during a local disaster.

CONCLUSION

This chapter has provided an overview to the student as to the anticipated public health impacts and challenges posed by a nuclear detonation. It specifically addressed the impact on, and response by, the areas immediately outside the zone of greatest destruction. The scope of such an event highlights the need for high-level coordination and communication. It also illustrates, through a case study example, the complex tasks at all levels (frontline workers, supervisors and managers, and leadership) that face public health and its many partners (the healthcare system, law enforcement, emergency services management, community-based nongovernmental organizations) in this type of massive event. It further elucidates the governmental levels potentially involved (local, regional, state, national) in the preparedness, response, and mitigation efforts. This case study allows the student to become familiar with the issues and vocabulary surrounding a nuclear detonation and, thereby, should give the student some level of confidence of working as a member of a team that may have to deal with such a horrific event should it ever occur.

DISCUSSION QUESTIONS

1. In the event of a nuclear detonation, discuss the first steps that need to be taken by, and the challenges facing, public health officials and other first responders.
2. Discuss what might be the pros and cons of prepositioning prophylactic potassium iodide (KI) in peoples' homes and where it may be appropriate to do so.
3. What challenges do civic leaders and county/city departments face in the recovery phase of a nuclear detonation as compared to other public health emergencies?
4. Discuss how affected county/counties coordinate with state and national governmental agencies for resources (both personnel as well as supplies and equipment) in the face of a public health emergency such as that caused by a nuclear detonation.

SUMMARY

TABLE 13.3 Select Essential Services of Public Health Demonstrated in Nuclear Detonation Response

Essential Service # and Definition	Context in Chapter Case	Competency # It Ties to	Importance for Emergency Preparedness, Response, or Recovery
1. Assess and monitor population health status, factors that influence health, and community needs and assets (Assessment)	Teams coordinate environmental monitoring with specialized equipment to collect and analyze data on the type, amount, and extent of the release.	1, 2, 3, 4	This information is critical to be able to determine what geographic areas may be evacuated due to radiological contamination.
2. Investigate, diagnose, and address health problems and hazards affecting the population (Assessment)	Centers for Disease Control and Prevention helps create a registry of people who may have been exposed to radiation and monitor these people.	1, 2, 3, 4, 21	Monitoring of people exposed, or potentially exposed, to radiation will identify persons who are having health effects due to either radiation exposure or stress.
3. Communicate effectively to inform and educate people about health, factors that influence it, and how to improve it (Policy Development)	Planning section chief asked the public information officer to get information on external decontamination to the Emergency Alert System (EAS) stations for broadcasting.	18, 19, 20	It is important for the public to know that 99% of the fallout contamination can be safely removed from someone's body by going to the back of their dwelling, taking off their outer layer of clothing, double bagging it, leaving it at the rear property line, and coming into the house to shower and wash their hair.
4. Strengthen, support, and mobilize communities and partnerships to improve health (Policy Development)	Reception Centers (refugee shelters) set up by the Red Cross.	7, 9, 22	Mobilizing community partners (such as the Red Cross) and developing appropriate policies (such as where to establish Reception Centers and how to staff them) are important examples of systems thinking in looking at the totality of resources needed to meet the many needs of the population.
6. Utilize legal and regulatory actions designed to improve and protect the public's health (Policy Development)	A declaration of emergency from the county and a request from the county to the governor to do likewise is an important step in a disaster.	16, 21	Such declarations of emergency from an affected county and, in turn, a declaration of emergency by the governor are key steps to mobilize additional resources (manpower and materiel) in support of the county's efforts to respond and recover from a disaster.
7. Assure an effective system that enables equitable access to the individual services and care needed to be healthy (Assurance)	EOC Medical Branch deploys the National Disaster Medical System (NDMS), a nationwide mutual aid network including medical response, patient evacuation, and definitive medical care.	7, 9	The utilization of the NDMS is important in that it provides Disaster Medical Assistance Teams that can assist in the care of victims at the location of a disaster.
8. Build and support a diverse and skilled public health workforce (Assurance)	Planning Section within the Health Care Agency Departmental Operations Center sends medical information to clinics, hospitals, offices, and outposts where doctors and nurses are providing treatment.	18, 19, 21	"Just in time" training and information is important in educating the workforce during a radiological emergency by placing emphasis on disseminating medical information about radiation-related illness, injuries related to a nuclear detonation, and steps that health professionals can take to avoid radiation contamination.

(continued)

TABLE 13.3 Select Essential Services of Public Health Demonstrated in Nuclear Detonation Response *(continued)*

Essential Service # and Definition	Context in Chapter Case	Competency # It Ties to	Importance for Emergency Preparedness, Response, or Recovery
9. Improve and innovate public health functions through ongoing evaluation, research, and continuous quality improvement (Assurance)	Red Cross is constantly evaluating sheltering capacity against the volume of evacuees and creating more capacity as needed.	7, 15	Continuing evaluation and quality improvement of the actions being taken in a nuclear or other emergency incident with mass casualties are important to ensure safe and sufficient sheltering and that there is a means for linking people to needed personal health services

EOC, Emergency Operations Center

TABLE 13.4 Select CEPH Competencies Needed for Frontline Health Workers, Managers, and Leaders for Nuclear Emergency Preparedness, Response, and Recovery

Competency # and Definition	Context in Case/Chapter	Level	Importance for Emergency Preparedness, Response, and Recovery
1. Apply epidemiological methods to settings and situations in public health practice.	The Radiological Assistance Program (RAP) team is to arrive at the site of an emergency within 4 to 6 hours and conduct a radiological assessment of the area.	Level 1	Frontline workers in the RAP assigned to rapidly respond to a nuclear emergency have available radiation detectors and air-sampling equipment to measure contamination.
7. Assess population needs, assets and capacities that affect communities' health.	Trained counselors are on-site in the emergency departments, the hospitals, and at the Assessment Centers.	Level 1	These frontline counselors, briefed on radiological issues, are in an important position to use knowledge of trauma intervention strategies for the public in their counseling sessions.
9. Design a population-based policy, program, project, or intervention.	Long-term needs for federal and state resources must be determined. An after-action report on the event will be conducted with input from various partners and stakeholders.	Level 3	Leadership will need to design a multitude of interventions to ensure, among other things, hospital capacity, water and sewage system restoration, recovery of private property, and adequate food, fuel, and power.
16. Apply leadership and/or management principles to address a relevant health issue.	Elected officials, emergency medical services, the Office of Emergency Services personnel, and public health leadership will need to discuss the incident and the ethics in what and when to communicate with the public.	Level 3	Those in leadership positions, by giving credible direction to "Get Inside. Stay Inside. Stay Tuned" that reaches the public in a timely manner (within minutes after the explosion), has the potential to keep tens of thousands of people from fleeing their homes and avoiding what might otherwise be a chaotic and risky situation.
18. Select communication strategies for different audiences and sectors.	Planning section chief asks the public information officer to get information about external decontamination to the Emergency Alert System stations for broadcast to the public.	Level 2	The communication strategy needs both craft messages that can reach large segments of the population rapidly in a nuclear emergency as well as "tailored" messages that are targeted to populations with different language and cultural backgrounds through media channels that these groups use and trust.
21. Integrate perspectives from other sectors and/or professions to promote and advance population health.	Ventura County brings together a team of subject matter experts to form a plume mappers group.	Level 2	It is important that such a group have representation from a number of disciplines to create redundancy so that if the most reliable plume maps are not available, a backup plume map will be.

Key: Essential services of public health; CEPH competencies; Leadership levels.

REFERENCES

Becker, S. M. (2009). *Incorporating psychosocial and behavioral issues into radiological/nuclear exercises.* Southwest Center for Advanced Public Health Practice.

Benjamin, G. C., McGeary, M., & McCutchen, S. R. (Eds.). (2009). *Assessing medical preparedness to respond to a terrorist nuclear event.* National Academies Press. https://doi.org/10.17226/12578

Burkle, F. M., Potokar, T., Gosney, J. E., & Dallas, C. (2017). Justification for a nuclear global health workforce: Multidisciplinary analysis of risk, survivability and preparedness, with emphasis on the triage management of thermal burns. *Conflict and Health, 11*, Article 13. https://doi.org/10.1186/s13031-017-0116-y

Center For Drug Evaluation and Research. (2001). *Guidance: Potassium iodide as a thyroid blocking agent in radiation emergencies.* U.S. Department of Health and Human Services. https://www.fda.gov/media/72510/download

Davis, M., Reeve, M., & Altevogt, B. M. (Eds.). (2014). *Nationwide response issues after an improvised nuclear device attack: Medical and public health consequences for neighboring jurisdictions: Workshop summary.* National Academies Press. https://doi.org/10.17226/18347

Federal Emergency Management Agency. (2011). *Hazardous materials response: The Ventura County, California's plume mapping working group, lessons learned information sharing.* https://www.hsdl.org/?view&did=771103

Johns Hopkins Center for Health Security. (n.d.). *Rad Resilient City Initiative.* http://www.centerforhealthsecurity.org/resources/interactives/rad-resilient-city/index

Kisken, T. (2017, September 27). What to do in a nuclear explosion? Ventura County has a plan. *VC Star.* https://www.vcstar.com/story/news/local/2017/09/27/what-do-nuclear-explosion-ventura-county-has-plan/705170001

Levin, R. M. (2011). Ventura County nuclear explosion response plan, Version 3.0.

National Council on Radiation Protection and Measurements. (2011). *Responding to a radiation or nuclear terrorism incident: A guide for decision makers.* Author.

National Security Council Led Domestic Readiness Group. (2016). *Health and safety planning guide for planners, safety officers and supervisors for protecting responders following a nuclear detonation.* https://www.dhs.gov/sites/default/files/publications/IND%20Health%20Safety%20Planners%20Guide%20Final.pdf

Sokol, D. K. (2006). Virulent epidemics and scope of healthcare workers' duty of care. *Emerging Infectious Diseases, 12*(8), 1238–1241. https://doi.org/10.3201/eid1208.060360

U.S. Department of Homeland Security. (2006). *Preparedness directorate; Protective action guides for radiological dispersal device (RDD) and improvised nuclear device (IND) incidents.* https://www.federalregister.gov/documents/2006/01/03/05-24521/preparedness-directorate-protective-action-guides-for-radiological-dispersal-device-rdd-and

U.S. Department of Homeland Security. (2016). *Nuclear/radiological incident annex to the response and recovery federal interagency operational plans.* Federal Emergency Management Agency. https://www.fema.gov/sites/default/files/2020-07/fema_incident-annex_nuclear-radiological.pdf

U.S. Environmental Protection Agency. (2017). *PAG manual: Protective actions guides and planning guidance for radiological incidents* (EPA-400/R-17/001). https://www.epa.gov/sites/default/files/2017-01/documents/epa_pag_manual_final_revisions_01-11-2017_cover_disclaimer_8.pdf

CHAPTER 14

DISEASE OUTBREAKS AND PANDEMICS

COVID-19 AND OTHER CASE STUDIES

DAWN TERASHITA, MOON KIM, AND SHARON BALTER

KEY TERMS

Association for Professionals in Infection Control (APIC)
Botulism
California Code of Regulations (CCR)
Carbapenem-Resistant Enterobacteriaceae (CRE)
CDC Quarantine Station
Coccidioidomycosis
Division of Occupational Safety and Health (Cal/OSHA)
Doctor's First Report (DFR) of Occupational Injury or Illness
Health Officer Orders
Hospital Infection Prevention and Control (IPC)
Injury and Illness Prevention Program (IIPP)
Multidrug-Resistant Organism (MDRO)
Persons Under Investigation (PUI)
Public Health Nurses
Reportable Diseases and Conditions List
Society for Healthcare Epidemiology of America (SHEA)

INTRODUCTION

In 2020, with the spread of the COVID-19 pandemic, the epidemiology of communicable diseases became major news and terms like "R0," "risk factors," "sensitivity," and "specificity" became household words. As the virus spread across the world and daily case counts were projected in headlines, many health department spokespersons were called upon to explain the difference between daily case counts and overall trends, different tests and

---

The following icons, located in the margins throughout the chapter and within the summary tables, denote essential services of public health, CEPH competencies, and leadership levels: Essential services of public health; CEPH competencies; Leadership levels.

their sensitivities and specificities, and why it is important to follow the overall percent positivity. In 2021, the conversation shifted to vaccine effectiveness and virus variants. Although epidemiologists and Public Health staff were not quite the stars of cocktail parties (as they had all stopped), many of them were sought after to explain these concepts to friends, families, media, and the public.

At the same time, many pundits and others read the data and came to their own conclusions on what measures would be needed. Even trained epidemiologists could not clearly agree on what measures were needed and we saw a variation throughout the world, with Sweden insisting lockdowns were unnecessary, Australia and New Zealand locking down to a much greater degree than many countries, and other places falling in between. What became clear is that it is important in the setting of a pandemic for everyone to have some basic understanding of outbreak investigation and disease control to make informed decisions in their everyday lives about such things as where to go for testing, which test to use, when to seek medical attention, which mask to use, and even whether to allow their children to return to school.

Despite the development of molecular testing and genetic sequencing in the modern era, the basic steps of communicable disease investigation have changed little since 1854 when John Snow, the father of modern epidemiology, mapped cases of cholera, interviewed households that were sick and those that were not sick, and concluded that water flowing into the Broad Street pump was responsible for the terrible outbreak. He needed his communication skills to persuade local officials to remove the pump handle and therefore stop the outbreak. In 2020 public health officials were tracking COVID-19 through interviews and mapping, as well as making a similar case to communities to urge COVID-19 precautions. In addition to COVID-19, in this chapter we present three other communicable disease outbreaks to illustrate the basic steps that apply to all investigations. While we hope that our work may inspire others to enter the field of communicable disease epidemiology, we also hope that learning about outbreak investigation will be helpful and useful to all thoughtful readers.

COVID-19

In December 2019, China reported a cluster of cases of pneumonia of unknown etiology detected in Wuhan, Hubei Province, China. Subsequently identified as a novel coronavirus, the virus spread to a growing number of countries worldwide including the United States. On January 21, 2020, the first case of 2019 novel coronavirus was confirmed in the United States, and on January 26, 2020, the first case was identified in Los Angeles County. On February 2, 2020, the United States declared a public health emergency. On March 11, 2020, the World Health Organization (WHO) declared COVID-19 a pandemic.

Using this case study, we explore and identify the essential public health services, the CEPH competencies, and the level of personnel required for responding to this pandemic. All 10 of the essential services of Public Health were applied to this unprecedented event.

As a local public health department, we monitor health status in the community through core competencies including applying epidemiologic methods, data collection, analysis, and interpretation of results. Upon initial notification from the Centers for Disease Control and Prevention (CDC) regarding a cluster of cases of pneumonia in Wuhan, China, we began to implement nonetiologic methods to collect epidemiologic data, conduct surveillance for severe pneumonia as testing was initially unavailable, conduct case interviews, identify risk factors for infection, and, once testing became available, apply criteria for laboratory testing of the 2019 novel coronavirus based on criteria and guidance from the CDC. On January 8, 2020 (Los Angeles County Health Alert Network [LAHAN], 2020a), the CDC issued the initial health alert regarding an outbreak of pneumonia of unknown etiology (PUE) in Wuhan, China. The alert requested that healthcare providers ask patients with severe respiratory disease about travel history to Wuhan City, to use both contact and airborne isolation precautions, and to collect and save respiratory specimens as the etiology was unknown. Once the etiology was determined to be a novel coronavirus, a subsequent health alert was issued by the CDC on January 17, 2020 (LAHAN, 2020b), with criteria for testing. As testing was only being performed by the CDC, **persons under investigation (PUI)** who met criteria for testing were only those with lower respiratory illness and travel to Wuhan City, China, or persons who had close contact with a confirmed 2019-nCOV patient. Because surveillance, testing, analysis, and interpretation of data on suspected and confirmed cases conducted (Levels 1 and 2; Level 1/frontline, Level 2/supervisory, and/or Level 3/Executives and Leadership) initially focused on travel-associated risk factors, we coordinated (Levels 1 and 2) with the **CDC Quarantine Station** at the Los Angeles International Airport as screening of returning travelers from Wuhan City, China, was implemented as well as other ports of entry working with the CDC, U.S. Coast Guard, and U.S. Customs and Border Patrol. Additional surveillance methods for deaths and severe pneumonias requiring hospitalization were also developed, including reviewing reports of severe pneumonias requiring ICU admission, death certificates and reports, and coroner cases. Because testing was limited, surveillance for cases and the potential for disease spread was a challenge (CDC COVID-19 Response Team et al., 2020). As the number of cases began to increase and testing became more available in the community, monitoring the health status increasingly became a priority as control measures were needed to mitigate the impact of a healthcare system surge. During the pandemic a new syndrome was also identified in children post-COVID-19 infection called multisystem inflammatory syndrome in children (MIS-C) for which additional surveillance and case identification had to be developed utilizing a team consisting of a **public health nurse (PHN)**, an epidemiologist, and physicians (LAHAN, 2020d).

The capability to diagnose and investigate health problems and health hazards in the community was also essential as cases increased and outbreaks in the community started to become apparent. Health threats were identified in vulnerable populations with increased morbidity and mortality from COVID-19 including those living in congregate living settings such as skilled nursing facilities (SNFs) and assisted living facilities. Certain work sites, including clothing factories (Miller, 2020) and meat/poultry processing plants, were especially vulnerable due to their close working quarters (Dyal et al., 2020), and environmental health inspectors played a critical role in enforcing health officer orders and educating work sites on infection control. Outbreak investigation and management required coordination among epidemiologists, environmental health, PHNs, and physicians to interpret the data on spread of disease, physical assessment of work sites including ventilation, and implementing necessary infection control measures. Settings requiring intensive intervention on clusters and outbreaks also included schools as they reopened, colleges, worksites, correctional facilities, and in persons experiencing homelessness (PEH). In all these settings, knowledge of case and contact investigation, infection controls, and outbreak management were essential. Protocols and health officer orders for each of these settings and for businesses within the community were developed in order to control further spread of COVID-19. Although local health officer orders had been used on a limited basis for isolation and quarantine prior to the COVID-19 pandemic, this was the first time in the modern era that they were used to prevent transmission not only on an individual level (e.g., isolation/quarantine) but also on a wider scale, including restrictions and subsequent reopening orders for sectors including businesses, community events, sports, schools, places of worship, and gatherings (County of Los Angeles Public Health, n.d.).

Communication strategies for different audiences and sectors were utilized to inform and educate individuals about COVID-19. Information was disseminated through various methods including health alerts to providers, webinars, telebriefings for sector guidance updates, website updates, frequently asked questions, social media posts, press conferences, and sector protocols (County of Los Angeles Public Health, n.d.). Information on all aspects of COVID-19 signs and symptoms, isolation, quarantine, testing, and control and prevention measures were included in the various guidance documents. Development of materials and guidance was
1,2,3 an ongoing task based on updated evidence-based data and the state/CDC.

Mobilizing community partnerships to identify and solve health problems was another key essential service of Public Health's response to this pandemic. Partnerships and interventions to control further disease spread were necessary in all aspects of the community including with individuals, businesses, schools, congregate living facilities, healthcare systems, first responders, correctional facilities, and those working with PEH (e.g., use of hotels for isolation and quarantine). Staff at all levels played a role in activities including creating open communication channels, obtaining relevant case data on reporting, managing outbreaks, and ensuring adherence to health officer orders.

5 During this pandemic, Public Health was constantly updating and developing policies, plans, and health officer orders that supported individual and commu-
7,8,9 nity health efforts to control further spread of infections. Until vaccines could be developed and administered, control of disease relied upon individual and col-
2,3 lective use of behavioral and environmental controls including isolation, quarantine, use of face coverings, social distancing, hand hygiene, and environmental cleaning. Controlling spread of infections in indoor community settings was a challenge as the virus could spread more easily in these settings (e.g., places of worship, fitness centers, restaurants).

The enforcement of laws and regulations that protect health and ensure safety were a vital component of protection strategies during this pandemic. **Health officer orders** to control disease spread included quarantine and isolation, use of face coverings, restrictions on business and guidance on reopening, and restrictions on gatherings. Public Health compliance and enforcement activities were conducted by environmental health inspectors and public health investigators. Locations where citations were issued due to a lack of compliance with health officer orders were posted to our website to inform the public. In addition, the Los Angeles City mayor enforced health officer orders by turning off utilities
16 at houses identified to violate orders regarding gatherings by hosting parties (https://www.latimes.com/california/story/2020-08-05/residents-holding
3 -large-parties-may-have-their-water-and-power-shut-off-garcetti-says).

Linking people to needed personal health services and assuring the provision of healthcare was critical during this pandemic because of the need for isolation and quarantine of cases and their exposed close contacts. A county information 211 line was set up to answer questions on where individuals could access healthcare and where they could get needed services, including food or mental health services. Elective surgeries and nonessential healthcare services also had to be delayed due to healthcare surge planning. Early in the pandemic, and currently, use of telehealth visits became more common. Health alerts were disseminated to keep healthcare providers updated on surge planning guidance.

Assuring a competent public health workforce was essential in responding 8
to this pandemic. Skills required included skills in interviewing patients and making connections (including collecting risk factors, identifying commonalities, and noting potential sources of disease acquisition). Staff also needed 1
experience in developing protocols for investigation, interview tools, key messages for staff trainings, key variables to collect on data collection tools, 2
and working across systems (e.g., healthcare, congregate living, schools, cor- 1,2,3,4,18, 19,20
rectional facilities, workplaces, PEH).

There was a consistent need to evaluate effectiveness, accessibility, and 1,2
quality of personal and population-based health services. Trends in data (hospitalization, deaths, risk factors, disparities) were posted on a publicly avail- 9
able dashboard (http://publichealth.lacounty.gov/media/Coronavirus/ 4
data/index.htm). Decisions based on data included health officer closure of businesses and activities (e.g., gatherings) and healthcare system surge plan- 2,3
ning (e.g., mass fatality planning, crisis care standards). An unprecedented amount of data was collected and shared during this pandemic, including data on cases, testing, testing positivity rate, hospitalizations, deaths, death rate, recovery metrics, and contact tracing dashboard (e.g., total number of cases assigned to interviewer, cases that had follow-up initiated within 1 day of assignment, assigned cases that completed the interview, number of contacts identified through case interview). Locations and names of where outbreaks were reported to Public Health were posted to our website. The cumulative case rate and recent trends by city/community were also posted to our website as well as locations of outbreaks in worksites, schools, residential congregate and acute healthcare settings, homeless service settings, educational settings, and correctional and law enforcement settings. Specific SNF data including, for example, the 7-day average daily total and skilled nursing facility-associated COVID-19 laboratory confirmed cases and deaths by date were posted to our website and a dashboard that provided self-reported weekly information on 340 SNFs on the number of COVID-19 tests performed and persons diagnosed with COVID-19 was publicly posted to our website. As vaccines became available, data on the percent vaccinated by city/community were posted on our website (http://publichealth.lacounty.gov/media/Coronavirus/locations.htm). Large teams of personnel including the electronic laboratory reporting team, epidemiology team, outbreak management team, sector teams (e.g., education, healthcare, worksite, homeless service, corrections), environmental health, and information technology worked tirelessly to analyze, interpret, and maintain the immense amount of data during this pandemic. There was also a strong emphasis on equity, using data to identify the communities that were most impacted by the pandemic and subsequently using that information to implement protective measures at

worksites and educational campaigns. Once the vaccine became available, data were used in an effort to target the most heavily affected communities.

Although our focus was on responding to the pandemic, research for new insights and efforts at sharing our data, experience, and findings were important. As time permitted, we contributed to the research literature on public health findings, data on cases and contact investigations, and other epidemiologic studies (e.g., healthcare workers, multisystem inflammatory syndromic in children, deaths among persons younger than 21 years).

The COVID-19 pandemic continues to provide public health with additional new challenges including the identification of variants (LAHAN, 2020c) and equitable distribution of vaccines (County of Los Angeles Public Health, 2021). Although our experiences as a local health department are not exhaustive, we hope our experiences and actions described provide perspective into the essential services needed at the local level to prepare, respond, and recover from this pandemic.

CARBAPENEM-RESISTANT ENTEROBACTERIACEAE DUODENOSCOPES

Carbapenem-resistant Enterobacteriaceae (CRE) are **multidrug-resistant organisms (MDROs)** that often cause healthcare-associated infections. Infections and outbreaks associated with endoscopic retrograde cholangiopancreatography (ERCP) procedures have been reported. Previous investigations have identified breaches in cleaning protocols and subsequent bacterial contamination of the ERCP duodenoscope as the mechanism of transmission in the outbreaks (Wendorf et al., 2015). Other investigations report finding no breach in cleaning and reprocessing protocols or defects in the implicated duodenoscopes (Epstein et al., 2014). The duodenoscope's design has been implicated as a source of potential contamination due to the complexity of the elevator channel and the difficulty in ensuring adequate cleaning and disinfection (Rutala & Weber, 2015).
6 In Los Angeles County, the health officer added CRE in acute care hospitals and
skilled nursing facilities to the **California Code of Regulations (CCR)**, Title 17,
1 §2500 to the **Reportable Diseases and Conditions list**. Additionally, the CCR,
Title 17, §2500 requires healthcare providers to report outbreaks of any disease to
2 the local health officer.

In January 2015, the hospital infection preventionist (IP) notified the Los Angeles County Department of Public Health (LAC DPH) Acute Communicable Disease Control (ACDC) of a cluster of patients who were carbapenem-resistant Klebsiella pneumoniae (CRKP) culture positive after undergoing an ERCP procedure. The ACDC frontline staff began an investigation. In mid-December 2014, an infectious disease physician alerted the **hospital Infection Prevention and Control (IPC)** to an unusual case of CRKP bacteremia in a patient shortly after undergoing an ERCP procedure. An investigation was initiated by the IPC, who requested a list of all 2014 CRE isolates identified by the laboratory. The laboratory identified 33 CRE-positive patients in 2014, of which 23 had CRKP. Hospital staff conducted a comprehensive investigation including extensive chart review of each case to identify potential risk factors, room locations, and

IPC direct observation of duodenoscope reprocessing. The microbiology laboratory did further molecular testing on a subset of the CRKP isolates to determine genetic relatedness.

Molecular results were reviewed by IPC and further investigation was performed to determine the point source. Multiplex real-time PCR assay, which detect carbapenemases, was negative for several CRKP.

A total of 15 patients met the case definition. A case was defined as a patient who was CRKP OXA-232 culture positive, infected, or colonized at any site, and had an ERCP procedure between October 2014 and January 2015. Of these cases, three died during their hospitalization.

Initially, eight patients met the case definition, with clinical culture positive sites including blood (n = 4) and abdominal sources including aspirate, drainage, or abscess (n = 4). Seven isolates had identical sensitivity patterns and were resistant to carbapenems, aminoglycosides, penicillins, cephalosporins, and fluoroquinolones, as well as susceptible to colistin. One multiplex-negative CRKP isolate underwent whole genome sequencing that identified the OXA-232 carbapenemase. Additional molecular testing by repetitive sequence-based polymerase chain reaction (repPCR) and high-resolution melt analysis (HRM) was conducted by the hospital's laboratory on CRE isolates from 17 patients in 2014 to determine relatedness. The unique carbapenemase OXA-232 strain was identified in CRKP isolates from ERCP-related patients (n = 8). RepPCR and HRM results showed OXA-232 strains from all cases to be almost identical. When focusing on the strains that were highly related to each other, the only commonality among patients was ERCP during their hospitalization.

An index patient who was CRKP OXA-232 positive prior to their ERCP procedures in October 2014 was identified. This patient underwent multiple procedures with two duodenoscopes (duodenoscope 1 and duodenoscope 2).

Once ERCP with duodenoscopes 1 and 2 was established as a risk factor for transmission of CRKP, patient notification was initiated by the hospital. In total, 186 patients had ERCP with the implicated duodenoscopes between October 2014 and January 2015. Notification included phone calls and mailed letters informing of possible CRE exposure and offers to screen for CRE by rectal swab of all patients notified; 150 patients were screened, and seven (5%) were positive for CRKP. Isolates from the surveillance cases were also identified as OXA-232.

The hospital implemented many control measures including ceasing all ERCP procedures during the investigation, sequestering the two implicated duodenoscopes (1 and 2), training on and assessing the duodenoscope cleaning and disinfection process, culturing all seven adult ERCP duodenoscopes, reprocessing following manufacturer's guidelines, and sending duodenoscopes to a private company for additional ethylene oxide gas sterilization. A Manufacturer and User Facility Device Experience report was submitted by the hospital to the U.S. Food and Drug Administration (FDA). All seven duodenoscopes were cultured and all were negative for CRE.

A site visit was conducted by ACDC staff in February 2015, 5 days after the outbreak was reported. During this visit, duodenoscope cleaning and high-level disinfection procedures were observed. Reprocessing was done by gastrointestinal (GI) reprocessing technicians or GI registered nurses (RNs), both trained in reprocessing. Precleaning was performed immediately after the procedure in the procedure room. The facility used an automated endoscope reprocessor. No breaches in cleaning and disinfection techniques were observed. Duodenoscopes were stored appropriately according to manufacturer instructions. Several consultations with the California Department of Public Health (CDPH), the CDC, and the FDA were conducted. In late February 2015, ACDC sent an email to all acute care hospital IPs encouraging active surveillance for CRE infections following ERCP procedures, including a retrospective review. Additional clusters were identified and reported to LAC DPH.

The epidemiology and laboratory analyses of these investigations suggest that the cause of these outbreaks was multifactorial, including that the complex design of the scope may impede effective cleaning, disinfection, and reprocessing (Kim et al., 2016). In January 2016, the duodenoscope manufacturer initiated a recall of one scope model for replacement of the elevator mechanism. In addition, several nationally recognized experts have recommended several options to enhance reprocessing, including double high-level disinfection with periodic culturing of a sample of scopes and use of Eto sterilization after high-level disinfection. The CDC, FDA, and CDPH provided guidance to hospitals and providers on duodenoscope reprocessing after ERCP. Professional associations that provide infection prevention and related information, for example, the **Association for Professionals in Infection Control (APIC)** and the **Society for Healthcare Epidemiology of America (SHEA),** also provided reprocessing guidance.

Partnerships between hospitals performing ERCP procedures and LAC DPH are essential to ensuring optimal surveillance and coordination of prevention activities. The facilities experiencing CRE ERCP-associated outbreaks were large, prestigious hospitals with robust infection prevention and control programs. Due to the design flaw of this instrument, hospitals could follow manufacturer guidelines and standard practices correctly and still experience duodenoscope-related MDRO transmission. In addition, there may be other facilities with duodenoscope-related transmission of MDROs that may not have the expertise to conduct a complex investigation and implement effective prevention and control strategies. The involvement of LAC DPH in this issue is key to address these problems on a larger policy scale that will improve the safety of the patients these hospitals treat.

BOTULISM

In 2008, a wound **botulism** outbreak occurred in injection drug users. Botulism is a rare but serious and potentially fatal paralytic illness most commonly caused by the neurotoxin produced by the bacterium *Clostridium botulinum* and is considered a medical emergency. Suspected cases are mandated to be reported immediately to local and state public health authorities.

While most commonly associated with food, the wound botulism associated with illicit drug use (e.g., black tar heroin) is a far more common cause in Los Angeles County. In Los Angeles County, the 5-year average number of wound botulism cases is 3.2 cases/year. Between June and August 2018, there were six cases of wound botulism identified. In addition, four of the six cases were reported from a single acute care hospital, and two were reported within 1 hour of each other. This sudden increase above baseline in wound botulism cases warranted an outbreak investigation.

Using this case study, we explore and identify the essential public health services required for responding to this outbreak. Several essential services of public health were applied to this particular outbreak.

As a local public health department, we monitor health status in the community through core competencies including applying epidemiologic methods, data collection, analysis, and interpretation of results. Although botulism is rare, a doubling of the annual average number of cases within a 3-month period triggered a further detailed look to diagnose and investigate health problems occurring in the community. Frontline staff consisting of nurses and epidemiologists need to have basic knowledge of botulism including signs and symptoms, as well as the ability to conduct surveillance and analysis, identify epidemiologic risk factors for botulism, know the types of laboratory testing utilized, and know preventive measures. This includes how those components apply to the different types of botulism and distinguishing case definitions: wound, foodborne, adult intestinal, and infant forms. Public health supervisory-level staff roles include the ability to draw conclusions based on the data analysis, allocating resources to take action based on the data (e.g., additional field response staff, outreach activities needed, laboratory testing capacity/capability, availability of botulism antitoxin that is a limited resource), developing strategies to control disease based on risk factors identified, and determining the need for additional protocols for response (e.g., field deployment and trainings).

As the investigation for this cluster of botulism cases further revealed that cases were occurring in persons who inject drugs, public health had to develop a strategy to inform and educate those at risk in the community and those who provide medical, mental health, and social services to those at risk in the community. This included strategies for different audiences and sectors (e.g., healthcare providers, homeless outreach workers, community public health center staff education, and police). Frontline level staff consisting of PHNs and health educators developed presentation materials for training field teams that included PHNs, health educators, and mental health and homeless outreach workers, and developed posters/educational flyers for individuals and community stakeholders (to see the poster, visit http://publichealth.lacounty.gov/acd/docs/BotWarningPoster.pdf). Supervisory-level staff reviewed and approved the key messages that they determined were necessary for the trainings and community flyers and for health alerts (the primary method of sharing about urgent public health incidents to healthcare providers; to see the health alert sent to healthcare providers during this outbreak, visit http://publichealth.lacounty.gov/eprp/Health%20Alerts/DPH%20HAN%20Alert%20Wound%20Botulism%20070218%20FINAL.pdf) in identifying suspected cases, as cases of botulism are rare; specific guidance regarding treating with botulism antitoxin for clinically suspected botulism before testing results were included. Supervisory staff also reviewed messages for press releases (County of Los Angeles Public Health, 2018) and applied any relevant evidence-based strategies effective in communicating with this challenging at-risk population, persons who inject drugs (Trayner et al., 2018), and messages that were used in other situations (Scottish Drugs Forum, 2017).

Mobilizing community partnerships to identify and solve health problems was another key essential service of Public Health responding to this outbreak. Persons who inject drugs may also have other conditions where access to the healthcare system or other community programs is needed. We collaborated with stakeholders including substance abuse treatment centers, mental health workers, community homeless outreach teams, needle exchange programs, and police community outreach teams in order to implement strategies to provide education to prevent further botulism cases. A challenging aspect for this outbreak was messaging to those persons who inject drugs regarding the risks of botulism associated with injecting drugs while acknowledging that persons who use these drugs would be unlikely to stop injecting drugs in the near short term. Frontline staff, which included community workers and PHNs, provided feedback on their experiences with the at-risk group, their input from the field on the limitations and benefits of community outreach, and provided insight on tactics
1 to best conduct field outreach. Supervisory-level staff led discussions on strategies and tactics and had to consider the structural bias toward persons who use drugs and social inequities that could cause challenges in our response to this outbreak; they also reviewed organization policies for alignment with the goals and objectives for this community field response.

While responding to this outbreak and as a result of collaborations with the specific stakeholders, the at-risk individuals were linked to personal health ser-
7 vices and offered healthcare. The field outreach teams consisted of Public Health workers, homeless outreach teams, and local police community outreach officers
3 who were knowledgeable about the locations of persons who use drugs, many of whom were homeless or frequented certain locations in the community. The
18,19,20 police community outreach officers functioned on the teams predominantly for safety versus an enforcement role and provided invaluable guidance on
1 geographic locations or "hang outs" where targeted education could be beneficial. Frontline staff including public health community workers and PHNs had knowledge of the resources that existed in the community for assistance with substance abuse and treatment programs, mental health referral networks, and social services resources. Supervisory staff explored further connections in the community; for example, assistance with meals or other social services that could be helpful for this community response and coordinated with management at those other organizations/agencies to facilitate coordination and further education about botulism.

Assuring a competent public health workforce was essential in responding to this outbreak. Frontline staff consisting of PHNs and community workers required skills in interviewing patients and making connections, including collecting risk factors and identifying commonalities, potential sources of disease acquisition, and skills in developing just-in-time training for stakeholders for a rare disease. Supervisory-level staff roles included providing key input into developing protocols for investigation, interview tools, key messages for staff trainings, and key variables to collect with a data collection tool used by deployed field staff. As time in the field, including engagement of the individual being educated, is limited, priority elements to collect in the field needed to be decided upon to further evaluate effectiveness of the response. For this response, final data collection elements included the number of individuals reached, number who were homeless,
2 language used for education (e.g., English, Spanish), whether the individual had previously heard of botulism, and assessment of the individual's level of engage-
1,2 ment/willingness to receive education (e.g., engaged verbally, accepted written material, asked questions, refused, referred for services).

In order to evaluate the effectiveness of this outbreak response, we measured the response times to both releasing botulism antitoxin and time to conducting patient interviews to determine epidemiologic links (Figure 14.1). We also analyzed data elements collected from the field, as well as conducting surveillance for additional botulism cases. Frontline staff included PHNs and epidemiology analysts who reviewed reports about suspected botulism expeditiously and deployed into the field to interview cases to determine epidemiologic links before the patient clinically became worse (Rao et al., 2018). Public Health staff conducting the interview also had to engage individuals with compassion as these patients were ill and hospitalized at the time the staff was gathering the key pieces of epidemiologic information. Timely recognition and response is critical because the potential exists for rapid clinical progression of botulism, and respiratory deterioration can occur in many patients within 2 days of illness onset. In one review by the CDC, a total of 184 (46%) of 402 patients with botulism were reportedly intubated during their hospitalization. Of these, 154 had the hospital day of intubation (intubation is a medical procedure in which a tube is inserted in the airway and connected to a ventilator to assist a patient with breathing; in botulism, this is due to respiratory muscle paralysis) reported, and 134 (87%) were intubated during the first 2 hospital days (Chatham-Stephens et al., 2018). Supervisory-level staff had to make decisions based on data obtained about the case quickly as well as adjust the case interview tool to capture and expand on any relevant epidemiologic links. Interviews were delayed during our outbreak because three cases became clinically unstable, so we revised protocols to interview cases in the hospital as soon as possible upon receipt of the report of a suspected case while botulism antitoxin was being coordinated for delivery; three of the

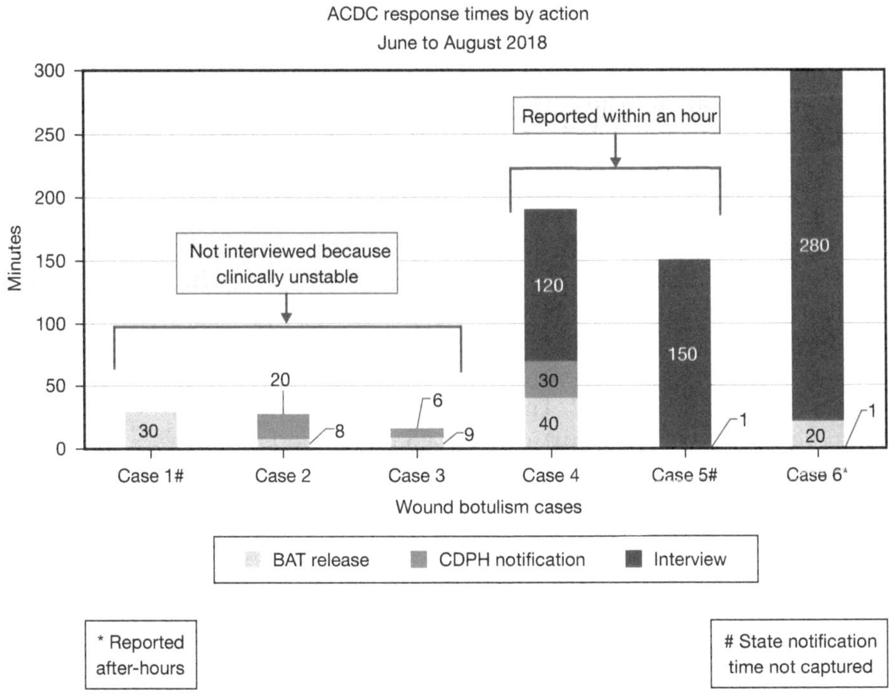

Figure 14.1 Acute Communicable Disease Control (ACDC) program response times to both releasing botulism antitoxin and time to conducting patient interviews.

BAT, Botulism antitoxin; CDPH, California Department of Public Health.

six cases were interviewed before paralysis progressed to the patient requiring intubation. Eventually all cases were interviewed.

After each targeted community outreach activity, an evaluation of the field data collected showed that 80.3% of individuals (those who may inject drugs but who are not ill with botulism) who were recipients of public health educational outreach engaged verbally, 88.3% accepted written educational material, and 11.7% were referred for other services. Another notable point is that throughout the targeted outreach effort, new at-risk individuals began to indicate that they had previously heard of botulism associated with injection drug use, suggesting they had received the educational materials previously from their peers who had been educated on previous team outreach days. Public health surveillance conducted for the remainder of 2018 did not identify any further clusters of botulism cases.

COCCIDIOIDOMYCOSIS

Coccidioidomycosis, also known as valley fever, is a fungal disease transmitted through the inhalation of Coccidioides immitis spores that reside in soil. The fungus is endemic in the northern part of Los Angeles County and much of the Central Valley of California. Most infected individuals exhibit no or mild respiratory symptoms, but a few develop severe symptoms such as pneumonia or dissemination of the fungus to other parts of the body such as the meninges, skin, or bone. Exposure occurs when soil is disturbed, and the spores become aerosolized. The disease is often found to be associated with occupational activities that move soil. The CCR, Title 17, §2500 requires healthcare providers to report cases of coccidioidomycosis to the local health officer for the jurisdiction where the patient resides. Additionally, CCR, Title 8, § 9785(e) requires that all emergency, urgent care, and new primary treating physicians must each submit a **Doctor's First Report (DFR) of Occupational Injury or Illness** form within 5 working days of the injured worker's initial examination to the employer or their workers' compensation insurance carrier, who will forward it to the California Department of Industrial Relations. DFRs are provided to the CDPH for occupational injury and disease surveillance purposes.

In March 2013, LAC DPH frontline staff were notified by the CDPH about
1 two DFRs in individuals who had been diagnosed with coccidioidomycosis and
were involved in filming a popular television series episode at an outdoor set
1 in an adjacent county (Wilken et al., 2014). The suspected location of exposure
was a ranch located in Simi Valley, which is an area also considered high risk for
1 coccidioidomycosis. The cluster involved the crew from a TV show, and an on-
location shoot in January 2012. The filming event involved construction of sets and filming of the episode occurring over a 5-day period.

LAC DPH frontline staff conducted an outbreak investigation that included review of medical records, employer rosters, CDPH-provided occupational surveillance records, social media, and interviews with cases, the employer, and the site manager. Investigators also reviewed the LAC DPH Acute Communicable Disease Control surveillance database, which includes all reported coccidioidomycosis cases with demographics, risk factors, laboratory results, and initial case interview notes.

A confirmed case was defined as an individual with laboratory confirmation of coccidioidomycosis and a clinical presentation that included an influenza-like illness, pneumonia or pulmonary lesion, erythema nodosum or erythema multiforme rash, or extrapulmonary disease (Council of State and Territorial Epidemiologists, 2014) that occurred in a person who was present at the filming event. A probable case was a clinically compatible illness in a person present at the filming event. In total, there were five confirmed and five probable cases linked to this filming event.

Of the 10 confirmed and probable cases, eight cases were identified through review of DFRs. A simple internet search that consisted of terms such as "Valley Fever" and the show's name identified one case, wherein the patient had posted details about his hospitalization on Twitter. Subsequent interview of this case identified an additional case who was a visitor on-site during the filming event. Of 10 persons identified, seven were interviewed; three could not be contacted. The employee roster indicated 655 workers were associated with the television episode. The attack rate for all identified cases was 1.5%.

Seven cases were male; median age was 37 years (range 23–58). Half (5) of the cases were actors, three were sound/camera operators, one was involved in construction of the sets and another was a visitor to the set. The mean time to symptom onset was 7 days (range 3–26 days; Table 14.1). Of the 10 cases identified during the investigation, only two engaged in soil-disrupting activities during or immediately preceding the filming event. However, interviews with cases indicated that substantial manual digging and operating of heavy machinery was required for set construction, including erecting an amusement park and a large stage, and digging a large mud pit. Several cases indicated they were shuttled up to the set location from the main parking area of the ranch, and these shuttles generated a lot of dust up and down the roads. Five of the seven interviewed cases reported dry dusty conditions during the filming event. Furthermore, the site manager reported to LAC DPH and CDPH that substantial dust from an adjacent mining company blew onto the site daily. There were no identified cases among employees of the mine.

This communicable disease outbreak highlights occupational risks to environmental pathogens. The outbreak involved staff and a visitor present at an outdoor Coccidioides-endemic area. Prevention and risk reduction consist of two parts. The first increases awareness through information and education. Public Health frontline staff work with clinicians to suspect coccidioidomycosis in patients with respiratory symptoms who were exposed to outdoor dusty and windy conditions in endemic areas. Informing clinicians to ask about occupational exposures for patients diagnosed with coccidioidomycosis will help to quickly identify outbreaks. Additionally, Public Health staff engage workers and public members to be aware of potential disease to inform decisions. The second focuses on occupational dust abatement. California has a complicated system of labor laws, **Division of Occupational Safety and Health (Cal/OSHA)** regulations, and worker's compensation to protect workers. Public Health frontline and management staff work with employers and occupational health through education and policy to limit exposure to outdoor dust at work sites by controlling dust generation at the source (e.g., continuous soil wetting), providing employee training, and consistently enforcing an **Injury and Illness Prevention Program (IIPP)**, which includes providing respiratory protection with particulate filters.

#1

#8

An innovative surveillance approach using a review of DFRs by CDPH identified this outbreak. Four of the five confirmed cases were reported to

TABLE 14.1 Coccidioimycosis Outbreak Case Characteristics

Case #	Confirmed/ Probable	Interviewed	Occupation	Exposure Period	Time to Illness	Hospitalized	Symptom Duration	Identification Source
1	Confirmed	Yes	Actor	3 days	5 days	4 weeks	4 weeks	Social media
2	Probable	No	Actor	3 days	26 days	No	Unknown	DFR
3	Confirmed	Yes	Actor	3 days	4 days	No	1 week	DFR
4	Probable	Yes	Actor	3 days	3 day	No	3 weeks	DFR
5	Probable	No	Actor	3 days	unk	No	unk	DFR
6	Probable	No	Sound tech	3 days	13 days	No	unk	DFR
7	Confirmed	Yes	Camera operator	3 days	20 days	No	6 mos	DFR
8	Probable	Yes	Construction manager	4 days	7 days	No	3 weeks	DFR
9	Confirmed	Yes	Prop Maker/built sets	3 days	2 days	No	4 weeks	DFR
10	Confirmed	Yes	N/A (visitor)	3 days	13 days	2 days	3 weeks	Patient interview

DFR, Doctor's First Report.

LAC DPH through traditional case report; however, the outbreak was only detected by use of a nontraditional database for occupational surveillance. This outbreak investigation identified occupations and an industry not previously known to be at risk. A limitation of this approach is the time lag from the patient presenting to a clinician to the review of DFRs.

Social media was useful in identifying two additional cases. Social media technology is a fast, easy, and convenient method of searching for information and is often indefinitely stored online. It is also a powerful method to share information with consumers.

DISCUSSION QUESTIONS

1. When faced with the emergence of a new communicable disease (such as COVID-19), describe the initial steps that public health agencies at international (e.g., World Health Organization), national (e.g., Centers for Disease Control and Prevention), state, and local levels take to better understand the disease and develop appropriate control strategies.
2. Disease surveillance is an important public health tool to identify outbreaks and determine the impact of control measures on the spread of disease. Discuss the types of disease surveillance and their relative strengths and weaknesses.
3. In what ways can local public health departments, elected officials, healthcare organizations, and community-based organizations work together to address public health communicable disease problems?
4. Discuss how environmental and occupational factors (such as those mentioned in the case example of coccidioidomycosis) have an effect on the risks of infectious disease and their transmission.

SUMMARY

TABLE 14.2 Select Essential Services of Public Health Demonstrated in Disease Outbreaks and Pandemics

Essential Service # and Definition	Context in Chapter Case	Competency # It Ties to	Importance for Emergency Preparedness, Response, or Recovery
1. Assess and monitor population health status, factors that influence health, and community needs and assets (Assessment)	Los Angeles County Department of Public Health frontline staff notified of two Doctor's First Reports in individuals who were diagnosed with coccidioidomycosis–innovative surveillance approach identified the outbreak	1	The outbreak was only detected by use of a nontraditional database for occupational surveillance and it identified occupations and an industry not previously known to be at risk.
2. Investigate, diagnose, and address health problems and hazards affecting the population (Assessment)	Following spike in botulism cases, investigation into number of individuals reached, number that were homeless, language used for education, knowledge of botulism, and assessment of the individual's level of willingness to receive education	1, 2	Because time in the field, including engagement of the individual being educated, is limited, priority elements to collect in the field needed to be decided upon to further evaluate effectiveness of the response.
3. Communicate effectively to inform and educate people about health, factors that influence it, and how to improve it (Policy Development)	The field outreach teams for botulism included public health workers, homeless outreach teams, and local police community outreach officers who were knowledgeable of locations of persons who use drugs.	18, 19, 20	Implementing effective strategies to provide education is critical to preventing further botulism cases.
5. Create, champion, and implement policies, plans, and laws that impact health (Policy Development)	During the COVID-19 pandemic, public health was constantly updating and developing policies, plans, and health officer orders that supported individual and community health efforts to control further spread.	7, 8, 9	Before vaccines could be developed and administered, control of disease relied upon individual and collective use of behavioral and environmental controls including isolation, quarantine, use of face coverings, social distancing, hand hygiene, and environmental cleaning.
6. Utilize legal and regulatory actions designed to improve and protect the public's health (Policy Development)	In Los Angeles County, health officer added CRE in acute care hospitals and skilled nursing facilities to the Reportable Diseases and Conditions list of the California Code of Regulations, Title 17, §2500.	1	This requirement for healthcare providers to report any CRE disease to the local health officer helps to identify outbreaks.
7. Assure an effective system that enables equitable access to the individual services and care needed to be healthy (Assurance)	While responding to a botulism outbreak and as a result of collaborations with the specific stakeholders, at-risk individuals were linked to personal health services and offered healthcare.	7, 9, 14	Field outreach teams (consisting of public health workers, homeless outreach teams, and a local police community outreach officer) were able to use their knowledge about the locations of persons who use drugs to reach out and link persons to needed health services.
8. Build and support a diverse and skilled public health workforce (Assurance)	Informing clinicians to ask about occupational exposures for patients diagnosed with coccidioidomycosis helps to quickly identify outbreaks.	3	Increased suspicion to consider the possibility of coccidioidomycosis in patients with respiratory symptoms who were exposed to outdoor dusty and windy conditions in endemic areas led to identification of outbreaks.

(continued)

TABLE 14.2 Select Essential Services of Public Health Demonstrated in Disease Outbreaks and Pandemics *(continued)*

Essential Service # and Definition	Context in Chapter Case	Competency # It Ties to	Importance for Emergency Preparedness, Response, or Recovery
9. Improve and innovate public health functions through ongoing evaluation, research, and continuous quality improvement (Assurance)	Consistent need to evaluate effectiveness, accessibility, and quality of personal and population-based health services for COVID-19 infection.	4	Trends in data (hospitalization, deaths, risk factors, disparities) that were posted on a publicly available dashboard helped to inform decisions based on data–including health officer closure of businesses and activities and healthcare system surge planning.

CRE, carbapenem-resistant enterobacteriaceae.

TABLE 14.3 Select CEPH Competencies Needed for Frontline Health Workers, Managers, and Leaders for Disease Outbreak Preparedness, Response, and Recovery

Competency # and Definition	Context in Case/Chapter	Level	Importance for Emergency Preparedness, Response, or Recovery
1. Apply epidemiological methods to settings and situations in public health practice.	Health officer added carbapenem-resistant enterobacteriaceae (CRE) in acute care hospitals and skilled nursing facilities to the Reportable Diseases and Conditions list of the California Code of Regulations (CCR), Title 17, §2500.	Level 2	By including CRE as a reportable disease, it added an epidemiological tool to assess the magnitude of disease burden, pattern, and risk factors for CRE.
2. Select quantitative and qualitative data collection methods appropriate for a given public health context.	Staff needed to be experienced in developing protocols for investigation, interview tools, key messages for staff trainings, key variables to collect on data collection tools, and working across systems.	Level 1	Assuring a competent public health workforce is working on the frontline is essential to ensure sufficient experience is available to perform these critical tasks.
4. Interpret results of data analysis for public health research, policy, or practice.	Decisions based on data included health officer closure of businesses and activities and healthcare system surge planning.	Level 2	An unprecedented amount of data was collected during the COVID-19 pandemic and, most important, these data need to be analyzed and interpreted by supervisors and managers on which to base public health decisions regarding control and response measures.
8. Apply awareness of cultural values and practices to the design, implementation, or critique of public health policies or programs.	Required skills for a competent workforce include skills in interviewing patients and making connections (collecting risk factors, identifying commonalities, and potential sources of disease acquisition).	Level 1	It is critical that frontline staff consisting of such staff as public health nurses (PHNs) and community workers be competent to interview patients and their contacts for such activities as contact tracing.
16. Apply leadership and/or management principles to address a relevant health issue.	Los Angeles City mayor enforced health officer orders by turning off utilities at houses identified to violate orders regarding gatherings.	Level 3	The close collaboration between the leadership of departments of public health and elected civil leaders to identify locations where health officer orders are not being complied with, issue citations, and take actions against violators (such as fines, closing business establishments, or turning off utilities) can improve overall compliance in the community.
18. Select communication strategies for different audiences and sectors.	Development of materials and guidance was an ongoing task based on updated evidence-based data and the state/CDC.	Level 3	Communication strategies (types of materials, methods of distribution, cultural sensitivities, etc.) need to be "tailored" and "nuanced" for different audiences and sectors to inform and educate communities and individuals about COVID-19. Importantly, such strategies and materials need to account for changing approaches based on new scientific information as it evolves or occurs when faced with a new disease.

Key: Essential services of public health; CEPH competencies; Leadership levels.

CDC, Centers for Disease Control and Prevention.

REFERENCES

CDC COVID-19 Response Team, Jorden, M. A., Rudman, S. L., Villarino, E., Hoferka, S., Patel, M. T., Bemis, K., Simmons, C. R., Jespersen, M., Iberg Johnson, J., Mytty, E., Arends, K. D., Henderson, J. J., Mathes, R. W., Weng, C. X., Duchin, J., Lenahan, J., Close, N., Bedford, T., . . . Chung, J. R. (2020). Evidence for limited early spread of COVID-19 within the United States, January-February 2020. *Morbidity and Mortality Weekly Report, 69*(22), 680–684. https://doi.org/10.15585/mmwr.mm6922e1

Chatham-Stephens, K., Fleck-Derderian, S., Johnson, S. D., Sobel, J., Rao, A. K., & Meaney-Delman, D. (2018). Clinical features of foodborne and wound botulism: A systematic review of the literature, 1932–2015. *Clinical Infectious Diseases, 66*(Suppl. 1), S11–S16. https://doi.org/10.1093/cid/cix811

Council of State and Territorial Epidemiologists. (2014). *Position statement 10-ID-04. Coccidioidomycosis (valley fever) (Coccidioides spp.) 2011 case definition.* U.S. Department of Health and Human Services, Centers for Disease Control and Prevention. https://wwwn.cdc.gov/nndss/conditions/coccidioidomycosis/case-definition/2011

County of Los Angeles Public Health. (n.d.). *Reopening LA County: All the information you need to stay safe, stay healthy, & get vaccinated.* http://publichealth.lacounty.gov/media/Coronavirus/reopening-la.htm#orders

County of Los Angeles Public Health. (2018, July 3). *Public Health warns heroin may be contaminated and cause wound botulism.* http://publichealth.lacounty.gov/phcommon/public/media/mediapubhpdetail.cfm?prid=1865

County of Los Angeles Public Health. (2021, February 19). *Public Health continues work to address vaccination inequities: 150 new deaths and 2,459 new confirmed cases of COVID-19 in Los Angeles County* [News Release]. http://publichealth.lacounty.gov/phcommon/public/media/mediapubdetail.cfm?unit=media&ou=ph&prog=media&cur=cur&prid=2976&row=25&start=1

Dyal, J. W., Grant, M. P., Broadwater, K., Bjork, A., Waltenburg, M. A., Gibbins, J. D., Hale, C., Silver, M., Fischer, M., Steinberg, J., Basler, C. A., Jacobs, J. R., Kennedy, E. D., Tomasi, S., Trout, D., Hornsby-Myers, J., Oussayef, N. L., Delaney, L. J., Patel, K., . . . M. A. Honein (2020). COVID-19 among workers in meat and poultry processing facilities—19 States, April 2020. *Morbidity and Mortality Weekly Report, 69*, 557–561. https://doi.org/10.15585/mmwr.mm6918e3

Epstein, L., Hunter, J. C., Arwady, M. A., Tsai, V., Stein, L., Gribogiannis, M., Frias, M., Guh, A. Y., Laufer, A. S., Black, S., Pacilli, M., Moulton-Meissner, H., Rasheed, J. K., Avillan, J. J., Kitchel, B., Limbago, B. M., MacCannell, D., Lonsway, D., Noble-Wang, J., . . . Kallen, A. J. (2014). New Delhi Metallo-β-lactamase-producing carbapenem-resistant *Escherichia coli* associated with exposure to duodensoscopes. *JAMA, 312*(14), 1447–1455. https://doi.org/10.1001/jama.2014.12720

Kim, S., Russell, D., Mohamadnejad, M., Makker, J., Sedarat, A., Watson, R. R., Yang, S., Hemarajata, P., Humphries, R., Rubin, Z., & Muthusamy, V. R. (2016). Risk factors associated with the transmission of carbapenem-resistant enterobacteriaceae via contaminated duodenoscopes. *Gastrointestinal Endoscopy, 83*(6), 1121–1129. https://doi.org/10.1016/j.gie.2016.03.790

Los Angeles County Health Alert Network. (2020a, January 8). *CDC health advisory: Outbreak of pneumonia of unknown etiology (PUE) in Wuhan, China.* http://publichealth.lacounty.gov/eprp/lahan/alerts/CDCPneumoniaChina010820.pdf

Los Angeles County Health Alert Network. (2020b, January 17). *CDC health update: Update and interim guidance on outbreak of 2019 novel coronavirus (2019-nCoV) in Wuhan, China.* http://publichealth.lacounty.gov/eprp/lahan/alerts/CDCUpdateCoronaVirus011720.pdf

Los Angeles County Health Alert Network. (2020c, December 24, 2020). *LAC DPH health advisory: SARS-CoV-2 virus variant.* http://publichealth.lacounty.gov/EPRP/lahan/alerts/LAHANCOVIDVvariant122420.pdf

Los Angeles County Health Alert Network. (2020d, May 12). *LAC DPH health alert: Pediatric multi-system inflammatory syndrome potentially associated with COVID-19.* http://publichealth.lacounty.gov/eprp/lahan/alerts/LAHANPediatricMultiSystemInfl ammation051220.pdf

Miller, L., (2020, July 17). Workers vanished as coronavirus swept through L.A. apparel. Colleagues struggled for answers. *Los Angeles Times.* https://www.latimes.com/california/story/2020-07-17/la-me-la-apparel-outbreak-safety-protections

Rao, A. K., Lin, N. H., Griese, S. E., Chatham-Stephens, K., Badell, M. L., & Sobel, J. (2018). Clinical criteria to trigger suspicion for botulism: An evidence-based tool to facilitate timely recognition of suspected cases during sporadic events and outbreaks. *Clinical Infectious Diseases, 66*(Suppl. 1), S38–S42. https://doi.org/10.1093/cid/cix814

Rutala, W. A., & Weber, D. J. (2015). ERCP Scopes: What can we do to prevent infections? *Infection Control & Hospital Epidemiology, 36*(6), 643–664. https://doi.org/10.1017/ice.2015.98

Scottish Drugs Forum. (2017). *Wound botulism and drug use: What workers need to know.* http://www.sdf.org.uk/wp-content/uploads/2017/03/Botulism_Booklet.pdf

Trayner, K. M. A., Weir, A., McAuley, A., Godbole, G., Amar, C., Grant, K., Penrice, G., & Roy, K. (2018). A pragmatic harm reduction approach to manage a large outbreak of wound botulism in people who inject drugs, Scotland 2015. *Harm Reduction Journal, 15,* Article 36. https://doi.org/10.1186/s12954-018-0243-9

Wendorf, K. A., Kay, M., Baliga, C., Weissman, S. J., Gluck, M., Verma, P., D'Angeli, M., Swoveland, J., Kang, M. G., Eckmann, K., Ross, A. S., & Duchin, J. (2015). Endoscopic retrograde cholangiopancreatography-Associated AmpC *Escherichia coli* outbreak. *Infection Control & Hospital Epidemiology, 36*(6), 634–642. https://doi.org/10.1017/ice.2015.66

Wilken, J. A., Marquez, P., Terashita, D., McNary, J., Windham, G., & Materna, B. (2014). Coccidioidomycosis among cast and crew members at an outdoor television filming event—California, 2012. *Morbidity and Mortality Weekly Report, 63*(15), 321–324. https://www.cdc.gov/mmwr/preview/mmwrhtml/mm6315a1.htm

CHAPTER 15

WATER SUPPLY HAZARDS AND PUBLIC HEALTH

DRINKING WATER *CRYPTOSPORIDIUM* RESPONSE PLAN

JUNE E. BANCROFT, TAYLOR S. PINSENT, ANN LEVY, JONATHAN S. YODER, AND JOHN PERSON

KEY TERMS

Aqueous Ammonia
Chloranime
Cryptosporidium
Immunocompromised
Listeria
Oocyst
Protozoan
Salmonella
Sodium Hydroxide
Watershed
Whole Genome Sequencing

INTRODUCTION

Turning on a kitchen faucet and filling a cup with clean and safe drinking water is something many people take for granted. Safe drinking water and wastewater treatment are routine public health services that many benefit from without much thought. However, providing safe drinking water requires continually addressing threats to clean water and its availability. Drinking water emergencies are a by-product of natural or intentional events. Flooding, earthquakes, large-scale power outages, or chemical events can

The following icons, located in the margins throughout the chapter and within the summary tables, denote essential services of public health, CEPH competencies, and leadership levels: Essential services of public health; CEPH competencies; Leadership levels.

result in contamination of drinking water. Additionally, although a drinking water emergency affects everyone in the community, it's important to understand that it may affect people differently based on their access to healthcare and language resources. Genuine, preexisting community partnerships are essential to understand what barriers or challenges exist for accessing bottled water or understanding a boil water alert during a drinking water emergency.

This case study highlights the steps public health agencies and drinking water utilities can take to prepare for a water contamination event. The Portland Water Bureau (PWB) supplies drinking water to approximately 1 million Oregonians—almost one-quarter of the population of Oregon. Portland's drinking water is primarily surface water supplied from the Bull Run **Watershed** in the Mount Hood National Forest and is not filtered. The raw water is disinfected with chlorine, then travels to a facility where aqueous ammonia is added to form chloramine and the pH is adjusted. Unfiltered water systems such as PWB are required by the Long-Term 2 (LT2) Enhanced Surface Water Treatment Rule (2006) to treat source water for *Cryptosporidium* and use at least two disinfectants.

Cryptosporidium is a **protozoan** parasite that can be found in surface waters worldwide. In the environment, *Cryptosporidium* exists as a thick-walled **oocyst** that can withstand harsh conditions and protect it from chlorine disinfection. When ingested, *Cryptosporidium* can cause a gastrointestinal illness that is potentially severe and sometimes fatal in people with weakened immune systems. *Cryptosporidium* contamination in drinking water can come from any source of fecal matter, such as domestic animals (e.g., cattle), infected humans, wastewater treatment plant discharges, and wild animals.

The Safe Drinking Water Act permits a state to issue a variance to the LT2 rule regarding source water treatment requirements if a water system can demonstrate that it can protect public health without treatment for *Cryptosporidium* due to the nature of its raw water source. PWB obtained a variance in 2012; however, a series of detections of *Cryptosporidium* at low levels in 2017 resulted in revocation of the variance and requires PWB to build a treatment plant no later than September 30, 2027.

The detections in raw water beginning in 2017 and the need to identify possible gaps in capabilities for detection and investigation of a drinking water contamination event prompted the development of a tabletop exercise in 2018. This multiagency project resulted in a gap analysis, procedures, and potential enhancements for responding to water contamination events.

CASE BACKGROUND

CRYPTOSPORIDIUM BASICS

Cryptosporidium is a protozoan parasite that can be found in surface waters worldwide. In the environment, *Cryptosporidium* exists as a thick-walled oocyst that can withstand harsh conditions and is partially resistant to chlorine disinfection. When ingested, certain types of *Cryptosporidium* can cause cryptosporidiosis, a gastrointestinal illness that is potentially severe and sometimes fatal in people with weakened immune systems. According to the Centers for Disease Control and Prevention (CDC), the average time from consumption of oocysts to illness onset is 7 days and ranges from 2 to 12 days. Symptoms include watery diarrhea, abdominal pain, nausea, vomiting, and weight loss. In most people with healthy immune systems, the illness is self-resolving. However, persons with weakened immune systems may have extended and severe illness. Some people might be asymptomatically infected, and they can transmit the infection. People can shed the parasite in their feces for 2 weeks or more after their symptoms resolve, and some people become chronically infected (CDC, n.d.).

Cryptosporidium lives and reproduces in its host and is excreted in feces. Figure 15.1 outlines the life cycle of *Cryptosporidium*. Transmission occurs through direct or indirect contact with infected people or animals or through consumption of food or water contaminated with feces from infected people or animals. A review of *Cryptosporidium* outbreak investigations reported between 2009 and 2017 (Gharpure et al., 2019) indicated that exposure to treated recreational water (e.g., pools, water playgrounds) was associated

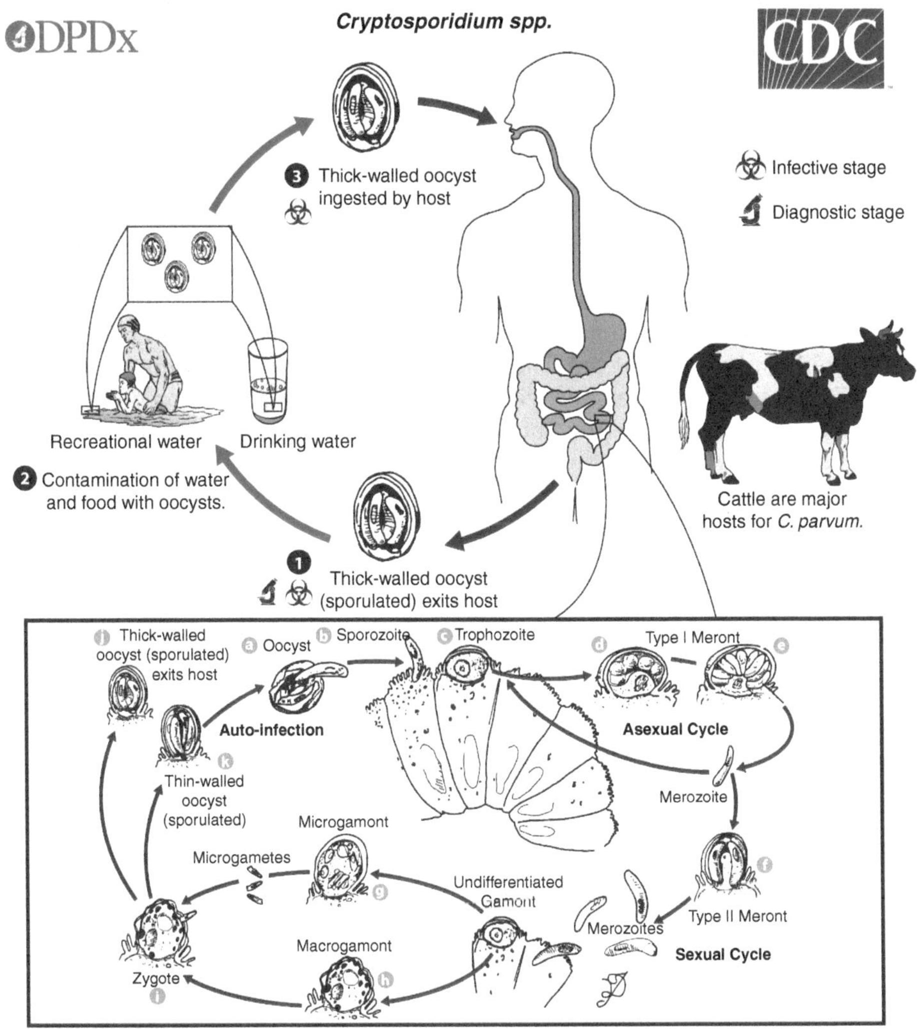

Figure 15.1 *Cryptosporidium* life cycle.

Source: From Centers for Disease Control and Prevention. (n.d.) *Cryptosporidiosis.* DPDx – Laboratory Identification of Parasites of Public Health Concern. https://www.cdc.gov/parasites/images/crypto/cryptosporidium_lifecycle.gif

with 35.1% of outbreaks, followed by contact with cattle (14.6%) and contact with infected persons in childcare settings (12.8%).

Cryptosporidium contamination in drinking water can come from any source of fecal matter, such as domestic animals (e.g., cattle), infected humans, wastewater treatment plant discharges, and wild animals. Although many species of *Cryptosporidium* have been identified, only a few are known to cause human infection. Approximately 95% to 99% of cryptosporidiosis cases in humans are caused by two well-described species: *C. parvum,* which particularly infects humans and cattle, and *C. hominis,* which infects primarily humans (Alves et al., 2006; Chalmers, Elwin, et al., 2009; Elwin, Hadfield, Robinson, & Chalmers, 2012; Elwin, Hadfield, Robinson, Crouch, et al., 2012; Feltus et al., 2006; Jex et al., 2007, 2008; Ng et al., 2008; O'Brien et al., 2008; Soba & Logar, 2008; Waldron et al., 2009; Xiao, 2010; Xiao & Ryan 2004; Zintl et al., 2009). One study (Chappell et al., 2011) demonstrated that other species, like *C. meleagridis,* can cause human gastrointestinal infections. *C. cuniculus* was associated with one waterborne outbreak in the United Kingdom in 2008 (Chalmers, Robinson, et al., 2009). A handful of species have been documented in infected humans at very low levels (fewer than 5% *Cryptosporidium* cases) but have not been associated with waterborne outbreaks. These include *C. ubiquitum, C. felis, C. canis,* and *C. viatorium* (Cama et al., 2007, 2008; Chalmers, Elwin, et al. 2009; Gatei et al., 2002; Xiao & Feng, 2008; Xiao et al., 2007).

Because *Cryptosporidium* has a low infectious dose (DuPont et al., 1995) and is chlorine-tolerant (Shields et al., 2008), it is ideally suited for transmission through chlorinated drinking water systems. There have also been large drinking water outbreaks associated with filtered water supplies. For example, one of the largest documented *Cryptosporidium* drinking water outbreaks occurred in 1992 in Milwaukee, Wisconsin. The prevalence of illness was estimated to range from 370,000 to 435,000 persons with an estimated 69 deaths. (Corso et al. 2003; Mac Kenzie et al., 1994). To prevent cryptosporidiosis transmission through public drinking water systems, the Environmental Protection Agency (EPA) implemented multiple regulatory changes designed to protect surface water supplies and enhance the treatment (e.g., filtration) of water to remove *Cryptosporidium.*

PORTLAND WATER BUREAU

This case study highlights the Portland Water Bureau (PWB) and its collaborative work with public health agencies to develop a *Cryptosporidium* response plan. The PWB is the municipal utility supplying drinking water to approximately 1 million Oregonians—almost one-quarter of the population of Oregon (Figure 15.2). In addition to the more than 610,000 customers throughout the City of Portland, PWB serves approximately 342,000 customers through regional wholesale providers. Portland's drinking water is primarily surface water supplied from the Bull Run Watershed, located 26 miles from downtown Portland in the Sandy River basin in the Mount Hood National Forest. Groundwater from the Columbia South Shore Well Field is used as an emergency backup and for supply augmentation during the summer high-demand and low-precipitation season.

The Bull Run Watershed has an area of 102 square miles (26,400 hectares) of heavily forested land upstream of the intake for the PWB drinking water supply. The watershed typically receives 80 to 170 inches (203–432 cm) of rainfall a year, with the heaviest rains falling from late fall through spring. Two reservoirs located on the Bull Run River store more than 17 billion gallons (64 billion liters) of water

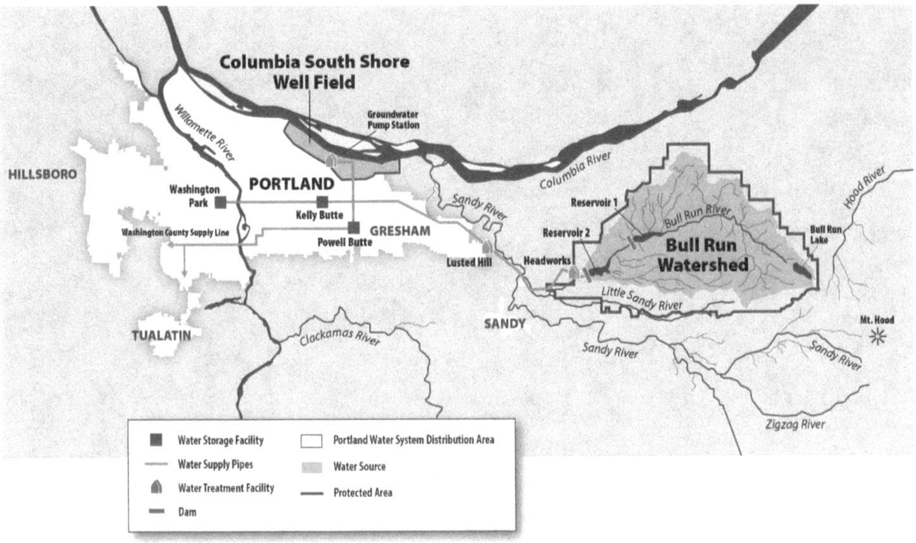

Figure 15.2 Portland Water Bureau supply system and watershed map.

Source: Reproduced with permission from the Portland Water Bureau.

for producing drinking water. PWB disinfects the raw water with chlorine before it enters conduits and travels to the Lusted Hill Treatment Facility where **aqueous ammonia** is added to form **chloramine** and pH is adjusted using **sodium hydroxide**.

Protecting a water source by keeping humans and agricultural and commercial activities away is one strategy for reducing the load of microbial pathogens in the water. The Bull Run Watershed has long been a protected source of drinking water. President Benjamin Harrison first established the Bull Run Reserve in 1892, and a 1977 act of Congress (Public Law 95-200) formally established the Bull Run Watershed Management Unit (BRWMU) and closed it to public entry. The BRWMU covers 147 square miles (38,000 hectares) of land. An additional 1.3 square miles (340 hectares) of city-owned land on the western edge of the unit adds to the protected area and forms what is known as the Bull Run Watershed Closure Area. About 95% of the BRWMU is federal land administered by the U.S. Forest Service; 4% is owned by the City of Portland; and 1% is federal land administered by the U.S. Bureau of Land Management. The land in the Bull Run Watershed is protected through a variety of federal, state, and local legal controls, which limit access to certain federal, state, and city employees. Tree logging in the BRWMU is prohibited. No recreational, residential, or commercial uses occur within the unit boundaries.

PWB monitors water quality and quantity in the Bull Run Watershed (Figure 15.3) to ensure that the Bull Run source water meets state and federal standards, provides information for making operational decisions, and tracks long-term trends. The Oregon Health Authority (OHA) Drinking Water Services regularly inspects the watershed and the related treatment and distribution facilities. The Bull Run supply complies with state and federal regulations for source water, including the 1989 Surface Water Treatment Rule (SWTR; EPA, 1989) filtration-avoidance criteria.

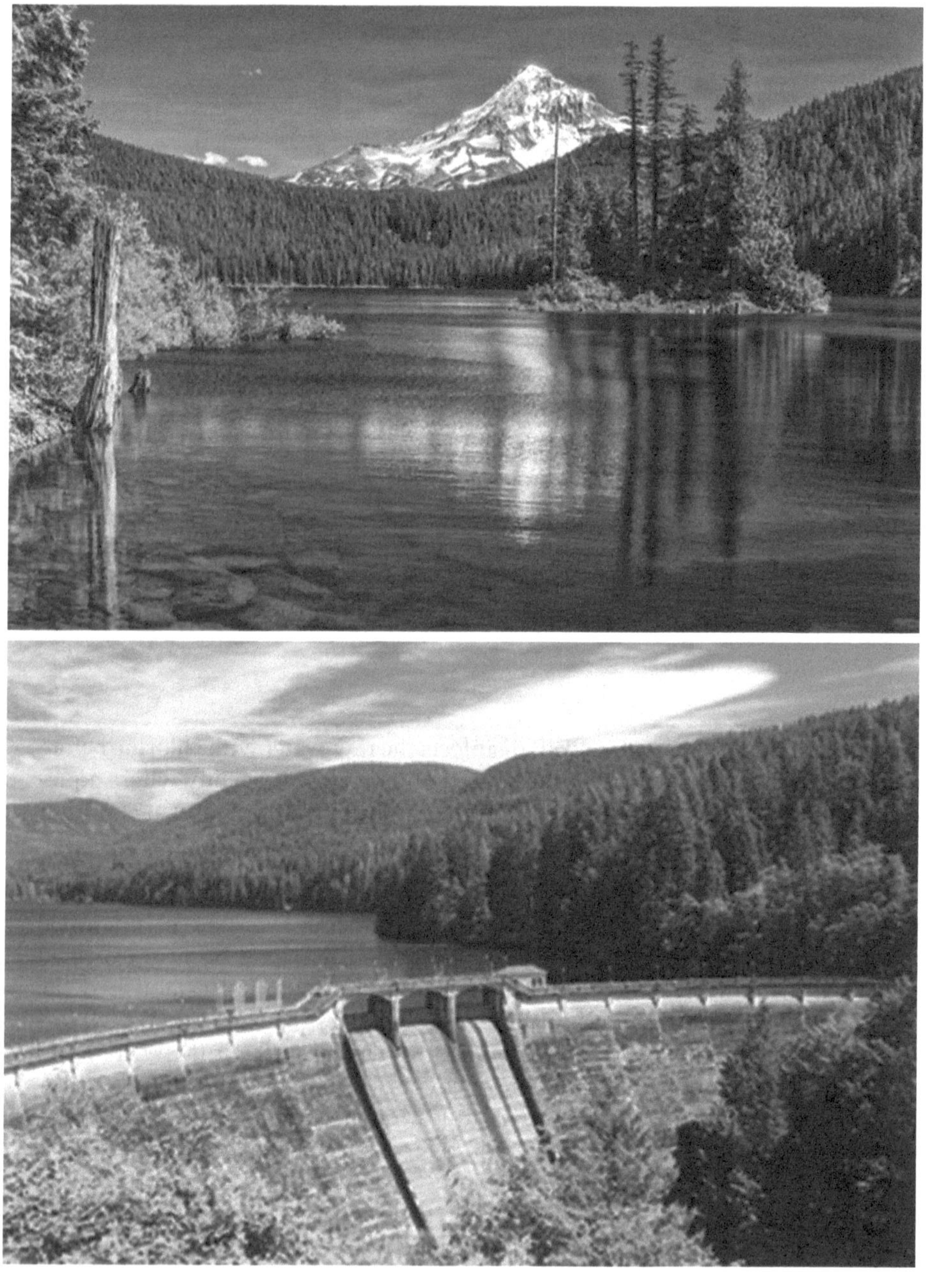

Figure 15.3 Bull Run Lake inside the Bull Run Watershed looking southeast toward Mount Hood, Oregon (top) and Bull Run Reservoir No. 1 and Dam 1, within the Bull Run Watershed, Oregon (bottom).

Source: Reproduced with permission from the Portland Water Bureau.

Filtration is another way water suppliers can remove pathogens (including those resistant to disinfectants) from drinking water. The SWTR (EPA, 1989) was established to ensure public health protection against microbial pathogens when using drinking water from surface water supply systems. The rule requires all surface water suppliers to filter the water they deliver unless the source water meets strict criteria for water quality and watershed protection. Water quality is achieved through the monitoring of turbidity and fecal coliform bacteria.

Turbidity must not exceed 5 nephelometric turbidity units (NTUs) and fecal coliform bacteria in raw water must not exceed 5% of samples with more than 20 colonies per 100 mL in any 6-month period.

Disinfection is a third way to reduce the number of infectious pathogens in water. Unfiltered water systems such as PWB are required by the LT2 Enhanced Surface Water Treatment Rule (2006) to treat source water for *Cryptosporidium* and use at least two disinfectants. However, the Safe Drinking Water Act permits a state to issue a variance from a treatment technique if a water system can demonstrate that it can protect public health without such a technique due to the nature of its raw water source. PWB demonstrated that its source water meets these criteria due to stringent source water monitoring and watershed protection and was granted a variance from the treatment requirements of the LT2 rule in 2012 (OHA, 2012). The Multnomah County Health Department (MCHD) supported PWB's request for a variance using local public health data.

PWB met the conditions of its treatment variance for 5 years. However, after a series of detections of *Cryptosporidium* at low levels in early 2017, OHA revoked the variance in December 2017 and entered into a Bilateral Compliance Agreement with PWB. The agreement requires that PWB treat for *Cryptosporidium* no later than September 30, 2027. PWB is planning to meet this requirement by using filtration. Until treatment is in place, PWB must continue to monitor for *Cryptosporidium* at the intake twice weekly. If *Cryptosporidium* is detected in any sample, sampling increases to four times a week and a press release must be issued. In addition, PWB must carry out monthly and quarterly reporting of results, public health outreach to vulnerable populations, semiannual watershed inspections, and environmental sampling of tributary water and wildlife scat and report annually to the OHA's Drinking Water Services. No association with health effects was detected during the *Cryptosporidium* detections in 2017 or during subsequent seasonal detections in the following years. Testing and routine review of data with the OHA, the MCHD, and PWB will continue until the water filtration plant is functioning.

HEALTH DATA

Health Hazards and Risks

Cryptosporidium can cause severe disease and chronic sequelae in children and people with weakened immune systems (Sparks, 2015). Those with a weakened immune system include those with cancer, those with HIV/AIDS, and transplant patients who are taking certain immunosuppressive drugs. According to the CDC, the risk of developing severe disease may differ depending on a person's degree of immune suppression. Infection in these populations can result in more severe and prolonged illness, like chronic diarrhea. Prolonged diarrhea can lead to rapid loss of fluids, which can be life-threatening for some populations.

After the series of low-level detections of *Cryptosporidium* in early 2017, the MCPH and PWB began annual messaging to healthcare providers who work with **immunocompromised** patients as directed by the OHA. This messaging includes information on diagnosis and testing for cryptosporidiosis, that Bull Run is not treated for *Cryptosporidium*, and actions providers should consider. Mailed materials include educational brochures (Figure 15.4) and posters that can be displayed in clinics.

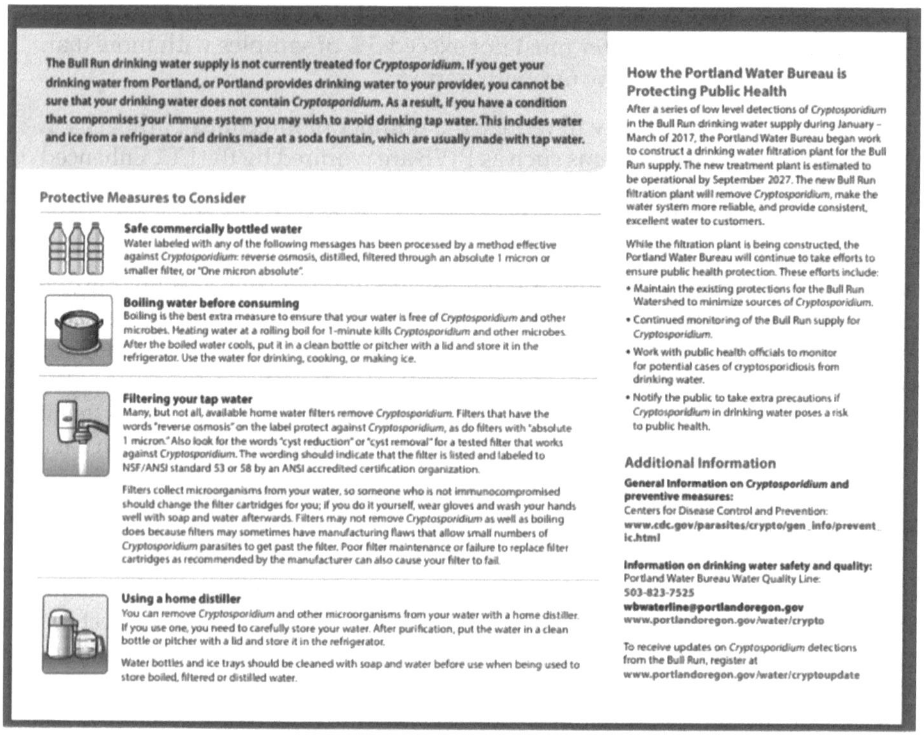

The Bull Run drinking water supply is not currently treated for *Cryptosporidium*. If you get your drinking water from Portland, or Portland provides drinking water to your provider, you cannot be sure that your drinking water does not contain *Cryptosporidium*. As a result, if you have a condition that compromises your immune system you may wish to avoid drinking tap water. This includes water and ice from a refrigerator and drinks made at a soda fountain, which are usually made with tap water.

Protective Measures to Consider

Safe commercially bottled water
Water labeled with any of the following messages has been processed by a method effective against *Cryptosporidium*: reverse osmosis, distilled, filtered through an absolute 1 micron or smaller filter, or "One micron absolute".

Boiling water before consuming
Boiling is the best extra measure to ensure that your water is free of *Cryptosporidium* and other microbes. Heating water at a rolling boil for 1-minute kills *Cryptosporidium* and other microbes. After the boiled water cools, put it in a clean bottle or pitcher with a lid and store it in the refrigerator. Use the water for drinking, cooking, or making ice.

Filtering your tap water
Many, but not all, available home water filters remove *Cryptosporidium*. Filters that have the words "reverse osmosis" on the label protect against *Cryptosporidium*, as do filters with "absolute 1 micron." Also look for the words "cyst reduction" or "cyst removal" for a tested filter that works against *Cryptosporidium*. The wording should indicate that the filter is listed and labeled to NSF/ANSI standard 53 or 58 by an ANSI accredited certification organization.

Filters collect microorganisms from your water, so someone who is not immunocompromised should change the filter cartridges for you; if you do it yourself, wear gloves and wash your hands well with soap and water afterwards. Filters may not remove *Cryptosporidium* as well as boiling does because filters may sometimes have manufacturing flaws that allow small numbers of *Cryptosporidium* parasites to get past the filter. Poor filter maintenance or failure to replace filter cartridges as recommended by the manufacturer can also cause your filter to fail.

Using a home distiller
You can remove *Cryptosporidium* and other microorganisms from your water with a home distiller. If you use one, you need to carefully store your water. After purification, put the water in a clean bottle or pitcher with a lid and store it in the refrigerator.

Water bottles and ice trays should be cleaned with soap and water before use when being used to store boiled, filtered or distilled water.

How the Portland Water Bureau is Protecting Public Health

After a series of low level detections of *Cryptosporidium* in the Bull Run drinking water supply during January – March of 2017, the Portland Water Bureau began work to construct a drinking water filtration plant for the Bull Run supply. The new treatment plant is estimated to be operational by September 2027. The new Bull Run filtration plant will remove *Cryptosporidium*, make the water system more reliable, and provide consistent, excellent water to customers.

While the filtration plant is being constructed, the Portland Water Bureau will continue to take efforts to ensure public health protection. These efforts include:

- Maintain the existing protections for the Bull Run Watershed to minimize sources of *Cryptosporidium*.
- Continued monitoring of the Bull Run supply for *Cryptosporidium*.
- Work with public health officials to monitor for potential cases of cryptosporidiosis from drinking water.
- Notify the public to take extra precautions if *Cryptosporidium* in drinking water poses a risk to public health.

Additional Information

General Information on *Cryptosporidium* and preventive measures:
Centers for Disease Control and Prevention:
www.cdc.gov/parasites/crypto/gen_info/prevent_ic.html

Information on drinking water safety and quality:
Portland Water Bureau Water Quality Line:
503-823-7525
wbwaterline@portlandoregon.gov
www.portlandoregon.gov/water/crypto

To receive updates on *Cryptosporidium* detections from the Bull Run, register at
www.portlandoregon.gov/water/cryptoupdate

Figure 15.4 Portland Water Bureau's educational brochure about *Cryptosporidium* in drinking water for immunocompromised individuals.

Source: Reproduced with permission from the Portland Water Bureau.

Active and Passive Disease Surveillance System

Laboratories, physicians, and others providing healthcare are required by Oregon law to report confirmed or presumptive cryptosporidiosis cases to the local public health authority (LPHA). The LPHA attempts to interview patients in all reported cases to identify potential sources of exposure and provide education regarding disease transmission. Questions routinely asked by LPHA include source of drinking water, potential recreational water exposures (e.g., pools, lakes, rivers), livestock and other animal exposures, attendance or work at a childcare or assisted living facility (regarding contact with incontinent persons), and consumption of uncooked, ready-to-eat produce or unpasteurized products (e.g., raw milk; see Figure 15.5).

Infected persons are also educated about disease transmission and prevention of continued spread (e.g., proper cleaning and handwashing messaging). The information collected during the interview is entered manually into Oregon's statewide integrated communicable disease surveillance database, called the Oregon Public Health Epi User System or "Orpheus." This database allows local and state epidemiologists to conduct analyses to identify trends and detect outbreaks or geographic clusters. If public health officials identify an outbreak or an increase above an established local baseline within the same time and space, active surveillance is initiated. Unlike passive surveillance, active surveillance involves additional outreach to find cases in the community. Examples of active case finding might be alerts to urgent cares, emergency departments, or providers and notifying the public via a press release. However, it is important to note that outbreaks associated with drinking water can be difficult to detect through passive surveillance. For example, in one drinking water outbreak in Baker City, Oregon,

RISKS Provide details as appropriate.

yes	no	ref	unk	
☐	☐	☐	☐	travel outside home area (specify place, reason, transportation mode (car) travel companions____________________
☐	☐	☐	☐	visitor/refugee/immigrant from endemic area
☐	☐	☐	☐	foreign travel by household member
☐	☐	☐	☐	raw/unpasteurized milk
☐	☐	☐	☐	other raw milk product
☐	☐	☐	☐	eat any soft cheese made with raw milk
☐	☐	☐	☐	unpeeled fruits or vegetables
☐	☐	☐	☐	raw or other unpasteurized product (circle one) (dairy, milk, fruit juice, veg juice, cider, other, unk)
☐	☐	☐	☐	unpasteurized apple juice/cider
☐	☐	☐	☐	restaurants, fast food, vendors
☐	☐	☐	☐	eating at other gatherings (potlucks, events)
☐	☐	☐	☐	attends or works in daycare center/nursery
☐	☐	☐	☐	diapered children or adults
☐	☐	☐	☐	contact with farm animals
☐	☐	☐	☐	contact with household pets, esp puppies and kittens
☐	☐	☐	☐	*if yes*, did the pet have loose stools
☐	☐	☐	☐	work with animal products, research, slaughter house, veterinary medicine
☐	☐	☐	☐	contact with other people sick with diarrhea
☐	☐	☐	☐	drinking untreated surface water
☐	☐	☐	☐	recreational water (pools, water slides, lakes)
☐	☐	☐	☐	*if yes circle type:* fresh water, hot spring, hot tub or whirlpool, interactive fountain, recreational water part, sea, swimming pool, other ____________________

Figure 15.5 Excerpt from Oregon *Cryptosporidium* exposure questions, source of drinking water.

Source: Reproduced with permission from June Bancroft.

only five laboratory confirmed cases were reported. That was the total signal detected through passive surveillance. In contrast, active surveillance through a community survey indicated 2,780 cases might have occurred (DeSilva, 2013).

Syndromic Surveillance System

An early detection tool used in public health is "syndromic surveillance," for which Oregon uses the ESSENCE application for syndromic surveillance. Syndromic surveillance provides close to real time data on patients presenting at emergency departments or urgent care centers. Specific keyword queries are developed to search triage notes and chief complaint fields. The detection of continual, low-level, naturally occurring contaminants, like *Cryptosporidium*, is challenging because cryptosporidiosis generally produces nonspecific symptoms like abdominal pain and diarrhea, making it difficult to distinguish it from other gastrointestinal infections. People rarely seek care for cryptosporidiosis unless they experience more severe disease (e.g., dehydration due to diarrhea lasting several weeks); however, syndromic surveillance does provide situational awareness and could detect an outbreak if a dramatic increase in emergency department visits due to community-wide infection occurred.

Informatics and Biostatistics

Access to complete and timely communicable disease data is extremely important for detection and tracking of drinking water outbreaks. Leveraging informatics and building a robust data governance infrastructure allow for a more modern and efficient data system. This allows the state and the LPHA to create innovative ways to access data for routine and ad hoc analyses. Building this kind of infrastructure also allows a variety of nontraditional data sources to incorporate during a public health emergency.

Data collected from case investigations are available for local and statewide review. Public health officials routinely analyze these data to identify infection trends by age, sex, race, location, and risk factors. Examples of risk factors for this disease include international travel, exposure to recreational water, and contact with infected animals. Public health also has a 24/7 telephone system to respond to reports of illness from the public or providers who notice an increase in illness within clinics or emergency departments. These stories and reports can also trigger public health investigations and additional review of laboratory data. A goal of these efforts is to quickly identify an increased disease burden in a community and to implement public health interventions to stop the spread.

Laboratory data are the backbone of communicable disease surveillance. Public health officials learn of most infections based on a clinical specimen that is tested at a laboratory. Laboratories identify *Cryptosporidium* with a variety of tests including microscopy, the detection of a cell antigen, or the detection of the parasite's genetic material via polymerase chain reaction. Laboratories can also speciate *Cryptosporidium,* which can be an important clue as to the source of infection. A novel technique for public health surveillance includes **whole genome sequencing**. This type of genetic analysis is often utilized during enteric disease outbreaks, for pathogens such as ***Salmonella*** or ***Listeria***. CryptoNet (cdc.gov/parasites/crypto/cryptonet.html) is a CDC laboratory-based network to create a reference genetic database for *Cryptosporidium.* All sequence data are uploaded to the National Center for Biotechnology Information (NCBI) database that can be mined by analysts to determine whether specific infections are genetically similar. However, use of the NCBI database has limitations for a waterborne outbreak of *Cryptosporidium* since the genetic typing of parasitic infections is not as mature as those for bacterial pathogens. Using genetic typing, public health agencies can link animal and human infections; however, these data are delayed and not available in real time.

Communication

Crisis and risk communications that include specific, consistent, clear, and transparent information are extremely important during any drinking water emergency. Developing key talking points and educational materials prior to the emergency is essential. As a public health department, it is also important to build relationships with hospitals, community-based organizations, elected officials, and water utilities before the emergency. Including local businesses in these conversations will allow LPHAs to understand their needs and concerns during a boil water notice. Such businesses include hospitals, dialysis centers, ambulatory care centers, restaurants, food manufacturing facilities, and other businesses that use water in their operations. Often these places require culturally specific or custom messaging. The CDC's Drinking Water Advisory Toolkit is a good place to start, but it should be customized for the situation and location. Alerts and information in different languages and via multiple channels or different formats of media are required to address local needs (Figure 15.6).

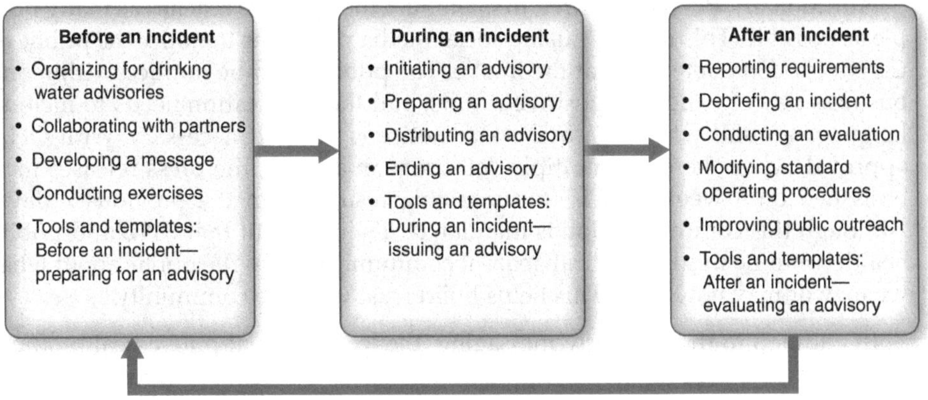
Before an incident
• Organizing for drinking water advisories
• Collaborating with partners
• Developing a message
• Conducting exercises
• Tools and templates: Before an incident—preparing for an advisory
During an incident
• Initiating an advisory
• Preparing an advisory
• Distributing an advisory
• Ending an advisory
• Tools and templates: During an incident—issuing an advisory
After an incident
• Reporting requirements
• Debriefing an incident
• Conducting an evaluation
• Modifying standard operating procedures
• Improving public outreach
• Tools and templates: After an incident—evaluating an advisory

Figure 15.6 Centers for Disease Control and Prevention drinking water advisory toolkit.

Source: Centers for Disease Control and Prevention. (2016). *Drinking water advisory communication toolbox.* https://www.cdc.gov/healthywater/emergency/pdf/DWACT-2016.pdf

Currently, we are in the "before an incident" stage that includes more routine notification of risk to PWB customers; specifically, quarterly notifications to the public that its drinking water is not treated for *Cryptosporidium*, the potential associated risk, and Portland's plans to filter Bull Run drinking water. This notification is mandated under the Bilateral Compliance Agreement. The public notice may be in the form of a press release or part of other annual reports (i.e., the Consumer Confidence Report). A template is used for this notification to ensure clear and consistent messaging.

> The Portland Water Bureau does not currently treat for *Cryptosporidium*, but is required to do so under the drinking water regulations. Portland is working to install filtration by 2027 under a compliance schedule with the Oregon Health Authority. In the meantime, Portland Water Bureau is implementing interim measures such as watershed protection and additional monitoring to protect public health [*Insert actions customers should take, and what steps PWB is taking to correct the situation.*]
>
> Exposure to *Cryptosporidium* can cause cryptosporidiosis, a serious illness. Symptoms can include diarrhea, vomiting, fever, and stomach pain. People with healthy immune systems recover without medical treatment. According to the Centers for Disease control and Prevention (CDC), people with severely weakened immune systems include those with AIDS, those with inherited diseases that affect the immune system, and cancer and transplant patients who are taking certain immunosuppressive drugs.
>
> The Environmental Protection Agency has estimated that a small percentage of the population could experience gastrointestinal illness from *Cryptosporidium* and advises that customers who are immunocompromised and receive their drinking water from the Bull Run Watershed consult with their health care professional about the safety of drinking the tap water. [*Insert list of water suppliers that serve Bull Run water*] receive all or part of their drinking water supply from Bull Run. To learn if your drinking water comes from Bull Run, please contact your local drinking water provider.

Additionally, PWB is required to make sure the message reaches as many people as possible. This includes using social media platforms to notify the public of *Cryptosporidium* detections at the intake. The public must be notified within one business day of validated positive results, and the notification needs to include language around whether a boil water notice is deemed necessary. With OHA approval, when there are multiple detections in a week, the press releases may be issued on a weekly basis, summarizing results from the previous 7 days. Although this communication is mandated, it's important that PWB and public health continue this kind of transparent communication to the public about what we may or may not know. This helps build trust with the community.

In addition to the quarterly messaging, the lead regional public health officer for the three counties where Portland serves water, Clackamas, Multnomah, and Washington Counties, annually issues a clinician update to medical providers who care for immunocompromised patients. The update contains background on *Cryptosporidium*, diagnosis recommendations, health effects of cryptosporidiosis, laboratory methods, and how to register for PWB notification of detections, and it encourages patients to sign up at https://publicalerts.org to receive emailed emergency notices such as drinking water advisories. The email list allows concerned customers and medical providers to receive notification whenever public notifications of *Cryptosporidium* detections are issued. The availability of the email list for notification is shared in the clinician update and is posted on PWB's website.

Another important component to public notification is ensuring that public health officials have culturally appropriate messaging. Cultural competency within our public health systems is important during any event and making sure we are meeting the communication needs of our communities should be a priority for public health. Although a drinking water emergency affects everyone in the community, it's important to understand that it may affect people differently based on their access to healthcare and language resources. Building genuine community partnerships is a good first step to understanding what barriers or challenges exist within the community when accessing bottled water or understanding a boil water alert. Depending on the local population, translated materials that include clear instruction on boiling water might be necessary. Public health agencies should partner with community leaders to ensure culturally appropriate messaging during the crisis.

POLICY

Turning on a kitchen faucet and filling a cup with clean and safe drinking water is something many people take for granted. Safe drinking water and wastewater treatment are routine public health services from which most people in the United States benefit without much thought. However, providing safe drinking water requires continually addressing threats to clean water and its availability. National regulations legally require water providers to adhere to specific standards and processes. The Safe Drinking Water Act (SDWA) was passed by Congress in 1974 and amended in 1986 and 1996. This national policy was established to ensure and protect the quality of Americans' drinking water. The SDWA mandates that all public water systems in the United States follow standards and regulations set by the EPA. However, individual primacy agencies can set and enforce state-specific standards if they are at least as stringent as the SDWA. In 1998 the Consumer Confidence Report Rule was enacted to improve public health protection by providing educational material to enable consumers

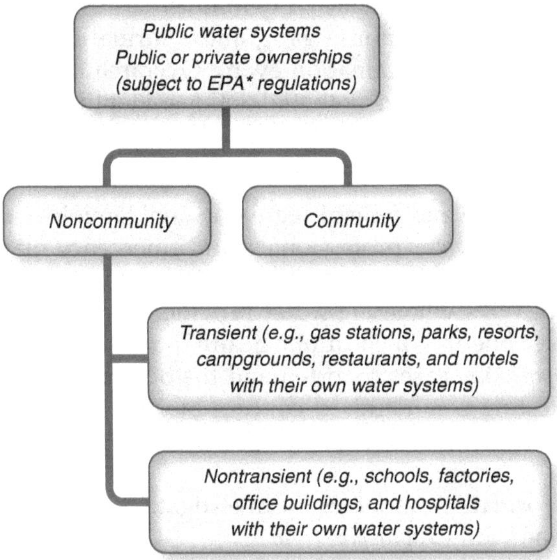

Figure 15.7 Public water system structure.

to make educated decisions regarding any potential health risks pertaining to the quality, treatment, and management of their drinking water supply. This rule applies to all community water systems (Figure 15.7). Included in the rule is a specification that water systems with a large proportion of non-English-speaking residents must include information in the appropriate language(s) as determined by the state or the EPA. The legally enforceable standards are part of the National Primary Drinking Water Regulations. These rules and regulations are in place to protect public health.

National, state, and local agencies play specific enforcement and regulation roles while working in partnership to provide this essential service of safe, clean drinking water. The EPA oversees the SDWA through partnership and oversight of the State Drinking Water program, which, in Oregon, resides in the OHA (Figure 15.7). State drinking water programs monitor, inspect, and advise individual water systems, and local environmental health staff perform this work for smaller systems using groundwater sources. State and local public health authorities collaborate with these regulatory programs to decrease morbidity related to drinking water. The role of the CDC includes providing subject matter expertise and specialty laboratory testing capacity for affected jurisdictions in the case of a drinking water emergency.

Preparedness and Response

Since the approval of the variance to treat Portland's water for *Cryptosporidium* in 2012, PWB, the OHA, and the MCHD continued to meet regularly to share relevant environmental and public health data. The increase in water sample *Cryptosporidium* detections in 2017 and the need to identify possible gaps in capabilities for detection and investigation of a drinking water contamination event prompted the development of a tabletop exercise in 2018. This multiagency project resulted in a gap analysis, procedures, and potential enhancements for responding to water contamination events. The project included an environmental and public health surveillance capabilities assessment, a workshop with key partners to identify response gaps, and a formal tabletop exercise focused on a *Cryptosporidium* contamination event. Overarching goals included confirming and clarifying roles and potential actions, identifying all stakeholders, building coalitions and partnerships for influencing public health outcomes, and identifying areas to enhance the existing systems.

Tabletop participants included state and federal regulators, epidemiologists, public health professionals, drinking water professionals, and emergency managers from agencies such as the EPA, PWB, the CDC, the OHA, the MCHD, the Oregon Poison Center, and PWB's wholesale water providers. Participants exercised two different scenarios: one in which public health surveillance data detected an increase in *Cryptosporidium* cases reported and the other a scenario where Bull Run source water testing results raised concern of *Cryptosporidium* water contamination. The tabletop exercise objectives are as follow.

1. Evaluate procedures and information resources for investigating possible drinking water contamination with *Cryptosporidium.*
   a. Evaluate whether the steps in the draft procedure accurately represent the investigative activities to be implemented and information resources to be consulted to assess the magnitude of public health risk to PWB's customers in response to an elevation in case counts and/or increases in detections in the source water.
   b. Identify gaps in existing data sources and new or novel data streams to supplement existing data.

2. Evaluate procedures and plans for responding to credible/confirmed drinking water contamination with *Cryptosporidium.*
   a. Discuss the factors that influence the decision to switch to the groundwater source when there is a potential increased risk of cryptosporidiosis in PWB's service area suspected or confirmed to have originated in the Bull Run source.
   b. Discuss the factors that influence the decision to issue a boil water notice, when there is an increased risk of cryptosporidiosis in PWB's service area.
   c. Discuss considerations (e.g., operation of healthcare facilities, public services for which boiling is not practical) for an extended boil water notice, longer than 24 hours and potentially longer than a week, in response to suspected or confirmed drinking water contamination with *Cryptosporidium*.
   d. Evaluate the capacity of public health agencies to identify and interview cases during a long-term investigation as well as laboratory capacity for clinical samples (e.g., when would the CDC be needed to help with sample analyses?).
   e. Discuss environmental control measures for *Cryptosporidium* (e.g., dishwashers, soda fountain machines, breweries, food manufacturing).

3. Identify incident command structure and communication protocols during credible/confirmed drinking water contamination with *Cryptosporidium.*
   a. Determine which agencies would be part of an Incident Command System (ICS)/Unified Command during an extended boil water notice.

b. Identify, describe, and document notification processes and communication pathways within and between organizations.
c. Identify, describe, and document processes and procedures for communicating with key stakeholders, beyond the public at large, during an extended boil water notice. This would include customers with special needs related to water quality who may not have been previously identified.
d. Anticipate and plan for customer expectations during a *Cryptosporidium* contamination incident and resulting extended boil water notice (e.g., water testing, filters in homes).

The main output of the tabletop exercise included a comprehensive written report and a set of diagrams that would help guide each agency during an actual event. Each diagram identified which agencies and what factors are considered or communicated during a response to an actual incident. The actions practiced and discussed during the tabletop exercise used existing communication tools and relationships to work through what a response might look like if there was an actual drinking water contamination incident involving *Cryptosporidium*. Every situation is different, and actions taken by utilities and public health agencies would depend on the information available during the incident. The report detailed the two scenarios and documented processes, leadership, governance, and incident management. The exercise also focused on fostering collaboration and multiagency decision-making. As the water filtration plant is constructed for Portland, the OHA will continue its work to improve the overall capacity and identify and respond to drinking water contamination events.

Case Summary

Safe drinking water is essential to public health and is critical community infrastructure. Regulations have been developed to address water contamination threats, including those caused by *Cryptosporidium*. When a public water system is threatened with contamination, it is a public health emergency with the potential to affect the health of the entire community. This requires a timely public health response, utilizing multiple public health competencies and engaging with multiple response partners.

Key messages to be learned from Portland's drinking water case study include the importance of using the available tools to prevent and control public health threats. This includes: (a) understanding the applicable regulations that protect public health, (b) timely access to complete communicable disease data for detection and tracking of drinking water outbreaks, (c) crises and risk communication that includes specific, consistent, clear, and transparent information throughout the emergency, and (d) learning from water-related emergencies and outbreaks to evaluate and update public health policies to effectively protect public health.

Protecting our communities requires continued work to respond to waterborne disease outbreaks and water-related emergencies. This can be achieved through careful planning and collaboration between public health professionals in every step of the process.

DISCUSSION QUESTIONS

1. Describe the following water treatment rules: (1) The Surface Water Treatment Rule, (2) Long-Term 2 Enhanced Surface Water Treatment Rule.
2. What entities participate in providing safe drinking water?
3. What are the key messages summarized in the chapter that were learned from this case study?
4. Describe some important partners and local businesses that should be included in the planning process before a water emergency. Why is it important to build a relationship with these entities prior to an emergency?
5. Describe what steps are taken if *Cryptosporidium* is detected in any raw water sample from the Bull Run.

SUMMARY

TABLE 15.1 Select Essential Services of Public Health Demonstrated in the *Cryptosporidium* Response

Essential Service # and Definition	Context in Chapter Case	Competency # It ties to	Importance for Emergency Preparedness, Response, or Recovery
1. Assess and monitor population health status, factors that influence health, and community needs and assets (Assessment)	Laboratories, physicians, and others providing healthcare are required by Oregon law to report confirmed or presumptive *Cryptosporidium* cases to local public health authority (LPHA).	3, 4	Early detection of pathogenic outbreaks is critical for immediate response. Syndromic surveillance systems capture hospital reports of symptomatic cases and can aid in spotting the first signs of an outbreak to thwart massive exposure.
2. Investigate, diagnose, and address health problems and hazards affecting the population (Assessment)	Laboratories identify *Cryptosporidium* with tests including microscopy, detection of a cell antigen, or detection of the parasite's genetic material.	1, 2, 3, 4	Testing of water sources periodically to ensure proper protocols for sterilization are adhered to and maintained are essential activities for water safety in communities. Rapid testing of water sources after an exposure event (e.g., broken water main) can ensure appropriate strategies are immediately enforced.
3. Communicate effectively to inform and educate people about health, factors that influence it, and how to improve it (Policy Development)	Lead regional public health officer for Clackamas, Multnomah, and Washington Counties annually issues a clinician update to providers who care for immunocompromised patients.	18, 19, 20	When a potential contamination of water occurs, timely, transparent, and clear communication to affected communities is essential. In addition, there needs to be bidirectional messaging and coordination with local businesses, hospitals, and CBO's. Healthcare providers must also be updated regularly by the health department for testing and isolation recommendations.
4. Strengthen, support, and mobilize communities and partnerships to improve health (Policy Development)	The Portland Water Bureau, the Oregan Health Authority, and Multnomah County Health Department meet regularly to share relevant environmental and public health data. It's important to build relationships with hospitals, CBO's, water utilities, and elected officials before the water emergency.	5, 13, 14, 21	Safe water practices should involve community and organizational support. Health department staff should have close bidirectional relationships with community leaders, health agencies, hospitals, public utilities, and others to promote synergy for clean water.
5. Create, champion, and implement policies, plans, and laws that impact health (Policy Development)	Consumer Confidence Report Rule enacted to improve public health protection by informing consumers to make educated decisions regarding any potential health risks pertaining to their drinking water supply.	13, 21	Health department staff can use community stories, data reports, after-action reports, and program evaluation data to advocate for policies to protect community water sources.
6. Utilize legal and regulatory actions designed to improve and protect the public's health (Policy Development)	Safe Drinking Water Act was passed by Congress in 1974 and amended in 1986 and 1996 to ensure and protect drinking water.	11	Health department staff must be up-to-date and knowledgeable on government regulations regarding safe and clean water.

CBO, community-based organization.

TABLE 15.2 Select CEPH Competencies Needed for Frontline Health Workers, Managers, and Leaders for Water Supply Emergency Preparedness, Response, and Recovery

Competency # and Definition	Context in Case/Chapter	Level	Importance for Emergency Preparedness, Response, or Recovery
1. Apply epidemiological methods to settings and situations in public health practice.	Local public health authority interviews patients in all reported cases to identify potential sources of exposure and provide education regarding transmission.	Level 1	At this level, data on contaminated water, outbreaks of waterborne diseases, and morbidity and mortality are collected and analyzed, and reports are produced.
3. Analyze quantitative and qualitative data using biostatistics, informatics, computer-based programming, and software, as appropriate.	Public health officials routinely analyze case investigations to identify infection trends by age, sex, race, location, and risk factors.	Level 1	At this level, when an increase in cases is detected, additional case investigations can be conducted to understand risk factors and provide public health interventions. Quantitative data and qualitative data from interviews or focus groups can be used to understand risk factors and/or differences in exposures. Reports are produced to inform next steps.
4. Interpret results of data analysis for public health research, policy, or practice.	State and LPHAs to create innovative ways to access data for routine and ad hoc analyses through leveraging informatics.	Level 2	At this level, the mid-level manager may review many data reports and summary findings to provide data-driven guidance for elected officials and public health leadership.
13. Propose strategies to identify stakeholders and build coalitions and partnerships for influencing public health outcomes.	Portland Water Bureau, Oregon Health Authority, and Multnomah County Health Department meet regularly to share relevant data.	Level 3	Based on lessons learned from outbreaks and data reports, Level 3 leaders can advocate for policies to protect community water sources and build coalitions with communities, stakeholders, and other leaders to make the case for improved water safety practices.
18. Select communication strategies for different audiences and sectors.	Portland Water Bureau carries out monthly and quarterly reporting of results, public health outreach to vulnerable populations, and semiannual inspection reports.	Level 3	Level 3 leaders may be the spokespersons for communicating information to the public about potential water hazards and disease outbreaks. They may appear in the media to provide a summary of what is currently known and to issue boil water notices to affected communities.
19. Communicate audience-appropriate (i.e., non-academic, non-peer audience) public health content, both in writing and through oral presentation.	Lead regional public health officer annually issues a clinician update to medical providers who care for immunocompromised patients.	Level 3	Level 3 leaders may issue guidance for clinicians for treatment of affected populations, as well as recommendations for public utilities on best practices.

Key: Essential services of public health; CEPH competencies; Leadership levels.

DISCLAIMER

This chapter was prepared by Jonathan S. Yoder and John Person in his/her personal capacity. The opinions expressed in this article are the author's own and do not reflect the view of the Centers for Disease Control and Prevention, the Department of Health and Human Services, or the United States government.

REFERENCES

Alves, M., Xiao, L., Antunes, F., & Matos, O. (2006). Distribution of *Cryptosporidium* subtypes in humans and domestic and wild ruminants in Portugal. *Parasitology Research, 99*, 287–292. https://doi.org/10.1007/s00436-006-0164-5

Cama, V. A., Bern, C., Roberts, J., Cabrera, L., Sterling, C. R., Ortega, Y., Gilman, R. H., & Xiao, L. (2008). *Cryptosporidium* species and subtypes and clinical manifestations in children, Peru. *Emerging Infectious Diseases, 14*, 1567–1574. https://doi.org/10.3201/eid1410.071273

Cama, V. A., Ross, J. M., Crawford, S., Kawai, V., Chavez-Valdez, R., Vargas, D., Vivar, A., Ticona, E., Navincopa, M., Williamson, J., Ortega, Y., Gilman, R. H., Bern, C., & Xiao, L. (2007). Differences in clinical manifestations among *Cryptosporidium* species and subtypes in HIV-infected persons. *Journal of Infectious Diseases, 196*, 684–691. https://doi.org/10.1086/519842

Centers for Disease Control and Prevention. (n.d.). Parasites – *Cryptosporidium* (also known as "Crypto"). https://www.cdc.gov/parasites/crypto

Chalmers, R. M., Elwin, K., Thomas, A. L., Guy, E. C., & Mason, B. (2009). Long-term *Cryptosporidium* typing reveals the aetiology and species specific epidemiology of human cryptosporidiosis in England and Wales, 2000 to 2003. *EuroSurveillance, 14*, 19086. https://doi.org/10.2807/ese.14.02.19086-en

Chalmers, R. M., Robinson, G., Elwin, K., Hadfield, S. J., Xiao, L., Ryan, U., Modha, D., & Mallaghan, C. (2009). *Cryptosporidium* rabbit genotyped, a newly identified human pathogen [Letter]. *Emerging Infectious Diseases, 15*, 829–830. https://doi.org/10.3201/eid1505.081419

Chappell, C. L., Okhuysen, P. C., Langer-Curry, R. C., Akiyoshi, D. E., Widmer, G., & Tzipor, S. (2011). *Cryptosporidium meleagridis:* Infectivity in healthy adult volunteers. *The American Journal of Tropical Medicine and Hygiene, 85*(2), 238–242. https://doi.org/10.4269/ajtmh.2011.10-0664

Corso, P. S., Kramer, M. H., & Blair. K. A. (2003). Costs of illness in the 1993 waterborne cryptosporidium outbreak, Milwaukee, Wisconsin. *Emerging Infectious Diseases, 9*(4), 426–431. https://doi.org/10.3201/eid0904.020417

DeSilva, M. S. (2013). Communitywide cryptosporidiosis outbreak associated with a surface water-supplied municipal water system – Baker City, Oregon. *Epidemiology and Infection, 144*(2), 274–284. https://doi.org/10.1017/S0950268815001831

DuPont, H. L., Chappell, C. L., Sterling, C. R., Okhuysen, P. C., Rose, J. B., & Jakubowski, W. (1995). The infectivity of *Cryptosporidium parvum* in healthy volunteers. *The New England Journal of Medicine, 332*, 855–859. https://doi.org/10.1056/NEJM199503303321304

Elwin, K., Hadfield, S. J., Robinson, G., & Chalmers, R. M. (2012). The epidemiology of sporadic human infections with unusual cryptosporidia detected during routine typing in England and Wales, 2000–2008. *Epidemiology and Infections, 140*, 673–683. https://doi.org/10.1017/S0950268811000860

Elwin, K., Hadfield, S. J., Robinson, G., Crouch, N. D., & Chalmers, R. M. (2012). *Cryptosporidium viatorum* n. sp. (*Apicomplexa: Cryptosporidiidae*) among travelers returning to Great Britain from the Indian subcontinent, 2007–2011. *International Journal of Parasitology, 42*, 675–682. https://doi.org/10.1016/j.ijpara.2012.04.016

Environmental Protection Agency. (1989). *Surface Water Treatment Rule.* https://www.epa.gov/dwreginfo/surface-water-treatment-rules

Feltus, D. C., Giddings, C. W., Schneck, B. L., Monson, T., Warshauer, D., & McEvoy, J. M. (2006). Evidence supporting zoonotic transmission of *Cryptosporidium* in Wisconsin. *Journal of Clinical Microbiology, 44*, 4303–4308. https://doi.org/10.1128/JCM.01067-06

Gatei, W., Suputtamongkol, Y., Waywa, D., Ashford, R. W., Bailey, J. W., Greensill, J., Beeching, N. J., & Hart, C. A. (2002). Zoonotic species of *Cryptosporidium* are as prevalent as the anthroponotic in HIV-infected patients in Thailand. *Annals of Tropical Medicine and Parasitology, 96*, 797–802. https://doi.org/10.1179/000349802125002202

Gharpure, R., Perez, A., Miller, A. D., Wikswo, M. E., Silver, R., & Hlavsa, M. C. (2019). Cryptosporidiosis Outbreaks—United States, 2009–2017. *Morbidity and Mortality Weekly Report, 68*, 568–572. http://doi.org/10.15585/mmwr.mm6825a3external icon

Jex, A. R., Pangasa, A., Campbell, B. E., Whipp, M., Hogg, G., Sinclair, M. I., Stevens, M., & Gasser, R. B. (2008). Classification of *Cryptosporidium* from sporadic cryptosporidiosis cases in humans employing sequence-based multilocus analysis following mutation scanning. *Journal of Clinical Microbiology, 46*, 2252–2262. https://doi.org/10.1128/JCM.00116-08

Jex, A. R., Whipp, M., Campbell, B. E., Caccio, S. M., Stevens, M., Hogg, G., & Gasser, R. B. (2007). A practical and cost-effective mutation scanning-based approach for investigating genetic variation in *Cryptosporidium*. *Electrophoresis, 28*, 3875–3883. https://doi.org/10.1002/elps.200700279

Mac Kenzie, W. R., Hoxie, N. J., Proctor, M. E., Gradus, M. S., Blair, K. A., Peterson, D. E., Kazmierczak, J. J., Addiss, D. G., Fox, K. R., & Rose, J. B. (1994). A massive outbreak in Milwaukee of cryptosporidium infection transmitted through the public water supply. *The New England Journal of Medicine, 331*, 161–167. https://doi.org/10.1056/NEJM199407213310304

Ng, J., Eastwood, K., Durrheim, D., Massey, P., Walker, B., Armson, A., & Ryan, U. (2008). Evidence supporting zoonotic transmission of *Cryptosporidium* in rural New South Wales. *Experimental Parasitology, 119*, 192–195. https://doi.org/10.1016/j.exppara.2008.01.010

O'Brien, E., McInnes, L., & Ryan, U. (2008). *Cryptosporidium* GP60 genotypes from humans and domesticated animals in Australia, North America and Europe. *Experimental Parasitology, 118*, 118–121. https://doi.org/10.1016/j.exppara.2007.05.012

Oregon Health Authority. (2012). *Drinking water program*. https://yourwater.oregon.gov/portland/variancefinalorder.pdf

Shields, J. M., Hill, V. R., Arrowood, M. J., & Beach, M. J. (2008). Inactivation of *Cryptosporidium parvum* under chlorinated recreational water conditions. *Journal of Water and Health, 6*, 513–520. https://doi.org/10.2166/wh.2008.068

Soba, B., & Logar, J. (2008). Genetic classification of *Cryptosporidium* isolates from humans and calves in Slovenia. *Parasitology, 135*, 1263–1270. https://doi.org/10.1017/S0031182008004800

Sparks, H. N.-G. (2015). Treatment of cryptosporidium: What we know, gaps, and the way forward. *Current Tropical Medicinereports, 2*(3), 181–187. https://doi.org/10.1007/s40475-015-0056-9

Waldron, L. S., Ferrari, B. C., & Power, M. L. (2009). Glycoprotein 60 diversity in *C. hominis* and *C. parvum* causing human cryptosporidiosis in NSW, Australia. *Experimental Parasitology, 122*, 124–127. https://doi.org/10.1016/j.exppara.2009.02.006

Xiao, L. (2010). Molecular epidemiology of cryptosporidiosis: An update. *Experimental Parasitology, 124*, 80–89. https://doi.org/10.1016/j.exppara.2009.03.018

Xiao, L., & Feng, Y. (2008). Zoonotic cryptosporidiosis. *FEMS Immunology and Medical Microbiology, 52*, 309–323. https://doi.org/10.1111/j.1574-695X.2008.00377.x

Xiao, L., & Ryan, U. M. (2004). Cryptosporidiosis: An update in molecular epidemiology. *Current Opinions in Infectious Diseases, 17*, 483–490. https://doi.org/10.1097/00001432-200410000-00014

Xiao, L., Zhou, L., Santin, M., Yang, W., & Fayer, R. (2007). Distribution of *Cryptosporidium parvum* subtypes in calves in eastern United States. *Parasitology Research, 100*, 701–706. https://doi.org/10.1007/s00436-006-0337-2

Zintl, A., Proctor, A. F., Read, C., Dewaal, T., Shanaghy, N., Fanning, S., & Mulcahy, G. (2009). The prevalence of *Cryptosporidium* species and subtypes in human faecal samples in Ireland. *Epidemiology and Infection, 137*, 270–277. https://doi.org/10.1017/S0950268808000769

PART III

SPECIAL CONSIDERATIONS

CHAPTER 16

PUBLIC HEALTH LAW

FOUNDATIONS AND APPLICATIONS DURING EMERGENCIES

LAUREN T. DUNNING, JENNIFER L. PIATT, AND JAMES G. HODGE, JR.

KEY TERMS

Defense Production Act
Homeland Security Act of 2002
Isolation
Medical Countermeasures
Model State Emergency Health Powers Act (MSEHPA) of 2001
National Emergencies Act (NEA)
Pandemic and All-Hazards Preparedness Act (PAHPA) of 2006
Parens Patriae Power
Police Power
Preemption
Public Health Emergency of International Concern (PHEIC)
Public Health Law
Public Health Service Act (PHSA)
Public Readiness and Emergency Preparedness (PREP) Act
Quarantine
Robert T. Stafford Disaster Relief and Emergency Assistance Act (Stafford Act)

INTRODUCTION

Law is the foundation for action to promote public health, laying out the powers, duties, and limitations of governments and their partners to prevent and respond to health risks and threats. When faced with emergencies, public health agencies and other governmental entities utilize legal and regulatory

The following icons, located in the margins throughout the chapter and within the summary tables, denote essential services of public health, CEPH competencies, and leadership levels: Essential services of public health; CEPH competencies; Leadership levels.

actions in concert with other essential public health services to protect human lives and promote healthy conditions. Different types of emergencies—disease outbreaks, natural disasters, environmental contamination events, and other urgent health threats—require tailored responses using available legal tools, such as declarations and orders, authorized under existing federal, state, territorial, tribal, and local laws. This chapter introduces public health law and the legal basis for government action, describes the legal landscape for responses to public health emergencies (PHEs), and shares case studies applying legal interventions to protect the public's health during emergencies.

FOUNDATIONS OF PUBLIC HEALTH IN LAW

This text provides numerous examples of public health law in action, although not always with accompanying references to specific laws or regulations. The same is true in everyday public health practice. From reporting by physicians for specific infectious diseases to required face coverings to stymie the spread of COVID-19 to testing, remediation, and authorization to reinhabit properties impacted by wildfires, public health interventions rely on legal authorizations. Statutes, regulations, and judicial decisions enable public health workers at all levels to respond to emergencies, fund public health agencies, and enable manifold interventions, such as screening, testing, treatment, and social distancing (Hodge, 2018).

The range of potential issues impacting communal health necessitates broad legal authorities to promote and protect health, safety, and welfare. Understanding and wielding these powers across the scope of routine and emergency public health services centers around the following definition proffered by Professors Lawrence O. Gostin and Lindsay F. Wiley:

> **Public health law** is the study of the legal powers and duties of the state, in collaboration with its partners (e.g., healthcare, business, the community, the media, and academe), to ensure the conditions for people to be healthy (to identify, prevent, and ameliorate risks to health in the population), and of the limitations on the power of the state to constrain for the common good the autonomy, privacy, liberty, proprietary, and other legally protected interests of individuals. The prime objective of public health law is to pursue the highest possible level of physical and mental health in the population, consistent with the values of social justice. (Gostin & Wiley, 2016)

Two key aspects of this definition guide public health response to emergencies: (a) legal powers and duties to advance public health and (b) limitations on constraining individual liberties for the common good.

LEGAL POWERS AND DUTIES TO ADVANCE PUBLIC HEALTH

As the source of federal authority to act in the interests of the public's health (Gostin, 2001), the U.S. Constitution (a) delineates the powers of the federal government; (b) reserves sovereign powers to states, territories, and tribes (i.e., federalism); and (c) divides powers among the three branches of government—legislative, executive, and judicial (i.e., separation of powers; U.S. Const. art. I; U.S. Const. amend. X; U.S. Const. art. II; U.S. Const. art. III.). In addition to the

U.S. Constitution, each state and territory has its own constitution that provides legal authority for public health within state or territorial boundaries (Leonard, 2010). These authorities may be delegated to local governments as well, which bear significant independent responsibility for public health depending on the degree of "home rule" powers states allow (National Association of County & City Health Officials, 2020).

Federalism

Constitutional principles of federalism distribute power between the national government and the states (Federalism, 2019). The federal government has limited powers specifically enumerated in the U.S. Constitution (Nolan et al., 2018). They range from the operational, like the ability to coin money and establish post offices, to the more expansive, like the powers to tax and spend and to regulate commerce (U.S. Const. art. I). In terms of public health, these powers enable such critical measures as regulating clean air and clean water (Clean Air Act, 2018; Clean Water Act, 2018), preventing the spread of communicable diseases at national borders and between states (Public Health Service Act, 2018), and providing federal funding to states for emergency preparedness and planning (Centers for Disease Control & Prevention [CDC], n.d.-b, n.d.-c).

While constitutionally limited in their scope, federal laws are the "supreme law of the land" (U.S. Const. art. IV). This means federal law preempts, or supersedes, conflicting state laws. Though the applications of federal **preemption** are extensive and complicated, in general, preemption prevents states from taking contradictory action whenever the federal government has the sole authority to act or chooses to act in areas of overlapping authority with states. For example, the federal government, through the Atomic Energy Act (1954), expressly preempts states from regulating aspects of nuclear power plants related to radiologic safety. Preemption operates across all levels of government—legislative, executive, and judicial. Accordingly, a decision of the U.S. Supreme Court preempts conflicting decisions of state courts. Just as the federal government may preempt state laws, state governments can preempt local laws within their jurisdictions (Hodge et al., 2018).

Powers not granted to the federal government are reserved to the states or territories by the 10th Amendment: "the powers not delegated to the United States by the Constitution, nor prohibited by it to the States, are reserved to the States respectively, or to the people" (U.S. Const. amend. X.). Reserved powers include the "**police power**," which refers to the inherent authority of states to provide for the health, safety, morals, and general welfare of their citizens, including constraining private actions for the benefit of the public good (Gostin & Wiley, 2016).

State Police Powers

Manifestations of state-based police powers are extensive, especially in furtherance of protecting the public's health. For example, state police powers authorize school vaccination requirements for infectious diseases like measles, mumps, and rubella (MMR) and varicella. Businesses may be required to engage in specific food safety practices to prevent foodborne illness. Patrons of commercial entities like bars or restaurants may be prohibited from smoking in public (Parmet et al., 2005). In some states, smoking bans may even extend to personal residences in multi-unit complexes. Case studies in the second half of this chapter explore police powers in the context of public health emergencies (PHEs). Though extensive, exercises of state police powers—through the passage and enforcement of laws, promulgation of regulations, and issuance of orders in support of public health—have limits. Public health interventions must often make trade-offs between individual rights and communal goods due to constitutional constraints (Gostin & Wiley, 2020).

Adjacent to the police power is the ***parens patriae* power**, which enables states to protect individuals who lack the capacity to do so on their own behalf (Hodge, 2018). This power is most often invoked in relation to child custody, civil commitment, and treatment decisions for incapacitated individuals. The *parens patriae,* literally "parent of the nation," doctrine also allows states to litigate on behalf of citizens to preserve their welfare (*Alfred L. Snapp & Son, Inc. v. Puerto Rico,* 1982). For example, states and tribes have filed lawsuits against opioid manufacturers, distributors, and retailers citing a variety of public harms via their *parens patriae* powers to enjoin specific actions and seek damages (Ausness, 2014).

Separation of Powers

The constitutional separation of powers between the three branches of government—legislative, executive, and judicial—provides checks and balances on government actions to prevent centralization of power and the potential for tyranny and oppression (Chemerinsky, 2015; Hodge, 2018). Generally, the legislative branch creates the law, the executive branch executes it, and the judicial branch interprets it, resulting in legal precedents (or a series of binding judicial decisions on which other branches may rely). While laws enacted by legislatures are an essential component of the public health framework and judicial decisions provide critical guidance on the legal limits of public health authority, the executive branch is involved in the day-to-day practice of public health and emergency responses. Multiple federal agencies have critical public health roles, such as the Department of Health and Human Services (HHS), the CDC, and the Federal Emergency Management Agency (FEMA).

State constitutions similarly separate powers across state entities, with corresponding state-based health agencies responsible for public health in their jurisdictions (National Association of County & City Health Officials, 2020). As discussed later, emergency preparedness and response requires extensive coordination between all levels and branches of government with complementary roles and areas of oversight (Rose et al., 2017).

CONSTITUTIONAL LIMITS ON GOVERNMENT ACTION

The first 10 amendments to the U.S. Constitution, otherwise known as the "Bill of Rights," enshrine the rights of citizens in relation to the federal government, and the Fourteenth Amendment makes those protections applicable to the states (U.S. Const. amend. I-X; U.S. Const. amend. XIV). These rights include freedom of religion, speech, and assembly (First Amendment; U.S. Const. amend. I); the right to keep and bear arms (Second Amendment; U.S. Const. amend. II); and freedom from unreasonable searches and seizures (Fourth Amendment; U.S.

Const. amend. IV). Furthermore, the Fifth and Fourteenth Amendments prevent the deprivation of individual life, liberty, or property without procedure (procedural due process) and without adequate rationale (substantive due process; U.S. Const. amend. V; U.S. Const. amend. XIV; Chemerinsky, 2015), and the Fourteenth Amendment protects individuals from arbitrary or discriminatory government action (equal protection; U.S. Const. amend. XIV). Many challenges to public health laws are based on claims citing these and other core individual rights.

JUDICIAL REVIEW OF GOVERNMENT ACTION

Constitutional limits require government to justify its actions in the interests of the public's health when they may inhibit individual rights. Thus, when government public health interventions infringe on individual liberty or other constitutionally protected interests, courts may require government to show at least a rational relationship between the action taken and the proposed public health outcome (Gostin, 2010). Fairness of public health interventions is key. In *Jew Ho v. Williamson* (1900), for example, a discriminatory *cordon sanitaire* ("roping off") of most of San Francisco's Chinatown district to prevent the spread of bubonic plague was struck down by the court in 1900 as the result of "an evil eye and an unfair hand" (*Jew Ho v. Williamson*, 1900). Heightened levels of scrutiny requiring a compelling or substantial public interest and use of least restrictive means to advance them may be applied by modern courts to prevent overreach when fundamental rights or interests of individuals are infringed (Chemerinsky, 2015).

During the COVID-19 pandemic in 2020 to 2021, courts across the country analyzed many public health measures implemented by federal, state, and local governments designed to prevent disease spread, preserve hospital capacities, and ultimately save lives (Parmet, 2020b). For example, Los Angeles County's temporary ban on outdoor dining at restaurants in response to COVID-19 was challenged in November 2020. A local trial court found that the county's order lacked a rational relationship to a legitimate end, as the county could not support the order with specific epidemiologic data on outdoor dining and the spread of COVID-19 (*California Restaurant Association, Inc. v. County of Los Angeles Department of Public Health*, 2020). The decision was later overturned when an appellate court found a sufficient rational basis supporting the government's intrusion on restaurants' proprietary interests even without specific studies or data on transmission of COVID-19 through outdoor dining (*County of Los Angeles Department of Health v. Superior Court*, 2021). This decision demonstrates the deference courts generally afford to public health when responding to emergencies and other health threats (*County of Los Angeles Department of Health v. Superior Court*, 2021). State and local restrictions impacting attendance at religious services during the COVID-19 pandemic, however, have been struck down by the U.S. Supreme Court using higher levels of scrutiny (*Roman Catholic Diocese of Brooklyn v. Cuomo*, 2020).

JACOBSON V. MASSACHUSETTS

The foundational case affirming the basic power of government to protect the public's health is *Jacobson v. Massachusetts* (1905). This case involved a challenge to a local implementation of a state law allowing vaccinations to halt smallpox outbreaks (*Jacobson v Massachusetts*, 1905). Vaccinations for smallpox, a deadly disease without any effective treatment, were demonstrated to be effective despite risks to those vaccinated (*Jacobson v. Massachusetts*, 1905). Facing recurring smallpox outbreaks, Massachusetts passed a law requiring that all adults be vaccinated or pay a fine of five dollars, unless an individual could provide a valid medical exemption to this mandate (Hodge, 2018; Parmet, 2020a). Failure to pay the fine could result in incarceration. Reverend Henning Jacobson refused vaccination and challenged the law on multiple constitutional grounds, appealing lower court decisions to the U.S. Supreme Court. Ultimately, the court decided against Jacobson, upholding the Massachusetts law and recognizing the validity of public health action to constrain individual liberty for the common good (*Jacobson v. Massachusetts*, 1905). Justice Harlan, writing for the court's majority, stated "the liberty secured by the Constitution of the United States . . . does not import an absolute right in each person to be . . . wholly freed from restraint. There are manifold restraints to which every person is necessarily subject for the common good" (*Jacobson v. Massachusetts*, 1905).

The court outlined a floor of constitutional protections to prevent governmental overreach and protect individual rights through four constitutionally grounded standards: public health necessity, reasonable means, proportionality, and harm avoidance (*Jacobson v. Massachusetts*, 1905). Public health necessity requires that exercise of police power be based on the "necessity of the case" and cannot be "beyond what [i]s reasonably required for the safety of the public" (*Jacobson v. Massachusetts*, 1905). Reasonable means describes the need for a "real or substantial relation" between the intervention being implemented and the public health goal (*Jacobson v. Massachusetts*, 1905). Public health interventions also must follow the standard of proportionality in that the burdens imposed by interventions cannot be entirely disproportionate to their benefits. Finally, public health measures cannot impose known health risks on individuals. For example, if Jacobson could have proved administration of smallpox vaccination would have harmed him directly, the government could not require him to be vaccinated. He would be deemed an "unfit candidate." If the law failed to offer such exemptions to those presenting evidence of a medical contraindication to vaccination, the government would have failed to meet the standard of harm avoidance (Gostin, 2005). While jurisprudence has evolved, particularly concerning judicial standards of review (Gostin, 2005), *Jacobson* remains central to the history and foundations of public health law through its balancing of civil liberties and the common good (970 F.3d 174, 189, 2020; Hodge et al., 2021).

SPECIFIC LEGAL TOOLS FOR PUBLIC HEALTH

Public health officials and lawmakers have a set of legal tools to draw from when responding to health threats and emergencies. These include interventions impacting individuals and groups, such as testing, screening, vaccination, and social distancing powers like quarantine and isolation (Hodge, 2018). **Quarantine** entails separation of persons who are reasonably believed to have been exposed to a communicable disease but who are not known to be ill from others during the incubation period of the disease to prevent disease spread should they develop the disease. **Isolation** refers to the separation of individuals who are known to be ill and contagious from those who are well for the period of infectiousness. Public health interventions also include a variety of actions focused on businesses and environments, such as closures, evacuations, and abatements (Burris et al., 2020), among multiple other powers.

Statutes authorizing these interventions may be general and apply throughout a jurisdiction, meaning they are not directed at a specific individual or business. Noncompliance can result in civil or criminal penalties. Regulations promulgated by executive agencies with delegated legislative authority provide more specific guidance. Public health orders issued by government officials provide real-time responses to urgent risks or emergencies, and can apply to individuals and groups, businesses, or the entire population. For example, California law authorizes local health officers to "take any preventive measure that may be necessary to protect and preserve the public health from any public health hazard during any 'state of war emergency,' 'state of emergency,' or 'local emergency'" (Cal. Health & Safety Code § 101040, 1995). Local health officers in California also have broad authority to respond to communicable disease cases to prevent outbreaks, even without a specific emergency declaration (Cal. Health & Safety Code § 120175, 1996). Specific public health actions are informed by available scientific information and data, public health practice, and the law. Many states, for example, provide detailed laws governing isolation and treatment of individuals with tuberculosis (Cabrera et al., 2008). Within this legal framework, there is still significant decision-making authority for public health officials who must comport with public health ethics and principles of equity.

PUBLIC HEALTH EMERGENCY LAW

Within the larger U.S. legal infrastructure grounded in constitutional principles like federalism, separation of powers, and protection of individual rights exist specific laws governing PHEs. PHE statutes, regulations, and cases encompass an evolving body of laws at all levels of government that empower public and private sectors to plan for, prevent, and respond to emerging infectious diseases (e.g., COVID-19), catastrophic events (e.g., hurricanes), and other crises (e.g., opioid addiction) seriously impacting communal health (Hodge, 2016). High-impact, sudden-onset events, such as bioterrorism, may justify immediate national emergency declarations (Sunshine et al., 2019). More localized PHEs, like chemical spills, food contaminations, or limited disease outbreaks, may warrant state- or local-based declarations. Seminal events like the COVID-19 pandemic entail PHE declarations of every type and at every governmental level for months on end.

Throughout most of the 20th century, legal responses to PHEs followed an "all hazards" approach framed around general declarations of "emergency" or "disaster" (Sunshine, 2018) managed typically by federal, state, tribal, or local emergency management agencies. PHEs were legally indistinguishable from other hazards that led to emergency declarations. After the terrorist acts on September 11, 2001, and ensuing anthrax attacks, however, the legal environment surrounding PHEs changed dramatically. Government leaders engaged in a series of legislative and regulatory reforms to (a) specifically classify and define PHEs, (b) clarify and authorize public- and private-sector responses, and (c) coordinate efforts across federal and state governments.

The resulting legal environment supporting national, state, and local emergency declarations and powers is assessed next.

FEDERAL EMERGENCY LAWS, DECLARATIONS, AND POWERS

While national powers via principles of federalism are narrower than the aforementioned state-based *police* and *parens patriae* powers, federal emergency laws are extensive, detailed, and supreme. Congress has authorized vast federal emergency powers and regulatory authorities in the president, HHS, CDC, FEMA, and other federal agencies. General emergency authorities are derived primarily through the **Robert T. Stafford Disaster Relief and Emergency Assistance Act** (**Stafford Act**; 42 U.S.C.A. § 5121 *et seq.*), **National Emergencies Act** (**NEA**; 50 U.S.C.A. §§ 1601, 1621, 1622, 1631, 1641, 1651, West 2020), and (c) **Public Health Service Act** (**PHSA**; 42 U.S.C.A. § 201 *et seq.*, 2020).

Collectively, these laws authorize federal declarations of "emergency," "disaster," and "PHE," each of which has been issued in response to manifold events, including the COVID-19 pandemic. Declarations of emergency or disaster are made by the president via the Stafford Act or the NEA. Stafford Act emergencies can be declared typically after a state governor requests federal assistance "to save lives and to protect property and public health and safety, or to lessen or avert the threat of a catastrophe" (42 U.S.C.A. §§ 5170, 5122(1) West, 2020). Emergencies issued pursuant to the NEA trigger a litany of federal executive agency authorities to enable real-time responses (Elsea et al., 2020). The president may also declare states of disaster often in response to substantial natural calamities (e.g., tornadoes, earthquakes, snowstorms, or droughts) affecting specific localities, states, or regions. These declarations mobilize federal aid and assistance through FEMA among other entities.

In addition to presidential states of emergency or disaster, the HHS secretary can declare a federal PHE whenever "a disease or disorder presents a [PHE]" or in response to "significant outbreaks of infectious diseases or bioterrorist attacks" (42 U.S.C.A. § 247d(a), West, 2020). Pursuant to these declarations under the PHSA, which last 90 days subject to reauthorization, HHS can issue grants, authorize contracts, cover expenses, conduct and support disease investigations, and access emergency funds. Some Medicare and Medicaid requirements can be temporarily waived to facilitate national response efforts. Emergency use authorizations (EUAs) of nonapproved drugs, vaccines, tests, or devices may be conducted through the Food and Drug Administration (FDA, 2017). During the COVID-19 pandemic, FDA's real-time issuance of EUAs allowed for widespread distributions of vaccines not otherwise approved through time-consuming, extensive reviews.

Additional statutory laws guide national emergency preparedness and response efforts. The **Homeland Security Act of 2002** (Homeland Security Act, 2002) empowers the Department of Homeland Security (DHS) to coordinate and manage key federal responses. Federal deployments of rapid response teams through the National Disaster Medical System are allowed via the Public Health Security and Bioterrorism Preparedness and Response Act of 2002. The Project BioShield Act of 2004 establishes the Strategic National Stockpile (SNS) to collect and distribute essential medicines and supplies nationally. The **Pandemic and All-Hazards Preparedness Act (PAHPA) of 2006** streamlines federal public health responses, requires states to engage in emergency planning, facilitates medical voluntarism, and encourages the rapid development of **medical countermeasures (MCMs**; e.g., medicines, vaccines, or supplies) through the HHS's Biomedical Advanced Research and Development Authority (BARDA).

The **Public Readiness and Emergency Preparedness (PREP) Act** (42 U.S.C. § 247d–6d, 2012) supports distribution and implementation of federally approved MCMs. Subject to a specific PREP Act declaration by the HHS secretary, liability protections may be extended to officials, manufacturers, distributors, health workers, and others involved in developing or administering MCMs. A compensation fund supports claims of individuals injured directly by the administration or use of MCMs. HHS Secretary Alex Azar's PREP Act declaration in response to COVID-19 in March 2020, which was subsequently amended multiple times (85 Fed. Reg. 15,198, 2020), featured broad, preemptive language overriding conflicting state laws and policies related to medical licensure, scope of practice limitations, and more. During the COVID-19 pandemic in 2020 to 2021, a new slate of real-time legislative enactments provided extensive economic relief for Americans and supplemented federal emergency powers. The Families First Coronavirus Response Act (2020), for example, assured greater access to no-cost COVID-19 tests and limited paid sick leave benefits. The CARES Act (2020) explicitly protected volunteer health workers from liability and instituted a limited eviction moratorium of qualified residential properties. Substantial funding for hospitals and providers and support for testing and contact tracing efforts were secured via the Paycheck Protection Program and Healthcare Enhancement Act (2020). The Consolidated Appropriations Act (2020) expanded Medicare access to telemedicine mental health services and enhanced payments for physician services. Finally, the American Rescue Plan Act (2021) substantially funded subnational COVID-19 response efforts based on expanded public health priorities in President Biden's national strategic plan (The White House, 2021).

STATE AND LOCAL EMERGENCY POWERS AND ROLES

Federal emergency classifications are similarly reflected in state/territorial/tribal and local level declarations. Post-9/11 transformations of these authorities centered on detecting, preventing, and responding to bioterrorism incidents and other emerging disease threats. Substantial reforms extended from the **Model State Emergency Health Powers Act (MSEHPA) of 2001** (Gostin et al., 2002), adopted in whole or part by 39 states (Center for Law and the Public's Health, 2006). MSEHPA introduced an original, structured, and cohesive series of model provisions triggered by a declared PHE. PHE was defined generally via the model act as an occurrence or imminent threat of a health condition from any of a number of sources that "poses a high probability of" substantial deaths, disabilities, or future health harms via exposure to infectious or toxic agents (Model State Emergency Health Powers Act, 2001).

Declarations of PHEs limited in their duration (to protect against misuses) authorized a menu of expedited public health powers including (a) real-time testing, screening, vaccination, and treatment for affected persons; (b) social distancing measures including isolation and quarantine to reduce disease transmission; (c) temporary business or road closures to limit public health impacts; (d) mass evacuations where needed to prevent excess morbidity and mortality; (e) culturally appropriate public communications; (f) abatement of hazardous materials or nuisances threatening the public's health; (g) seizing and using private property (with compensation) to acquire needed resources or space; (h) controlling essential supplies via procurement, rationing, prioritization, and price gouging limits; (i) collection, analyses, and safe handling of lab specimens from persons or animals; (j) licensure reciprocity for out-of-state healthcare workers or volunteers in good standing; and (k) limited liability protections against unscrupulous or unwarranted legal claims.

Nearly all these powers were wielded in response to COVID-19, but not all PHEs merit their extensive use. Over the last two decades, for example, some jurisdictions have declared PHEs to address differing events and conditions, such as water contamination, domestic violence, food insecurity, homelessness, vaping, and medical cannabis (Hodge et al., 2019). These novel uses extend the concept beyond its initial conceptions.

MSEPHA and similar enactments across states/territories/tribes/localities protect against unnecessary or abusive uses of public health powers through explicit measures supporting constitutional protections (e.g., respect for autonomy, liberty, due process, and equal protection) and political limits. For example, the model act allows governors or other politically accountable actors to temporarily waive routine statutory, regulatory, or judicial laws that inhibit PHE responses. Widespread implementation of these waiver authorities via emergency declarations dominated states' responses to COVID-19. However, the emergency ability to waive conflicting laws for a limited duration does not apply to constitutional requirements. Efforts that look past or are directly contrary to constitutional norms are unwarranted even in PHEs.

During the COVID-19 pandemic, for example, some governors proposed sealing their state borders to outsiders, which directly contravenes federal interstate commerce authority. Select courts issued decisions suggesting that certain constitutional rights are not implicated or can be set aside during crises (Hodge et al., 2021). There is little judicial support for these findings. What is permissible, however, are judicial interpretations entailing recalibrations of constitutional rights against the backdrop of governments' compelling interests in quelling emerging and deadly infectious diseases. In the end, balancing emergency public health powers and societal or individual rights and ethics is a necessary part of effective response efforts.

CASE STUDY 1: FEDERAL AND STATE AUTHORITY TO RESPOND TO PUBLIC HEALTH EMERGENCIES

In late 2019, the World Health Organization (WHO) received reports of a novel coronavirus in a cluster of patients in Wuhan, Hubei Province, China (Phelan et al., 2020). The highly transmissible virus, later designated COVID-19, spread rapidly across the globe, resulting in a worldwide pandemic by March 2020 (WHO, 2020). COVID-19's spread throughout the United States during 2020 to 2021 set off emergency declarations and responses at all levels of government to prevent transmission in the hopes of lowering morbidity and mortality (Hodge et al., 2021). Differences in legal authorities among states and the public health strategies applied across jurisdictions resulted in an amalgam of approaches.

FEDERAL GOVERNMENT RESPONSES

During PHEs, the federal government has traditionally acted to support state/territorial/tribal/local governments confronting crises on the front lines, as

PHEs are not always national in their scope and state powers provide broad authority to respond (Hodge, 2018). While the federal government can place appropriate conditions on the receipt of federal funds and regulate interstate commerce, it cannot step beyond its constitutionally enumerated powers (Hodge, 2018). The federal government also cannot order state actors to enforce federal law under principles of federalism (*New York v. United States*, 1992; *Printz v. United States*, 1997). These limitations illustrate why certain uniform federal COVID-19 responses, including implementation of federal mask mandates or intrastate quarantines and business closures, are difficult to justify and enforce.

Despite these limitations, national emergency powers enabled the issuance of several federal emergency declarations at the inception of the pandemic, authorizing expedited emergency responses. On January 31, 2020, HHS Secretary Alex Azar declared a national PHE (HHS, 2020) allowing for the provision of emergency funding, waiver of specific federal laws, support of social distancing via telehealth services, and more (42 U.S.C. § 247d; Elsea et al., 2020). Shortly thereafter, Secretary Azar issued a PREP Act Declaration effective February 4, paving the way for specific MCMs and immunizing from liability certain persons involved in their provision (85 Fed. Reg. 15,198, 2020).

President Donald Trump declared national emergencies via the Stafford
Act and NEA on March 13, 2020 (85 Fed. Reg. 15,337, 2020; Trump, 2020b).
The NEA declaration enabled the HHS secretary to waive certain program
requirements (including Medicare and Medicaid) and the Health Insurance
Portability and Accountability Act (HIPAA) Privacy Rule as necessary. The
Stafford declaration allowed FEMA to provide additional assistance to states. 6
President Trump also invoked the **Defense Production Act** via a March 18
executive order, opening avenues to require American companies to engage 15
in certain necessary manufacturing (e.g., personal protective equipment and
ventilators; Trump, 2020a). 3

The federal government also implemented specific social distancing
actions to curb COVID-19's spread. On September 30, 2020, CDC's director banned cruise ships from allowing new passengers on board until 6
November 1, 2020 (Thaler, 2020). On January 20, 2021, President Joe Biden
issued an executive order requiring mask wearing and social distancing on 16
federal lands and in federal buildings (Biden, 2021). Nevertheless, the primary actors in issuing social distancing orders to prevent COVID-19 trans- 3
mission, including mask mandates, curfews, and more, were state and local
governments (Blum, 2020).

STATE GOVERNMENT RESPONSES

As noted earlier, state governments have primary authority to protect the public's health through their *police* and *parens patriae* powers (Berman, 2020). However, emergency powers and responses differ across states as per their statutes, regulations, and court decisions (Blum, 2020). These legal distinctions, when paired with varying strategic or political approaches, resulted in contrasting state responses (Gordon, 2020).

State-level PHE declarations generally permit state and local officials to issue public health orders including the following: isolation, quarantine,

curfews, and other social distancing measures; screening, testing, and vaccinating persons; closing businesses; and more (Hodge, 2018). From the outset of the COVID-19 pandemic, states utilized these emergency powers differently. Several
6 states, including California and Oregon, employed more restrictive approaches, issuing mandatory shelter in place or stay-at-home orders by March 23, 2020.
9 Other states, including Florida and South Dakota, implemented advisory, rather than mandatory, orders. A few states, including Arkansas, Nebraska, and North
3 Dakota, did not implement any form of stay-at-home order. Between March 1 and May 31, 2020, 42 jurisdictions, including states and U.S. territories, had implemented mandatory stay-at-home orders, eight others had issued advisory stay-at-home orders, and six had not issued stay-at-home orders (Moreland et al., 2020).

State jurisdictions diverged in their approaches to additional social distancing requirements, including mask mandates, curfews, and business closures (Leatherby & Harris, 2020). Some states were quick to reopen, while others implemented extended social distancing measures, at times resulting in litigation (Hodge et al., 2020, 2021). Some local governments implemented requirements in the absence of state orders, or alternatively refused to comply with state directives, provoking further legal action (Haddow et al., 2020; Hodge et al., 2020). States diverged even on administrative details, including reporting terminology and mechanisms (Kettl, 2020).

Significant public health repercussions arose rapidly, with differences in cases and deaths noted among states. An analysis of the early months of the pandemic comparing states with and without stay-at-home orders found that the epidemic doubling time was significantly increased in states with orders (Lurie et al., 2020). By November 2020, states implementing fewer restrictions were experiencing more severe outbreaks (Leatherby & Harris, 2020). According to April 2021 data, North and South Dakota, two of the states employing the least restrictive COVID-19 responses in the nation, possessed the highest per capita death rates (*New York Times*, n.d.). Numerous additional variables, including the presence of sprawling metropolitan areas, also impacted results (Hamidi, 2020). The relationship between the restrictiveness of state responses and morbidity and mortality is not linear, and additional analysis is needed to understand the effects of orders, as demonstrated by converging per capita death rates in California and Florida in early 2021 despite differing approaches (Curley, 2021).

Responses to COVID-19 illustrate the federal government's ability to support state and local frontline actions during PHEs. Nevertheless, postpandemic critical analyses include the potential for more active federal interventions in future PHEs, particularly given widely contrasting state strategies (Hodge, 2021).

CASE STUDY 2: PUBLIC HEALTH POWERS AND INDIVIDUAL RIGHTS

On March 23, 2014, the WHO reported cases of Ebola Virus Disease (EVD) in Guinea, which marked the commencement of the largest epidemic of the disease in history (CDC, n.d.-h). EVD is a severe, often fatal illness spread through direct contact with body fluids of a person who is sick with or has died from EVD. At the time of the outbreak, there was no vaccine or specific treatment for EVD. The virus quickly spread to Sierra Leone and Liberia, with cases reported in dense, urban areas, including the capitals, a marked departure from previous outbreaks in rural areas. The WHO declared a **Public Health Emergency of International Concern (PHEIC)** on August 8, 2014. International resources were marshalled for a coordinated response (WHO, 2014). The CDC deployed workers to West Africa to support the effort, and international medical aid workers, including those from the United States, provided care to the sick.

While the WHO worked to stem the spread of EVD in West Africa, the U.S. federal government and states mounted domestic public health responses to prevent cases from being introduced domestically via travel. The federal government routed flights from areas with active EVD outbreaks through specific airports and screened thousands of travelers for EVD exposure risk and symptoms (CDC, n.d.-h). The CDC also issued guidance to states on isolation for cases and quarantine for exposed individuals identified through federal screening. This guidance provided for a tiered approach to quarantine, with the types of movement restrictions imposed on individuals tailored to their specific level of risk for becoming ill, based on history of exposure (CDC, 2014). States prepared quarantine orders directed to individual travelers and set up monitoring systems. Against this backdrop, Kaci Hickox, an American nurse who volunteered with Médecins Sans Frontières treating patients with EVD in Sierra Leone, returned home to the United States in October 2014.

On October 22, New Jersey Governor Chris Christie signed Executive Order 164, which created a statewide Ebola Preparedness Plan that included provisions for isolation and quarantine (Christie, 2014). On October 24, Hickox flew into Newark Liberty International Airport. Upon arrival, she was screened for symptoms and assessed for contact with known EVD cases. Initial screening showed an elevated temperature. She was immediately transferred to an isolation tent outside of University Hospital in Newark. An order was issued by the state health commissioner quarantining Hickox in New Jersey (*Hickox v. Christie*, 2016).

1,2,5,6 9 3

Hickox remained in the isolation tent, which lacked amenities beyond a portable toilet, handwashing station, and bed, while the state monitored her symptoms and awaited results from her tests over 3 days. After a negative blood test and 24 hours without symptoms, Hickox was transported to her home state of Maine by emergency medical technicians. Later she filed a lawsuit challenging her original quarantine measures in New Jersey, asserting individual liberties infringements in violation of due process (*Hickox v. Christie*, 2016). An agreement was reached between Hickox and the State of New Jersey in 2017 that placed binding requirements in place for the state to only impose quarantine for EVD when medically and epidemiologically necessary, use the least restrictive means necessary to prevent the spread of EVD, and provide detailed orders that include information on the medical and legal basis of the order and the right to appeal it (American Civil Liberties Union of New Jersey, 2017).

Upon her arrival in Maine on October 27, 2014, Hickox, although asymptomatic, was placed under a home quarantine order that substantially restricted her public movement. After indicating her intent not to comply with quarantine, the state filed a court order seeking to impose specific conditions (Dexter, 2016). The quarantine conditions were in part a product of the tiered approach contained in CDC guidance, which prescribed additional monitoring and restrictions for those having had close contact with known EVD cases, such as healthcare workers (CDC, 2014).

The court recognized the importance of protecting the public from EVD but denied the state's request for what amounted to a full quarantine. It found that the State of Maine did not prove by clear and convincing evidence that it was "necessary to protect other individuals from the dangers of infection" by imposing such movement restrictions (*Mayhew v. Hickox*, 2014). EVD is not spread by aerosols or casual contact, and asymptomatic transmission is uncommon. As a result, comprehensive movement restrictions are not supported by the epidemiology of the disease. The court did uphold the requirement to submit to direct active monitoring, coordinate travel with health officials, and inform them of any symptoms—the least restrictive alternative available for preventing spread of the disease (*Mayhew v. Hickox*, 2014). Hickox subsequently agreed to comply with the terms of the court's order through the remainder of her 21-day monitoring period.

Some public health lawyers supported Hickox's challenges of her quarantines, especially given the important role of international medical workers in responding to PHEICs and the potential chilling effect of quarantines (Gostin, 2014). As of July 2017, the CDC has retired its "Interim U.S. Guidance for Monitoring and Movement of Persons With Potential Ebola Virus Exposure," which represented an evolution in quarantine by providing a graded series of restrictions based on individualized assessments (CDC, 2017). The guidance, together with the Hickox cases, demonstrate the importance of decision-making by state and local public health officials during emergencies using available data, legal guidance, and ethical principles to prevent government overreach. Public health officials must carefully weigh options when imposing restrictions on individuals that potentially infringe upon their individual liberty for the common good.

CASE STUDY 3: LOCAL RESPONSE TO EMERGING THREATS

Overdose deaths in the United States have quadrupled since 1999 due to abuse of prescription and illicit opioids (CDC, n.d.-f). Over 841,000 individuals have perished in overdoses so far (CDC, n.d.-g). States and localities have taken innovative actions to reduce these alarming statistics. Many local responses have demonstrated successful reductions in opioid-related deaths (CDC, n.d.-e).

Arizona's opioid crisis statistics drove innovation in state and local responses. In 2016 alone, 431 million pills were prescribed in the state with a population just under 7 million (The Arizona Opioid Epidemic Act, 2018). Arizona's Department of Health Services (ADHS) published a 2016 report cataloguing 51,473 opioid-related hospital encounters that year, indicating that 790 deaths (more than two per day) could be directly attributed to opioids (ADHS, 2017b). From 2009 to 2015, ADHS estimated over $1.6 billion in costs for opioid-related hospital encounters (ADHS, 2017b).

1,2,5,6 These concerning public health trends spurred Arizona's Governor Doug
Ducey to declare a state of emergency on June 5, 2017 (Ducey, 2017a) consis-
4,9 tent with the state's adoption of key provisions of the aforementioned MSEHPA
(Hodge et al., 2017). Other states including Massachusetts, Virginia, Alaska,
3 Maryland, and Florida issued similar declarations (Rutkow & Vernick, 2017). On
October 27, 2017, the federal government declared the opioid crisis a national
PHE (HHS, 2017). Arizona's declaration directed control and coordination of
state assets through ADHS, whose director was authorized to issue an Enhanced

Surveillance Advisory, initiate emergency rulemaking on opioid prescribing and treatment, report on additional needs and recommendations for legislative action, and develop prescribing practice guidelines and protocols/training relating to naloxone. ADHS (2017b) completed a 50-state review of opioid policy in August 2017 to better understand best practices across the nation. By virtue of an additional executive order, Governor Ducey compelled agency reporting, within 24 hours, of suspected overdoses and fatalities, naloxone administrations, and overdose trends by county through a novel, publicly accessible ADHS data dashboard (ADHS, 2021; Ducey, 2017b). ADHS also utilized its emergency rulemaking authority to implement stricter prescribing/treatment practices in health facilities in the state (Opioid Prescribing and Treatment, 2019). In January 2018, the state legislature passed the Arizona Epidemic Act of 2018, which, among other requirements, placed limits both on dosage and length of opioid prescriptions (S.B. 1001, 53rd Leg, 1st Spec. Sess, 2018).

1,2,9
11
1,2,3
5
14
3

The declaration made available $500,000 in the emergency public health fund, allowing for increased naloxone distribution in local communities (Locke & Dedon, 2019). County public health agencies used the state database to compare local trends to statewide information (Coconino County Public Health Services District, 2017; Weisman, 2019). The City of Tempe (2021) created its own online opioid dashboard, tracking EMS calls. Pima County developed a strategic action plan as a complement to ADHS's report and recommendations (City of Tempe, 2021; Healthy Pima, 2018). Maricopa County worked to coordinate with the governor's office and implemented an award-winning program targeting misuse and addiction in the jail system (Maricopa County, 2017, 2021).

1,2
3,4
2,3

Arizona's emergency declaration and subsequent actions on a state and local level produced significant results. The year following the declaration witnessed a 44% reduction in reported opioid overdoses (Sunshine et al., 2019). Arizona's dispensed opioid prescriptions per month dropped by 23% from July 2017 to November 2019. In roughly that same period, naloxone dispensations increased by 185% (ADHS, 2020). Arizona's opioid-related emergency declaration allowed implementation of best practices, spurred innovative responses, and opened emergency options, fueling more rapid progress at state and local levels.

CASE STUDY 4: LEGAL RESPONSE TO ENVIRONMENTAL CONTAMINATION

Lead is a potent neurotoxin with acute and long-term health impacts. Lead dust from industrial pollution, and the historic use of lead in paint and gasoline, persists in the environment and remains hazardous until remediated. In children, lead exposure can cause persistent cognitive deficits and psychological impairments (Ettinger et al., 2019), even at low levels of exposure and without obvious symptoms (CDC, n.d.-a). Annually, preventable childhood lead exposure is estimated to cost $50.9 billion in lost economic productivity stemming from reduced cognitive potential (Trasande & Liu, 2011). In adults, lead exposure can increase risk for high blood pressure, heart disease, kidney disease, and cancer (CDC, n.d.-d). Consequently, sustained initiatives enabled by federal and state laws aim to prevent lead poisoning and remove lead in the environment.

In Vernon, California, south of downtown Los Angeles, a battery recycling plant, Exide Technologies, Inc. (Exide), polluted communities across multiple cities with lead for decades. The eventual closure of this plant and subsequent efforts to address the contamination demonstrate the challenges of responding to health crises that are many years in the making. The response to the lead contamination caused by Exide included community advocacy for cleanup and resources, technical assessments to characterize the scope of the contamination, public health agency support for the health of residents, interagency engagement to implement response and remediation plans, and, ultimately, litigation aimed at recovering costs. But, diverging from the previous case studies in this chapter, the Exide response importantly did not include the declaration of a PHE. Efforts to fund and complete the lead cleanup of the site and the surrounding communities are still ongoing, even though the Exide facility closed in 2015.

Prior to its closure, the Exide facility operated under interim status authorization from the California Department of Toxic Substances Control (DTSC), a state agency with primary oversight authority over the facility (County of Los Angeles Department of Public Health, 2016). Stacks at the facility emitted lead at levels exceeding federal standards, as monitored by the Southern California Air Quality Management District (AQMD; South Coast Air Quality Management District, n.d.), and various DTSC investigations identified widespread soil contamination at the site (Barboza, 2015). Facing prosecution for the illegal disposal, storage, shipment, and transportation of hazardous waste by the U.S. Department of Justice (DOJ, 2015), Exide agreed to close down its operations.

The areas surrounding Exide are home to approximately 100,000 residents, the majority of whom are Latino (Johnston et al., 2020). Environmental assessments identify the areas as some of the most environmentally burdened in California (Johnston et al., 2020). Lead contamination produced by Exide impacted homes, schools, and community facilities within a 1.75-mile radius of the facility, posing a risk for elevated blood lead levels in children (County of Los Angeles Department of Public Health, 2016). A study by the California Department of Public Health found children living closer to the Exide facility had higher blood lead levels than those living further away (Barboza, 2016). Following closure of the Exide facility, the process of identifying and prioritizing the most affected properties and removing lead-contaminated soil progressed slowly, hampered by the magnitude of the funding needed and the challenges posed by the administration of a cleanup spanning multiple cities and thousands of properties. Community members,
4 advocates, and representatives, along with the Los Angeles County Department of Public Health, continually called attention to the major environmental justice
13 and health equity issues at stake (Los Angeles Times Editorial Board, 2016).

In contrast to Arizona's response to the opioid epidemic, during which a PHE
1,2,3 declaration hastened coordination and provided access to increased funding, the lead contamination of the neighborhoods surrounding Exide was never declared a PHE. California's state government did not take steps to support residential cleanup efforts with emergency declarations of any kind, though it was a topic of political debate and community outcry (Mason, 2016). In addition, no emergency actions were taken at the federal level by the Environmental Protection Agency (EPA), HHS, or otherwise. Despite multiple local government entities and agencies characterizing the lead contamination as an emergency or a disaster (County of Los Angeles, Chief Executive Officer, 2017; Los Angeles City Council, 2017), the DTSC stated early on that the level of lead contamination associated with Exide was not a PHE despite the documented public health impacts (Florido,

2014; Garrison, 2014), and did not revisit this decision as additional data 1,2
became available. Over the ensuing years, environmental assessments more
fully characterized the threat, which found that nearly 8,000 homes reached 4
lead contamination levels hazardous to health and requiring remediation
(Auditor of the State of California, 2020). 1,2

Contemporaneous with the initiation of Exide cleanup efforts in California, the Flint water crisis was developing in Michigan. In response to this incident involving lead contamination of the water supply in Flint, Michigan, federal, state, and local PHEs were declared to mobilize resources and restore safe water to residents (HHS, 2021). These declarations, while delayed in their making (Flint Water Advisory Task Force, 2016), brought federal technical assistance, funding, and response supplies, including filters and testing kits (The White House, 2016), to Flint—a majority-Black city of 90,000 where about 40% of residents live below the federal poverty level (Kennedy, 2016). After a significant and sustained response, along with infrastructure investments, the water system's lead levels were brought back within EPA thresholds (EPA, n.d.). However, the health harms to residents, which included a doubling in the number of children with elevated blood lead levels during the water crisis, will persist into the future through cognitive impacts and increased chronic disease risks (Hanna-Attisha et al., 2016). In comparison to Flint, progress of the Exide cleanup in California is slower, and a resolution for impacted communities has not yet been reached.

The effort to remove lead contamination from the communities around Exide is the state's largest environmental undertaking of this kind, with an average cost to remediate a lead-contaminated yard of $45,000 (Barboza & Poston, 2018), and total estimates for the cleanup as high as $630 million (Auditor of the State of California, 2020). In complicated and costly situations like this, local public health orders for lead abatement are insufficient, especially when the responsible entity is bankrupt, as is the case with Exide. Moving forward, the state is seeking to recover its costs for cleaning up the lead contamination from other potentially contributory companies through litigation, but such efforts can take years (Barboza, 2020).

Thus far, California has allocated $260 million of its own funds for the cleanup (Auditor of the State of California, 2020). The DTSC sought to reach 3,200 of the most contaminated properties by June 2021, but projections indicated this benchmark was unlikely to be met (Auditor of the State of California, 2020). The pace of cleanup has been widely criticized by community members (Barboza, 2020), and additional funds will be needed to address the remaining balance of the affected properties (Auditor of the State of California, 2020). Commentary from a recent bankruptcy court decision allowing Exide to abandon the property and turn over cleanup responsibility to the state demonstrates remaining preconceptions about the nature of PHEs. Because "the entire property is not . . . a seething, glowing toxic lead situation," the court found no immediate threat to the public in allowing the abandonment (*In re Exide Holdings, Inc.*, 2020).

Response to PHEs and the application of declarations have evolved and expanded, potentially encompassing environmental issues that develop over time but result in emergent health threats (Sunshine et al., 2019). Failure to implement emergency declarations when needed can prolong response efforts to the detriment of public health and compound the burdens of environmental injustices in communities already harmed by health inequities.

CONCLUSION

The law provides the tools and the parameters for responses to multifarious PHEs. Consistent with constitutional design and principles, federal and state laws direct and allocate authority to act in response to health risks and threats. Public health agents and other government officials have significant decision-making power to protect the health, safety, and welfare of communities and apply available epidemiologic and scientific information, best practices, and ethical norms to lead PHE responses.

DISCUSSION QUESTIONS

1. Making and implementing public health laws, even in a PHE, must balance the duties to advance public health with the limits on constraining individual liberties for the common good. Describe factors determined by the U.S. Supreme Court to be a "floor" of constitutional protections to prevent governmental overreach and protect individual rights.
2. Describe the concept of "preemption" and the interplay between the roles and responsibilities of the federal and state governments to make and enforce laws and regulations.
3. Discuss some of the legal tools and interventions that public health departments can use in a declared PHE.
4. What are some of the federal emergency laws that the U.S. Congress has authorized that provide federal emergency powers and general emergency authorities?

SUMMARY

TABLE 16.1 Select Essential Services of Public Health Demonstrated in Public Health Law Foundations and Applications During Emergencies

Essential Service # and Definition	Context in Chapter Case	Competency # It Ties to	Importance for Emergency Preparedness, Response, or Recovery
6. Utilize legal and regulatory actions designed to improve and protect the public's health (Policy Development)	Invoking the Defense Production Act, opening avenues to require American companies to engage in certain necessary manufacturing during the COVID-19 pandemic	15	Shortages of personal protective equipment and ventilators required an evaluation of policies to protect public health and health equity.
6. Utilize legal and regulatory actions designed to improve and protect the public's health (Policy Development)	Issuing mandatory shelter in place or stay-at-home orders during the COVID-19 pandemic	9	To prevent or reduce high levels of disease transmission in the community.
5. Create, champion, and implement policies, plans, and laws that impact health (Policy Development)	Creating a statewide Ebola Preparedness Plan that includes provisions for isolation and quarantine	9	Provides a framework for coordinated action throughout the state.
1. Assess and monitor population health status, factors that influence health, and community needs and assets (Assessment)	Monitoring the opioid crisis statistics and public health trends	4	Documented the public health crisis to call attention to the need for action.
5. Create, champion, and implement policies, plans, and laws that impact health (Policy Development)	Placing limits both on dosage and length of opioid prescriptions	14	Restrictions on opioid prescriptions may prevent addiction.
4. Strengthen, support, and mobilize communities and partnerships to improve health (Policy Development)	Community members, advocates, and representatives, along with the County Department of Public Health, continually called attention to the major environmental justice and health equity issues at stake related to environmental lead contamination.	13	The role of an informed community and their leaders strengthens the voice of public health in dealing with community emergencies

TABLE 16.2 Select CEPH Competencies Needed for Frontline Health Workers, Managers, and Leaders for Public Health Law Foundations and Applications During Emergencies

Competency # and Definition	Context in Case/Chapter	Level	Importance for Emergency Preparedness, Response, or Recovery
16. Apply leadership and/or management principles to address a relevant health issue.	The U.S. president issued an executive order requiring mask wearing and social distancing on federal lands and in federal buildings.	Level 3	Puts into place and demonstrates the actions needed at all levels to prevent the transmission of COVID-19.
11. Select methods to evaluate public health programs.	Completed a 50-state review of opioid policy to better understand best practices across the nation.	Levels 1, 2, 3	Provided a mechanism to evaluate public health actions to identify best approaches to address the opioid crisis. Persons at all levels were needed to collect data, analyze data, and make policy decisions based on data.
4. Interpret results of data analysis for public health research, policy, or practice.	County public health agencies used the state database to compare local trends to statewide information.	Levels 2, 3	Local data analysis and interpretation at both supervisory and leadership levels allows for local public health agencies and elected leaders to better understand how their local policies are impacting the opioid crisis.
4. Interpret results of data analysis for public health research, policy, or practice.	Environmental assessments more fully characterized the threat, which found that nearly 8,000 homes reached lead contamination levels hazardous to health and requiring remediation.	Levels 1, 2	Data analysis of environmental threats provides a documentation and quantification of the threat that can identify specific areas where remedial actions are needed.

Key: Essential services of public health; CEPH competencies; Leadership levels.

REFERENCES

Alfred L. Snapp & Son, Inc. v. Puerto Rico, 458 US 592, 603 (1982).

American Civil Liberties Union of New Jersey. (2017). *Victory: Detained nurse's Ebola suit secures due process.* https://www.aclu-nj.org/news/2017/07/27/victory-detained-nurses-ebola-suit-secures-due-process

American Rescue Plan Act, Pub. L. No. 117-2, 135 Stat. 2 (2021).

Arizona Department of Health Services. (2017a). *50 state review on opioid related policy.* https://azdhs.gov/documents/prevention/womens-childrens-health/injury-prevention/opioid-prevention/50-state-review-opioid-related-policy.pdf

Arizona Department of Health Services. (2017b). *2016 Arizona opioid report.* https://www.azdhs.gov/documents/audiences/clinicians/clinical-guidelines-recommendations/prescribing-guidelines/arizona-opioid-report.pdf

Arizona Department of Health Services. (2020). *Opioid update & surveillance data summary,* July 1, 2017–December 31, 2019. https://www.azdhs.gov/documents/prevention/health-systems-development/epidamic/update-adhs-opioid-response-2017-2019.pdf

Arizona Department of Health Services. (2021). *Opioid interactive dashboard.* https://www.azdhs.gov/prevention/womens-childrens-health/injury-prevention/opioid-prevention/opioids/index.php#dashboard

The Arizona Opioid Epidemic Act: Protecting individuals with chronic pain. (2018). https://azgovernor.gov/sites/default/fi les/related-docs/chronicpainweb_0.pdf

Atomic Energy Act of 1954, 42 U.S.C. § 2011 *et seq.*

Auditor of the State of California. (2020). *The state's poor management of the Exide cleanup project has left Californians at continued risk of lead poisoning.* http://auditor.ca.gov/pdfs/reports/2020-107.pdf

Ausness, R. C. (2014). The role of litigation in the fight against prescription drug abuse. *West Virginia Law Review, 116,* 1117. https://researchrepository.wvu.edu/wvlr/vol116/iss3/12

Barboza, T. (2015). Exide's troubled history: Years of pollution violations but few penalties. *Los Angeles Times.* https://graphics.latimes.com/exide-battery-plant

Barboza, T. (2016). Exide's troubled history: Years of pollution violations but few penalties. *Los Angeles Times.* https://www.latimes.com/local/lanow/la-me-exide-children-blood-lead-levels-20160408-story.html

Barboza, T. (2020). California sues to recover costs for Exide lead cleanup, but community still wants justice. *Los Angeles Times.* https://www.latimes.com/california/story/2020-12-19/state-lawsuit-to-recover-exide-cleanup-cost-targets-past-operators

Barboza, T., & Poston, B. (2018). The Exide plant in Vernon closed 3 years ago: The vast majority of lead-contaminated properties remain uncleaned. *Los Angeles Times.* https://www.latimes.com/local/lanow/la-me-exide-cleanup-20180426-story.html

Berman, E. (2020). The roles of the state and federal governments in a pandemic. *Journal of National Security Law & Policy, 11*(16), 63. https://doi.org/10.2139/ssrn.3617058

Biden, J. R., Jr. (2021). *Executive order on protecting the federal workforce and requiring mask-wearing.* https://www.whitehouse.gov/briefing-room/presidential-actions/2021/01/20/executive-order-protecting-the-federal-workforce-and-requiring-mask-wearing

Blum, S. C. (2020). Federalism: Fault or feature: An analysis of whether the United States should implement a federal pandemic statute. *Washburn Law Journal, 60*(1), 1–61. https://contentdm.washburnlaw.edu/digital/collection/wlj/id/7276

Burris, S., de Guia, S., Gable, L., Levin, D.E., Parmet, W.E., & Terry, N.P. (Eds.). (2020). *Assessing legal responses to COVID-19.* Public Health Law Watch. https://static1.squarespace.com/static/5956e16e6b8f5b8c45f1c216/t/5f4d6578225705285562d0f0/1598908033901/COVID19PolicyPlaybook_Aug2020+Full.pdf

Cabrera, O., Hodge, J. G., Jr., & Gostin, L. O. (2008). *Express tuberculosis control laws in selected U.S. jurisdictions: A report to the Centers for Disease Control and Prevention.* https://www.cdc.gov/phlp/docs/Centers_Report-Express_TB_Control_Laws-Final.pdf

Cal. Health & Safety Code § 101040. (1995).

Cal. Health & Safety Code § 120175. (1996).

California Restaurant Association, Inc. v. County of Los Angeles Department of Public Health, et al. No. 20STCP03881 (2020). https://www.courthousenews.com/wp-content/uploads/2020/12/CRA_LACounty-RULING_compressed.pdf

CARES Act, Pub. L. No. 116-136, 134 Stat. 281 (2020).

Center for Law and the Public's Health. (2006). *MSEHPA state legislative activity table.* http://www.publichealthlaw.net/MSEHPA/MSEHPA%20Leg%20Activity.pdf

Centers for Disease Control and Prevention. (n.d.-a). *Blood lead levels in children.* https://www.cdc.gov/nceh/lead/prevention/blood-lead-levels.htm

Centers for Disease Control and Prevention (n.d.-b). *CDC's Public Health Emergency Preparedness Program: Every response is local.* https://www.cdc.gov/cpr/whatwedo/phep.htm

Centers for Disease Control and Prevention. (n.d.-c). *Emergency Preparedness funding.* https://www.cdc.gov/cpr/epf/index.htm

Centers for Disease Control and Prevention. (n.d.-d). *Health Problems Caused by Lead: Information for workers.* https://www.cdc.gov/niosh/topics/lead/health.html

Centers for Disease Control and Prevention. (n.d.-e). *Opioid overdose: State successes.* https://www.cdc.gov/drugoverdose/policy/successes.html

Centers for Disease Control and Prevention. (n.d.-f). *Opioids: Understanding the epidemic.* https://www.cdc.gov/drugoverdose/epidemic/index.html

Centers for Disease Control and Prevention. (n.d.-g). *The drug overdose epidemic: Behind the numbers.* https://www.cdc.gov/drugoverdose/data/index.html

Centers for Disease Control and Prevention. (n.d.-h). *2014-2016 Ebola outbreak in West Africa.* https://www.cdc.gov/vhf/ebola/history/2014-2016-outbreak/index.html

Centers for Disease Control and Prevention. (2014). Announcement: Interim U.S. guidance for monitoring and movement of persons with potential Ebola virus exposure. *Morbidity and Mortality Weekly Report, 63*(43), 984. https://www.cdc.gov/mmwr/preview/mmwrhtml/mm6343a5.htm

Centers for Disease Control and Prevention. (2017). *Notes on the interim U.S. guidance for monitoring and movement of persons with potential Ebola virus exposure.* https://www.cdc.gov/vhf/ebola/exposure/monitoring-and-movement-of-persons-with-exposure.html

Chemerinsky, E. (2015). *Constitutional law: Principles and policies 1* (5th ed.). Wolters Kluwer Law & Business.

Christie, C. (2014). *Executive Order No. 164.* https://nj.gov/infobank/circular/eocc164.pdf

City of Tempe. (2021). *Opioid abuse probable EMS call dashboard.* https://tempegov.maps.arcgis.com/apps/opsdashboard/index.html#/374b80b6ab65483e8ea4d30bf0100c23

Clean Air Act, 42 U.S.C. § 7401 *et seq.* (2018).

Clean Water Act, 33 U.S.C. §§ 1251-1388 (2018).

Coconino County Public Health Services District. (2017). *Opioid poisoning and abuse among Coconino County residents.* https://www.coconino.az.gov/DocumentCenter/View/17695/Opioid-Report-6-9-17-

Consolidated Appropriations Act, Pub. L. No: 116-260 (2020). https://www.congress.gov/116/bills/hr133/BILLS-116hr133enr.pdf

County of Los Angeles, Chief Executive Officer. (2017). *Semi-annual report on board priorities.* http://file.lacounty.gov/SDSInter/bos/bc/1016629_SemiAnnualReportonBoardPriorities010417.pdf

County of Los Angeles Department of Health v. Superior Court, 61 Cal. App. 5th 478, 478 (2021).

County of Los Angeles Department of Public Health. (2016). *Status report on issues related to Exide.* http://file.lacounty.gov/SDSInter/bos/bc/240684_StatusReportonIssuesRelatedtoExide.PDF

Curley, C. (2021). Why do California and Florida have similar COVID-19 case rates? The answer is complicated. *Healthline.* https://www.healthline.com/health-news/why-do-california-and-florida-have-similar-covid-19-case-rates-the-answer-is-complicated

Declaration Under the Public Readiness and Emergency Preparedness Act for Medical Countermeasures Against COVID-19, 85 Fed. Reg. 15,198 (March 17, 2020).

Declaring a National Emergency Concerning the Novel Coronavirus Disease (COVID-19) Outbreak, 85 Fed. Reg. 15,337 (March 18, 2020).

Dexter, B. W. (2016). Mayhew v. Hickox: Balancing Maine's public health with personal liberties during the Ebola "Crisis." *Maine Law Review, 68,* 263–285. https://digitalcommons.mainelaw.maine.edu/cgi/viewcontent.cgi?article=1023&context=mlr

Ducey, D. A. (2017a). *Declaration of emergency and notification of enhanced surveillance advisory, opioid overdose epidemic.* https://azgovernor.gov/sites/default/files/related-docs/opioid_declaration.pdf

Ducey. D. A. (2017b). *Executive order 2017-04: Enhanced surveillance advisory.* https://azgovernor.gov/sites/default/files/eo_2017-04_0.pdf

Elsea, J. K., Sykes, J. B., Lampe, J. R., Lewis, K. M., & Adkins, B. L. (2020). *Emergency authorities under the National Emergencies Act, Stafford Act, and Public Health Service Act.* Congressional Research Service. https://fas.org/sgp/crs/natsec/R46379.pdf

Ettinger, A., Leonard, M. L., & Mason, J. (2019). CDC's Lead Poisoning Prevention Program: A long-standing responsibility and commitment to protect children from lead exposure. *Journal of Public Health Management and Practice, 25,* S5–S12. https://doi.org/10.1097/PHH.0000000000000868

Families First Coronavirus Response Act, Pub. L. No. 116–127, 134 Stat. 178 (2020).

Federalism. (2019). *Black's law dictionary* (11th ed., p. 755). Thomson West.

50 U.S.C.A. §§ 1601, 1621, 1622, 1631, 1641, 1651 (West, 2020).

Flint Water Advisory Task Force. (2016). *Flint Water Advisory Task Force–Final report*. https://www.michigan.gov/documents/snyder/FWATF_FINAL_REPORT_21March2016_517805_7.pdf

Florido, A. (2014). *Free blood tests for Exide neighbors are still more than 2 weeks off*. Southern California Public Radio. https://www.scpr.org/news/2014/03/20/42916/regulators-tell-exide-neighbors-to-keep-kids-out-o/

42 U.S.C. § 247d

42 U.S.C. § 247d–6d (2012).

42 U.S.C.A. § 201 et seq. (2020).

42 U.S.C.A. § 247d(a) (West, 2020).

42 U.S.C.A. § 5121 et seq.

42 U.S.C.A. §§ 5170, 5122(1) (West, 2020).

Garrison, J. (2014). Lead found in soil of homes near Exide plant; health alert issued. *Los Angeles Times*. https://www.latimes.com/local/lanow/la-xpm-2014-mar-10-la-me-ln-exide-lead-homes-20140310-story.html

Gordon, S. H. (2020). What federalism means for the US response to coronavirus disease 2019. *JAMA Health Forum*. https://jamanetwork.com/channels/health-forum/fullarticle/2766033

Gostin, L. O. (2001). Public health theory and practice in the constitutional design. *Health Matrix Clevel, 11*(2), 265–326. https://scholarlycommons.law.case.edu/cgi/viewcontent.cgi?article=1559&context=healthmatrix

Gostin, L. O. (2005). *Jacobson v. Massachusetts* at 100 years: Police power and civil liberties in tension. *American Public Health Association, 95*, 576–581. https://doi.org/10.2105/AJPH.2004.055152

Gostin, L. O. (2008). *Public health law: Power, duty, restraint* (2nd ed.). University of California Press.

Gostin, L. O. (2010). *Public health law & ethics: A reader*. University of California Press.

Gostin, L. O. (2014). The United States' misguided self-interest on Ebola. *Health Affairs Blog*. https://www.healthaffairs.org/do/10.1377/hblog20141031.042420/full/

Gostin, L. O., & Wiley, L. F. (2016). *Public health law: Power, duty, restraint* (3rd ed., pp. 3–38). University of California Press.

Gostin, L. O., & Wiley, L. F. (2020). Governmental public health powers during the COVID-19 pandemic. *JAMA, 323*, 2137–2138. https://doi.org/10.1001/jama.2020.5460

Gostin, L. O., Sapsin, J. W., Teret, S. P., Burris, S., Mair, J. S., & Hodge, J. G. (2002). The Model State Emergency Health Powers Act: Planning and response to bioterrorism and naturally occurring infectious diseases. *JAMA, 288*, 622–628. https://doi.org/10.1001/jama.288.5.622

Haddow, K., Carr, D., Winig, B. D., & Adler, S. (2020). Preemption, public health, and equity in the time of COVID-19. In S. Burris, S. de Guia, L. Gable, D. E. Levin, W. E. Parmet, & N. P. Terry (Eds.), *Assessing legal responses to COVID-19* (pp. 71–76). https://papers.ssrn.com/sol3/papers.cfm?abstract_id=3675884

Hamidi, S. (2020). Does density aggravate the COVID-19 pandemic? *American Journal of Planning Association, 86*, 495–509. https://doi.org/10.1080/01944363.2020.1777891

Hanna-Attisha, M., LaChance, J., Sadler, R. C., & Schnepp, A. C. (2016). Elevated blood lead levels in children associated with the flint drinking water crisis: A spatial analysis of risk and public health response. *American Journal of Public Health, 106*, 283–290. https://doi.org/10.2105/AJPH.2015.303003

Healthy Pima. (2018). *2018 action plan: Goals, objectives, and strategies*. https://www.naccho.org/uploads/downloadable-resources/44-46-Healthy-Pima-Action-Plan-Project-Description-and-Alliance-Roster.pdf

Healthy Pima. (2021). *Substance misuse*. https://healthypima.squarespace.com/substance-misuse-mental-health

Hickox v. Christie, 205 F. Supp. 3d 579 (D.N.J. 2016).

Hodge, J. G., Jr. (2016). Public health emergency legal and ethical preparedness. In G. Cohen, A. K. Hoffman & W. M. Sage (Eds.), *The Oxford handbook of American health law* (pp. 1008–1030). Oxford University Press.

Hodge, J. G., Jr. (2018). Source & scope of public health legal powers. In *Public health law in a nutshell* 35, 90 (3rd ed., pp. 29–63, 34–35, 53–54, 57–58, 97–134, 361–362). West Academic Publishing.

Hodge, J. G., Jr. (2021). Nationalizing public health emergency legal preparedness and response. *Journal of Law, Medicine, and Ethics, 49*. Advanced online publication. http://doi.org/10.2139/ssrn.3806811

Hodge, J. G., Jr., Chronister, D., Hess, A., Morcelle, M., Piatt, J., & Wetter, S. A. (2018). Public health preemption plus: Constitutional affronts to public health innovations. *Ohio State Law Journal, 79*(4), 685–703. https://kb.osu.edu/bitstream/handle/1811/87397/OSLJ_V79N4_0685.pdf

Hodge, J. G., Jr., Reinke, H., Carey, E., & Piatt, J. (2021). COVID's constitutional conundrum: Assessing individual rights in public health emergencies. *Tennessee Law Review, 88*(1). http://dx.doi.org/10.2139/ssrn.3802045

Hodge, J., Wetter, S., Carey, E., Pendergrass, E., Reeves, C., & Reinke, H. (2020). Legal "tug-of-wars" during the COVID-19 pandemic: Public health v. economic prosperity. *Journal of Law, Medicine & Ethics, 48*(3), 603–607. https://doi.org/10.1177/1073110520958888

Hodge, J. G., Jr., Wetter, S. A., & White, E. N. (2017). Redefining public health emergencies: The opioid epidemic. Journal of Jurimetrics, 58(1). https://papers.ssrn.com/sol3/papers.cfm?abstract_id=3073193

Hodge, J. G., Wetter, S. A., & White, E. N. (2019). Legal crises in public health. *Journal of Law, Medicine, and Ethics, 47*, 778–782. https://doi.org/10.1177/1073110519897792

Homeland Security Act of 2002, Pub. L. No. 107-296, 116 Stat. 2135 (2002).

In re Exide Holdings, Inc., No. 20-11157-CSS (BANKR. D. DEL. October 16, 2020).

Jacobson v. Massachusetts, 197 US 11, 12, 26, 28, 31, 38 (1905).

Jew Ho v. Williamson, 103 F. 10 (C.C.N.D. Cal. 1900).

Johnston, J. E., Lopez, mark!, Gribble, M. O., Gutschow, W., Austin, C., & Arora, M. (2020). A collaborative approach to assess legacy pollution in communities near a lead-acid battery smelter: The "Truth Fairy" project. *Health Education and Behaviour, 46*(Suppl. 1), 71S–80S. https://doi.org/10.1177/1090198119859406

Kennedy, M. (2016). *Lead-laced water in Flint: A step-by-step look at the makings of a crisis*. National Public Radio. https://www.npr.org/sections/thetwo-way/2016/04/20/465545378/lead-laced-water-in-flint-a-step-by-step-look-at-the-makings-of-a-crisis

Kettl, D. F. (2020). States divided: The implications of American federalism for COVID-19. *Public Administration Review, 80*, 595–602. https://doi.org/10.1111/puar.13243

Leatherby, L., & Harris, R. (2020). States that imposed few restrictions now have the worst outbreaks. *New York Times*. https://www.nytimes.com/interactive/2020/11/18/us/covid-state-restrictions.html

Leonard, E. W. (2010). State constitutionalism and the right to health care. *Journal of Constitutional Law, 12*, 1325–1406. https://scholarship.law.upenn.edu/cgi/viewcontent.cgi?article=1135&context=jcl

Liberian Cmty. Ass'n of Connecticut v. Lamont, 970 F.3d 174, 189 (2d Cir. 2020) (relying on *Jacobson* to uphold the Connecticut governor's authority to mandate a quarantine following a trip to Africa during the Ebola epidemic).

Locke, J., & Dedon, L. (2019). The role of state emergency powers in curbing the opioid epidemic: A case study in lessons learned. *Arizona State Law Journal, 51*, 629–673. https://arizonastatelawjournal.org/wp-content/uploads/2019/08/05-Locke-Final.pdf

Los Angeles City Council. (2017). *Motion 16-0181* (March 3, 2016). https://clkrep.lacity.org/onlinedocs/2016/16-0181_mot_02-12-2016.pdf

Los Angeles Times Editorial Board. (2016). Why does affluent Porter Ranch get more urgent environmental relief than working-class Boyle Heights? *Los Angeles Times*. https://www.latimes.com/opinion/editorials/la-ed-exide-20160131-story.html

Lurie, M. N., Silva, J., Yorlets, R. R., Tao, J., & Chan, P. A. (2020). Coronavirus disease 2019 epidemic doubling time in the United States before and during stay-at-home restrictions. *Journal of Infectious Diseases, 222*(10), 1601–1606. https://doi.org/10.1093/infdis/jiaa491

Maricopa County. (2017). *Maricopa County works to combat opioid epidemic*. https://www.maricopa.gov/CivicAlerts.aspx?AID=334&ARC=600

Maricopa County. (2021). *Award-winning programs, harm reduction: A response to the opioid epidemic in a large urban county jail*. https://www.maricopa.gov/5616/Award-Winning-Programs

Mason, M. (2016). L.A.-area and state officials call for quicker cleanup of Exide plant contamination. *Los Angeles Times*. https://www.latimes.com/politics/la-pol-sac-exide-cleanup-legislators-20160126-story.html

Mayhew v. Hickox, No. CV-2014-36 (Me. Dist. Ct., Fort Kent, October 31, 2014).

Model State Emergency Health Powers Act § 104(m). (2001). *Center for Law and the Public's Health at Georgetown and Johns Hopkins Universities*. http://www.publichealthlaw.net/MSEHPA/MSEHPA.pdf

Moreland, A., Herlihy, C., Tynan, M. A., Sunshine, G., McCord, R. F., Hilton, C., Poovey, J., Werner, A. K., Jones, C. D., Fulmer, E. B., Gundlapalli, A. V., Strosnider, H., Potvien, A., García, M. C., Honeycutt, S., Baldwin, G. (2020). Timing of state and territorial COVID-19 stay-at-home orders and changes in population movement—United States, March 1–May 31, 2020. *Morbidity and Mortality Weekly Report, 69*, 1198–1203. http://dx.doi.org/10.15585/mmwr.mm6935a2

National Association of County & City Health Officials. (2020). *2019 National profile of local health departments. Author. https://www.naccho.org/uploads/downloadable-resources/Programs/Public-Health-Infrastructure/NACCHO_2019_Profile_final.pdf*

New York Times. (n.d.). Coronavirus in the U.S.: Latest map and case count. Accessed April 2021. https://www.nytimes.com/interactive/2020/us/coronavirus-us-cases.html?action=click&module=Top%20Stories&pgtype=Homepage

New York v. United States, 505 U.S. 144, 188 (1992).

Nolan, A., Lewis, K. M., Sykes, J. B., & Hickey, K. J. (2018). *Federalism-based limitations on congressional power: An overview* (R45323). Congressional Research Service.

Opioid Prescribing and Treatment. Title 9, Arizona Administrative Code § R9-10-120. (2019).

Pandemic and All-Hazards Preparedness Act, Pub. L. No. 109-417, 120 Stat. 2831 (2006).

Parmet, W. E. (2020a). Rediscovering *Jacobson* in the era of COVID-19. *100 Boston University Law Review, 110*, 117–133. https://www.bu.edu/bulawreview/files/2020/07/PARMET.pdf

Parmet, W. E. (2020b). The COVID cases: A preliminary assessment of judicial review of public health powers during a partisan and polarized pandemic. *San Diego Law Review, 57*, 999–1038. https://digital.sandiego.edu/cgi/viewcontent.cgi?article=3394&context=sdlr

Parmet, W. E., Goodman, R. A., & Farber, A. (2005). Individual rights versus the public's health—100 years after *Jacobson v. Massachusetts. The New England Journal of Medicine, 352*, 652. https://doi.org/10.1056/NEJMp048209

Paycheck Protection Program and Healthcare Enhancement Act Pub. L. No: 116-139, 134 Stat. 620 (2020).

Phelan, A., Katz, R., & Gostin, L. O. (2020). The novel coronavirus originating in Wuhan, China: Challenges for global health governance. *Journal of American Medical Association, 323*, 709–710. https://doi.org/10.1001/jama.2020.1097

Printz v. United States, 521 U.S. 898, 900 (1997).

Project BioShield Act of 2004, Pub. L. No. 108-276, 118 Stat. 835 (2004).

Public Health Security and Bioterrorism Preparedness and Response Act of 2002, Pub. L. No. 107-188, 116 Stat. 594 (2002).

Public Health Service Act, 42 U.S.C. §§ 264-272 (2018).

Roman Catholic Diocese of Brooklyn v. Cuomo, 592 U.S. __ (2020).

Rose, D. A., Murthy, S., Brooks, J., & Bryant, J. (2017). The evolution of public health emergency management as a field of practice. *American Public Health Association, 107*(Suppl. 2), S126–S133. https://doi.org/10.2105/AJPH.2017.303947

Rutkow, L., & Vernick, J. S. (2017). Emergency legal authority and the opioid crisis. *The New England Journal of Medicine, 377*, 2512–2514. https://doi.org/10.1056/NEJMp1710862

S.B. 1001, 53rd Leg, 1st Spec. Sess. (Ariz. 2018).

South Coast Air Quality Management District. (n.d.). *Exide technologies: Ambient monitoring and source tests.* https://www.aqmd.gov/home/news-events/community-investigations/exide-updates/ambient-monitoring-and-source-tests

Sunshine, G. (2018). The case for streamlining emergency declaration authorities and adapting legal requirements to ever-changing public health threats. *Emory Law Journal, 67*(3), 397–414. https://scholarlycommons.law.emory.edu/cgi/viewcontent.cgi?article=1054&context=elj

Sunshine, G., Barrera, N., Corcoran, A. J., & Penn, M. (2019). Emergency declarations for public health issues: Expanding our definition of emergency. *Journal of Law, Medicine and Ethics, 47*, 95–99. https://doi.org/10.1177/1073110519857328

Thaler, J. (2020). The next surges are here: What can American governments lawfully do in response to the ongoing COVID-19 pandemic? *Mitchell Hamline Law Journal of Public Policy and Practice, 42*, Article 5. https://open.mitchellhamline.edu/policypractice/vol42/iss1/5

Trasande, L., & Liu, Y. (2011). Reducing the staggering costs of environmental disease in children, estimated at $76.6 billion in 2008. *Health Affairs, 30*(5), 863–870. https://doi.org/10.1377/hlthaff.2010.1239

Trump, D. J. (2020a). *Executive order on prioritizing and allocating health and medical resources to respond to the spread of COVID-19.* https://trumpwhitehouse.archives.gov/presidential-actions/executive-order-prioritizing-allocating-health-medical-resources-respond-spread-covid-19

Trump, D. J. (2020b). *Letter from President Donald J. Trump on emergency determination under the Stafford Act.* https://trumpwhitehouse.archives.gov/briefings-statements/letter-president-donald-j-trump-emergency-determination-stafford-act

U.S. Const. amend. I.

U.S. Const. amend. II.

U.S. Const. amend. IV.

U.S. Const. amend. I-X

U.S. Const. amend. V.

U.S. Const. amend. X.

U.S. Const. amend. XIV.

U.S. Const. art. I.

U.S. Const. art. II.

U.S. Const. art. III.

U.S. Const. art. IV.

U.S. Department of Health and Human Services. (2017). *Determination that a public health emergency exists.*

U.S. Department of Health and Human Services. (2020, January 31). *Secretary Azar declares public health emergency for United States for 2019 novel coronavirus.*

U.S. Department of Health and Human Services. (2021). *State and federal emergency declarations for Flint contaminated water.* https://www.phe.gov/emergency/events/Flint/Pages/declarations.aspx

U.S. Department of Justice. (2015). *Exide Technologies admits role in major hazardous waste case and agrees to permanently close battery recycling facility in Vernon.* https://www.justice.gov/usao-cdca/pr/exide-technologies-admits-role-major-hazardous-waste-case-and-agrees-permanently-close

U.S. Environmental Protection Agency. (n.d.). *Flint drinking water response.* https://www.epa.gov/flint

U.S. Food & Drug Administration. (2017). *Emergency use authorization of medical products and related authorities: Guidance for industry and other stakeholders.* https://www.fda.gov/regulatory-information/search-fda-guidance-documents/emergency-use-authorization-medical-products-and-related-authorities

Weisman, J. (2019). *Data driven approaches to fighting the opioid crisis.* Institute for Excellence in Government. https://scholar.harvard.edu/files/janewiseman/files/data_driven_approaches_to_fighting_the_opioid_crisis_jane_wiseman_april_2019.pdf

The White House. (2016). *Federal support for the Flint water crisis response and recovery.* https://obamawhitehouse.archives.gov/the-press-office/2016/05/03/fact-sheet-federal-support-flint-water-crisis-response-and-recovery

The White House. (2021). *National strategy for the COVID-19 response and pandemic preparedness.* https://www.whitehouse.gov/wp-content/uploads/2021/01/National-Strategy-for-the-COVID-19-Response-and-Pandemic-Preparedness.pdf

World Health Orgnization. (2014). *Statement on 1st meeting of the IHR emergency committee on the 2014 Ebola outbreak in West Africa.* https://www.who.int/mediacentre/news/statements/2014/ebola-20140808/en/

World Health Organization. (2020). *WHO director-general's opening remarks at the media briefing on COVID-19–11 March 2020.* https://www.who.int/director-general/speeches/detail/who-director-general-s-opening-remarks-at-the-media-briefing-on-covid-19---11-march-2020

CHAPTER 17

ACCESS AND FUNCTIONAL NEEDS

I Am My Brother's Keeper

TANYA TELFAIR LEBLANC

KEY TERMS

Access and Functional Needs
Chronic Disease
C-MIST
Cognitive Disabilities
Dialysis
Disability
Health Equity
Rugged Individualism
Social Determinants of Health

INTRODUCTION: ACCESS AND FUNCTIONAL NEEDS SCOPE

Man-made and natural disasters create unique challenges for persons with access and functional needs (U.S. Department of Health and Human Services, 2021). Persons with **access and functional needs** cover a huge swath of the American population, representing all ages and socioeconomic statuses.

The Federal Emergency Management Agency (FEMA, 2021) contends that

> people with access and functional needs includes individuals who need assistance due to any condition (temporary or permanent) that limits their ability to act. To have access and functional needs does not require that the individual have any kind of diagnosis or specific evaluation. Individuals having access and functional needs may include, but are not limited to, individuals with disabilities, seniors, and populations having limited English proficiency, limited access to transportation, and/or limited access to financial resources to prepare for, respond to, and recover from the emergency. (paras. 2–3)

Persons with access and functional needs are those who have physical or structural restrictions, limitations, or other barriers to self-protection and will require assistance before, during, and after an emergency. The list of persons to whom this will apply includes (but is not limited to) children, pregnant women, cultural and linguistic groups, older adults, unhoused persons, persons with chronic medical conditions, the impoverished, the geographically isolated, and persons without access to transportation, as well as persons with physical or **cognitive disabilities**. By one estimate, persons with access and functional needs (calculated to include children younger than 15 years; the elderly—ages 65 years and older; noninstitutionalized disabled individuals, and nonproficient English speakers only) represent approximately 50% of the general population (Kailes & Enders, 2007). Add to that assessment people who are poor, without access to transportation, on medication for chronic conditions, and so on, the scope of the problem should become clear. Within any jurisdiction or organization planning emergency operations, medical responses, or citizen security/safety measures, leaders should consider that not everyone will be able to simply evacuate, shelter in place, or follow recommendations to acquire a home cache of medical supplies, food, and water to survive until the situation is abated. There are likely to be many people in any community with a variety of access and functional needs during a medical or other emergency. In addition, some hidden populations may not be informed of impending dangerous circumstances that may put their lives in peril.

PERSONS WITH DISABILITIES

The World Health Organization (WHO, n.d.-a) sorts disabilities into three general categories:

Impairment in body structure or function, or mental functioning; for example, restricted vision due to cataracts

Activity limitation, such as difficulty walking or problem-solving

(Restrictions in) Participation, such as having challenges carrying on daily activities including self-care, working, engaging in recreational activities, and obtaining healthcare and preventive services

According to the Centers for Disease Control and Prevention (CDC), 61 million adults, 26% of the American population, or one in four persons, live with a **disability** (CDC, n.d.-c). Globally, over 1 billion people live with a disability, representing 15% of the world's population (WHO, 2021). The 2018 American Community Survey report classifies disabilities as having difficulty with hearing, vision, being ambulatory, self-care, cognitive processes, and independent living (U.S. Census Bureau, 2020a). Moreover, persons with disabilities are likely to have additional health challenges, including **chronic diseases**, such as diabetes and kidney disease. During the life course, almost anyone may experience a temporary or permanent disability (WHO, 2021). In July of 1990, the American Disabilities Act (ADA) was signed into law by then president George H. W. Bush. The law prohibited discrimination against persons with disabilities in housing, hiring, education, transportation, and other aspects of public life. In addition, the law required employers to offer reasonable accommodations to applicants with disabilities for improving access to job recruitment opportunities and to employees to support job performance.

In planning for public health emergency responses, the concept of providing reasonable accommodations to persons with disabilities should figure significantly into strategic thinking. Ultimately, persons with disabilities should be provided knowledge of and access to the same local emergency preparedness programs, training, services, communication plans, and community activities as persons without disabilities, but reasonably modified to fit the need of specific disabilities. Some states have disability registries (www.jik.com/d-rgt-links.html) to aid planners and responders in locating persons with disabilities during an emergency, but as with most voluntary registries, some people may be reluctant to provide information or may not know of its existence. In addition, addresses or other contact information may be out of date in a registry. Registries should serve as a component of emergency planning and not be considered a panacea. However, knowledge of the number of likely persons with disabilities in a community, where these people are located, if they have a designated caregiver, or if they live alone may contribute to lives saved during an emergency event.

To ensure that planners are aware of persons with disabilities in their communities and are aware of specific requirements for providing evacuation plans that include transportation if required, contingency plans to continue vital medical services, communication strategies for the deaf or blind, and provision of appropriate equipment at shelters, persons with disabilities and their caregivers, advocates of persons with disabilities, community-based organizations serving persons with disabilities, and other providers of medical and support services must be involved in planning for emergencies and involved in practical exercises, communications, strategic planning, and tabletop exercises. Sustainable engagement with the community with disabilities should be a priority for public health emergency planners in public and private sectors.

FEMA issued guidance for emergency preparedness planning to integrate functional needs support services in shelters designed for populations during an evacuation. The guidance offers practical strategies for accommodating persons with disabilities in shelters including communication protocols for the deaf or blind, personal care and hygiene, dietary concerns, toilet facilities, support animals, wheelchair access, staffing, special equipment, and medications. In addition, the comprehensive guide offers considerations for spacing of shelter inhabitants, transportation to and from facilities, and plans for transitioning persons with disabilities back to the community post-disaster (FEMA, 2010).

CHRONIC DISEASES

Diseases or conditions that last 1 year or longer and require medical treatment or restrict activity are considered chronic (CDC, n.d.-a). An estimated 6 in 10 American adults live with a chronic disease, and 4 in 10 have two or more chronic diseases, including the following major ailments: heart disease, cancer, chronic lung disease, stroke, Alzheimer disease, diabetes, and kidney disease (CDC, n.d.-a). In addition, an estimate based on 2015 to 2016 survey data indicates that 45.8% of the American population used one or more prescription drugs in the 30 days before completing the survey. The estimate included adults and children, with 85% of adults ages 60 and older reporting the use of at least one prescription medication (C. Martin et al., 2019). During emergencies in which access to pharmacies may be restricted or prevented, the CDC recommends creating an emergency supply of prescribed medicines expressly for use during disasters or prolonged societal disruption (CDC, n.d.-e). This information should be conveyed and emphasized to the general public. Citizens who use prescription medications must, if financially possible, maintain a supply of medicines to take with them if evacuation is necessary or to maintain treatment protocols while sheltering in place. However, states have emergency prescription laws that authorize pharmacies to fill prescriptions for some vital medications, the specifics of which vary by state. Emergency planners should be apprised of the legislation that applies to their catchment areas and develop plans to access emergency medications to serve persons with chronic diseases who are without supplies, in shelters or in other locations.

The growth of obesity, diabetes, hypertension, and other chronic diseases and conditions in the American population have contributed to soaring rates of kidney disease. An estimated 786,000 people in the United States are currently living with end-stage renal disease (ESRD), and among that number 71% are on **dialysis** (CDC, 2021). Dialysis patients pose additional challenges during national, regional, or local emergencies. In response to the burgeoning disease rates, dialysis clinics, both public and private, have proliferated all over the country. The National Kidney Foundation website offers instructional materials for persons with kidney disease and emergency preparedness planners (www.kidney.org/help) to aid in preparing for potential disruptions in routine services, including emergency contact information for the major dialysis service companies and survival guides if dialysis services are interrupted. In addition, the Kidney Community Emergency Response coalition (www.kcercoalition.com), under a contract sponsored by the Centers for Medicare and Medicaid Services, provides timely information, training, and technical assistance for preparedness activities to ESRD networks, kidney organizations, and others with the goal of saving lives and reducing complications among kidney patients during disasters.

SENIOR CITIZENS

The U.S. Census Bureau has documented growth in the nation's 65-and-older population since 2010. Baby boomers, persons born between 1946 and 1964, the large demographic that generated much interest in the past 50 years, are entering into senior citizenry and changing the age structure of the nation from a median of 37.2 in 2010 to 38.4 in 2019 (U.S. Census Bureau, 2020c). The American Community Survey estimates that 54,074,028 members of the American population, currently standing at 328,239,523, are 65 and older, representing 16.5% of the country's people (Figure 17.1 and Table 17.1). Roughly one-third live in poverty, with few programs or services to meet their needs as they age (U.S. Census Bureau, 2021). An important point should be made that over 10.6 million older adults live in geographic areas designated as rural according to a 2016 census report (Smith & Trevelyan, 2019).

Older people are more likely to have chronic diseases and more likely to have disabilities. Seniors are also more likely to be isolated from local preparedness awareness activities. It is important that emergency planning includes building capacity for training senior citizens individually, in community groups, in nursing and other care homes, and in assisted living facilities; and building capacity for training care providers, senior citizen service providers, houses of worship, and others to emphasize the importance of being ready for a disaster among senior citizens, their families, and their caregivers. The American Red Cross

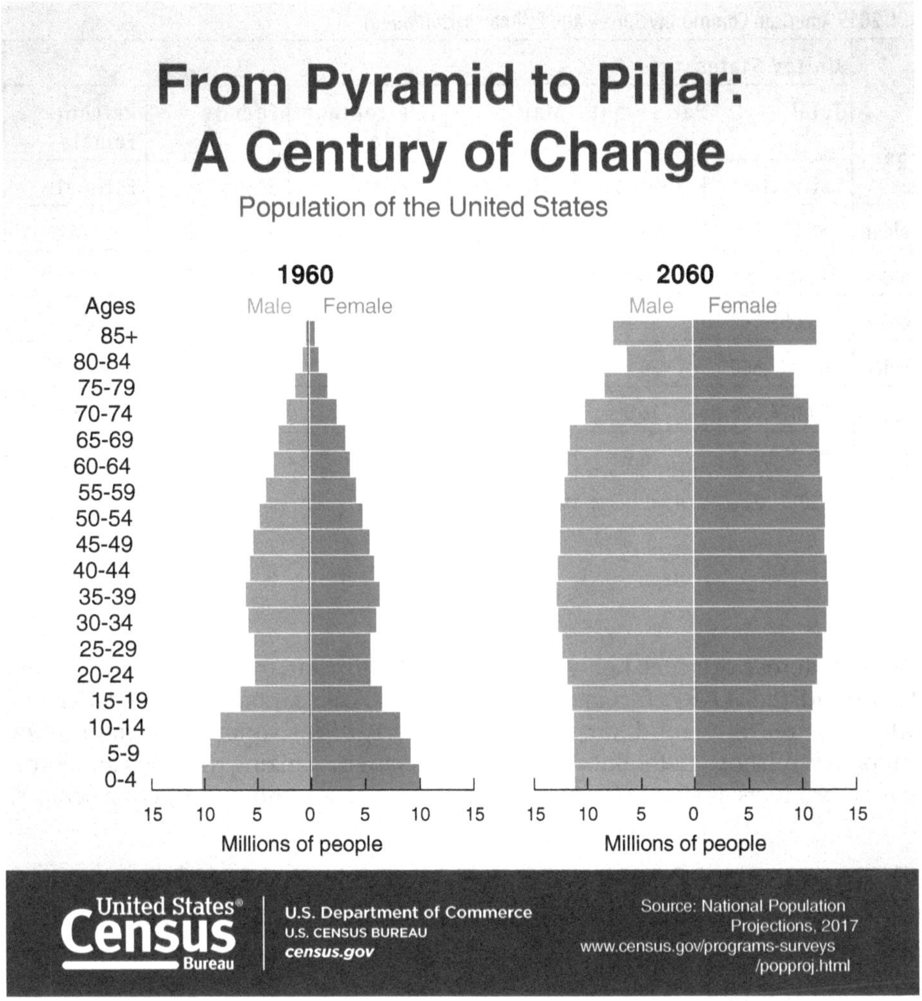

Figure 17.1 Change in age structure of the American population.

TABLE 17.1 2019 American Community Survey Age Estimates

Selected Age Categories	United States					
	Total	Percentage	Male	Percentage Male	Female	Percentage Female
	Estimate	Estimate	Estimate	Estimate	Estimate	Estimate
5 to 14 years	41,113,916	12.5	21,020,831	13.0	20,093,085	12.1
15 to 17 years	12,449,034	3.8	6,361,859	3.9	6,087,175	3.7
Under 18 years	72,967,785	22.2	37,321,627	23.1	35,646,158	21.4
18 to 24 years	30,373,170	9.3	15,556,254	9.6	14,816,916	8.9
15 to 44 years	130,315,524	39.7	65,938,127	40.8	64,377,397	38.6
16 years and older	263,534,161	80.3	128,496,159	79.5	135,038,002	81.0

(*continued*)

TABLE 17.1 2019 American Community Survey Age Estimates (*continued*)

Selected Age Categories	United States					
	Total	Percentage	Male	Percentage Male	Female	Percentage Female
	Estimate	Estimate	Estimate	Estimate	Estimate	Estimate
18 years and older	255,271,738	77.8	124,267,346	76.9	131,004,392	78.6
21 years and older	241,886,206	73.7	117,407,269	72.7	124,478,937	74.7
60 years and older	75,058,081	22.9	34,095,451	21.1	40,962,630	24.6
62 years and older	66,395,660	20.2	29,927,016	18.5	36,468,644	21.9
65 years and older	54,074,028	16.5	24,044,281	14.9	30,029,747	18.0
75 years and older	22,498,467	6.9	9,323,252	5.8	13,175,215	7.9

Source: U.S. Census Bureau. (2021). *Older Americans Month: May 2021*. https://www.census.gov/newsroom/stories/older-americans-month.html

(www.redcross.org/get-help/how-to-prepare-for-emergencies/older-adults.html) and the AARP, formerly the American Association of Retired Persons (https://createthegood.aarp.org/volunteer-guides/operation-emergency-prepare.html?how-to-toolkit=1), have toolkits for organizing trainings and information products available for planning preparedness seminars targeting seniors.

THE C-MIST FRAMEWORK FOR DEVELOPING EMERGENCY PREPAREDNESS AND RESPONSE PLANS FOR PEOPLE WITH ACCESS AND FUNCTIONAL NEEDS

Catastrophic weather events that have a long-lasting impact on a community, such as a major hurricane, can be especially challenging for persons with disabilities as they try to maintain optimum conditions for health. According to a report from the National Council on Disability, Hurricanes Katrina and Rita in 2005 affected approximately 155,000 persons older than the age of 5 with physical, developmental, and cognitive disabilities in impact zones. Deaf and blind persons suffered from communication issues and could not receive information regarding evacuation procedures. Neither evacuation transportation nor shelters were equipped to accommodate many persons requiring wheelchairs, walkers, and service animals. Many hurricane survivors with disabilities had chronic health conditions, complicating provision of basic care. A disproportionate number of fatalities associated with the storms were among persons with disabilities (National Council on Disability, 2006).

In response to the results of the 2005 hurricane season, June Isaacson Kailes and Alexandra Enders (2007) developed a function-based approach for comprehensively including considerations for persons with disabilities in disaster planning initiatives. Their approach eschews unhelpful and limiting medical terminology that focuses on "specialness," in favor of a structural application emphasizing the complexity and diversity of persons with access and functional needs. For Kailes and Enders, persons with access and functional needs may require Communication Needs, Medical Needs, (maintaining functional) Independence Needs, Supervision Needs, and Transportation Needs; thus, their framework has been dubbed C-MIST. The **C-MIST** framework's use is extended and applied to persons other than those designated as "disabled," for example, persons with chronic diseases who may require medication or medical equipment or pregnant women and older adults. The C-MIST framework is flexible to include people who experience social or economic restrictions that limit the ability to protect themselves or their families in an emergency situation (Kailes & Enders, 2007). The framework was adopted by the Assistant Secretary for Preparedness and Response (ASPR), FEMA, and the National Association for County and City Health Officials, realizing its potential for preparedness planning and its consistency with the whole-community approach. Having the capacity to reach and protect every member in a community during emergencies is a central goal for public health emergency preparedness planning leaders and responders. Understanding specific needs of populations is critical to this effort. Examples of persons with access and functional needs applying C-MIST definitions include the following:

Communications—Persons requiring documents formatted for the blind, sign language for the deaf, or methods for hard-to-reach populations without access to telephone service and internet access

Medical—Pregnant women may require morning sickness comfort, appropriate diets, and protection from environmental hazards that would harm a pregnancy. Persons with chronic diseases may need medicines and/or access to dialysis, oxygen, nebulizers, and breathing medications. Persons with mental health issues may require access to counseling, medications, and protocols to prevent stress or emotional triggers.

Independence—Persons who require equipment to promote independence, including wheelchairs, canes, walkers, portable oxygen, or service animals

Supervision—Persons with mental illness or anxiety issues, unaccompanied children, persons under detention, or those with Alzheimer disease

Transportation—Nondrivers of all ages or persons without access to transportation

From the preceding examples, clearly some individuals may have multiple or seemingly unlimited needs during an emergency. The C-MIST is a useful planning tool to ensure emergency planners are aware of the dynamics and breadth of access and functional needs among members of communities and helps planners think through how they will accommodate persons with access and functional needs in responses. In a rural North Carolina, Appalachian community covering three counties, the C-MIST framework was utilized by the district health department serving the area (2016–2018) to build an all-inclusive all-hazards preparedness plan designed to reach the whole community. Diverse community partners from various sectors worked together on the plan and conducted tabletop and full-scale exercises to evaluate the operational functionality of plans. The C-MIST criteria enabled the team to identify and prepare for community members with access and functional needs, including unaccompanied children, persons requiring language translation services, and persons with symptoms indicating illness (Schroeder & Bouldin, 2019).

SPECIAL CONSIDERATIONS

Women and Children Last? The Status of Women and Children in Public Health Emergency Preparedness

Whatever happened to the noble 19th-century aphorism "women and children, first"? Women, infants, and children are among the least considered by male-dominated planners of national responses to natural or man-made disasters. Though women are capable and often resilient in the face of multiple life challenges, gendered concerns associated with the female sex during emergency situations can be complex. Problems experienced by women, girls, and dependent children facing disasters are under-researched, rarely considered, and inadequately acted upon. In the United States, the status of women has changed dramatically in the past 50 years. The benefits incurred through greater access to career opportunities have come with a huge price tag. In 2019, women's labor force participation was 57.4%, representing 47% of the total workforce. Among unmarried mothers, 78.2% were in the workforce. Women are more likely than men to be among the working poor, 4.5% and 3.5%, respectively. Minority women are more likely to be among the working poor; for example, Black women, 8.9%, and Hispanic women, 7.1%, compared with White women (3.7%; U.S. Bureau of Labor Statistics [BLS], 2021c). Women are also more likely than men to be employed in jobs with pay at or below the minimum wage (BLS, 2021a). Women, whether married or unmarried, often bear the majority of responsibility for their children, the children of others, and older adults as well. However, national efforts to prepare for catastrophic events continue to have gender bias toward men. As the events following Hurricanes Katrina and Rita in 2005 demonstrated, women, infants, and children are particularly vulnerable during disasters (Callaghan et al., 2007). During the flooding and dislocation associated with the hurricanes, prenatal care was interrupted for pregnant women, and premature infants were sent to alternative hospitals without their mothers. Women in shelters were sexually assaulted. Emergency contraception was not available (Burnett, 2005; Thornton & Voigt, 2007). In addition, accusations of sexual assault and rape have been the subject of draconian and archaic interpretations by some policy makers. Taking these issues into consideration, women have specific needs during emergencies.

Going further, women face additional challenges when disasters interrupt their vital function as breadwinners. In February 2020, women's participation in the labor force peaked at 59.2%. When the COVID-19 pandemic descended upon the United States, in March and April 2020, women's nonfarm employment declined by 12.5 million jobs, representing 55% of the total job loss at the time (BLS, 2021b). Greater job losses occurred among the service sectors, which employ more women than men. When businesses in the hospitality industries, food service, childcare, education, and other jobs that require close people contact shut down, women were left with no alternatives to continue working. In addition, shuttering schools and childcare centers created additional barriers for women with children to continue working. Given women's roles as mothers, breadwinners, caregivers, and support structure for families and social groups, women leaders should be included in emergency planning activities in any community to leverage their knowledge of critical issues and experiences for implementing a whole-community approach to preparedness planning.

CHILDREN

In recent years, the way children experience childhood has dramatically changed. Marriage rates are declining, and divorce rates have increased. In 2019, the percentage of births to unmarried women was 40%, and the proportion of children younger than 18 years living in single-parent households was 34% (Annie E. Casey Foundation, 2021; J. A. Martin et al. 2021). Based on 2019 data, the U.S. population has 73 million children (persons younger than the age of 18) or 22% of the total population, with an estimated 10,000,000 American children, or 14.4%, living in poverty (Children's Defense Fund, 2021). During the 2017–2018 school year, an estimated 1.5 million children enrolled in public schools experienced homelessness (Children's Defense Fund, 2021). Taking the state of America's children a step further, nationally 656,000 victims of child abuse and neglect were reported in 2019, with a rate of 8.9 victims per 1,000 children in the population. The first year of a child's life, when they are most vulnerable, appears to be the most hazardous, with a victimization rate of 25.7 per 1,000 same-age children in the national population. The victimization rate for girls is 9.4 per 1,000 girls in the population, which is higher than boys at 8.4 per 1,000 boys in the population. The most common form of child maltreatment was neglect, representing 61.0% of cases, with physical abuse representing 10.3% of reported cases. In 2019, 877 victims of sex trafficking were identified in 29 states; 88.5% were girls and 10.6% were boys (Children's Bureau, 2021).

Beyond the issues of poverty, abuse, and neglect, many children in middle-class homes are being "managed" to accommodate their parents' careers, ever-changing relationships, and other priorities (Palmer, 2007). Even children in stable married-couple homes can be stressed due to the multiple responsibilities and careers of two working parents. Management can take the form of being medicated for behavior control (Palmer, 2007); plopped down in front of a television set, computer, tablet, or mobile device for "human" interaction; or overscheduled with programmatic extracurricular activities outside the home (Palmer, 2007). Recent studies have shown that American children eat too much fast food and junk food, with 36.3% of children ages 2 to 19 consuming fast food on a given day (Fryar et al., 2020); are becoming obese (31% of 10- to 17-year-old children are overweight or obese; Annie E. Casey Foundation, 2021); and are not getting enough sleep for proper growth and development (American Academy of Pediatrics, 2019). Moreover, based on 2019 prevalence estimates, 5,104,410 children younger than the age of 18 had asthma (CDC, n.d.-d).

Emergency planners and leaders should comprehend the lives of children in today's changing world as they face planning for them in emergencies. Simply planning for reuniting with caregivers if children are separated during a catastrophic event may not be sufficient. Critical awareness and knowledge of possibilities, problems, and protection of children encountered during emergencies are important. It is acknowledged that planners are not able to address or solve all the complex problems some children experience and are not expected to take on that daunting task during an emergency, but knowing what to look for to protect children in a shelter or to identify a situation requiring an intervention may contribute to saving a life or sparing a child harm.

Tribes

Human beings inhabited the landmass now known as the Americas, stretching from Canada in the north to the southern tip of South America, for thousands of years before European settlers arrived. Pre-Columbian civilizations were sophisticated, possessing permanent dwellings and cities, agriculture, architecture, art, and complex social and religious institutions, with thousands of miles of roads and administrative and trading centers throughout the region. Their descendants, American Indian/Alaska Natives (AI/ANs), make up 574 federally recognized tribes in 35 states. AI/ANs represent 2% of the U.S. population, or 6.9 million people (Bureau of Indian Affairs. n.d.; U.S. Census Bureau, 2020b). Tribes deserve special consideration due to their unique history and status as sovereign within a sovereign nation. This means that tribes have the right to govern themselves, though they are still classified as U.S. citizens. Thus, AI/ANs are citizens of three sovereigns: tribes, the state in which they reside, and the United States. Disasters may have a unique impact on these communities, with response and recovery efforts complicated by multiple statuses. Going further, many AI/ANs live in poverty, experience health disparities, and may live in rural areas with limited internet access, all of which challenge response to disasters. Emergency planners should include members of tribal communities in planning sessions and in preparedness drill activities and engage with tribal leaders to be confident that tribes are in the communication channels to receive lifesaving information and protection strategies.

Challenges to Protecting Persons with Access and Functional Needs During Emergencies

Rugged Individualism and Its Consequences

On the surface, the perspective of **rugged individualism** undergirds much of the social, economic, and political life in America (Eppard et al., 2020; Landress, 2021). As a country, the general default perspective is that individuals are autonomous and self-reliant and have free will to make decisions appropriate for themselves, and that success in life is due to individual effort, talent, and one's choices and behaviors (Eppard et al., 2020). The belief in individual "freedom" has in many cases precluded the country's ability to take collective action to solve social and economic problems that, in the long run, would be beneficial to all. Prime examples of the belief in personal freedom over collective responsibility are the rejection of nonpharmaceutical interventions, including mask wearing and social distancing, during the initial phases of the COVID-19 pandemic among nearly half of the American populous (Bazzi et al., 2021) and the rejection of medical interventions in the later phases of the pandemic, evidenced by vaccine hesitancy, reflected in only about 48.8% of the population being fully vaccinated against the virus as of July 2020 (CDC, n.d.-b). Vaccine hesitancy is driven by complex social factors, which include the spread of misinformation and disinformation, fear among minority populations based on historic ethical misconduct in public health initiatives, mistrust of government motives, and belief in rugged individualism and the right to reject any action, even if that action may contribute to the well-being of the whole society.

Rugged individualism can easily be seen in our national employment policies, which are based on assumptions that everyone can function nearly 100% of the time with minimal need for vacations, sick leave, maternity-paternity leave, or time to care for families and self and are indeed, in my view, appropriate for robots, not human beings. Though I would argue that even robots need downtime to care for their working systems. However, the proverbial American Dream ideology conveys that with hard work and determination, anyone can "pull themselves up by the bootstraps" and succeed in building a decent life. The facts of the matter are in stark contrast to this contention. In the last 50 years, it has become more difficult for Americans to achieve middle-class status and stay there. The wealth gap has widened, with greater proportions of economic benefits and resources channeled upward to the top 1% of the population (Mishel & Bivens, 2021). And with these changes, the health and well-being of Americans have declined over time.

Though the United States of America is a wealthy country, it ranks poorly compared with other wealthy countries in important quality of life and health measures, including poverty, childhood poverty, economic inequality, worker benefits, maternal and child health, and healthcare access (Tikkanen & Abrams, 2020; Woolf & Aron, 2013). The United States spends twice as much on healthcare but has the lowest life expectancy and the highest suicide rate compared with 11 nations in the Organisation for Economic Co-operation and Development (OECD). In addition, the United States has the highest chronic disease burden and twice the obesity rate as other countries. It is no wonder that the health of Americans has declined. Between 1979 and 2017, in America, the productivity of average workers, representing approximately 80% of the private-sector workforce, rose, while compensation for that productivity dramatically decreased by 43% (Mishel & Bivens, 2021). Simply put, workers are paid less but working more hours to survive. In most average jobs, employees are treated as expendable or interchangeable. In the United States, most average jobs provide 12 weeks of unpaid maternity leave, compared with much more generous leave, with pay, in other developed countries (Finland, 161; Japan, 58; Germany, 58; Canada, 52; and Ireland, 26 weeks paid maternity leave, respectively.) In addition, other developed countries provide employees 20 to 30 paid holidays annually (World Economic Forum, 2018). Paid holidays are not required by the federal government, but according to the BLS (2017), on average employees receive eight paid holidays and up to 14 days vacation in the United States. Higher wage workers have access to more generous leave policies in their professions (BLS, 2017). Disparities in leave policies, which are likely to contribute to ill health, are politically defended in the rugged individualist perspective. To top it all, the United States is the only Western country that does not have a healthcare plan to cover all of its citizens, regardless of age or employment status.

During the COVID-19 pandemic, it became clear that people employed in work without sick or other leave policies, health insurance, or other benefits were at an extreme disadvantage, and many of those jobs, grocery store and pharmacy clerks, for example, must be done in person, risking exposure to the disease.

Going further, the indicators of high quality of life and health are not evenly distributed in the population. If you and your loved ones are wealthy or superwealthy, your life in America is, on average, excellent. However, persons of average or below-average means are likely to experience struggles and stressors pursuing the rugged individualism approach to establishing a stable and healthy life.

FINAL WORDS: THE IMPORTANCE OF RECOGNIZING SOCIAL DETERMINANTS OF HEALTH AND EMBRACING STRATEGIES FOR HEALTH EQUITY

People with access and functional needs are likely to be poor, marginalized, and sometimes isolated from larger communities due to structural and functional limitations. In the past 40 or more years, significant evidence has emerged in the scientific literature demonstrating that population health outcomes are influenced by complex, integrated, and overlapping social structures and economic systems that position human beings in a social status hierarchy (Marmot & Allen, 2014). One's place in this hierarchy influences the conditions that expose one to disease morbidity and mortality, and access to healthcare. One of the simplest examples used to explain the social gradient in health outcomes is the class disparities among *Titanic* survivors. The *Titanic* was a British passenger ship that sank in the North Atlantic Ocean on April 15, 1912. More first-class passengers survived this tragic accident at sea, compared with second-class passengers. And more second-class passengers survived compared with third-class passengers, and so on (Marmot & Wilkinson, 1999). A more recent example of the role the social hierarchy plays in determining health outcomes is the death, disease, and dislocation of the most disadvantaged population subgroups in the aftermath of hurricanes Katrina and Rita along the U.S. Gulf Coast in 2005. Persons most likely to suffer sickness and death or become homeless or dislocated after the devastating hurricanes were overwhelmingly among the poor and among ethnic minorities (Gault et al., 2005). **Social determinants of health** then are the conditions in the social, economic, and physical environments into which people are born, live, are educated, work, play, worship, and age that contribute significantly to health and life outcomes (WHO, n.d.-b). From the two earlier examples that involve major disasters, social determinants of health can determine who survives and who perishes. Firmly understanding that the social gradient in which we all live renders preferential treatment to those with more social and economic resources, public health emergency planners at all levels should embrace the aspirational goal of **health equity** to ensure that everyone in their jurisdiction or community has an equal opportunity to be prepared for a disaster and an equal opportunity to be protected from harm, regardless of social status, or requirements for access and functional needs.

DISCUSSION QUESTIONS

1. Plan and conduct a mock tabletop preparedness activity for your class. How would you use the C-MIST framework to help identify and plan for persons with access and functional needs in a community?
2. Discuss a whole community approach for addressing access and functional needs. What kinds of organizations would you include in your community outreach?
3. Develop a strategy to contact disabled persons who do not have access to internet or telephone.
4. How does rugged individualism influence preparedness activities? What should we do about it?

DISCLAIMER

This chapter was prepared by Tanya Telfair LeBlanc in his/her personal capacity. The opinions expressed in this article are the author's own and do not reflect the view of the Centers for Disease Control and Prevention, the Department of Health and Human Services, or the United States government.

RESOURCES

https://www.ada.gov/shleterck.htm

A Guide to Disability Laws: https://www.ada.gov/cguide.htm

Civil Rights Requirements for Persons With Disabilities: https://www.hhs.gov/civil-rights/for-individuals/special-topics/needy-families/persons-with-disabilities/index.html

https://www.disasterassistance.gov

https://asprtracie.hhs.gov/technical-resources/62/access-and-functional-needs/0

https://training.fema.gov/programs/emischool/el361toolkit/assets/preparingpeoplewithdisabilities.pdf

https://training.fema.gov/programs/emischool/el361toolkit/assets/bestpractices_evacuating_special_needs.pdf

https://www.fema.gov/disaster/coronavirus/best-practices/exercise-starter-kit-preparedness-pandemic

https://www.kidney.org/sites/default/files/11-10-0807_IBD_disasterbrochure.pdf

NACCHO Health and Disability Learning Community: *Ways to enhance emergency planning and preparedness activities that engage and include people with disabilities:* www.naccho.org/topics/hpdp/healthdisa/eplearncomm.cfm

Department of Justice: *ADA best practices toolkit for state and local government:* www.ada.gov/pcatoolkit/toolkitmain.htm#pcatoolkitch7

Department of Justice: *ADA checklist for emergency shelters:* www.ada.gov/pcatoolkit/chap7shelterchk.htm

NACCHO Advanced Practice Centers: *Easy-to-use pocket translator and pictogram tools:* http://apc.naccho.org/products/apc20071675/pages/overview.aspx

https://www.ready.gov/disability

https://www.ready.gov/seniors

https://www.redcross.org/get-help/how-to-prepare-for-emergencies/inclusive-preparedness-resources.html

https://www.redcross.org/content/dam/redcross/atg/PDF_s/Preparedness___Disaster_Recovery/Disaster_Preparedness/Disaster_Preparedness_for_Srs-English.revised_7-09.pdf

http://www.jik.com/disaster.html

https://createthegood.aarp.org/volunteer-guides/operation-emergency-prepare.html?how-to-toolkit=1

https://www.phe.gov/Preparedness/planning/abc/Pages/older-adults.aspx

REFERENCES

American Academy of Pediatrics. (2019). *Only half of U.S. children get enough sleep: Why that's a serious problem.* https://www.healthline.com/health-news/children-lack-of-sleep-health-problems

Annie E. Casey Foundation. (2021). *Kids count data book.* https://www.aecf.org/resources/2021-kids-count-data-book

Bazzi, S., Fiszbein, M., & Gebresilasse, M. (2021). Rugged individualism and collective (in)action during the COVID-19 pandemic. *Journal of Public Economics, 195.* https://doi.org/10.1016/j.jpubeco.2020.104357

Bureau of Indian Affairs. (n.d.) *Frequently asked questions: What is a federally recognized tribe.* https://www.bia.gov/frequently-asked-questions

Burnett, J. (2005). *More stories emerge of rapes in post-Katrina chaos.* National Public Radio Report. https://www.npr.org/templates/story/story.php?storyId=5063796

Callaghan, W. M., Rasmussen, S., Jamieson, D., & Ventura, S. (2007). Health concerns of women and infants in times of natural disasters: Lessons learned from Hurricane Katrina. *Maternal and Child Health, 11,* 307–311. https://doi.org/10.1007/s10995-007-0177-4

Centers for Disease Control and Prevention. (n.d.-a). *About chronic diseases*. https://www.cdc.gov/chronicdisease/about/index.htm

Centers for Disease Control and Prevention. (n.d.-b). *COVID data tracker weekly review*. https://www.cdc.gov/coronavirus/2019-ncov/covid-data/covidview

Centers for Disease Control and Prevention. (n.d.-c). *Disability and health overview*. https://www.cdc.gov/ncbddd/disabilityandhealth/disability.html

Centers for Disease Control and Prevention. (n.d.-d). *Most recent national asthma data*. https://www.cdc.gov/asthma/most_recent_national_asthma_data.htm

Centers for Disease Control and Prevention. (n.d.-e). *Prepare your health: Prescriptions*. https://www.cdc.gov/prepyourhealth/takeaction/prescriptions

Centers for Disease Control and Prevention. (2021). *Chronic kidney disease in the United States, 2021*. https://www.cdc.gov/kidneydisease/pdf/Chronic-Kidney-Disease-in-the-US-2021-h.pdf

Children's Bureau. (2021). *Child maltreatment 2019*. https://www.acf.hhs.gov/sites/default/files/documents/cb/cm2019.pdf

Children's Defense Fund. (2021). *The State of America's Children* ® 2021. https://www.childrensdefense.org/state-of-americas-children/soac-2021-housing

Eppard, L. M., Rank, M. R., & Bullock, H. E. (2020). *Rugged individualism and the misunderstanding of American inequality*. Lehigh University Press.

Federal Emergency Management Agency. (2010). *2010 Guidance on planning for integrational of functional needs support services in general population shelters*. https://www.fema.gov/sites/default/files/2020-07/fema_functional-needs-support-services-guidance.pdf

Federal Emergency Management Agency. (2021). *FEMA reaches out to people with disabilities, and access and functional needs* (Release # NR 012). https://www.fema.gov/press-release/20210318/fema-reaches-out-people-disabilities-access-and-functional-need

Fryar, C. D., Carroll, M. D., Ahluwalia, N., & Ogden, C. L. (2020). *Fast food intake among children and adolescents in the United States, 2015–2018* (NCHS Data Brief No. 375). https://www.cdc.gov/nchs/data/databriefs/db375-h.pdf

Gault, B., Hartmann, H., Jones-DeWeever, A., Werschkul, M., & Williams, E. (2005). *The women of New Orleans and the Gulf Coast: Multiple disadvantages and key assets for recovery part I. Poverty, race, gender and class*. Institute for Women's Policy Research. https://iwpr.org/wp-content/uploads/2020/11/D464.pdf

Kailes, J. I., & Enders, A. (2007). Moving beyond "special needs": A function-based framework for emergency management and planning. *Journal of Disability Policy Studies, 17*(4), 230–237. https://doi.org/10.1177/10442073070170040601

Landress, S. (2021, March 31). Rugged individualism in American political thought. *CUREJ: College Undergraduate Research Electronic Journal*. https://repository.upenn.edu/curej/257

Marmot, M., & Allen, J. (2014). Social determinants of health equity. *American Journal of Public Health, 104*(Suppl. 4), S517–S519. https://doi.org/10.2105/AJPH.2014.302200

Marmot, M., & Wilkinson, R. (Eds.). (1999). *Social determinants of health*. Oxford University Press.

Martin, C., Hales, C., Gu, Q., & Ogden, C. (2019). *Prescription drug use in the United States, 2015–2016* (NCHS Data Brief, No. 334). Department of Health and Human Services. https://www.cdc.gov/nchs/data/databriefs/db334-h.pdf

Martin, J. A., Hamilton, B., Osterman, M., & Driscoll, A. (2021, March 23). *Births: Final data for 2019* (Vital Statistics Report, Vol. 20, No. 2). National Center for Vital Statistics. https://www.cdc.gov/nchs/data/nvsr/nvsr70/nvsr70-02-508.pdf

Mishel, L., & Bivens, J. (2021). *Identifying the policy levers generating wage suppression and inequality*. Economic Policy Institute. https://www.epi.org/unequalpower/publications/wage-suppression-inequality/

National Council on Disability. (2006). *The impact of Hurricanes Katrina and Rita on people with disabilities: A look back and remaining challenges*. https://ncd.gov/publications/2006/Aug072006

Palmer, S. (2007). *Toxic childhood: How the modern world is damaging our children and what we can do about it*. Orion Books.

Schroder, J., & Bouldin, E. (2019). Including public health preparedness program to promote resilience in rural Appalachia (2016–2018). *American Journal of Public Health, 109*(S4), S283–S285. http://doi.org/10.2105/AJPH.2019.305086

Smith, A. S., & Trevelyan, E. (2019). *The older population in rural America: 2012–2016* (American Community Survey Report ACS-41). https://www.census.gov/content/dam/Census/library/publications/2019/acs/acs-41.pdf

Thornton, W. E., & Voigt, L. (2007). Disaster rape: Vulnerability of women to sexual assault during Hurricane Katrina. *Journal of Public Management and Social Policy, 13*(2), 23–49. http://www.jpmsp.com/volume-13/vol13-iss2

Tikkanen, R., & Abrams, M. K. (2020). *U.S. health care from a global perspective, 2019: Higher spending, worse outcomes?* https://collections.nlm.nih.gov/catalog/nlm:nlmuid-101761886-pdf

U.S. Bureau of Labor Statistics. (2017). Workers in private industry received an average of 8 paid holidays in 2017. *The Economics Daily*. https://www.bls.gov/opub/ted/2018/workers-in-private-industry-received-an-average-of-8-paid-holidays-in-2017.htm

U.S. Bureau of Labor Statistics. (2021a). *Characteristics of minimum wage workers 2020*. https://www.bls.gov/opub/reports/minimum-wage/2020/pdf/home.pdf

U.S. Bureau of Labor Statistics. (2021b). *COVID-19 ends longest employment expansion in CES history, causing unprecedented job losses in 2020*. https://www.bls.gov/opub/mlr/2021/article/covid-19-endslongest-employment-expansion-in-ces-history.htm

U.S. Bureau of Labor Statistics. (2021c). *Women in the labor force: A data book*. https://www.bls.gov/opub/reports/womens-databook/2020/home.htm

U.S. Census Bureau. (2020a). *Anniversary of Americans With Disabilities Act: July 26, 2020* (Release Number CB20-FF.06). https://www.census.gov/newsroom/facts-for-features/2020/disabilities-act.html

U.S. Census Bureau. (2020b). *Facts for features: American Indian and Alaska Native Heritage Month: November 2020* (Release Number CB20-FF.08). https://www.census.gov/newsroom/facts-for-features/2020/aian-month.html

U.S. Census Bureau. (2020c). 65 and older population grows rapidly as baby boomers age (Release Number CB20-99). https://www.census.gov/newsroom/press-releases/2020/65-older-population-grows.html

U.S. Census Bureau. (2021). *Older Americans month: May 2021* (Release Number CB21-SFS.057). https://www.census.gov/newsroom/stories/older-americans-month.html

U.S. Department of Health and Human Services. (2021). *Topic collections: Access and functional needs*. https://asprtracie.hhs.gov/technical-resources/62/access-and-functional-needs/0

Woolf, S. H., & Aron, L. (Eds.). (2013). *U.S. health in international perspective: Shorter lives, poorer health*. National Academies Press. https://www.ncbi.nlm.nih.gov/books/NBK115854

World Economic Forum. (2018). *People in these countries get the most paid vacation days*. https://www.weforum.org/agenda/2018/08/average-paid-vacation-time-days-by-country

World Health Organization. (n.d.-a). *International classification of functioning disability and health*. https://www.who.int/standards/classifications/international-classification-of-functioning-disability-and-health

World Health Organization. (n.d.-b). *Social determinants of health*. https://www.who.int/health-topics/social-determinants-of-health#tab=tab_1

World Health Organization. (2021). *Disability and health*. https://www.who.int/news-room/fact-sheets/detail/disability-and-health

CHAPTER 18

CHILDREN AND DISASTERS

NANCY T. BLAKE AND CATHERINE J. GOODHUE

KEY TERMS

Catheters
Endotracheal Tube
Kawasaki Disease
Memorandum of Understanding
Misinformation
Moulage
Multisystem Inflammatory Syndrome
Myocardial Infarction
Nasogastric Tube
Social Determinants of Health
Telehealth
Toxic Shock Syndrome

INTRODUCTION

Children comprise approximately 23% of the U.S. population (U.S. Census Bureau, 2020). They have many unique characteristics that make them extremely vulnerable in the event of a disaster or public health emergency. Disaster planners may overlook different aspects of the needs of children in the event of a crisis event, resulting in additional harms to pediatric victims. Facilities that do not typically care for children may become overwhelmed with a surge of pediatric victims. Elements of disaster planning that need additional considerations include unaccompanied minors; triage and assessment of pediatric victims; medications, equipment, and supplies; decontamination; shelter setup; and reunification. Once a pediatric disaster plan is created, a disaster drill must be conducted. If there are deficits observed, the disaster plan should be revised and then tested again to ensure that the plan is adequate to meet the needs of pediatric victims. Children at times respond differently to diseases and recently, during the COVID-19 crisis, had a different disease process than adults did. Children didn't appear to have the same symptoms at first but a new multisystem inflammatory state was soon identified as **multisystem inflammatory syndrome** in children (MIS-C; Centers for Disease Control and Prevention [CDC], n.d.).

UNIQUE CHARACTERISTICS OF CHILDREN

Although children represent almost 25% of the population, there is little preparation for children in disasters. Children are especially vulnerable during disasters or public health emergencies. Adult models of disaster response do not work because children have unique needs. State and federal plans do not consistently have provisions for pediatric patients, and some communities may not have the appropriate response plans, supplies, equipment, and education to care for children. If they do have the supplies, they may not have the quantities that are needed because many communities have not drilled for pediatric patients (Ray et al., 2018). Children have developmental, physiological, and psychological differences. These differences make them especially vulnerable in disasters both from physical and mental health perspectives. Children are also more at risk because of these vulnerabilities from a physical standpoint in traumatic disasters and those related to nuclear, biological, or chemical terrorism (Blake, 2019).

DEVELOPMENTAL CHARACTERISTICS

Developmentally, children, depending on their age, are different from adults. Table 18.1 addresses the differences based on developmental levels.

Children with special healthcare needs (CSHCN) are especially vulnerable in the event of a disaster or public health emergency. For those with medical equipment requiring electricity, disaster planning is essential for this patient population. Their care is very complex and may include ventilators, **tracheostomies**, feeding tubes, parenteral nutrition, and oxygen. When their power goes out it is a public health emergency for them. They have voluminous medical records, and if the care team does not have access to their records, essential components of their care may be overlooked or missed. These families should be encouraged to have their healthcare provider complete an Emergency Information Form (EIF) for them. The EIF is a summary of the most important aspects of their medical records and care needs in the event they do not present to their home facility (American Academy of Pediatrics, 2010).

TABLE 18.1 Child Developmental Levels

Infant Birth to 1 year of age	Total dependence on their adult caregiver for all aspects of care; fear of strangers
Toddlers 1–2 years of age	Develop their ability to control their bodies and seek independence; egocentric view of life; view death as a temporary event
Preschoolers 3–5 years of age	They have a strong need to explore; they have inappropriate thoughts and are magical thinkers and have a vivid imagination; they fear separation from their loved ones
School age 6–12 years of age	They need to develop a sense of achievement and are eager to cooperate; rules, rituals, and conformity are very important to them; early school-aged children also believe death is temporary, but older children understand it is not.
Adolescents 13–18 years of age	Teenagers are very concerned about their physical appearance; they are very emotional; struggle for independence; unlike other age levels, they become logical thinkers; they may want to be with their family during a disaster, but otherwise want to be away from their family and more independent.

Source: From Pate, M. F., & Mullen, J. (2019). Caring for critically Ill children and their families. In M. C. Slota (Ed.), *AACN core curriculum for pediatric high acuity, progressive, and critical care nursing* (3rd ed., pp. 3–8). Springer Publishing.

PHYSIOLOGICAL CHARACTERISTICS

Children are not small adults and should not be treated as such. It is important that the community have drills in advance to educate all possible care team members and to ensure the appropriate resources are available. Because of the conditions that come with disaster events, children are more vulnerable to complications. There are some unique differences that are very important to understand in disaster situations. The important differences in children are listed in Table 18.2 and Figure 18.1.

TABLE 18.2 Unique Physiological Differences in Children Important to Disaster

Physiological Differences	Implications
Children have larger heads, thermoregulation	• In an explosion, their head can propel them forward and could increase the injuries to their heads. • Children (especially infants) have large surface area-to-volume ratio (and less subcutaneous tissue) and lose heat to the environment. • Cold stress causes energy consumption, increased oxygen need, and metabolism. • Can get hypoglycemic and deteriorate.
Tracheal diameter is smaller	• During traumatic events blood or vomitus can block their airway. • In children under 8 years of age the cricoid cartilage is the narrowest portion of the airway.
Thinner skin, larger body surface area	• They are more susceptible to the effects of radiological exposure. • Risk for burns • Increased absorption of chemical agents
Breathing	• Diaphragm is positioned more horizontally–they rely on the diaphragm to assist with breathing. • Air in stomach can cause the diaphragm to elevate and compromise lung capacity. • Chest wall is more pliable in children.
Circulation	• Children can compensate for blood or fluid loss by increasing their heart rate. • Blood volume depends on the size of the child.
Neurological	• Skull is thin and offers little protection to the brain of the infant/ young child. • More prone to head trauma • Head circumference can be increased with head trauma. • Shear hemorrhage and diffuse brain injury from swelling are more common in kids.
Abdominal	• Protruding abdomen • Most common injured organs are liver and spleen. • Pelvic fractures are uncommon because the pelvis is more anterior. • Abdominal muscles are thinner and weaker.
Stature (Lower to the ground)	• High risk for bioterrorism as they will get ill early
Bones are more pliable	• Injuries may not be obvious on the surface because the bones are not broken.
Vital signs vary by age	• Providers who are not familiar with pediatrics may not notice abnormalities.

Source: From Blake, N. (2019). Disaster preparedness and response. In M. C. Slota (Ed.), *AACN core curriculum for pediatric high acuity, progressive, and critical care nursing* (3rd ed., pp. 829, 830) Springer Publishing.

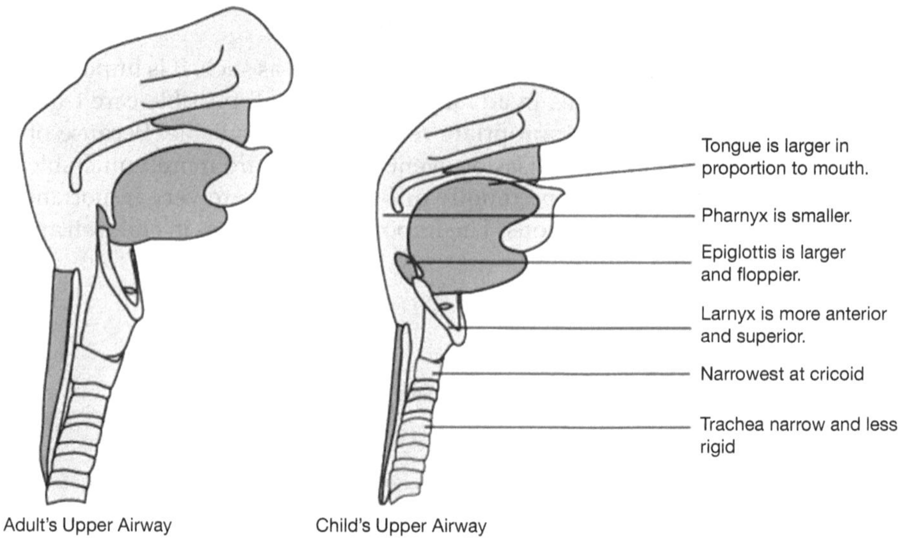

Figure 18.1 Airway differences in children.

Source: Reproduced with permission from Fuhrman, B. P., & Zimmerman, J. J. (2016). *Pediatric critical care* (5th ed.). Elsevier.

Ensuring providers have the education to care for pediatric patients in a disaster is essential. The resources may be sparse in a disaster; it is important to address issues immediately, as disaster triage is very different from usual care.

PSYCHOLOGICAL CHARACTERISTICS

In addition to their medical health needs, children have additional mental health needs that were listed earlier, and they do not follow the standard development chart milestones. Children are also at risk for child abuse and neglect as they cannot protect themselves from predators and/or neglect due to an overwhelming natural disaster in which their caregivers might be dead or otherwise injured and incapacitated. These issues make them high risk for developing posttraumatic stress disorder, and they need community resources (social workers, psychologists, etc.) to help keep them safe and address their psychosocial needs, which are addressed later.

Because of developmental issues, children do not understand what is going on and they may be scared. They may not have the ability to comprehend and escape a dangerous situation. They can sense the stress of adults who are around them, and it is important that there are resources to deal with their stress as well as distractors to keep them busy. They may fall back into an earlier developmental level and regress. Children who have been toilet-trained may start wetting the bed again or having accidents. Also, children may not talk when asked questions because they are scared, and it may be difficult for the healthcare providers to know if they have a medical condition or if they are just being silent.

DISASTER PLANNING FOR CHILDREN

Disaster planners in the past have not considered the needs of children in their disaster plans. Original disaster plans were developed around the needs of the military, so they were focused on adults. Recent disasters have highlighted the need for pediatric disaster planning. Once disaster plans are developed, they need to be tested to ensure there are no gaps or issues with implementing the plans. A study by Ferrer et al. (2009) reviewed after-action reports from healthcare facilities in Los Angeles County. They found that most facilities did not include children in their disaster drills or exercises.

The disaster drills can be tabletop drills, but live drills can more realistically test the plans. Using children in the drills can truly test the procedures. Groups such as the Girl Scouts and the Boy Scouts and various sports teams can be recruited to be "disaster victims" in facility drills. The children can be **moulaged** and follow scripts on "victim cards" to provide healthcare workers with more realistic victims. Any gaps in the disaster plans or areas needing improvement can then be revised and undergo further drill testing to ensure that best practices and procedures adequately cover the needs of pediatric victims.

INVOLVE COMMUNITY STAKEHOLDERS

The U.S. Hospital Preparedness Program (HPP) was started in 2002 to plan for and respond to public health emergencies and bioterrorism (Kim, 2016). Then, in 2004, the emphasis moved to an all-hazards approach and collaboration to conduct a hazard vulnerability assessment (Kim, 2016). In 2012, the HPP combined with the U.S. Public Health Emergency Preparedness (PHEP) program to remove identical goals (Kim, 2016). In 2013, the Institute of Medicine (Wizemann et al., 2014) recommended broadening community stakeholders who are invested in children following its workshop on preparedness, response, and recovery considerations for children.

It is important in public health and disaster preparedness planning that the needs of children are considered in the planning phase as most of the time children are not included in the planning phase and their needs are not addressed until the disaster strikes. These needs include child care, spiritual and religious needs for families, and that youth are prepared to be resilient and deal with the issues. The IOM recommends that stakeholders should include nontraditional partners beyond pediatric clinicians and child-focused organizations and include stakeholders from all sectors that work or interact with children, including schools, religious organizations, and youth groups (Wizemann et al., 2014). This allows for better community buy-in, improved risk communication, and message dissemination.

It is important to include various stakeholders in the community when developing disaster plans. This may include fire, emergency medical services, police, local hospitals, public health departments, schools, child-care centers, faith-based organizations, and coalitions. Each stakeholder representative should share disaster plans to ensure there are no gaps or significant overlaps in the existing plans. Roles and responsibilities should be determined in the preparation phase of the disaster continuum. A **memorandum of understanding** should be created between various stakeholders before a disaster strikes.

UNACCOMPANIED MINORS

In the event of a disaster or public health emergency, children may present to the emergency department (ED) without a parent or guardian. An event involving a large number of children—for example, a mass shooting at a school—who may be unresponsive or unable to communicate due to a medical condition may not be accompanied by an adult caregiver who can identify the child. Younger unaccompanied children may not be able to provide the name of their parents as the child calls them "mom" and "dad"; they may not know their address or telephone number. CSHCN may not be able to communicate identifying information, and obviously, infants will not have any appropriate verbal skills.

Healthcare facilities and agencies must have plans and procedures in place on how to (a) identify the unaccompanied minors (injured/ill and uninjured/well), (b) contact/attempt to contact the parent/guardian, (c) track the child in the facility, (d) house the uninjured/well child, and (e) reunify the child with the correct parent/guardian (more discussion on this topic is found further in this chapter). An intake form should include as much information on the unaccompanied minor as possible: description of the child including clothing, identifying features such as birthmarks, location where child was found, anything the child may have said, and so on. Take photographs of each child to aid in the identification and reunification process. There should be a system in place for logging all of this information. The Unaccompanied Minors Registry is a national registry overseen by the National Center for Missing and Exploited Children (NCMEC); the unaccompanied minors should be entered into the system. The facility then provides an identification number, such as a wristband, for the unaccompanied minor. The wristband should not be easily removed so that the child can be tracked in the facility or if transferred to another facility. If the unaccompanied minor must be transferred to another facility, it is crucial that adequate information be provided to the receiving facility so that eventual reunification can take place. Unaccompanied minors who are uninjured/well need to be housed in a safe area until they can be reunited with their families. Facilities must identify an area within for these minors; adequate staff must be vetted ahead of time to ensure they do not have criminal records and the like. Ideally, the area would have only one entrance that can be monitored by security. The area must be childproofed and adequately staffed to ensure the safety of the minors. There should be age-appropriate activities for the children such as board games, puzzles, books, arts and crafts, and child-friendly movies. Snacks, drinks, and different-sized clothing should be available. Infants will also require cribs, diapers, and formula as well as age-appropriate toys that can be easily disinfected after use. Staff should also ensure that the children are not exposed to media covering the incident. Please refer to the section on reunification for those considerations (Federal Emergency Management Agency et al., 2013).

TRIAGE AND ASSESSMENT

An area for triaging or sorting disaster victims must be identified. Triage supplies should be readily available including tents, cots, identification/medical records packets, and medical supplies. Most triage systems are color coded: green, yellow, red, and black. Green is for minor injuries that can wait for treatment. Yellow is for injuries that are urgent but not life-threatening. Red indicates life-threatening injuries, and black indicates nonsalvageable injuries. The black area should be in a separate area and out of sight from the treatment areas.

Facilities and agencies should identify the triage protocol that will be followed in the event of a surge of patients. It is critical that life-threatening injuries are not missed (undertriaged) and that non-life-threatening injuries are not considered serious (overtriaged). START is the most commonly used mass casualty triage tool for adults, and JumpSTART was developed specifically for children (Figure 18.2). JumpSTART triage is applied to victims who are children, not infants. Appearance, breathing, and circulation are rapidly assessed using this triage algorithm. Staff must be trained in using JumpSTART, and, once triaged,

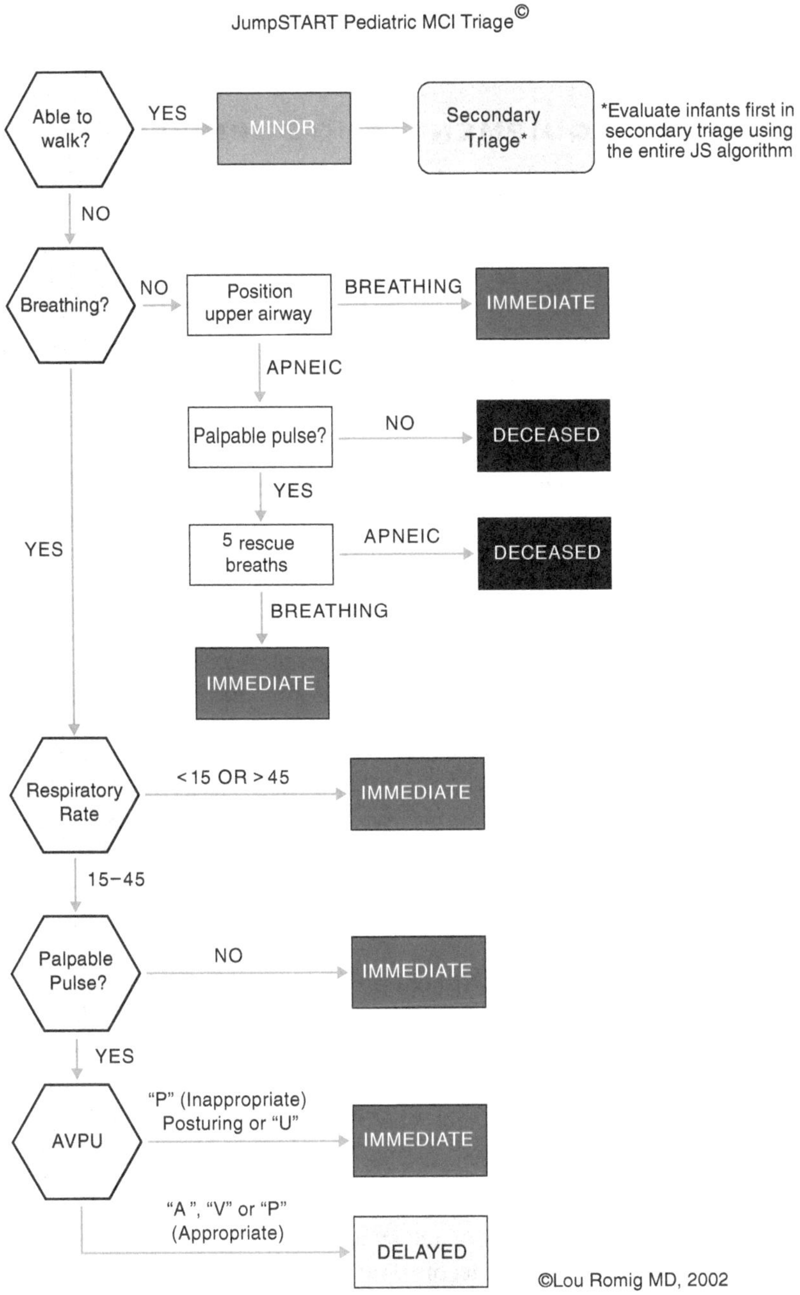

Figure 18.2 JumpSTART Pediatric MCI Triage©.

Source: Reproduced with permission from Lou Romig, MD.

JS, JumpSTART; MCI, Multicasualty Incident

healthcare workers must continually reassess pediatric victims as they can decompensate quickly.

Children can be difficult to assess as they may be frightened or in pain, making it hard for them to communicate. Infants cannot verbally express themselves; they may be crying because they are hungry, in pain, tired, or afraid. Providers not accustomed to or comfortable assessing pediatric patients may overlook injuries or incorrectly triage them. Pediatric-specific education is important for all healthcare workers.

MEDICATIONS, EQUIPMENT, AND SUPPLIES

A nationwide survey of ED preparedness for pediatric emergencies was conducted in 2003. The response rate was 29%, and a mere 6% of those EDs had all the recommended supplies and equipment. The researchers also calculated an overall pediatric-preparedness score, and the median score was 55 (Gausche-Hill et al., 2007). A follow-up study in 2013 demonstrated an improvement in the recommended pediatric supplies and equipment, and the median pediatric-preparedness score rose to 70. However, persistent gaps still exist (Gausche-Hill et al., 2015).

In pediatrics, medication is dosed based on the child's weight. As children vary in size and weight, it can be difficult to rapidly estimate their body weight, especially in life-threatening situations. The Boselow tape can be a very useful tool for facilities and providers who do not typically care for children. This is a length-based tape with appropriately dosed packs of emergency medications color coded to the length of the child.

Besides medications, children require smaller medical equipment such as **endotracheal tubes**, blades for intubation, face masks, urinary **catheters, nasogastric tubes**, and intravenous catheters. Younger children will also need cribs, gowns, and diapers. There are many resources available online with pediatric-specific equipment and supplies including the Emergency Medical Services for Children Innovation and Improvement Center website: https://emscimprovement.center/education-and-resources/toolkits/pediatric-equipment-toolkit.

DECONTAMINATION

Decontamination is very different with children as small children cannot understand instructions, and it is a very intimidating experience for them. Because of this, it is important to keep families together. Provided the parents are not very ill and injured, they can assist in getting the children through the decontamination process. The processes are very similar in general, but how these processes are followed is what are different in order to allow the family to be decontaminated together. The key differences are dependent on the child's age and developmental level. Obviously, infants will require total care from disrobing to showering them off. As babies are very slippery when wet, it is advisable to put them in a plastic laundry basket and then accompany them through the decontamination shower. Once decontaminated, infants must be rapidly dried and dressed to avoid hypothermia. They do not understand what they need to do to assist during decontamination. Staff and families need to hold them and assist with disrobing. They also may be scared and not understand what is going on. They need to keep warm as they can get cold stress if they are exposed to cold or not kept covered. There is also a very high risk for children when they are exposed to hazardous materials because of the issues mentioned earlier in the physiological differences section. Because of these differences, children can absorb the contaminated agents faster than adults, and being low to the ground they have a higher exposure level. Figure 18.3 is an example of a decontamination trailer that can accommodate children and families (Blake, 2019).

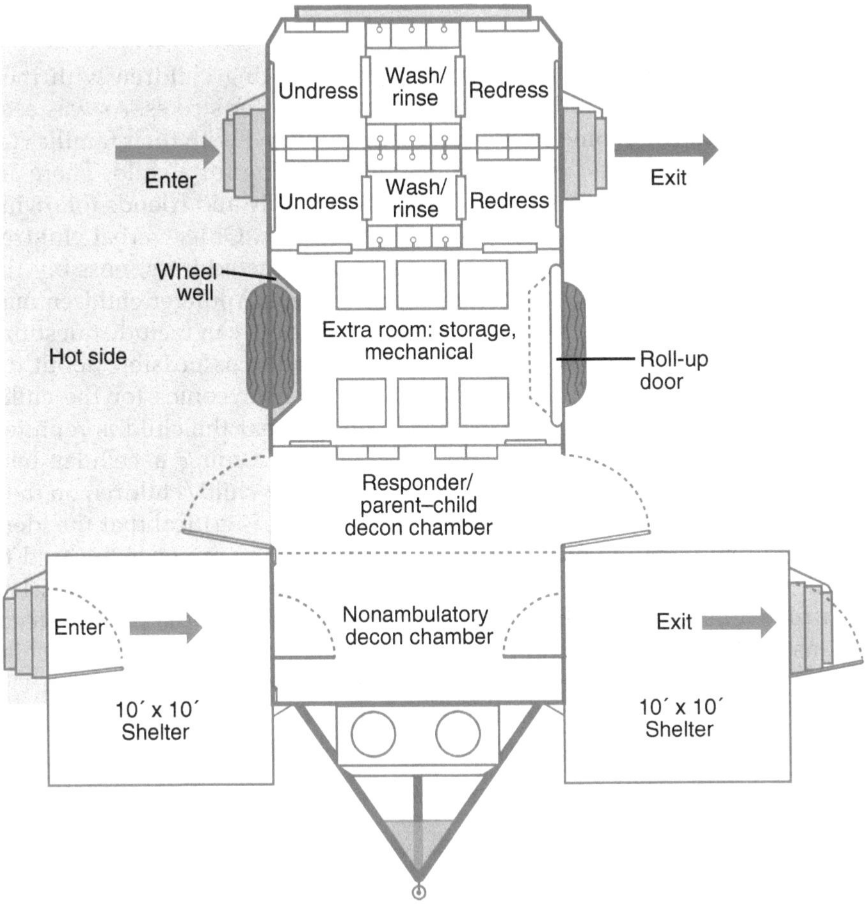

Figure 18.3 Decontamination trailer.

Source: Reproduced from Slota, M. C. (2018). *AACN core curriculum for pediatric high acuity, progressive and critical care nursing* (3rd ed.). Springer.

SHELTER SETUP/FAMILY ASSISTANCE CENTER

Children may come from a variety of settings when a disaster strikes and may end up in a shelter without their parents. They could come from child-care centers, school, or even their home. During Hurricane Katrina, children were airlifted from homes and some of their parents ended up in shelters in other states. One of the most important things to do is to ensure these children are in a safe place and not being cared for by volunteers who have not been appropriately vetted. These shelters or Family Information Centers (FICs) may be deployed by the local resources. Los Angeles County EMS Agency has put together a plan for an FIC planning guide that can be found at https://www.calhospitalprepare.org/FIC.

If the parents are present, it is important to keep the family together. In addition, there needs to be activities so the children can be distracted and not focus on the disaster that just happened. Many will not understand and could have increased stress. The activities should be age-appropriate to alleviate their stress and normalize their time.

REUNIFICATION

Facilities and agencies must develop plans for reuniting children with their parents. These plans need to be in place before a disaster strikes. As was seen with Hurricane Katrina, some children were not reunited with their families for many months. This can be very emotionally devastating for a child. There are different social media websites for tracking down family and friends following a disaster, but finding children is much more difficult. Older verbal children will be able to provide their parent's name, their home address, possibly the parent's place of employment, and telephone numbers. Younger children may not know this information. Procedures for older children can include questions and answers—a facilitator obtains as much information as possible about the family from the child. When a possible family member comes for the child, the facilitator asks a number of questions to ensure that the child is reunited with the parent/legal guardian. With most people owning a cellular telephone, many parents have current photographs of their child/children on their phones, and this can aid in the reunification process. It is critical that the identity of the parent/legal guardian is confirmed before the minor is released to them. For nonverbal children, the process may become more cumbersome. The disaster planner should also have a contingency plan in case the parents/legal guardians are seriously injured or killed in the incident. Social services/child protective custody services in the city or state may need to be involved. The NCMEC is the national agency tasked with reunifying unaccompanied minors with their families (Federal Emergency Management Agency et al., 2013).

CASE STUDY

In late December 2019, a statement was issued from the Wuhan Municipal Health Commission in China reporting a clustering of pneumonia cases in the Hubei Province of Wuhan, China (World Health Organization [WHO], n.d.). A new virus was identified soon thereafter, coronavirus, which is similar to the severe acute respiratory syndrome (SARS) that emerged in 2003. Initially limited to Asia, the first case in the United States was confirmed January 21, 2020. On January 30, 2020, the WHO declared a global health emergency. On February 29, 2020, the United States had its first death. On March 13, a national emergency was declared by President Trump. Schools were closed and nonessential workers were instructed to shelter in place (*New York Times Journal*, n.d.) It was initially thought that children were not impacted by the virus; however, soon researchers learned that the children were reacting to the virus differently than adults did. In China, 82% of the children had household contact with another infected person; however, only 10% of the children who tested positive were symptomatic (Zimmerman & Curtis, 2020).

A number of pediatric issues have been identified:

1. Schools were immediately closed to prevent the spread of the virus. Those who were economically disadvantaged had limited resources for online school. There was also an inconsistent school structure for online education, so schools varied in how they provided instruction. Different grading programs and different processes were implemented for whether there was a set time to go online to be taught by the teacher or not. With schools being closed, many disadvantaged children did not have access to breakfast and lunch; new processes were developed in order to serve those families.

2. For younger children, parents needed to work from home, provide some sort of day/child care, or juggle their job(s) with helping children with school and schoolwork. This created an additional stressor on the household and a potential financial impact if one or more parents needed to stay home on a regular basis.
3. Because of the stressors in the home, such as parents who lost their job altogether, there was a potential for an increase in child abuse and domestic violence with quarantine (Fry-Bowers, 2020).
4. There was an increase in anxiety and depression in the community from the stay-at-home orders and social distancing, but the immediate family caused an increase in social needs, especially for teenagers.
5. The cancellation of organized activities, including a lack of sports practices/team practices, created an increased social isolation for children and adolescents.
6. Because people were encouraged to stay at home, many clinics and doctor's offices were closed, causing a delay or decrease in immunizations and ensuring more children were at risk for developing those diseases.
7. There was a significant decrease of inpatient census in children's hospitals; early on, adult hospitals were running out of personal protective equipment (PPE) and ventilators. Hospitals had their workers reuse face masks. Then healthcare workers started dying from contracting the virus. Healthcare workers who were also parents stayed away from their families to prevent the virus' spread.
8. The disease didn't appear to affect children at first, but a new multisystem inflammatory state with overlapping features of **toxic shock syndrome** and atypical **Kawasaki disease** was soon identified as MIS-C (CDC, n.d.).
9. Definitive treatment is unclear, especially for adults, but more treatments are being identified every day.
10. It is unclear if people who are infected with COVID-19 will remain immune and for how long they will be immune.
11. There is a race to create a new vaccine, but it is unknown if it will be protective, its long-term effects, and its side effects.

While it has been determined that there is an issue with certain demographics and ethnic groups, children are more vulnerable and certain low-income areas of the demographic regions are considered more prone to be diagnosed. The local health departments have assigned staff to conduct contact tracing for the patients who are positive to determine if there are outbreaks in certain neighborhoods and demographic areas so they can target community education. Schools in these neighborhoods have been closed since the governor's stay-at-home order. The local health departments are collating their statistics and developing after-action reports to report out to the CDC.

SYMPTOMS OF MULTISYSTEM INFLAMMATORY SYNDROME IN CHILDREN RELATED TO COVID-19

MIS-C is a condition in which different body parts have an inflammatory response, including the heart, lungs, kidneys, brain, skin, eyes, or gastrointestinal organs. The cause is yet unknown; however, it is known that many children with MIS-C test positive for COVID-19 or have been exposed to someone with COVID-19. MIS-C can be serious, even deadly, but most children who were diagnosed with this condition have recovered. Symptoms are similar to those associated with COVID-19: fever, fatigue, nausea, and vomiting. In addition, there is a rash that is very different in children that is similar to the symptoms of Kawasaki disease (CDC, n.d.).

Care and Treatment of Multisystem Inflammatory Syndrome in Children

Symptoms that require immediate treatment are the following:

- Trouble breathing
- Pain or pressure in the chest that does not go away
- New confusion
- Inability to awaken or stay awake
- Bluish lips or face
- Severe abdominal pain

Diagnostic testing may include the following:

- Blood tests
- Chest x-ray
- Heart ultrasound (echocardiogram)
- Abdominal ultrasound
- Some children, depending on their symptoms, will be admitted for observation (CDC, n.d.).

Treatment is mainly supportive care depending on the symptoms.

ESSENTIAL SERVICES IN PUBLIC HEALTH

1. *Monitor health status* to identify and solve community health problems: Local health departments were monitoring for cases of pneumonia and follow-up whether or not COVID-19 was involved. Health departments should also be aware of an increase in resurgence of vaccine-preventable diseases due to primary care offices being closed and families not wanting to attend well-child care visits.
    a. Relevant Public Health Competencies
        i. Apply epidemiological methods to the breadth of settings and situations in public health practice.
        ii. Quantitative data collection
    b. Roles
        i. Frontline Staff
            a. Collect data on cases of pneumonia in the community and determine if COVID-19 is a consideration or not.
            b. Monitor for resurgence of vaccine-preventable diseases.

ii. Program Management
    a. Monitor the WHO and the CDC for updates on the situation.
    b. Develop and monitor surveillance systems and contact tracing policies.
    c. Communicate local surveillance results to federal agencies.

2. Diagnose and investigate health problems and health hazards in the community: Local public health departments initiated contact tracings for patients testing positive for COVID-19. Public health departments also monitored the community for any vaccine-preventable disease outbreaks.
    a. Relevant Public Health Competencies
        i. Apply epidemiological methods to the breadth of settings and situations in public health practice.
        ii. Select quantitative and qualitative data collection methods appropriate for a given public health context.
        iii. Interpret results of data analysis for public health research, policy, or practice.
    b. Roles
        i. Frontline Staff
            a. Initiate contact tracing for COVID-19-positive patients in the community.
            b. Monitor the community for vaccine-preventable diseases.
        ii. Program Management
            a. Develop and monitor surveillance systems and contact tracing policies.
            b. Communicate findings to state and federal agencies.
3. Inform, educate, and empower people about health issues: Public service announcements to socially distance and to wear face coverings were developed and disseminated via television and signs in the community. The messages were translated into many different languages. The term "face mask" was changed to "face covering." School districts disseminated announcements to students and families. School districts halted in-person learning and moved to online learning. Universities closed and sent students home to participate in online learning. With upcoming holidays, people were encouraged to continue social distancing. Community forums and lectures regarding COVID-19 were conducted through schools, faith communities, and other agencies.
    a. Relevant Public Health Competencies
        i. Select communication strategies for different audiences and sectors.
        ii. Communicate audience-appropriate public health content, both in writing and through oral presentation.
        iii. Describe the importance of cultural competence in communicating public health content.
    b. Roles
        i. Frontline staff
            a. Promote social distancing and the wearing of face coverings.
            b. Develop culturally appropriate public service announcements and signage.
        ii. Program Management
            a. Work with community leaders and school districts to disseminate consistent messages.

4. *Mobilize community partnerships* to identify and solve health problems: Schoolchildren who were receiving free meals at school are no longer receiving meals. Yet, programs and grants were developed to ensure that children and families received food through their schools. As a result, nonprofit organizations and faith-based organizations worked with school districts to provide meals. Food banks reported they are running low on donations and experiencing lines of cars waiting for hours to obtain food. Thus, solicitations for donations as well as volunteers to staff the food banks were initiated. Health departments reached out to librarians to assist with contact tracing of COVID-19–positive people.
    a. Relevant Public Health Competencies: Public Health and Healthcare Systems
        i. Propose strategies to identify stakeholders and build coalitions and partnerships for influencing public health outcomes.
        ii. Advocate for political, social, or economic policies and programs that will improve health in diverse populations.
    b. Roles
        i. Frontline staff
            a. Work with local school districts to identify families of need.
            b. Assist with distribution of food and services for those families.
        ii. Program Management
            a. Apply for federal grants to support the needs of at-risk families in the community.
            b. Work with governmental and nongovernmental agencies to provide services for at-risk families.
            c. Work with governmental agencies to ensure consistent messages.
5. *Develop policies and plans* that support individual and community health efforts: Local public health departments revised their pandemic policies and plans as the COVID-19 situation evolved. As statistics emerged, families in lower socioeconomic levels were found to be the hardest hit by the COVID-19 pandemic. Some health departments created tiered reopening plans once the situation subsided.
    a. Relevant Public Health Competencies
        i. Discuss multiple dimensions of the policymaking process, including the roles of ethics and evidence.
        ii. Propose strategies to identify stakeholders and build coalitions and partnerships for influencing public health outcomes.
    b. Roles
        i. Frontline staff
            a. Ensure that consistent messaging is released from the public health departments.
        ii. Program Management
            a. Identify new potential stakeholders as the pandemic evolves.
            b. Develop new policies and plans as new and updated knowledge is obtained for local, state, and federal agencies.
6. *Enforce laws and regulations* that protect health and ensure safety: Many healthcare facilities ran out of PPE and are promoting reusing disposable equipment. Healthcare workers have been fired for speaking out over some of these policies. Quarantine and stay-at-home orders were issued by public

health departments as well as city and state governments. Beaches and hiking trails were closed to enforce social distancing and stay-at-home orders.

a. Relevant Public Health Competencies
    i. Apply systems thinking tools to a public health issue.
    ii. Propose strategies to identify stakeholders and build coalitions and partnerships for influencing public health outcomes.
    iii. Advocate for political, social, or economic policies and programs that will improve health in diverse populations.
b. Roles
    i. Frontline Staff
        a. Assess the community for economic issues that may affect regulations and the health of the community.
    ii. Program Management
        a. Promote release of consistent public health messages.
        b. Continue to work with governmental and nongovernmental agencies to ensure regulations and laws are equitable and enforceable.
        c. Reinforce coalitions previously created to ensure the health and safety of the community.

7. *Link people to needed personal health services* and ensure the provision of healthcare when otherwise unavailable: People in the community are afraid to go to emergency departments for possible emergencies like **myocardial infarction**, stroke, and others. Families with lower socioeconomic levels are more adversely affected since many families have lost their jobs due to quarantine orders. Families have lost health benefits and many are unable to pay rent and are living in their cars.
    a. Relevant Public Health Competencies
        i. Compare the organization, structure, and function of healthcare, public health, and regulatory systems across national and international settings.
        ii. Discuss the means by which structural bias, social inequities, and racism undermine health and create challenges to achieving health equity at organizational, community, and societal levels.
    b. Roles
        i. Frontline Staff
            a. Work with local schools to identify families who may be in need of assistance.
            b. Promote well care in the community.
        ii. Program Management
            a. Develop public service announcements encouraging people to continue with well care visits via **telehealth**.
            b. Develop messages encouraging people to seek prompt medical care when developing serious symptoms of COVID-19, as well as symptoms of myocardial infarction and stroke.
            c. Leverage partnerships with businesses and other agencies to ensure families can obtain food and shelter (**social determinants of health**).
            d. Leverage partnerships with businesses and other agencies to ensure that children of lower socioeconomic levels have access to computers and Wi-Fi in order to attend virtual school.
            e. Develop policies to address inequities for future events based on current lessons learned.

8. *Ensure a competent public and personal healthcare workforce*: Initially healthcare workers were exposed to COVID–19-affected patients, and many became ill and died. PPE use was implemented rapidly, and supplies ran low as the number of affected patients grew. Many healthcare workers self-isolated from their families to ensure the safety of their loved ones. Best practices were communicated between healthcare facilities and many webinars on safety and COVID-19 treatments were presented.
   a. Relevant Public Health Competencies
      i. Perform effectively on interprofessional teams.
      ii. Apply systems thinking tools to a public health issue.
   b. Roles
      i. Frontline Staff
         a. Work with local hospitals in the community to ensure adequate PPE.
         b. Support healthcare provider families as providers self-isolate.
      ii. Program Management
         a. Work with healthcare facility leadership to address identified needs in the various facilities.
         b. Leverage partnerships to ensure the health and well-being of healthcare workers.
9. *Evaluate* effectiveness, accessibility, and quality of personal and population-based health services: Many university public health departments were collecting data on the incidence of COVID-19, number of people tested, number of people testing positive, and number of deaths due to COVID-19. Other organizations monitored the number of provider visits for well-care as well as ill-care. As different tests for COVID-19 evolved, differences in the various test results emerged and a lot of **misinformation** and misinterpretation of statistics were communicated. Mixed messages were also communicated regarding social distancing, the wearing of face coverings, and social gatherings. Social media platforms started fact-checking various posts.
   a. Relevant Public Health Competencies
      i. Interpret results of data analysis for public health research, policy, or practice.
      ii. Evaluate policies for their impact on public health and health equity leadership.
      iii. Apply principles of leadership, governance, and management, which include creating a vision, empowering others, fostering collaboration, and guiding decision-making.
   b. Roles
      i. Frontline Staff
         a. Encourage local communities to continue with social distancing and face covering.
      ii. Program Management
         a. Continue to provide accurate health information to the community.
         b. Support telehealth visits and drive through vaccination clinics, especially for influenza.
         c. Work with governmental leaders to provide consistent messaging and public service announcements.
10. *Research* for new insights and innovative solutions to health problems: Due to the high morbidity and mortality associated with COVID-19, and no

specific treatment, many treatment modalities were employed more or less haphazardly. As more details emerged on the pathophysiology of COVID-19, more focused treatments are being researched. Healthcare facilities are communicating results of these trials to other providers. Several biotechnology companies started research and development of a vaccine. Clinical trials of several vaccines with healthy volunteers commenced.

a. Relevant Public Health Competencies
    i. Analyze quantitative and qualitative data using biostatistics, informatics, and computer-based programming and software.
    ii. Interpret results of data analysis for public health research, policy, or practice.
b. Roles
    i. Frontline Staff
        a. Monitor vaccine trial results.
        b. Monitor communications regarding experimental treatments for COVID-19.
        c. Monitor for misinformation and unfounded treatments for COVID-19.
    ii. Program Management
        a. Develop vaccine distribution plans.
        b. Develop public service announcements for vaccine distribution.

PUTTING IT ALL TOGETHER

Disaster planners must incorporate children in their disaster and public health emergency plans. Children are not small adults and vary in size and developmental level, and these factors must be taken into account in the planning phase. Community preparedness must start at the family level. Families should be encouraged to

- create a family emergency plan and include the child in the planning process
- create or purchase an emergency kit
    - include favorite toy/comfort item for child
    - include activities for child
    - include pet items if family has a pet
- teach their children the home address, parent name(s), and phone numbers
- obtain a completed EIF from their healthcare provider if the child has special healthcare needs
- practice home disaster/emergency drill at least annually
- practice good hand hygiene
- get annual influenza vaccine
- keep children at home if they have fever and/or illness
- enroll their teenagers in a Community Emergency Response Team (CERT) class

Healthcare organizations and facilities must also incorporate pediatric factors into their disaster plans and disaster drills. All community stakeholders should be involved in community disaster planning including schools and day-care sites. Disaster and public health emergency plans including pediatric considerations will help in protecting one of our most vulnerable populations, our children.

DISCUSSION QUESTIONS

1. On January 28, 2014, Atlanta, Georgia, experienced a snowstorm that caused significant trauma to many schoolchildren. Ninety-nine school buses, full of children, were stuck in traffic, under freezing conditions, until midnight, and approximately 2,000 children were stranded overnight in schools.
2. Discuss a citywide public health strategy or strategies to avoid this situation in the future. What could be done to avoid having children stranded and separated from families? What could be some of the barriers to getting children evacuated and safely home before weather conditions precluded safe travel?
3. Discuss issues that schools housing children overnight would face, including communication concerns. What could schools do to improve capacity when caring for children in an emergency situation?
4. During the COVID-19 pandemic, school policies varied widely regarding shutting down in-person classes completely and using online teaching formats. Some schools developed hybrid teaching plans, with some online classes and some in-person learning continuing. Discuss issues that would determine a school's policy for educating children during a pandemic.
5. Should the county plan alternative educational strategies in case of another pandemic or other emergency that would make traditional in-person schooling difficult? What are some of your ideas to continue education during an emergency situation lasting for months?
6. Children and parents are sometimes separated during emergencies. As a public health professional, develop a strategy for tracking and reuniting parents with children after an event.

REFERENCES

American Academy of Pediatrics, Committee on Pediatric Emergency Medicine, Council on Clinical Information Technology, American College of Emergency Physicians, & Pediatric Emergency Medicine Committee. (2010). Policy statement–emergency information forms and emergency preparedness for children with special health care needs. *Pediatrics, 125*(4), 829–837. https://doi.org/10.1542/peds.2010-0186

Blake, N. (2019). Disaster preparedness and response. In M. C. Slota (Ed.), *AACN core curriculum for pediatric high acuity, progressive, and critical care nursing* (3rd ed., pp. 829–830). Springer Publishing.

Centers for Disease Control and Prevention. (n.d.). *For parents: Multisystem inflammatory syndrome in children (MIS-C) associated with COVID-19.* https://www.cdc.gov/coronavirus/2019-ncov/daily-life-coping/children/mis-c.html

Federal Emergency Management Agency, U.S. Department of Health and Human Services, American Red Cross, & National Center for Missing and Exploited Children. (2013, November). *Post-disaster reunification of children: A nationwide approach.* http://www.nationalmasscarestrategy.org/wp-content/uploads/2014/07/post-disaster-reunification-of-children-a-nationwide-approach.pdf

Ferrer, R. R., Ramirez, M., Sauser, K., Iverson, E., & Upperman, J. S. (2009). Emergency drills and exercises in healthcare organizations: Assessment of pediatric population involvement using after-action reports. *American Journal of Disaster Medicine, 4*(1), 23–32. https://www.wmpllc.org/ojs/index.php/ajdm/article/view/1918

Fry-Bowers, E. K. (2020). Children are at risk from COVID-19. *Journal of Pediatric Nursing, 53*(2020), A10–A12. https://doi.org/10.1016/j.pedn.2020.04.026

Gausche-Hill, M., Ely, M., Schmuhl, P., Telford, R., Remick, K. E., Edgerton, E. A., & Olson, L. M. (2015). A national assessment of pediatric readiness of emergency departments. *JAMA Pediatrics, 169*(6), 527–534. https://doi.org/10.1001/jamapediatrics.2015.138

Gausche-Hill, M., Schmitz, C., & Lewis, R. J. (2007). Pediatric preparedness of US emergency departments: A 2003 survey. *Pediatrics, 120*(6), 1229–1237. https://doi.org/10.1542/peds.2006-3780

Kim, D. H. (2016). Emergency preparedness and the development of health care coalitions: A dynamic process. *Nursing Clinics of North America, 51*(4), 545–554. https://doi.org/10.1016/j.cnur.2016.07.013

New York Times Journal. (n.d.). *The COVID 19 pandemic.* https://www.nytimes.com/news-event/coronavirus

Ray, K. R., Olson, L. M., Edgerton, E. A., Ely, M., Gausche-Hill, M., Schmuhl, P., Wallace, D. J., & Kahn, J. (2018). Access to high pediatric-readiness emergency care in the United States. *Journal of Pediatrics, 194*, 225–232. https://doi.org/10.1016/j.jpeds.2017.10.074

U.S. Census Bureau. (2020). *ACS demographic and housing estimates.* https://data.census.gov/cedsci/table?q=United%20States&table=DP05&tid=ACSDP5Y2018.DP05&g=0100000US&lastDisplayedRow=44&vintage=2017&layer=state&cid=DP05_0001E

Wizemann, T., Reeve, M., & Altevogt, B. M. (Eds.). (2014). *Preparedness, response, and recovery considerations for children and families: Workshop summary.* National Academies Press. https://doi.org/10.17226/18550

World Health Organization. (n.d.). *Coronavirus disease (COVID-19) weekly epidemiological update and weekly operational update.* https://www.who.int/emergencies/diseases/novel-coronavirus-2019/situation-reports

Zimmerman, P., & Curtis, N. (2020). Coronavirus infections in children including COVID-19: An overview of the epidemiology, clinical features, diagnosis, treatment and prevention options in children. *Pediatric Infectious Disease, 39*(5), 355–368. https://doi.org/10.1097/INF.0000000000002660

CHAPTER 19

EVOLVING AND EMERGING THREATS

ESTHER D. CHERNAK

KEY TERMS

Aedes aegypti Mosquito
Avian Influenza
Beta-Lactum Antibiotics
Borrelia burgdorferi
Campylobacter Infection
Candida auris
Clostridioides difficile
Cryptosporidiosis
Culex Species
Ebola Virus Disease
Flaviviruses
Guillain-Barré Syndrome
Ixodes scapularis
MERS
Microcephaly
Mycoplasma Pneumonia
Nonpharmaceutical Control Measures
Novel Coronavirus
Pathogen
Plasmodium Species
Prognosis
Salmonella
SARS
Serological Studies

INTRODUCTION

Emerging or evolving threats pose new and unexpected challenges for public health agencies. Applying descriptors of emerging infectious diseases to hazards of any origin, emerging threats are disease entities that are recognized for the first time in humans. They may also be "reemerging," or threats that have historically affected human health but reappear in new populations and locations (Fauci & Morens, 2012; Morens et al., 2004). Most infectious disease threats emerge from animal reservoirs, through activities that bring humans into close contact with animals and allow pathogens to "spillover" and cross the species barrier. The modern forces of globalization, population growth, demographic and epidemiologic transitions, migration and population displacement, and climate change become subsequent drivers for emerging threats to human health (McMichael, 2013; Ryu et al., 2017). These trends, along with the use of new technologies including modern healthcare advances, create conditions that produce new threats to human health and lead to public health emergencies (World Health Organization [WHO], 2003). This chapter describes how these factors lead to new public health threats and review some recent examples that illustrate how the essential services of public health are critical for preparedness and response.

DRIVERS OF EMERGING THREATS

One Health

Human populations have always lived in close contact with wild and domestic animals. This phenomenon is especially common in countries where many people keep backyard chickens and fowl and purchase food at live animal markets where they may be exposed to exotic animals. In other parts of the world, this phenomenon occurs as human populations grow and expand into new geographic areas. Originally referred to as "One Medicine," the term "One Health" is now used to recognize that the health of humans and the health of animals are inextricably linked. They inhabit the same ecosystem and share susceptibility to many of the same diseases and environmental hazards. This coexistence has led to most of the emerging infectious disease of public health importance in the last century (Allen et al., 2017).

Diseases that are endemic among animals are called "zoonotic diseases," and they are the most common causes of emerging infections. Spillover events are transmission events in which a human becomes infected with an animal-associated or zoonotic disease. Humans can become ill through a variety of mechanisms, including direct contact with fluids or tissues from infected animals (e.g., rabies, **Ebola virus disease, avian influenza**), consumption of food products of animal origin that are contaminated with bacteria (e.g., *Escherichia coli* 0157:H7 infection, from poorly cooked hamburger), or indirect contact with objects or surfaces that are contaminated with microorganisms that animals shed (e.g., ***Salmonella*** infections from handling reptiles). Insect vectors such as ticks or mosquitoes are another mechanism of transmission from animal to human. Vectors can transmit viruses, parasites, or bacteria from an animal reservoir to humans (e.g., West Nile virus), or from human to human (e.g., Dengue virus, malaria) if large numbers of people harbor infection and an animal reservoir is no longer needed to contribute to the transmission cycle. Some pathogens, such as the H7N9 strain of avian influenza, may be transmitted from chickens to humans, but the pathogen is poorly adapted to humans, and there are no subsequent human-to-human infections. However, if the pathogen has the potential to become easily transmitted from human to human, the conditions for a major public health emergency, even a worldwide pandemic, may be satisfied (JAMA Author Interviews, 2020).

The capacity for sustained transmission cycles in populations that have no prior immunity to the pathogen is one of the most concerning features of emerging threats. The global epidemics of novel strains of influenza that result from recombination with human influenza and strains of avian or swine origin, **novel coronaviruses**, and **flaviviruses** like Dengue and Zika viruses are recent examples of this phenomenon (Cunningham et al., 2017; Gebreyes et al., 2014; Choffnes & Mack, 2015). In heavily populated countries like China, human transmission of zoonotic pathogens that are transmitted via respiratory routes is amplified by the high frequency of human interactions in crowded communities. In addition, the ease of international travel facilitates the spread of many infectious diseases, especially easily transmitted respiratory viruses such as coronaviruses and influenza (del Rio & Malani, 2020). This is certainly the story of the COVID-19 pandemic, caused by SARS-CoV-2, a novel beta-coronavirus that successfully made the species leap from bats to humans, via an intermediate animal host whose identity has not been confirmed. This virus has so successfully adapted to its human host that animal-to-human transmission is no longer needed for human infections and the virus is capable of spreading exponentially in human populations in the absence of control measures.

Demographic Trends

Population Growth, Aging, and the "Unfinished Agenda"

The modern age is characterized by social changes, demographic trends, and environmental factors that have significant impact on the global burden of disease and produce new public health challenges. See Figure 19.1. These changes have been described as a "syndrome" of interrelated factors that act together to produce new health challenges (McMichael, 2013). The world's population continues to grow: The United Nations projects that the global population will increase from 7.7 billion in 2019 to 11.2 billion by the end of the century, nearly triple the population of the early 1960s (Roser, 2014/2019). Most of this

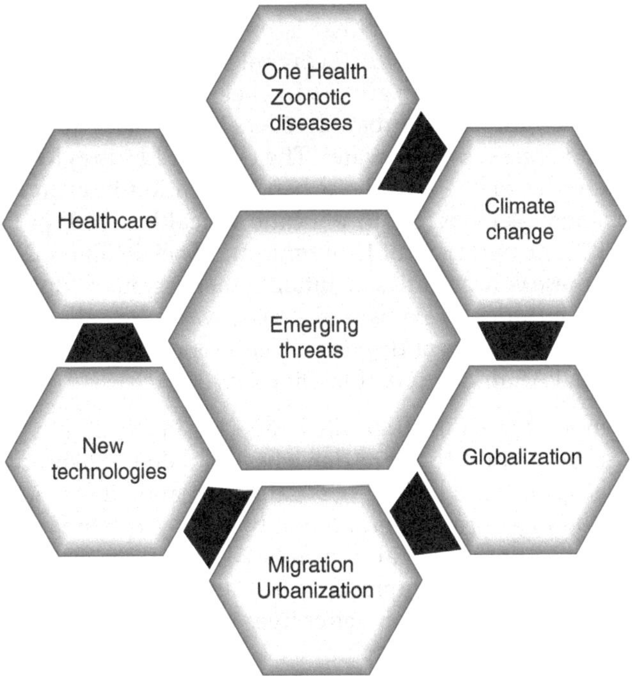

Figure 19.1 Drivers of emerging threats to public health.

Source: Data from McMichael, A. J. (2013). Globalization, climate change, and human health [Figure 1]. *New England Journal of Medicine, 368*(14), 1335–1343. https://doi.org/10.1056/NEJMra1109341

increase is occurring in the world's poorest countries where high fertility rates are resulting in a "youth bulge," or a greater proportion of young people (Jahan et al., 2014). At the same time, higher income countries have experienced demographic transitions: Declining fertility rates that result in stable or decreasing populations, in which a larger percentage of people are older adults. In a number of Western democracies, nearly 25% of the population is older than 60. This demographic transition is accompanied by an epidemiological transition: As the population ages and lives longer, the burden of disease evolves from infectious diseases and conditions affecting maternal and child health to chronic noncommunicable diseases that are more common later in life. However, even low-income countries with rising fertility rates are also seeing life expectancy gains as they experience economic development. As a result, they bear the burdens of disease in both young and older population segments—the so-called unfinished agenda, or diseases that result from inadequate sanitation and a lack of access to healthcare, as well as conditions that arise from tobacco use, obesity, and aging. These demographic changes are not public health emergencies in and of themselves. However, they strain healthcare and public health systems, especially in countries that devote few resources to them. Moreover, these vulnerable populations—children under the age of 5 years, and the increasingly larger proportion of the population of older adults—are more likely to experience significant health consequences from emerging threats and require special planning for response and control measures (Barrett et al., 2015).

Urbanization and Population Migration

Urbanization has accompanied economic and industrial development in many countries, resulting in significant population shifts into cities that offer greater potential for employment and economic security. Over one-half of the world's population lives in cities, a number that is projected to increase to two-thirds by the year 2050 (UN, Department of Economic and Social Affairs, Population Division, 2018). Much of this urban growth has been unplanned and unsupported by local governments, and many urban dwellers live in inadequate housing that lacks plumbing and access to clean water. The UN World Cities Report 2018 estimates that one-quarter of the world's urban population lives in overcrowded slums where residents lack access to education, healthy food, public services, and healthcare (UN, Department of Economic and Social Affairs, 2018). The living conditions in these communities facilitate transmission of contagious **pathogens**, as well as environmental exposures to toxic waste. So-called megacities are incubators for new epidemics of diseases (Neiderud, 2015; UN, Department of Economic and Social Affairs, Population Division, 2018).

The phenomenon of urbanization often reflects "internal" population shifts within countries, from rural to more densely populated urban areas. Another important demographic trend is the large-scale population migration that occurs from country to country, across international borders. An estimated 244 million people are considered international migrants (Wickramage et al., 2018). These are individuals who leave their home countries to flee conflict, escape drought conditions, or seek employment and better lives in countries that offer more economic opportunities. They may be asylum seekers, migrant laborers, or displaced persons. Often, these individuals are impoverished and marginalized in their new countries and lack fundamental services, adequate housing, and healthcare. They are highly vulnerable to health threats. Migrating populations may also introduce infectious diseases that are endemic in their countries of origin to new lands where they may not be recognized and where they may spread quickly among immunologically naïve populations. Finally, global travel and tourism has increased by 56-fold since 1950, and the UN World Tourism Organization estimates that there were over 1.4 billion international tourists in 2018 (Roser, 2017).

GLOBALIZATION

Modern transportation systems have facilitated a global economy where goods and services are bought and sold across the world. The global economy not only is a driver of migration and population movement but also impacts health in direct ways, perhaps best illustrated by the global food supply. In the United States, for example, the food supply is increasingly dependent on foreign imports. Much of the fresh produce and most of the fish consumed in this country comes from outside the United States, in countries with 12-month growing climates or active fishing economies. However, food production practices vary around the world and standards for manufacturing, processing, and food storage may allow for contamination of foods, a real concern for products that are consumed raw or without significant heating. Approximately 20% of food consumed in the United States is imported, including an estimated 97% of fish, 50% of fresh fruits, and 20% of fresh vegetables. Since 1996, the number of foodborne outbreaks in the United States related to consumption of imported food sources has increased by sixfold, from three per year between 1996 and 2000 to 18 per year between 2009 and 2014. Moreover, these outbreaks may be caused by new or emerging pathogens, such as unusual strains of *Salmonella*, **cryptosporidiosis**, and other parasitic infections (Gould et al., 2017).

Similarly, international commerce increases the availability of products across the globe and has contributed to a rise in noncommunicable diseases. Access to Western diets and to tobacco products now contribute to obesity, smoking, and hypertension in countries where these are relatively new risk factors and cause new health challenges. Globalization and a "nutrition transition" in countries where life expectancy is increasing and people are living longer are contributing to a "slow emergency" of cardiovascular disease and cancer that are now among the most significant global disease burdens (Ronto et al., 2018).

CLIMATE CHANGE

Human activities resulting from industrialization and use of combustible fuels have released large quantities of carbon dioxide and other greenhouse gases that trap heat in the lower atmosphere and affect the global climate. As a result, the world's average temperature has warmed by 0.85 °C in the last 130 years. The environmental consequences of our warming climate include rising sea levels, melting ice caps and glaciers, and changing weather and precipitation patterns. Extreme weather events have become more intense and common. Higher temperatures raise levels of air pollutants like ozone, particularly in urban areas. The changing climate impacts human health in ways that are both direct (primary) and indirect (secondary or tertiary; McMichael, 2013). High temperatures that occur during extreme heat waves are associated with increased mortality from hyperthermia and heat stroke, especially in older adult individuals living in "heat islands" in urban areas (McMichael, 2013). High temperatures also contribute to exacerbations of underlying cardiovascular and respiratory disease through heat stress and increased exposure to air pollutants (Guo et al., 2017). Weather-related natural disasters, which have more than tripled since the 1960s, are estimated to result in over 60,000 deaths annually, mainly in developing and low-income countries. Heavy rains contribute to flooding, injuries, and failure of sanitation and water treatment systems, which can lead to outbreaks of diarrheal disease from contaminated water. In the other extreme, climate change may also lead to water scarcity and drought, which leads to reduced farming capacity, food insecurity, and malnutrition. Reduced food yields and access to water may result in more diffuse effects: population displacement, mental health challenges, political conflict, and crises that lead to humanitarian emergencies (Intergovernmental Panel on Climate Change, 2014; McMichael, 2013).

Climate change also impacts vector-transmitted infections. Warmer temperatures increase the activity of vectors like ticks and mosquitoes and facilitate "overwintering" in climates that are increasingly less cold. Rising temperatures and humidity create new habitats for both host animal reservoirs and insect vectors, as well as the pathogens they transmit, resulting in expansion of diseases to new geographic areas. Rising temperatures also impact the viability of both the vector-borne pathogens and vectors themselves. The extension of Lyme disease, a bacterial infection caused by ***Borrelia burgdorferi*** and transmitted by the deer tick, ***Ixodes scapularis***, to northern climates is an example of how climate change contributes to the impacts of population migration as a driver of emerging diseases (Ogden & Gachon, 2019; B. L. Stone et al., 2017).

Modern Healthcare

Advances in healthcare in the last century have resulted in tremendous gains in health and improved outcomes from conditions that had for years been associated with poor **prognoses**. However, complications from procedures associated with modern healthcare have become a major source of morbidity and mortality worldwide and represent an emerging threat to human health. In the United States alone, an estimated 2 million people annually suffer from healthcare-associated infections, complications arising from the use of urinary and bloodstream catheters, and intubation with mechanical ventilation (P. W. Stone, 2009; WHO, 2011).

The use of antimicrobials in the healthcare environment creates selective pressure that contributes opportunistic infections such as ***Clostridioides difficile***, which causes healthcare-associated diarrheal disease, and ***Candida auris***, a highly drug-resistant fungus that causes untreatable systemic infections in compromised hosts. The use of broad-spectrum antimicrobials also contributes to the emergence of antibiotic resistance, a major public health threat. Healthcare facilities, especially hospitals, have facilitated "super-spreading" events that amplify transmission of emerging respiratory viruses, such as the **SARS** and **MERS** coronaviruses (Park et al., 2018; Wang et al., 2020), which result from insufficient infection control during the care of critically ill individuals with these infections.

In the community, immunosuppressive agents that are responsible for tremendous gains in the treatment of many malignancies and autoimmune diseases, and enable lifesaving organ transplantation, have created newly vulnerable populations who are uniquely susceptible to severe complications of both common and unusual infections. One survey identified that nearly 3% of the U.S. population self-report having a compromised immune system, due either to malignancies, the consequences of medication, or immunosuppressive medical conditions like

HIV infection. This increase in immunologic vulnerability in the general population has resulted in an increase in both common and unusual opportunistic infections. These at-risk individuals require targeted planning for health-protective measures during emergencies (Grossi, 2020; Harpaz et al., 2016; Miro et al., 2019).

Health Impacts of New Technology

New technologies used in modern transportation systems and industry, and for information storage and dissemination, create new vulnerabilities and hazards that threaten public health. Although not traditionally considered to be an emerging threat, injuries related to motor vehicle accidents are now a major cause of global morbidity and mortality; they are a phenomenon of the last 150 years of human history. Occupational injuries in workplace settings are another phenomenon of modern life; they are now estimated to result in over 300,000 deaths annually across the globe and contribute to 8.8% of global burden of mortality and 8.1% of disability-adjusted life years (DALYs; GBD 2017 Risk Factor Collaborators, 2018). Chemical spills and industrial accidents with exposures to toxic hazardous materials are now a recognized threat for which community-based emergency responders must be prepared (Federal Emergency Management Agency [FEMA], 2019).

Cyberterrorism—intentional attacks on computer systems with the goal of disrupting business operations, government, and overall societal functioning—may have the potential to cause the greatest human impacts and has emerged as a major concern with public health consequences. Direct attacks on public health and healthcare information systems can cause widespread damage to healthcare facilities, threatening the privacy of medical and financial records. They may compromise patient care, rendering electronic medical records inaccessible or unusable, and disrupt medical supply chains. Threats to public health and healthcare information systems require specific and costly investments to ensure their security and are now a major priority for healthcare systems and planners (Healthcare and Public Health Cybersecurity Working Group, 2017).

EXAMPLES OF EMERGING THREATS

This section presents several recent examples of emerging threats that illustrate how all these drivers contribute to their impact on human health. Each example will also include a description of how the public health response relies on the essential services of public health to contain or control the threat.

Arboviruses—The Evolving Epidemiology of Dengue and Zika Virus Infections

Globally, mosquito-borne infections, also known as "arboviruses," or arthropod-borne viruses, are the most significant contributor to the burden of vector-borne diseases, causing nearly 500,000 deaths annually worldwide. The parasitic infection, malaria (***Plasmodium* species**), accounts for most of the global burden of mosquito-transmitted disease and is responsible for over 400,000 deaths annually (WHO, 2020). Aggressive public health strategies including distribution of protective mosquito nets to high-risk communities, coupled with enhanced recognition and treatment of cases, has resulted in a significant decrease in malaria deaths in the last 15 years. Paradoxically, because of climate change, global travel and migration patterns, and urbanization, infections with two arthropod-borne flaviviruses have emerged as major threats to human health: Dengue virus and Zika virus (Sutherst, 2004).

Dengue Virus

The incidence of Dengue has grown nearly sixfold since 2010 and is now believed to be 390 million infections per year (WHO, 2021a) The WHO now estimates that nearly half of the world's population in over 128 countries is at risk, although Asia bears 70% of the actual burden of disease. Dengue is a flavivirus, an RNA virus that is transmitted from human to human via the bite of an infected mosquito. The infection produces a severe flu-like febrile illness associated with rash and severe headache. There are four major serotypes of Dengue virus. Infection with one serotype produces lifelong immunity against that strain, but reinfection with a new serotype after infection with another strain can lead to more severe symptoms known as "Dengue hemorrhagic fever," which is associated with shock, respiratory distress, and hemorrhage. In the absence of supportive care, mortality rate is as high as 20%, with younger children especially vulnerable.

The major mosquito vector for Dengue is the ***Aedes aegypti mosquito*** species. The mosquito is believed to have been introduced to "New World" countries by the European slave trade 500 years ago. The recent rise in infections has occurred as global travel and international trade has transported the *Aedes* mosquito to new parts of the world, especially to urban habitats where the mosquito thrives in small containers and collections of water that are common in crowded environments. The dramatic increase in Dengue virus infections has occurred in metropolitan areas of tropical and subtropical climates, where increasing temperatures associated with climate change have created newly hospitable regions for the mosquito to breed (Lwande et al., 2020; Powell & Tabachnick, 2013; Powell et al., 2018). Outbreaks of Dengue have occurred in Asian, Central American, and African countries. An outbreak of Dengue infections in Honduras in 2018 to 2019 illustrates how current demographic and environmental factors facilitate disease transmission, particularly in impoverished urban areas. This outbreak is one of the worst Dengue epidemics in Central America (Semple, 2019), resulting in over 400 deaths, 40% of all the Dengue deaths in the region. The factors believed to have contributed to this epidemic include drought conditions that alternated with periods of extreme rain, occurring in neighborhoods without reliable public water supplies. Residents store water inside and outside homes, creating potential breeding sites. Local flooding after heavy rains provides more breeding sites, particularly in areas that lack effective drainage systems. These meteorological events, occurring in densely populated areas that lack significant public and healthcare resources, contribute to devastating epidemics of Dengue fever in locations with limited ability to manage them (WHO, 2019).

Zika

The epidemic of Zika virus infections in the Western Hemisphere in 2014 to 2015 resulted from another "perfect storm" facilitated by the consequences of changing climate, international travel and trade, and urbanization in tropical and subtropical countries. Zika virus is a flavivirus that is related to Dengue virus. It was originally identified in the Zika forest of Uganda in 1947, where it was primarily a zoonotic infection with a primate reservoir. The first human cases were recognized in 1952 in individuals with direct exposure to the jungle environment. Only occasional human cases were recognized until 2007, when the first major human outbreak occurred on the Pacific island of Yap, likely introduced by travel or trade involving an infected mosquito or person. This outbreak was followed by a series of outbreaks in French Polynesia in 2013 to 2014 and ultimately pandemic spread of the virus to the Americas, the Caribbean, and Africa in 2015. The sporadic cases prior to these outbreaks occurred when mosquitoes transmitted the virus from Zika-infected primates to humans via a blood meal in rare "spillover" events. However, in the outbreaks of Yap, French Polynesia, and Central and South America, there were sufficient human infections to support direct transmission via mosquitoes from infected to uninfected persons. In South America, infected travelers introduced the virus into a geographic region with a competent mosquito vector (*Aedes*) and an immunologically naïve or susceptible population living in close proximity in populated areas, which resulted in explosive human-to-human transmission of this virus (Fauci & Morens, 2016; Musso et al., 2019). The transition from sylvatic, or primate-to-primate transmission, to an "urban" cycle of human-to-human transmission is depicted in Figure 19.2.

The symptoms of Zika virus infection in the first recognized cases was a mild, self-limited febrile illness. **Serological studies** completed after the outbreak suggested that nearly 80% of infections in a population are likely asymptomatic, although these individuals contribute to the reservoir for human-to-human transmission. However, new symptoms of infection were observed in the outbreak in Central and South America, particularly in Brazil, which infected over 60% of the exposed population and resulted in 200,000 cases. In addition to the relatively mild febrile illness, Zika virus infection was associated with congenital malformations, including infant microcephaly and neurologic abnormalities. This manifestation results from maternal–fetal

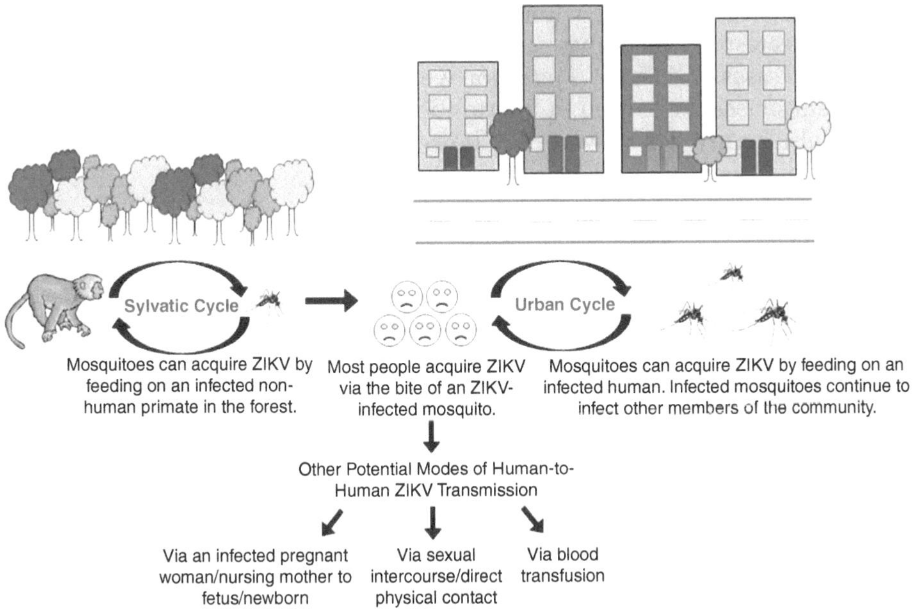

Figure 19.2 Sylvatic and urban transmission cycle.

Source: Reproduced from Sharma, A., & Lal, S. K. (2017). Zika virus: Transmission, detection, control, and prevention [Figure 3]. *Frontiers in Microbiology, 8*, 110. https://doi.org/10.3389/fmicb.2017.00110

transmission of the Zika virus during pregnancy, a phenomenon that was first recognized in this outbreak and had never before been described as a complication of a flavivirus infection. Indeed, it was the increase in cases of microcephaly and neurological disorders that prompted the WHO to declare a Public Health Emergency of International Concern in February 2016 (Heymann et al., 2016). In addition, sexual transmission, mainly male to female, was also recognized, and Zika virus has been detected in semen as well as blood and other body fluids. Transfusion-associated transmission has also occurred, raising important questions about how best to protect the blood supply in areas experiencing active Zika virus transmission. Infection was also associated with the occurrence of **Guillian-Barré syndrome** in adults (also recognized retrospectively after the French Polynesia outbreak), an immune-mediated condition that results in ascending paralysis and, rarely, respiratory failure due to paralysis of the diaphragm. This is a relatively uncommon complication of a number of other exposures to infectious diseases, including ***Campylobacter*** **infection, Mycoplasma pneumoniae**, influenza, hepatitis A, and Epstein-Barr virus, and a number of other viral and bacterial infections (Wijdicks & Klein, 2017).

In the United States, the incidence of vector-borne disease increased substantially between 2004 and 2016. Over 75% of this increase was due to tickborne diseases, mainly Lyme disease, which is now recognized in all of the continental United States but occurs mainly in the northeastern and Pacific states. Mosquito-borne disease has contributed to this increase, which is largely due to West Nile virus (WNV) infections. WNV infection was first recognized in the Western Hemisphere in 1999 in an outbreak affecting New York City, a result of a global importation of the virus into a new region with a competent mosquito vector, the **Culex species**. This virus has now become endemic throughout the United States and is now responsible for most endemic cases of mosquito-borne illness in this country. However, both Dengue and Zika virus infections cause substantial morbidity in the United States through sporadic epidemics. The subtropical states of Florida and Texas and the territories of Puerto Rico and the U.S. Virgin Islands bear the greatest impact of these events. During the 2015 to 2016 Zika pandemic, over 41,000 cases of Zika virus infection were reported in the United States. Most of this transmission occurred in Puerto Rico and the Caribbean, but local transmission also occurred in Brownsville, Texas, and Miami, Florida (Caminade et al., 2019; Kindhauser et al., 2016; Rosenberg et al., 2018).

Public Health Control Measures for Mosquito-Borne Infections

There are no specific antiviral treatments for Dengue or Zika virus infections; care of infected patients is generally supportive. Control measures for mosquito-borne disease in general and during major epidemics leverage all the essential services of public health and require the efforts of personnel at all levels in public health agencies. Population-based surveillance for human cases and disease investigation is critical for early recognition of community transmission. Surveillance for mosquito activity includes detection and speciation of circulating mosquitoes and identification of known arboviruses. This surveillance drives mosquito control activities that are targeted in geographic areas where there is high mosquito activity and include larviciding (measures to eliminate mosquito breeding) and adulticiding (spraying to kill adult mosquitoes), using insecticide agents that are specific for the species of mosquitoes that are identified. These control measures are generally authorized by government regulations to protect the health of the

BOX 19.1 Dengue and Zika Virus Infections (Emerging Flaviviruses)

Disease and Transmission Characteristics:

- Febrile illness may be complicated by hemorrhagic shock, death (Dengue), or congenital infections with fetal death, as well as microcephaly (Zika)
- Transmitted by bite of mosquito

Drivers:

- One Health; climate change, international travel and trade, urbanization, weak public health and healthcare systems

Public Health Response and Essential Services of Public Health

- Surveillance for human illness (monitoring health status, diagnosis and investigation, informing, and educating)
- Vector control measures (diagnosis and investigation, developing policies and plans, enforcing laws and regulations)
- Community education and education re: protective behaviors (informing and educating, mobilizing community partnerships, policy development)
- Treatment of infections (linking to personal health services)
- Research and evaluation

public. Vector control measures are supplemented by community education about personal protective measures and eliminating potential mosquito breeding sites (Association of State and Territorial Health Officials [ASTHO], 2005). Conducting research to understand the transmission characteristics and health outcomes related to these emerging threats and evaluating the impact of control programs are also critical components of the public health response to containing arbovirus epidemics. Importantly, research conducted during the Zika virus outbreak established the virus as a causal factor in infant **microcephaly**. Studies were also conducted for several candidate Zika vaccines (Musso et al., 2019). Although the outbreak subsided before any were approved for widespread usage, this research will facilitate the likelihood that a vaccine will be available during future outbreaks. Box 19.1 provides a summary of the transmission characteristics, drivers, and public health response measures for emerging flavivirus infections.

Ebola Virus Disease

Ebola virus is another infection that has emerged as a major global public health concern. The virus was first discovered in 1976 and has caused over 25 outbreaks of human illness since then. Like Zika, the virus was mainly a zoonotic infection, with a reservoir in fruit bats and nonhuman primates in rural regions of Central Africa. In humans, the virus causes "Ebola hemorrhagic fever," a syndrome that encompasses high fever, vomiting, rash, bleeding from the mouth and gastrointestinal tract, and kidney and liver failure. In many outbreaks, the case fatality rate is over 50%. Treatment has mainly been supportive, although there are new, promising antiviral therapies under evaluation (WHO, 2021b).

In all the reported outbreaks to date, the first or index case results from direct contact with an infected animal (often through hunting or preparation/consumption of bushmeat). The virus then spreads from person to person when other people have close contact with blood and body fluids from ill persons. These fluids contain high titers of virus, particularly during the late stages of the illness when people are critically ill. Prior to 2014, human outbreaks of Ebola virus were fairly limited, usually affecting between 10 to 25 people (although sometimes several hundred people). They were contained by limiting transmission through isolation of infected persons, identification and quarantine of contacts, and stringent infection control measures in healthcare settings. Community education and partnerships, along with strong healthcare and public health systems, were the mainstay of epidemic control of Ebola virus and Centers for Disease Control and Prevention [CDC] fact sheets), as outbreak control relies on rapid identification and isolation of Ebola patients (WHO, 2021b).

The largest Ebola outbreak in history began in West Africa in 2014. This epidemic began with cases in a rural region of Guinea. It is believed that multiple, unrecognized chains of human transmission occurred over a period of several months in rural Guinea and eventually spread to bordering regions of Liberia and Sierra Leone. The weak healthcare and public health systems in these three countries allowed the epidemic to spread to crowded urban areas where control measures became even more difficult to implement. Ritual burial practices in which surviving family members prepare bodies for burial were a cultural practice that facilitated spread of the virus. In addition, there was a great deal of mistrust of government and health officials in these countries, related to tribal culture and recent civil war and internal conflict. These factors complicated the implementation of the standard control measures that rely so heavily on community engagement and understanding of disease and its transmission.

Ultimately, over 28,652 cases of EVD were reported in this region, including 11,325 deaths, the largest EVD outbreak on record. Many of the cases (and fatalities) occurred in healthcare workers who lacked sufficient infection protection measures and became infected during the care of ill persons in poorly resourced settings. In the United States, a traveler from Liberia who was infected with Ebola was hospitalized in Dallas, Texas. He was critically ill and during the hospitalization transmitted the infection to a nurse who was taking care of him through a lapse in infection control practices. These two cases prompted major public health response measures in the United States: All travelers to the United States from Liberia, Guinea, and Sierra Leone during the outbreak period were required to undergo public health monitoring for 21 days postarrival. In addition, selected healthcare facilities throughout the country developed rigorous protocols for the care of highly contagious patients so that every region of the country had the capacity to care for new patients (Bell et al., 2016).

In 2018, another Ebola outbreak was recognized in the South Kivu region of the Democratic Republic of the Congo (DRC). Although the country has experienced over 10 outbreaks of Ebola since the virus's discovery in 1976, this most recent outbreak is now the second-largest outbreak of Ebola in the world, after the West African outbreak. A total of 3,000 cases have been reported, resulting in over 2,000 deaths. In the DRC, the epidemic is driven by internal conflict and violence, weak healthcare and public health systems, tribal practices, and distrust of government and health officials, all of which continue to stymie control efforts. However, two new vaccines, piloted during the 2014 to 2016 West African outbreak, are highly effective. They have supplemented the isolation/quarantine approach to disease containment and have been used to prevent infection in healthcare and public health workers, in contacts with recognized cases, and in the population of high-impact areas of the country. While this epidemic continues with low levels of transmission, there has been little spread outside the DRC to other African countries, or outside the continent (CDC, n.d.-b; WHO, 2021b)

Public Health Control Measures

Public health control measures for Ebola virus disease are challenging to implement as the disease has mainly emerged as a human pathogen in countries with weak public health and medical systems. Early recognition of initial cases is key to ensure clinical care and appropriate support for this serious medical condition, and to implement **nonpharmaceutical control measures** through isolation of cases and monitoring of close contacts to prevent subsequent cycles of person-to-person transmission. Infection control measures in healthcare facilities require the stringent observation of standard and contact precautions and the careful use of personal protective equipment to prevent infections in healthcare workers. Community education about this disease and its transmission characteristics has been an important and also the most difficult aspect of public health control measures when the disease has occurred in settings where government and public health systems are not trusted, and where political turmoil and violence interfere with effective public health response. New, recombinant vaccines are highly successful control measures, but their use requires strong public health infrastructure and acceptance of government and healthcare interventions in affected communities. Notably, health officials were able to conduct research that established the effectiveness of this vaccine during the West African outbreak response, demonstrating that it is both important and possible to conduct research during emergency situations (Kennedy et al., 2017; Lurie et al., 2013). Box 19.2 presents a summary of the transmission characteristics, drivers, and public health control measures for Ebola virus disease.

Antimicrobial Resistance

Antibiotic or antimicrobial resistance (AMR) has been described as the greatest global public health challenge of the modern age (Woolhouse et al., 2016). The term refers to infections that are resistant—unable to be killed—to antimicrobial drugs that are available to treat them. AMR has emerged as a major problem in virtually every type of microorganism that infects humans. Many of these infections are caused by drug-resistant bacteria that colonize the skin, mucosal surfaces, or gastrointestinal tract, but in the setting of severe underlying illness, they can become life-threatening causes of urinary tract, catheter-related, and surgical site infections and ultimately bloodstream infections and sepsis. The CDC estimates that 3 million antibiotic-resistant infections occur annually in the United States and result in over 35,000 deaths. An estimated 500,000 cases of drug-resistant tuberculosis occur globally. Moreover, antimicrobial resistance contributes to increased hospital stays and additional healthcare cost. It is estimated that in the United States, economic losses due

BOX 19.2 Ebola Virus Disease

Disease and Transmission Characteristics:

- Severe life-threatening febrile illness with hemorrhage, gastrointestinal symptoms; death in 50% of cases
- Transmitted person to person through direct contact with infected body fluids

Drivers:

- One Health, population mobility, urbanization, weak public health and healthcare systems

Public Health Response:

- Surveillance, investigation, and isolation of cases; contact tracing, quarantine, and monitoring (monitoring health status, diagnosis and investigation, informing and educating, developing policies and plans, enforcing laws and regulations)
- Isolation and treatment of cases, quarantine, and monitoring of contacts; vaccination (linking to personal health services)
- Community education and education re: protective behaviors (informing and educating, mobilizing community partnerships, policy development, enforcing laws and regulations)
- Research and evaluation

to antibiotic resistance range from $20 to $35 billion. One study estimates that the global economic burden from antimicrobial resistance might eventually be $120 trillion (CDC, 2019; Woolhouse et al., 2016).

Carbapenem-resistant and extended-spectrum beta-lactamase (ESBL)–producing enterobacteriaceae (CRE and ESBL, respectively) are examples of two important drug-resistant gram-negative bacterial infections. Methicillin-resistant *S. aureus* (MRSA) and vancomycin-resistant *Enterococci* (VRE) are examples of resistant gram-positive bacteria that can cause skin and soft tissue infections, urinary tract infections, infections of prosthetic joints and heart valves, and life-threatening bloodstream infections. Drug-resistant *Streptococcus pneumoniae* (DRSP) is a common cause of community-acquired pneumonia. Antimicrobial resistance has emerged in *Neisseria gonorrhea,* the sexually transmitted bacteria that causes urethritis and cervicitis, and in *Campylobacter, Salmonella,* and *Shigella,* common causes of gastroenteritis that are usually foodborne. AMR has emerged in *Mycobacterium tuberculosis,* the bacterium that causes tuberculosis. However, resistance has emerged in fungi such as *Candida auris,* which is a new cause of severe systemic infections in hospitalized, debilitated patients, and *Aspergillus,* which can cause pneumonia and systemic disease in immunocompromised patients. Drug resistance has also emerged in *Plasmodium falciparum,* the parasite that causes malaria, and in HIV, creating new treatment challenges in these global burdens of disease.

Antimicrobial resistance emerges during antibiotic use: It is thus a complication of modern medicine, in which selective pressure from antibiotic usage promotes the emergence of organisms with genetic mutations that permit them to survive in the presence of the antibiotic medication. While this may occur during indiscriminate or incorrect antibiotic usage (primary drug resistance), drug-resistant organisms can be transmitted to individuals without any antibiotic exposure (transmitted resistance, sometimes referred to as secondary resistance). Drug resistance is amplified in healthcare settings, where spread from person to person, via contaminated instruments or the hands of healthcare personnel, occurs frequently and easily. Infections with antibiotic-resistant organisms disproportionately affect sick hospitalized patients. Patient transfer across healthcare facilities, both long-term care and acute care hospitals, facilitates the spread of resistant organisms to other institutions (CDC, 2019).

Antibiotic resistance is another "One Health" challenge. Antimicrobial use in farm animals, specifically those bred for the food supply, has resulted in antibiotic-resistant organisms that colonize and cause disease in humans. Antimicrobial use in agriculture, specifically consumed by food-producing animals, may be an even more significant driver of antimicrobial resistance. Administered to livestock to prevent and treat infections and to promote growth, over 80% of antibiotics that are produced are used in agriculture. This widespread use contributes to resistant organisms in the global ecosystem, transmitted to humans via food chains and disseminated in the environment via animal waste (Holmes et al., 2016; Manyi-Loh et al., 2018).

Antibiotic resistance occurs through the molecular changes to bacterial genes that ultimately code for proteins that confer resistance to specific antibiotics. These resistance mechanisms result from the expression of genes that are transferred among bacteria by plasmids, transposons, and other genetic elements. They may code for a change in the protein that binds the antibiotic to the bacterial cell wall, preventing the antibiotic from attaching to the bacteria and doing its damage. Or they may code for enzymes (e.g., beta-lactamases) that hydrolyze a structural component of the antibiotic, rendering it ineffective. Resistance genes can also help to remove the antibiotic (e.g., through efflux pumps) or modify the target site for its activity so that it cannot work effectively (Aslam et al., 2018; Holmes et al., 2016).

While the main driver for antimicrobial resistance is antibiotic usage, human disease from resistant organisms is often facilitated by other aspects of modern healthcare. Infections with drug-resistant organisms are often introduced by the use of catheters or through invasive procedures. Patients who are debilitated or whose immune systems are weakened by the use of immune-modulating therapies are especially vulnerable to infections with resistant organisms. Additionally, global medical tourism contributes to the international spread of resistant organisms. A recent example is the New Delhi metallo-beta lactamase (NDM), a mechanism that produces resistance to virtually all **beta-lactam antibiotics**. It was first recognized in 2009 in a patient from Sweden who had been hospitalized in India. Organisms with the genes for NDM have been found to be very capable of transferring the genes that encode NDM, as well as other resistance genes. NDM has now spread globally to Europe, Asia, Central America, and the United States (Zmarlicka et al., 2015).

Public Health Control Measures of Antimicrobial Resistance

The public health management of antimicrobial resistance draws on the essential services of public health. Identification, diagnosis, and surveillance of resistant organisms are critical measures to characterize the problem both locally and globally and to implement control measures. Prevention relies on reduced antibiotic usage in medical care, through antimicrobial stewardship and judicious prescribing practices, as well as limits to antimicrobial use in agricultural settings (regulations). These accompany stringent transmission-based precautions in healthcare facilities (policy development). Community education and engagement regarding appropriate antimicrobial use is a necessary component of these control measures, as are partnerships with environmental health specialists and the agricultural community. Finally, public health control must entail evaluation of these interventions and research into best prevention practices and new antimicrobial drugs to combat resistant organisms (CDC, 2019). Box 19.3 provides a summary of the transmission factors and drivers of antimicrobial resistance, and the public health response needed to control this threat.

BOX 19.3 Antimicrobial Resistance

Disease and Transmission:

- Infections caused by microorganisms that are resistant to available antibiotics or antimicrobial agents
- May be transmitted person to person through direct contact with individuals who have drug-resistant organisms or from contact with contaminated environment

Drivers:

- Selection pressure due to antibiotic overuse in animals and in healthcare and One Health, population mobility and globalization, modern healthcare practices

Public Health Response:

- Detection, surveillance, and monitoring of antibiotic resistance; investigation of cases (monitoring health status, diagnosis and investigation, informing and educating, developing policies and plans, enforcing laws and regulations)
- Antibiotic stewardship in healthcare; elimination of unnecessary use in animals, community education and education re: correct and appropriate antibiotic use (informing and educating, mobilizing community partnerships, policy development, enforcing laws and regulations)
- Isolation, treatment of cases; transmission-based infection control precautions (linking to personal health services)
- Research and evaluation

Noninfectious Emerging Threats—E-Cigarette–Associated Lung Injury

Beginning in the summer of 2019, the United States experienced an outbreak of severe lung injury associated with use of electronic ("e-cigarette") or "vaping" products. Vaping refers to the heat-induced aerosolization of a liquid using a battery-powered device. Devices for nicotine vaping were developed as early as the 1960s; they were introduced to the United States in 2006 to 2007 and became popular in the decade following their introduction as an alternative to cigarette smoking and recreational habit (Consumer Advocates for Smoke-free Alternatives Association, 2020). Vaping technology is also used to consume cannabis and illicit substances such as methamphetamine and dimethyltryptamine.

By January 2020, over 2,669 cases and nearly 60 deaths related to e-cigarette–associated lung injury (EVALI, also called vaping-associated pulmonary injury or VAPI) were reported to the CDC from all 50 states, the District of Columbia, Puerto Rico, and the U.S. Virgin Islands. The syndrome is a noninfectious inflammatory disease of lung tissue, or chemical pneumonitis, resulting in shortness of breath and, in some cases, respiratory failure requiring respiratory mechanical ventilation. The syndrome can occasionally be fatal. The CDC investigated these cases to characterize the clinical manifestations of the respiratory illness, identify risk factors, and implement control measures. The majority of cases have reported using tetrahydrocannabinol (THC)–containing products, although some cases occurred in persons who reported exclusive use of nicotine-containing products. Laboratory testing of bronchoalveolar-lavage fluid samples from 51 patients with the EVALI syndrome revealed vitamin E acetate in all samples but did not identify this compound in control group samples, suggesting that exposure to this chemical is contributing to lung injury. Vitamin E acetate is used as a thickening agent in THC-containing vaping products; additional research is ongoing to determine if other chemicals are implicated in EVALI (Hooper & Garfield, 2019; King et al., 2020; Krishnasamy et al., 2020).

Public Health Control Measures

This outbreak has resulted from the larger epidemic of youth vaping among U.S. adolescents and young adults and was driven by the use of THC-containing products. Community education regarding the findings of this investigation, restriction of vaping products, and laws to limit the use of additives in THC-containing products have limited the occurrence of EVALI in the United States in the short term. Longer term health impacts of vaping and e-cigarette use remain an important area of public health inquiry (King et al., 2020; Krishnasamy et al., 2020). Box 19.4 provides a summary of vaping-associated pulmonary injury, its drivers, and the public health response measures used to control or limit its occurrence.

BOX 19.4 Vaping-Associated Pulmonary Injury

Disease and Etiology:

- Chemical pneumonitis, likely related to inhalation of vitamin E acetate, used in tetrahydrocannabinol (THC)-containing vaping products

Drivers:

- Novel technology for inhalation of nicotine, THC, and other products; epidemic of youth vaping

Public Health Response:

- Detection and surveillance of cases (monitoring health status, diagnosis, and investigation)
- Treatment of cases; community education related to use of vaping products, laws restricting access, and use of dangerous additives (linking to personal health services, informing and educating, developing policies and plans, enforcing laws and regulations)
- Research and evaluation

Respiratory Viruses With Pandemic Potential—SARS Coronaviruses and COVID-19

Novel strains of influenza A that emerge from nonhuman viruses and adapt to humans have caused pandemics throughout history. The influenza pandemic with the greatest global mortality occurred in 1918 (H1N1), but major pandemics of influenza A occurred in 1957 (H2N2), 1968 (H3N2), and, most recently, in 2009 (H1N1; CDC, 2021). However, another family of respiratory viruses, coronaviruses, have become a formidable emerging pathogen. Since 2003, several strains of coronavirus have successfully navigated the species jump from animal to human and caused significant epidemics, including SARS-CoV-2, the cause of COVID-19 and the largest pandemic to affect the world's population since the 1918 influenza pandemic.

Emerging Coronaviruses

Coronaviruses are a large family of respiratory viruses that infect both animals and humans. Named for the "crown" shape of their envelope as visualized through electron microscopy, these RNA viruses are a common cause of mild respiratory illness in humans that is transmitted from person to person via respiratory droplets. There are four major genera or subtypes of coronavirus—alpha, beta, gamma, and delta, although alpha and beta coronaviruses are the most common. Several alpha and beta coronaviruses have circulated among humans for many years and are responsible for what is recognized as the common cold; infections occur worldwide and usually during winter when other seasonal respiratory viruses are commonly transmitted. However, coronaviruses infect animals as well, and there have been three recognized epidemics of human illness due to novel or emergent beta coronaviruses that originated in an animal reservoir but resulted in human transmission cycles. In 2002, a novel coronavirus emerged in China and was associated with a "severe acute respiratory syndrome," usually meeting the criteria for the "acute respiratory distress syndrome," or ARDS (Ranieri et al., 2012). Bats are believed to be the reservoir for this virus, called the "SARS-coronavirus" (SARS-CoV-1), although the civet cat is believed to have been the intermediate host for the 2002 to 2003 outbreak. In late 2002, an outbreak of SARS-CoV-2 started in the Guangdong Province in southern China. Infection resulted in a severe atypical pneumonia. The first cases were related to animal exposure in live-animal markets; however, human-to-human transmission from these early cases resulted in a widespread outbreak that lasted nearly 6 months and spread to two dozen countries in North America, South America, Europe, and Asia. The outbreak ultimately caused over 8,000 cases and nearly 800 deaths until it ended in 2003. No new cases of SARS-CoV-2 infection have been reported since 2004 (Heaton, 2020; CDC, n.d.-a; Peiris et al., 2003).

In 2012, a new coronavirus causing severe respiratory illness was identified in Saudi Arabia. The syndrome, dubbed "Middle East Respiratory Syndrome," or MERS, became the second coronavirus to cross the species barrier and cause an epidemic of severe human illness. The MERS Co-V is thought to originate in animal sources. The original animal reservoir is believed to be bats, although several studies have identified exposures to camels (likely an intermediate host) as a risk factor for infection. However, the virus can also be transmitted from human to human through close contact, and respiratory transmission has been responsible for over 2,000 infections since then, all of them linked to exposures in the Arabian Peninsula. Like SARS-CoV-1, infection with the MERS Co-V is associated with a high case fatality rate (approximately 30%–40%) and represents a major concern for healthcare facilities, where the organism has been transmitted to healthcare workers and other patients. This epidemic continues to smolder at low levels in Middle Eastern countries where the virus is enzootic (del Rio & Malani, 2020; Heaton, 2020: JAMA Author Interviews, 2020; WHO, n.d.).

In late 2019, another novel beta coronavirus (SARS-CoV-2) emerged in Wuhan City, in Hubei Province, China. Like MERS Co-V and SARS-CoV-1, this strain appears to have emerged from a bat source, although it is believed to have jumped the species barrier via the pangolin, although this intermediate species has not been confirmed. SARS-CoV-2 is similar genetically to the SARS-CoV-1 that circulated in 2003 but is a distinct, different virus with different properties biologically and clinically (Paules et al., 2020). This virus is efficiently transmitted from human to human via the spread of respiratory droplets either through direct contact or inhalation of aerosols. The resulting respiratory infection, called COVID-19, ranges from a mild respiratory infection in most victims to a severe, life-threatening viral pneumonitis in approximately 20% of individuals. Severe disease occurs more commonly in older adults and in individuals with underlying comorbid conditions like obesity, diabetes, and cardiovascular disease. Children appear to have milder infections and are less likely to become infected, although serious illness including a severe, postinfectious multisystem inflammatory syndrome in children (MIS-C) can occur (Kim et al., 2020).

Up to 40% to 50% of individuals with COVID-19 are either asymptomatic or mildly symptomatic, but they are capable of transmitting the virus, and transmission has occurred in hospitals, churches, cruise ships, and other facilities where people congregate unknowingly with others who are infected (Gandhi et al., 2020). Infections in healthcare settings, particularly long-term care, are common. Healthcare workers must wear personal protective equipment, including face masks and respirators, to limit spread—these items quickly become depleted in the setting of a global pandemic (Karlsson & Fraenkel, 2020; Sim, 2020). The virus is highly contagious, and in the absence of effective control measures, the number of cases increase exponentially within a population. Global travel facilitated international spread of this disease early on and contributed to multiple outbreaks in other countries within Asia and across the world during 2020. Each of these outbreaks created opportunities for wider transmission globally. One year after this virus was recognized as a cause of human illness in China, over 61 million infections were recorded worldwide, resulting in nearly 1.5 million deaths. The United States has led the world in the number of infections (Johns Hopkins University, n.d.). In the United States, racial and ethnic minority groups have suffered the highest burden of disease, with both incidence rates and case fatality rates three to four times those of Whites. Inequities in social determinants of health, including discrimination, a lack of access to healthcare, a disproportionate representation in essential work settings with a higher risk of disease exposure, and a higher rate of underlying comorbidities that contribute to disease severity are all factors that contribute to this increased risk (CDC, 2021; Webb Hooper et al., 2020).

Asymptomatic infections and a lack of access to diagnostic testing (which relies on viral detection through either polymerase chain reaction or viral antigen detection assays) make COVID-19 disease recognition difficult and are major challenges to disease containment. The care for individuals with COVID-19 is largely supportive. Treatments like antivirals (e.g., remdesivir, which may accelerate the recovery of hospitalized adults) or antibody-based treatments such as monoclonal antibodies against the spike protein of the SARS-CoV-2 virus, are likely to be effective early in the disease when viral replication is high (Beigel et al., 2020; Gandhi et al., 2020). Immunosuppressing or anti-inflammatory medications (like dexamethasone, which has been shown to reduce mortality among individuals with respiratory failure on ventilators) are used in the later hyperinflammatory stage of infection when managing an overstimulated immune system is key to controlling symptoms (RECOVERY Collaborative Group, 2020).

Public Health Control Measures

Nonpharmaceutical control measures are the mainstay of public health interventions to contain COVID-19 without the use of a vaccine. These include the isolation of ill people until they are no longer contagious and tracing and quarantining their contacts for a period of 14 days, which is the incubation period for this virus. Universal wearing of face masks and social distancing are critical components of these measures, particularly when there are a large number of unrecognized infections in the community, making it difficult to recognize and isolate individuals who have the disease. Hand hygiene and environmental cleaning are also mitigating measures. These approaches have succeeded in containing transmission although their impact may take weeks to see in population transmission dynamics (Ferguson et al., 2020; Van Dyke et al., 2020). Societal approaches to social or physical distancing, long a mainstay of pandemic influenza planning, include closure of schools and nonessential businesses, and canceling congregate activities to limit person-to-person contact and reduce community transmission. Because these measures ultimately lead to fewer cases, they also reduce the load on the healthcare system, creating more capacity in hospitals including intensive care units and improving the care of critically ill individuals with and without COVID-19.

In 2021, control measures began to integrate vaccines that have demonstrated effectiveness against this pathogen. Like SARS-CoV-1 and MERS CoV, control of this pandemic has required global cooperation and coordination in the initial recognition and containment of this novel pathogen (del Rio & Malani, 2020) and for

BOX 19.5 SARS-CoV-2 Infection (COVID-19)

Disease and Transmission:

- Beta coronavirus, transmitted from person to person via airborne spread, perhaps direct contact with respiratory droplets

Drivers:

- One Health and exposures to infected animals in settings like live animal markets, globalization, evolution of coronaviruses with transmission related to travel, population growth and migration, aging population (increased risk for severe disease), intensive exposure in modern healthcare settings

Public Health Response:

- Detection and surveillance of cases, laboratory capacity for detection of infections (monitoring health status, diagnosis, and investigation)
- Isolation of cases, contact tracing and quarantine, social distancing, use of face masks; transmission-based infection control precautions in healthcare settings (linking to personal health services, developing policies and plans, enforcing laws and regulations)
- Community education related to disease recognition and transmission (informing and educating, mobilization of community [and global] partnerships)
- Vaccination (policy development, assurance functions)
- Research and evaluation

ongoing efforts to contain disease by limiting human contact. This pandemic has reinforced the need for effective cooperation within and between nations to track the disease and to implement and study both treatments as well as public health control measures, which will ultimately require the equitable distribution of vaccines to countries across the globe (Gostin et al., 2020). Box 19.5 provides a summary of SARS-CoV-2 infection transmission characteristics, the drivers that have promoted its spread, and the public health response measures needed to contain it.

EMERGING THREATS, THE ESSENTIAL SERVICES OF PUBLIC HEALTH, AND PUBLIC HEALTH PREPAREDNESS CAPABILITIES

Emerging threats have the potential to produce catastrophic events on a global scale. In 2011, the CDC established 15 Public Health Preparedness Capabilities (PHEP) to define national standards for state and local readiness. These capabilities inform public health agency preparedness planning at the state and local levels. They are intended to build capacity to respond to events that threaten the health of large populations and require specific public health actions and protective measures to reduce or prevent severe consequences. While these capabilities are specific to emergency preparedness, the functions and activities they encompass are geared to create response capacity for "all-hazards." They outline activities and functions that are relevant every day as well as during major disasters (CDC, 2018; Khan, 2011). As such, the PHEP capabilities lie squarely within the domains of Assessment, Policy Development, and Assurance that are the framework for the Essential Services of Public Health.

Perhaps the most important characteristic of emerging threats is that their scope is global, and the public health response must be global as well. For that reason, the WHO and country partners have created a framework intended to improve "global health security," based on the recognition that "threats have become a much larger menace in a world characterized by high mobility, economic interdependence, and electronic interconnectedness" (WHO, 2007, p. vi). The emerging threats described in this chapter are all examples of threats that do not respect national borders and require new tools for a "collective defense."

In 2005, in the wake of the global SARS-CoV-1 epidemic, the WHO reissued International Health Regulations (IHR) that were intended to provide a structure for countries to recognize threats that emerge within their own boundaries, address them, and control them. Instead of focusing on measures at airports and seaports to prevent the importation (or exportation) of disease, the IHR emphasizes the importance for every country to have a robust public health and healthcare system in place for recognizing and responding to threats, with the goal of containing them within countries and regions, before they threaten the health of the global public. They also emphasize transparency, or early sharing, of critical health information between countries and provide a mechanism for a coordinated response to international health emergencies, including the ability for the WHO to declare "Public Health Emergencies of International Concern" (Gostin & Katz, 2016). The IHR requires that all countries have the ability to do the following:

- detect—have surveillance systems to detect public health events in a timely manner
- assess and report—have the ability to assess a public health event and report to national and international systems, as needed
- respond—have capacity to respond to public health risks and emergencies

The WHO has defined IHR "core capacities" for countries, which are those required to be able to detect, assess, notify, and respond to health risks. Initially, eight capacities were outlined in the IHR 2005 update (WHO, 2008) and contain specific indicators within each capacity for monitoring within each country. An additional five capacities for countries to monitor were added in 2018, providing additional specificity for capacity-building for specific hazards (e.g., zoonoses, food safety, chemical and radionuclear threats) and vulnerabilities (e.g., points of entry). Most of the IHR core capacities pertain to every phase of detection, assessment, and response to health risks. The original eight capacities are explained briefly in the following (WHO, 2013):

National legislation and policy—countries must have adequate legal framework, policies, and financing to detect, assess, and respond to disease threats.

Coordination and communications with the national focal point—countries must have effective partnerships for response to disease threats across relevant sectors, and coordination of national resources through a national center or "focal point."

Surveillance—countries must have the capacity for rapid detection of health risks and prompt risk assessment.

Response—countries must have command, communications, and control operations to manage outbreak operations and response to public health emergencies. Includes establishment of Rapid Response Teams and capacity for case management, infection control, and decontamination.

Preparedness—countries must develop national, community-level response plans for relevant biological, chemical, radiological, and nuclear hazards. Includes risk assessment and resource identification.

Risk communication—countries must have the capacity for communicating health risks and vulnerabilities to stakeholders, as well as dissemination of public information.

Human resources—countries must strengthen the skills of the public health workforce to support capacities across all phases and response within health systems.

Laboratory—countries must have laboratory capacity for analysis of samples of infectious and other agents.

Table 19.1 presents a cross-walk of the Essential Services of Public Health, the PHEP capabilities, and IHR core capacities. The fundamental components of public health assessment, policy development, and assurance are present

TABLE 19.1 Cross-Walk–Essential Services of Public Health, Public Health Preparedness Capabilities, and International Health Regulations Core Capacities

Essential Services of Public Health	Public Health Emergency Preparedness Capabilities	International Health Regulations Core Capacities
Assessment: Monitor health status Diagnose and investigate	Public health surveillance and epidemiological investigation Public health laboratory testing	**Detect:** Surveillance Laboratory capacity
Policy Development: Inform, educate, and empower Mobilize community partnerships Develop policies	Community preparedness Community recovery Emergency public information and warning Information sharing	**Assess and report:** Response Risk communication Preparedness
Assurance: Enforce laws Link to/provide care Assure competent workforce Evaluate	Emergency operations coordination Medical surge Mass care Fatality management Medical countermeasure dispensing Medical materiel management and distribution Nonpharmaceutical interventions Responder safety and health Volunteer management	**Respond:** Legislation, policy, and financing Coordination and communication with national center Human resources

across each framework, although they are sometimes categorized or labeled in a slightly different way. Evaluation is not formally included as a PHEP capability or IHR capacity but is an important aspect of public health emergency preparedness. In the United States, the evaluation of public health emergency preparedness occurs through after-action reviews of actual events, and through the continuum of tabletop, functional, and field exercises that are so critical to preparedness planning. Similarly, the IHR (WHO, 2008) includes a component for monitoring and evaluating the public health capacities in UN member countries around the world through a process called the Joint External Evaluation process (JEE; WHO, 2016). A voluntary process, the JEE provides an independent, transparent, and multisectoral assessment of a country's preparation for infectious disease risks. The JEE is considered a collaborative effort between the external evaluation team and the country to identify and address any gaps in the health security. This effort, although not formally classified as research, is intended to provide new insights and innovative solutions to health problems.

DISCUSSION QUESTIONS

1. Discuss methods to reduce foodborne illnesses. Be sure to address the current complexities of food chains, which involve importation of products from global sources.
2. How can scientists and public health officials improve recommendations for use of antibiotics to reduce evolution of resistant strains of bacteria? What can be done to improve medical practices?
3. Have we lost the battle with microbes? Apply the "survival of the fittest" model to the survival of viruses and bacteria.
4. What can public health officials do to protect communities against emerging pathogens? What can you do in your community?

REFERENCES

Allen, T., Murray, K. A., Zambrana-Torrelio, C., Morse, S. S., Rondinini, C., Di Marco, M., Breit, N., Olival, K. J., & Daszak, P. (2017). Global hotspots and correlates of emerging zoonotic diseases. *Nature Communications, 8*(1), Article 1124. https://doi.org/10.1038/s41467-017-00923-8

Aslam, B., Wang, W., Arshad, M. I., Khurshid, M., Muzammil, S., Rasool, M. H., Nisar, M. A., Alvi, R. F., Aslam, M. A., Qamar, M. U., Salamat, M. K. F., & Baloch, Z. (2018). Antibiotic resistance: A rundown of a global crisis. *Infection and Drug Resistance, 11*, 1645–1658. https://doi.org/10.2147/IDR.S173867

Association of State and Territorial Health Officials. (2005). *Public health confronts the mosquito: Developing sustainable state and local mosquito control programs.* https://www.astho.org/Programs/Environmental-Health/Natural-Environment/confrontsmosquito

Barrett, B., Charles, J. W., & Temte, J. L. (2015). Climate change, human health, and epidemiological transition. *Preventive Medicine, 70*, 69–75. https://doi.org/10.1016/j.ypmed.2014.11.013

Beigel, J. H., Tomashek, I. M., Dodd, L. E., Mehta, A. K., Zingman, B. S., Kalil, A. C., Hohmann, E., Chu, H. Y., Luetkemeyer, A., Kline, S., Lopez de Castilla, D., Finberg, R. W., Dierberg, K., Tapson, V., Hsieh, L., Patterson, T. F., Paredes, R., Sweeney, D. A., Short, W. R., . . . Lane, H. C. (2020). Remdesivir for the treatment of COVID-19—Final report. *New England Journal of Medicine, 383*, 1813–1826. https://doi.org/10.1056/NEJMoa2007764

Bell, B. P., Damon, I. K., Jernigan, D. B., Kenyon, T. A., Nichol, S. T., O'Connor, J. P., & Tappero, J. W. (2016). Overview, control strategies, and lessons learned in the CDC response to the 2014–2016 Ebola epidemic. *MMWR Supplements, 65*(Suppl. 3), 4–11. http://doi.org/10.15585/mmwr.su6503a2

Caminade, C., McIntyre, K. M., & Jones, A. E. (2019). Impact of recent and future climate change on vector-borne diseases. *Annals of the New York Academy of Sciences, 1436*(1), 157–173. https://doi.org/10.1111/nyas.13950

Centers for Disease Control and Prevention. (n.d.-a). *CDC SARS response timeline.* https://www.cdc.gov/about/history/sars/timeline.htm

Centers for Disease Control and Prevention. (n.d.-b). *2018 Eastern Democratic Republic of the Congo Ebola outbreak (ongoing).* https://www.cdc.gov/vhf/ebola/outbreaks/drc/2018-august.html

Centers for Disease Control and Prevention. (2018). *Public health emergency preparedness and response capabilities.* U.S. Department of Health and Human Services. https://www.cdc.gov/cpr/readiness/00_docs/CDC_PreparednesResponseCapabilities_October2018_Final_508.pdf

Centers for Disease Control and Prevention. (2019). *Antibiotic resistance threats in the United States, 2019.* U.S. Department of Health and Human Services. https://www.cdc.gov/drugresistance/pdf/threats-report/2019-ar-threats-report-508.pdf

Centers for Disease Control and Prevention. (2021). *COVID-19: Health equity considerations and racial and ethnic minority groups.* https://www.cdc.gov/coronavirus/2019-ncov/community/health-equity/race-ethnicity.html#anchor_1595551060069

Choffnes, E. R., & Mack, A. (Eds.). *Emerging viral diseases: The One Health connection: Workshop summary.* National Academies Press. https://doi.org/10.17226/18975

Consumer Advocates for Smoke-free Alternatives Association. (2020). *Historical timeline of vaping & electronic cigarettes.* http://www.casaa.org/historical-timeline-of-electronic-cigarettes

Cunningham, A. A., Daszak, P., & Wood, J. L. N. (2017). One Health, emerging infectious diseases and wildlife: Two decades of progress? *Philosophical Transactions of the Royal Society B: Biological Sciences, 372*(1725). https://doi.org/10.1098/rstb.2016.0167

del Rio, C., & Malani, P. N. (2020). 2019 novel coronavirus—important information for clinicians. *JAMA, 323*(11), 1039–1040. https://doi.org/10.1001/jama.2020.1490

Fauci, A. S., & Morens, D. M. (2012). The perpetual challenge of infectious diseases. *New England Journal of Medicine, 366*, 454–461. https://doi.org/10.1056/NEJMra1108296

Fauci, A. S., & Morens, D. M. (2016). Zika virus in the Americas—yet another arbovirus threat. *New England Journal of Medicine, 374*(7), 601–604. https://doi.org/10.1056/NEJMp1600297

Federal Emergency Management Agency. (2019). *Hazardous materials incidents: Guidance for state, local, tribal, territorial, and private sector partners.* https://www.fema.gov/sites/default/files/2020-07/hazardous-materials-incidents.pdf

Ferguson, N. M., Laydon, D., Ndjati-Gilani, G., Imai, N., Ainslie, K., Baguelin, M., Bhatia, S., Boonyasiri, A., Cucunubá, Z., Cuomo-Dannenburg, G., Dighe, A., Dorigatti, I., Fu, H., Gaythorpe, K., Green, W., Hamlet, A., Hinsley, W., Okell, L. C., van Elsland, S., . . . Ghani, A. C. (2020). *Report 9: Impact of non-pharmaceutical interventions (NPIs) to reduce COVID-19 mortality and healthcare demand.* Imperial College COVID-19 Modeling Team, WHO Collaborating Centre for Infectious Disease Modeling. https://www.imperial.ac.uk/media/imperial-college/medicine/sph/ide/gida-fellowships/Imperial-College-COVID19-NPI-modelling-16-03-2020.pdf, November 27, 2020

Gandhi, R. T., Lynch, J. B., & del Rio, C. (2020). Mild or moderate Covid-19. *New England Journal of Medicine, 383*, 1757–1766. https://doi.org/10.1056/NEJMcp2009249

GBD 2017 Risk Factor Collaborators. (2018). Global, regional, and national comparative risk assessment of 84 behavioural, environmental and occupational, and metabolic risks or clusters of risks for 195 countries and territories, 1990–2017: A systematic analysis for the Global Burden of Disease Study 2017. *Lancet, 392*(10159), 1923–1994. https://doi.org/10.1016/s0140-6736(18)32225-6

Gebreyes, W. A., Dupouy-Camet, J., Newport, M. J., Oliveira, C. J., Schlesinger, L. S., Saif, Y. M., Saville, W., Wittum, T., Hoet, A., Quessy, S., Kazwala, R., Tekola, B., Shryock, T., Bisesi, M., Patchanee, P., Boonmar, S., & King, L. J. (2014). The global One Health paradigm: Challenges and opportunities for tackling infectious diseases at the human, animal, and environment interface in low-resource settings. *PLoS Neglected Tropical Diseases, 8*(11), e3257. https://doi.org/10.1371/journal.pntd.0003257

Gostin, L. O., & Katz, R. (2016). The International Health Regulations: The governing framework for global health security. *The Milbank Quarterly, 94*(2), 264–313. https://doi.org/10.1111/1468-0009.12186

Gostin, L. O., Moon, S., & Meier, B. M. (2020). Reimaging global health governance in the age of COVID-19. *American Journal of Public Health, 110*, 1615–1619. https://doi.org/10.2105/AJPH.2020.305933

Gould, L., Kline, J., Monahan, C., & Vierk, K. (2017). Outbreaks of disease associated with food imported into the United States, 1996–2014. *Emerging Infectious Diseases, 23*(3), 525–528. https://doi.org/10.3201/eid2303.161462

Grossi, P. A. (2020). Urban spread of flaviviruses: A new challenge in solid-organ transplant recipients. *Clinical Infectious Diseases, 70*(1), 149–151. https://doi.org/10.1093/cid/ciz390

Guo, Y., Gasparrini, A., Armstrong, B. G., Tawatsupa, B., Tobias, A., Lavigne, E., de Sousa Zanotti Staglior Coelho, M., Pan, X., Kim, H., Hashizume, M., Honda, Y., Guo, Y-L. L., Wu, C-F., Zanobetti, A., Schwartz, J. D., Bell, M. L., Scortichini, M., Michelozzi, P., Punnasiri, K., . . . Tong, S. (2017). Heat wave and mortality: A multicountry, multicommunity study. *Environmental Health Perspectives, 125*(8), 087006. https://doi.org/10.1289/ehp1026

Harpaz, R., Dahl, R., & Dooling, K. (2016). The prevalence of immunocompromised adults: United States, 2013. *Open Forum Infectious Diseases, 3*(Suppl. 1), 1439. https://doi.org/10.1093/ofid/ofw172.1141

Healthcare and Public Health Cybersecurity Working Group. (2017). *Healthcare and public health cybersecurity primer: Cybersecurity 101*. https://www.phe.gov/Preparedness/planning/cip/Documents/cybersecurity-primer.pdf

Heaton, P. (2020). Virology. In A. J. Spec, G. Escota, C. Chrisler, & B. Davies (Eds.), *Comprehensive review of infectious diseases* (pp. 51–72). Elsevier.

Heymann, D. L., Hodgson, A., Sall, A. A., Freedman, D. O., Staples, J. E., Althabe, F., Baruah, K., Mahmud, G., Kandun, N., Vasconcelos, P. F. C., Bino, S., & Menon, K. U. (2016). Zika virus and microcephaly: Why is this situation a PHEIC? *Lancet, 387*(10020), 719–721. https://doi.org/10.1016/s0140-6736(16)00320-2

Holmes, A. H., Moore, L. S., Sundsfjord, A., Steinbakk, M., Regmi, S., Karkey, A., Guerin, P. J., & Piddock, L. J. (2016). Understanding the mechanisms and drivers of antimicrobial resistance. *Lancet, 387*(10014), 176–187. https://doi.org/10.1016/s0140-6736(15)00473-0

Hooper, R. W., II, & Garfield, J. L. (2019). An emerging crisis: Vaping-associated pulmonary injury. *Annals of Internal Medicine, 172*(1), 57. https://doi.org/10.7326/m19-2908

Intergovernmental Panel on Climate Change. (2014). Summary for policymakers. In O. Edenhofer, R. Pichs-Madruga, Y. Sokona, E. Farahani, S. Kadner, K. Seyboth, A. Adler, I. Baum, S. Brunner, P. Eickemeier, B. Kriemann, J. Savolainen, S. Schlömer, C. von Stechow, T. Zwickel, & J.C. Minx (Eds.), *Climate change 2014: Mitigation of climate change. Contribution of Working Group III to the Fifth Assessment Report of the Intergovernmental Panel on Climate Change* (pp. 1–32). Cambridge University Press.

Jahan, N., Allotey, P., Arunachalam, D., Yasin, S., Soyiri, I. N., Davey, T. M., & Reidpath, D. D. (2014). The rural bite in population pyramids: What are the implications for responsiveness of health systems in middle income countries? *BMC Public Health, 14*(Suppl. 2), S8. https://doi.org/10.1186/1471-2458-14-s2-s8

JAMA Author Interviews. (2020). Coronavirus infections – more than just the common cold. *JAMA Network*. https://edhub.ama-assn.org/jn-learning/audio-player/18197306

Johns Hopkins University. (n.d.). *Coronavirus Resource Center: COVID-19 dashboard*. https://coronavirus.jhu.edu/map.html

Karlsson, U., & Fraenkel, C.-J. (2020). Covid-19: Risks to healthcare workers and their families. *BMJ* (Clinical research ed.), *371*, m3944. https://doi.org/10.1136/bmj.m3944

Kennedy, S. M., Bolay, F., Kieh, M., Grandits, G., Badio, M., Ballou, R., Eckes, R., Feinberg, M., Follmann, D., Grund, B., Gupta, S., Hensley, L., Higgs, E., Janosko, K., Johnson, M., Kateh, F., Logue, J., Marchand, J., Monath, T., . . . Lane, H. C. (2017). Phase 2 placebo-controlled trial of 2 vaccines to prevent Ebola in Liberia. *New England Journal of Medicine, 377*(15), 1438–1447. https://doi.org/10.1056/NEJMoa1614067

Khan, A. S. (2011). Public health preparedness and response in the USA since 9/11: A national health security imperative. *The Lancet, 378*(9794), 953–956. https://doi.org/10.1016/S0140-6736(11)61263-4

Kim, L., Whitaker, M., O'Halloran, A., Kambhampati, A., Chai, S. J., Reingold, A., Armistead, I., Kawasaki, B., Meek, J., Yousey-Hindes, K., Anderson, E. J., Openo, K. P., Weigel, A., Ryan, P., Monroe, M. L., Fox, K., Kim, S., Lynfield, R., Bye, E., . . . COVID-NET Surveillance Team. (2020). Hospitalization rates and characteristics of children aged <18 years hospitalized with laboratory-confirmed COVID-19 COVID-NET, 14 states, March 1–July 25, 2020. *Morbidity and Mortality Weekly Report, 69*, 1081–1088. https://doi.org/10.15585/mmwr.mm6932e3

Kindhauser, M. K., Allen, T., Frank, V., Santhana, R. S., & Dye, C. (2016). Zika: The origin and spread of a mosquito-borne virus. *Bulletin of the World Health Organization, 94*(9), 675–686. https://doi.org/10.2471/blt.16.171082

King, B. A., Jones, C. M., Baldwin, G. T., & Briss, P. A. (2020). The EVALI and youth vaping epidemics—Implications for public health. *New England Journal of Medicine, 382*(8), 689–691. https://doi.org/10.1056/NEJMp1916171

Krishnasamy, V. P., Hallowell, B. D., Ko, J. Y., Board, A., Hartnett, K. P., Salvatore, P. P., Danielson, M., Kite-Powell, A., Twentyman, E., Kim, L., Cyrus, A., Wallace, M., Melstrom, P., Haag, B., King, B. A., Briss, P., Jones, C. M., Pollack, L. A., Ellington, S., (Lung Injury Response Epidemiology/Surveillance Task Force. (2020). Update: Characteristics of a nationwide outbreak of e-cigarette, or vaping, product use-associated lung injury—United States, August 2019–January 2020. *Morbidity and Mortality Weekly Report, 69*(3), 90–94. https://doi.org/10.15585/mmwr.mm6903e2

Lurie, N., Manolio, T., Patterson, A. P., Collins, F., & Frieden, T. (2013). Research as a part of public health emergency response. *New England Journal of Medicine, 368*(13), 1251–1255. https://doi.org/10.1056/NEJMsb1209510

Lwande, O. W., Obanda, V., Lindström, A., Ahlm, C., Evander, M., Näslund, J., & Bucht, G. (2020). Globe-trotting *Aedes aegypti* and *Aedes albopictus*: Risk factors for arbovirus pandemics. *Vector-Borne and Zoonotic Diseases, 20*(2), 71–81. https://doi.org/10.1089/vbz.2019.2486

Manyi-Loh, C., Mamphweli, S., Meyer, E., & Okoh, A. (2018). Antibiotic use in agriculture and its consequential resistance in environmental sources: Potential public health implications. *Molecules, 23*(4), 795. https://doi.org/10.3390/molecules23040795

McMichael, A. J. (2013). Globalization, climate change, and human health. *New England Journal of Medicine, 368*(14), 1335–1343. https://doi.org/10.1056/NEJMra1109341

Miro, J. M., Grossi, P. A., & Durand, C. M. (2019). Challenges in solid organ transplantation in people living with HIV. *Intensive Care Medicine, 45*(3), 398–400. https://doi.org/10.1007/s00134-019-05524-1

Morens, D. M., Folkers, G. K., & Fauci, A. S. (2004). The challenge of emerging and re-emerging infectious diseases. *Nature, 430*(6996), 242–249. https://doi.org/10.1038/nature02759

Musso, D., Ko, A. I., & Baud, D. (2019). Zika virus infection – after the pandemic. *New England Journal of Medicine, 381*, 1444–1457. https://doi.org/10.1056/NEJMra1808246

Neiderud, C.-J. (2015). How urbanization affects the epidemiology of emerging infectious diseases. *Infection Ecology & Epidemiology, 5*, 27060. https://doi.org/10.3402/iee.v5.27060

Ogden, N. H., & Gachon, P. (2019). Climate change and infectious diseases: What can we expect? *Canada Communicable Disease Report, 45*(4), 76–80. https://doi.org/10.14745/ccdr.v45i04a01

Park, J. E., Jung, S., Kim, A., & Park, J.-E. (2018). MERS transmission and risk factors: A systematic review. *BMC Public Health, 18*(1), Article 574. https://doi.org/10.1186/s12889-018-5484-8

Paules, C. L., Marston, H. D., & Fauci, A. S. (2020). Coronavirus infections – more than just the common cold. *Journal of the American Medical Association, 323*(8), 707. https://doi.org/10.1001/jama.2020.0757

Peiris, J. S. M. , Yuen, K. Y., Osterhaus, A. D. M. E., & Stöhr, K. (2003). The severe acute respiratory syndrome. *New England Journal of Medicine, 349*, 2431–2441. https://doi.org/10.1056/NEJMra032498

Powell, J. R., Gloria-Soria, A., & Kotsakiozi, P. (2018). Recent history of *Aedes aegypti*: Vector genomics and epidemiology records. *BioScience, 68*(11), 854–860. https://doi.org/10.1093/biosci/biy119

Powell, J. R., & Tabachnick, W. J. (2013). History of domestication and spread of *Aedes aegypti*—a review. *Memorias do Instituto Oswaldo Cruz, 108*(Suppl. 1), 11–17. https://doi.org/10.1590/0074-0276130395

Ranieri, V. M., Rubenfeld, G. D., Thompson, B. T., Ferguson, N. D., Caldwell, E., Fan, E., Camporota, L., & Slutsky, A. S. (2012). Acute respiratory distress syndrome: The Berlin definition. *JAMA, 307*, 2526–2533. https://doi.org/10.1001/jama.2012.5669

RECOVERY Collaborative Group. (2020). Dexamethasone in hospitalized patients with Covid-19. *New England Journal of Medicine, 384*, 693–704. https://doi.org/10.1056/nejmoa2021436

Ronto, R., Wu, J. H., & Singh, G. M. (2018). The global nutrition transition: Trends, disease burdens and policy interventions. *Public Health Nutrition, 21*(12), 2267–2270. https://doi.org/10.1017/s1368980018000423

Rosenberg, R., Lindsey, N. P., Fischer, M., Gregory, C. J., Hinckley, A. F., Mead, P. S., Paz-Bailey, G., Waterman, S. H., Drexler, N. A., Kersh, G. J., Hooks, H., Partridge, S. K., Visser, S. N., Beard, C. B., & Petersen, L. R. (2018). Vital signs: Trends in reported vectorborne disease cases—United States and Territories, 2004–2016. *Morbidity and Mortality Weekly Report, 67*(17), 496–501. https://doi.org/10.15585/mmwr.mm6717e1

Roser, M. (2017). *Tourism*. https://ourworldindata.org/tourism

Roser, M. (2019). *Future population growth*. https://ourworldindata.org/future-population-growth. Original work published in 2014.

Ryu, S., Kim, B. I., Lim, J.-S., Tan, C. S., & Chun, B. C. (2017). One Health perspectives on emerging public health threats. *Journal of Preventive Medicine and Public Health, 50*(6), 411–414. https://doi.org/10.3961/jpmph.17.097

Semple, K. (2019, December 29). Climate change and political chaos: A deadly mix in Honduras Dengue epidemic. *New York Times*. https://www.nytimes.com/2019/12/29/world/americas/honduras-dengue-epidemic.html

Sim, M. R. (2020). The COVID-19 pandemic: Major risks to healthcare and other workers on the front line. *Occupational and Environmental Medicine, 77*(5), 281–282. https://doi.org/10.1136/oemed-2020-106567

Stone, B. L., Tourand, Y., & Brissette, C. A. (2017). Brave new worlds: The expanding universe of Lyme disease. *Vector-Borne and Zoonotic Diseases, 17*(9), 619–629. https://doi.org/10.1089/vbz.2017.2127

Stone, P. W. (2009). Economic burden of healthcare-associated infections: An American perspective. *Expert Review of Pharmacoeconomics & Outcomes Research, 9*(5), 417–422. https://doi.org/10.1586/erp.09.53

Sutherst, R. W. (2004). Global change and human vulnerability to vector-borne diseases. *Clinical Microbiology Reviews, 17*(1), 136–173. https://doi.org/10.1128/cmr.17.1.136-173.2004

United Nations, Department of Economic and Social Affairs. (2018, May 16). *68% of the world population projected to live in urban areas by 2050, says UN*. https://www.un.org/development/desa/en/news/population/2018-revision-of-world-urbanization-prospects.html

United Nations, Department of Economic and Social Affairs, Population Division. (2018). *The world's cities in 2018: Data booklet* (ST/ESA/ SER.A/417). Author. https://digitallibrary.un.org/record/3799524?ln=en

Van Dyke, M. E., Rogers, T. M., Pevzner, E. , Satterwhite, C. L., Shah, H. B., Beckman, W. J., Ahmed, F., Hunt, D. C., & Rule, J. (2020). Trends in county-level COVID-19 incidence in counties with and without a mask mandate Kansas, June 1–August 23, 2020. *MMWR. Morbidity and Mortality Weekly Report, 69*, 1777–1781. https://doi.org/10.15585/mmwr.mm6947e2

Wang, D., Hu, B., Hu, C., Zhu, F., Liu, X., Zhang, J., Wang, B., Xiang, H., Cheng, Z., Xiong, Y., Zhao, Y., Li, Y., Wang, X., & Peng, Z. (2020). Clinical characteristics of 138 hospitalized patients with 2019 novel coronavirus–infected pneumonia in Wuhan, China. *JAMA, 323*(11), 1061 –1069. https://doi.org/10.1001/jama.2020.1585

Webb Hooper, M., Nápoles, A. M., & Pérez-Stable, E. J. (2020). COVID-19 and racial/ethnic disparities. *Journal of the American Medical Association, 323*(24), 2466–2467. https://doi.org/10.1001/jama.2020.8598

Wickramage, K., Vearey, J., Zwi, A. B., Robinson, C., & Knipper, M. (2018). Migration and health: A global public health research priority. *BMC Public Health, 18*(1), Article 987. https://doi.org/10.1186/s12889-018-5932-5

Wijdicks, E. F., & Klein, C. J. (2017). Guillain-Barre syndrome. *Mayo Clinic Proceedings, 92*(3), 467–479. https://doi.org/10.1016/j.mayocp.2016.12.002

Woolhouse, M., Waugh, C., Perry, M. R., & Nair, H. (2016). Global disease burden due to antibiotic resistance - state of the evidence. *Journal of Global Health, 6*(1), 010306. https://doi.org/10.7189/jogh.06.010306

World Health Organization. (n.d.). *Middle East respiratory syndrome coronavirus (MERS-CoV)*. https://www.who.int/emergencies/mers-cov/en

World Health Organization. (2003). *Climate change and human health—risks and responses*. https://www.who.int/publications/i/item/climate-change-and-human-health---risks-and-responses

World Health Organization. (2007). *The world health report 2007. A safer future: Global public health security in the 21st century*. Author. https://www.who.int/whr/2007/whr07_en.pdf

World Health Organization. (2008). *International health regulations (2005)* (2nd ed.). Author. https://apps.who.int/iris/bitstream/handle/10665/43883/9789241580410_eng.pdf

World Health Organization. (2011). *Report on the burden of endemic health care-associated infection worldwide*. https://www.who.int/iris/bitstream/10665/80135/1/9789241501507_eng.pdf?

World Health Organization. (2013). *IHR core capacity monitoring framework: Checklist and indicators for monitoring progress in the development of IHR core capacities in states parties*. https://apps.who.int/iris/bitstream/handle/10665/84933/WHO_HSE_GCR_2013.2_eng.pdf?

World Health Organization. (2016). *Joint external evaluation tool: International Health Regulations (2005)*. https://apps.who.int/iris/handle/10665/204368

World Health Organization. (2020). *Vector-borne diseases*. https://www.who.int/en/news-room/fact-sheets/detail/vector-borne-diseases

World Health Organization. (2021a). *Dengue and severe dengue*. https://www.who.int/news-room/fact-sheets/detail/dengue-and-severe-dengue

World Health Organization. (2021b). *Ebola virus disease*. https://www.who.int/news-room/fact-sheets/detail/ebola-virus-disease

Zmarlicka, M. T., Nailor, M. D., & Nicolau, D. P. (2015). Impact of the New Delhi Metallo-beta-lactamase on beta-lactam antibiotics. *Infection and Drug Resistance*, *8*, 297–309. https://doi.org/10.2147/IDR.S39186

CHAPTER 20

GOING FORWARD

OTHER EMERGENCIES AND FUTURE CHALLENGES

ROBERT J. KIM-FARLEY

KEY TERMS

Complex Coordinated Terrorist Attacks (CCTAs)
Essential Public Health Services
Foundational Competencies
Incident Command System (ICS)
The President's National Infrastructure Advisory Council (NIAC)

INTRODUCTION

This book is a continuing effort to provide information on public health emergencies through a unique case study approach to emergencies through the combined perspective of both the 2020 **Essential Public Health Services** and the 2021 Master of Public Health (MPH) **Foundational Competencies**.

By studying this book, students and public health practitioners will develop and strengthen their practical knowledge and skills in addressing the complex task of preparing for, mitigating, responding to, and recovering from a variety of public health emergencies based upon case studies from actual emergency situations ranging from natural to man-made disasters.

This chapter reflects on how the student and public health professional put the learning from the book into practice, briefly examines other public health emergencies not specifically covered in this book, and looks into the future as to the new challenges that may be expected to arise in addressing public health emergencies in our changing world.

PUTTING THE LEARNING FROM THE BOOK INTO PRACTICE

The student who has consciously studied and absorbed the "lessons learned" from the three parts of the book—namely, (a) Fundamentals of Public Health Emergency Preparedness, (b) Lessons Learned From Actual Incidents, and (c) Special Considerations—should feel a sense of confidence that they are now equipped with the knowledge, vocabulary, tools, and insights into how to approach assessing public health risks and addressing public health emergencies. Such students are now sufficiently prepared to be members of a public health team, often organized into an **Incident Command System (ICS)** structure during an emergency response or preparedness drill.

Initially, as a newer public health professional, it is anticipated that readers will usually be working with, or under, a more experienced colleague or supervisor until they have had sufficient "on the job" training in acquiring the skills in needed to apply the knowledge gained from this book. It is only through the "crucible" of "trial by fire" and working on an actual emergency that we can develop and refine skills—as well as develop the emotional strength and temperament to handle the stress of emergency settings—to a level where one takes on increasing responsibilities, including supervising others.

In planning and drilling for emergencies, it will be helpful to refer to this book from time to time to refresh your understanding of the 10 Essential Public Health Services and the 22 MPH Foundational Competencies as a framework to analyze what actions need to be implemented for any particular emergency. No two emergencies are exactly the same—there are always nuances and conditions that vary from one disaster to another, and so the applications of the relevant Essential Services and Foundational Competencies may also need to be adjusted accordingly.

The authors and coeditors of this book are also very keen to receive any feedback that you have with respect to any additional information you feel should be included in future editions of the book that would assist in your learning of the materials. Equally important is hearing about "lessons learned" from your own experiences in planning and responding to public health emergencies, lessons that also could be incorporated into the book. As mentioned in the beginning, this book is not a theoretical exploration of public health emergencies—it is rather the distillation of practical advice derived from the hard-learned lessons forged from actual situations public health professionals have faced. It is now up to you, as an act of generativity, to help us pass along your wisdom to the next generation of students and public health workers.

OTHER PUBLIC HEALTH EMERGENCIES NOT SPECIFICALLY COVERED IN THIS BOOK

This book has strived to provide case studies from several real-life public health emergency preparedness, planning, and response situations, including

- local infectious disease outbreaks such as carbapenem-resistant enterobacteriaceae (CRE) in duodenoscopes in Los Angeles County to global pandemics such as COVID-19;
- natural disasters such as earthquakes, tornadoes, hurricanes, and floods;
- human-made public health emergencies such as chemical disasters and food and water supply hazards; and
- deliberate human-made disasters such as nuclear detonation and bioterrorism.

However, no book can cover all the public health emergencies that occur in the world. Students are encouraged to take the framework of the Essential Public Health Services and Foundational Competencies learned in this book and explore other public health emergencies that have occurred, are occurring, or may occur to further deepen their knowledge and understanding of preparing for, and responding to, disasters.

A few specific examples are worth explicitly mentioning (with suggested references for students who may wish to delve into the topics in greater depth) and may be considered for inclusion in future editions of this book.

Mass Shootings

There is no definitive definition of "mass shooting." The Federal Bureau of Investigation (FBI) has defined "mass murderer" as someone who "kills four or more people in a single incident (not including himself), typically in a single location," and the U.S. Congress has defined "mass killing" as "a single incident that leaves three or more people dead" (Smart & Schell, 2021, "What Is a Mass Shooting?"). It should be noted that these definitions do not cover those instances where many victims may have been nonfatally injured even though fewer than four persons were killed.

Due to such varying definitions and the source of data used, it is currently challenging to make precise generalizations about mass shootings. However, it is clear that when they occur, and depending on the magnitude of the event, they present as an emergency. The establishment of an ICS; the need for joint coordination of actions among local public health, healthcare, and law enforcement agencies; and the importance of communication with the public are all elements of responding to a mass shooting emergency that are shared with many of the case studies highlighted in this book.

Terrorism

In the United States, terrorism has been described by the Federal Emergency Management Agency (FEMA) as

> the use of force or violence against persons or property in violation of the criminal laws of the United States for purposes of intimidation, coercion, or ransom. Terrorists often use threats to: create fear among the public; try to convince citizens that their government is powerless to prevent terrorism; and get immediate publicity for their causes. Acts of terrorism include threats of terrorism; assassinations; kidnappings; hijackings; bomb scares and bombings; cyber-attacks (computer-based); and the use of chemical, biological, nuclear and radiological weapons. (n.d., p. 148)

This book contains chapters on the use of bioterrorism and nuclear detonation of a so-called dirty bomb as examples of terrorism resulting in actual, or potential, public health emergencies. However, given that there are many other forms of terrorism that can create a disaster or major public disruption, the student may wish to also explore such consummated or planned terrorist acts as

- *Explosions* due to conventional bombs, such as occurred in the 1995 bombing of the Oklahoma City Federal Building resulting in the death of 168 persons—the worst act of homegrown terrorism in the United States (FBI, n.d.-b);
- *Mass shootings*, as noted earlier, such as the 2015 San Bernardino, California, mass shooting that resulted in the death of 14 persons perpetrated by homegrown terrorists inspired by foreign terrorist groups (Wikipedia, 2021);

- ***Complex coordinated terrorist attacks (CCTAs)***, which FEMA considers "an evolving and dynamic terrorist threat, shifting from symbolic, highly planned attacks to attacks that could occur anywhere, at any time, with the potential for mass casualties" and, due to their complexities "(e.g., multiple teams, attack locations, and weapon types) may represent additional challenges to jurisdictions . . . and require the delivery of community capabilities and resources across a wide range of Core Capabilities" (2018, p. 1). The most famous example of a CCTA is the attacks of 9/11, the most lethal terrorist attacks in history. It resulted in the deaths of 2,996 people (including the hijackers) and injured more than 6,000 others in New York City, at the Pentagon, and in Shanksville, Pennsylvania. It ultimately led to "far-reaching changes in anti-terror approaches and operations in the U.S. and around the globe" (FBI, n.d.-a. para. 1); and
- *Chemical terrorist attacks* such as the one perpetrated in the 1995 subway system in Tokyo, Japan, using the nerve agent sarin. It killed 14 people, injured or affected some 5,000 other persons, and required a disaster management response. The United States also is vulnerable to such chemical terrorist attacks (Okumura et al., 1998).

War and Civil Unrest as a Public Health Emergency

Civilian populations are affected by armed conflict due to wars and civil unrest. Such populations may experience severe public health consequences resulting in an emergency due to not only war-related injuries and fatalities but also "population displacement, food scarcity, and the collapse of basic health services, giving rise to the term complex humanitarian emergencies. These public health effects have been most severe in underdeveloped countries in Africa, Asia, and Latin America" (Toole & Waldman, 1997).

Transportation Emergencies

Some transportation emergencies may be due to an incident involving chemical, biological, or radiological materials being transported by highway, railway, or airplanes. Such incidents become public health emergencies if there are significant impacts on human health and safety. The public health actions for response are covered under the topics in this book for the specific type of material involved in the incident.

However, there are also transportation emergencies that become public health emergencies in themselves because of the scope of human injuries and fatalities. Such events include subway fires, multicar pileups on freeways (often in times of impaired visibility such as dense fog and blizzard "whiteout" conditions), airplane crashes (especially if they occur in densely populated areas), and passenger ship and ferry capsizes and sinkings.

Tsunamis

Tsunamis can lead to large-scale disasters over wide-ranging areas. The 2004 Indian Ocean tsunami, for example, killed more than 174,000 persons. The CDC has provided guidelines for cleanup and safety, handling human remains; and so on in the aftermath of a tsunami (CDC, n.d.-c).

Tsunamis can even be trigger events to other public health emergencies. For example, the 2011 tsunami in Japan resulted in a nuclear accident at the Fukushima Daiichi Nuclear Power Plant, creating a nuclear meltdown of three reactor cores that ultimately led to the evacuation of some 154,000 persons.

Mudslides and Landslides

A landslide occurs "when masses of rock, earth, or debris move down a slope. Debris flows, also known as mudslides, are a common type of fast-moving landslide that tends to flow in channels." In the United States, such events result in 25 to 50 deaths each year, may result in displacement of persons, and disrupt roadways and railways (CDC, n.d.-b).

Volcanoes

Volcanoes are found on every continent, and "some 1,500 volcanoes are still considered potentially active around the world today; 161 of those—over 10 percent—sit within the boundaries of the United States." In addition to the danger of lava flows, there are also the "avalanches of hot rocks, ash, and toxic gas that race down slopes at speeds as high as 450 miles an hour," known as pyroclastic flows, as well as destructive volcanic mudflows known as lahars (Wei-Haas, 2018).

As an example, the May 18, 1980, volcanic eruption of Mount St. Helens in Washington State killed 57 persons and caused extensive damage to buildings, forests, recreation sites, and infrastructure such as bridges and roads. Many persons were left homeless. The CDC (n.d.-d) has noted that "some dangers from volcanos can be predicted ahead of time while others may occur with little or no notice after an eruption."

Infrastructure Failures

The scope of public health emergencies resulting from infrastructure failures is wide-ranging and includes the following:

- Building collapse—Aging buildings, especially if not properly structurally maintained, are at special risks. A recent example is the 2021 collapse of the 40-year-old Champlain Towers South condominium complex in Surfside, Florida, which claimed the lives of 98 persons.
- Dam failures—Human-made water reservoirs for drinking water and/or hydroelectric power are capable of highly destructive effects to life and the surrounding environment when they fail. An example is the 1963 breach of the Baldwin Hills Dam in Los Angeles, California, that resulted in the deaths of five persons and millions of dollars in damage.

- Bridge and overpass failures—Catastrophic failure of these structures may cause immediate deaths and injuries but can also result in a transportation-related emergency by cutting off the normal routes of egress and ingress for communities.
- Power grid failures—**The President's National Infrastructure Advisory Council** (2018) has provided recommendations for surviving a catastrophic power outage. Vulnerable populations, such as older adults, may be at special risks during power grid failure emergencies when heating and cooling systems may not be operating. Persons in special situations, such as those on home ventilators, and critical infrastructure, such as hospitals, are at risk during prolonged power outages.

LOOKING INTO THE FUTURE

There are emerging situations that have public health implications with the potential for increased impact in the future. Some are noted in the following text. The student can begin to "look forward" to evaluate possible emergencies they may be called on to prepare for and respond to in the future.

Cyberattacks. Cyberattacks can have important impacts on infrastructure, but may also have health and/or economic consequences (e.g., the many recent examples of cyber-criminals targeting healthcare institutions and food-processing plants to extort ransom money to retain access to their critical files and computer programs and storage). Cyberterrorists "seek to destroy, incapacitate, or exploit critical infrastructures in order to threaten national security, cause mass casualties, weaken the U.S. economy, and damage public morale and confidence. Terrorists may use phishing schemes or spyware/malware in order to generate funds or gather sensitive information" (Cybersecurity and Infrastructure Security Agency, 2021, "Terrorists").

Climate change. Climate change is becoming increasingly recognized as a global health emergency and encompasses a wide range of events, including heat waves; extreme weather events (e.g., rain, hurricanes, tornadoes, flooding); droughts (and the implications regarding safe water and food supplies); wildfires; sea-level rise; increases in ground-level ozone, airborne allergens, and other pollutants; and changes in the transmission of vector-, food-, and waterborne diseases. The CDC (n.d.-a) has provided policy recommendations and a scientific framework on climate and health. Although this book has individually addressed some of these events, comprehensive approaches to preparedness, mitigation, and both near- and long-term response actions need to be increasingly addressed at local, national, and global levels as a threat to all of us, especially the most vulnerable, on the planet.

Asteroid impact. "The United States spends about $4 million annually searching for near-Earth objects (NEOs) according to NASA [National Aeronautics and Space Administration]. The goal is to detect those that may collide with Earth" (p. 1)—such as asteroids. In the report *Defending Planet Earth* by the National Research Council of the National Academies, four types of mitigation were identified, namely, (a) *civil defense*—which may be the only option "feasible for warning times shorter than perhaps a year or two" (p. 4); (b) "*slow-push*" or "*slow-pull*" methods, whereby "the orbit of the target object would be changed so that it avoided collision with Earth" (p. 4); (c) *kinetic impactors* whereby "the target's orbit would be changed by the sending of one or more spacecraft with very massive payload(s) to impact directly on the target" (p. 4); and (d) *nuclear explosions*, which, as a last resort, "would be usable for objects up to a few kilometers in diameter" (p. 4). As noted in the report, for larger near-Earth objects "(more than a few kilometers in diameter), which would be on the scale that would inflict serious global damage and, perhaps, mass extinctions, there is at present no feasible defense" (p. 4). Fortunately, such events are extremely rare, and the last known impact of such a large object was approximately 65 million years ago. Planning for an asteroid impact is noted in the report as the "classic problem of the conflict between 'extremely important' and 'extremely rare'" (National Research Council, 2010, p. 6).

Zombie attack. The CDC perfected the art of "thinking outside the box" when the CDC Center for Preparedness and Response developed a campaign in 2011 on "Preparedness 101: Zombie Apocalypse." Although obviously somewhat "tongue-in-cheek," it did, however, excite the imaginations of students and educators teaching public health emergency preparedness. It is mentioned in this chapter as an example of creative approaches that may help us in the future to engage the public on important preparedness measures for real, likely emergency events such as those that have been mentioned in this book. Preparedness measures highlighted in the Zombie Apocalypse campaign included such practical actions as stocking drinking water and nonperishable foods; having an extra supply of critical medications, sanitation, and hygiene supplies; having clothing and bedding, and important documents; and having first aid supplies on hand (CDC, 2021).

CONCLUSION

It is hoped that the reader has enjoyed the learning process throughout the case examples used in this book and is also left reflecting on the wide-ranging scope of public health emergency preparedness actions from "A to Z" (i.e., from asteroids to zombies). Two "take-home lessons learned" from the case studies is that no two disasters are the same and that such forces as the increasing effects of climate change mean that the "mix" of emergencies will vary over time. There will always be the "expected–unexpected" events such as the COVID-19 pandemic, and we, in public health, need to be anticipating them, planning for them, stockpiling the needed supplies to address them (e.g., the National Strategic Stockpile with medicines to counter bioterrorist attacks, personal protective equipment, ventilators, field hospitals, and so on), drilling on them, and responding to them.

Just as the emergency department in a hospital is in a constant state of preparedness and response to the needs of their patients on an individual level (and on a mass casualty level in disasters), public health professionals in emergency preparedness are always at the ready to prepare for, drill, and respond to the community and the disasters that inevitably will affect it. We wish you well in taking your place on the front lines of defense of your community and jurisdictions through the application of public health emergency preparedness and response principles learned in this book.

DISCUSSION QUESTIONS

1. Briefly review the types of other public health emergencies mentioned in this chapter and in the case studies earlier in the book. What additional types of emergencies exist or have occurred in the past?
2. Take one of the other public health emergencies briefly mentioned in this chapter and further explore about that type of emergency in greater depth using the included references or other sources obtained through your own online search. How are the Essential Health Services and Foundational Competencies used in preparing or responding to that type of emergency?
3. Discuss how you plan to use the learning gleaned from this book into practice in your current or anticipated future work environment.
4. Briefly review the types of public health emergencies mentioned in the section "Looking Into the Future" in this chapter. What additional types of emergencies can you envision that may challenge public health workers in the future?

REFERENCES

Centers for Disease Control and Prevention. (n.d.-a). *Climate and health: CDC policy*. https://www.cdc.gov/climateandhealth/policy.htm

Centers for Disease Control and Prevention. (n.d.-b). *Landslides and mudslides*. https://www.cdc.gov/disasters/landslides.html

Centers for Disease Control and Prevention. (n.d.-c). *Response and cleanup after a tsunami*. https://www.cdc.gov/disasters/tsunamis/response.html

Centers for Disease Control and Prevention. (n.d.-d). *Volcanoes*. https://www.cdc.gov/disasters/volcanoes/index.html

Centers for Disease Control and Prevention. (2021). *Zombie preparedness*.

Cybersecurity and Infrastructure Security Agency. (2021). *Cyber threat source descriptions*. https://us-cert.cisa.gov/ics/content/cyber-threat-source-descriptions

Federal Bureau of Investigation. (n.d.-a). *9/11 investigation*. https://www.fbi.gov/history/famous-cases/911-investigation

Federal Bureau of Investigation. (n.d.-b). *Oklahoma City bombing*. https://www.fbi.gov/history/famous-cases/oklahoma-city-bombing

Federal Emergency Management Agency. (n.d.). *Terrorism*. https://www.fema.gov/pdf/areyouready/terrorism.pdf

Federal Emergency Management Agency. (2018). *Planning considerations: Complex coordinated terrorist attacks*. https://www.fema.gov/sites/default/files/2020-07/planning-considerations-complex-coordinated-terrorist-attacks.pdf

National Research Council. (2010). *Defending planet Earth: Near-Earth-objects and hazard mitigation strategies*. National Academies Press. https://doi.org/10.17226/12842

Okumura, T., Suzuki, K., Fukuda, A., Kohama, A., Takasu, N., Ishimatsu, S., & Hinohara, S. (1998), The Tokyo Subway Sarin attack: Disaster management, Part 1: Community emergency response. *Academic Emergency Medicine*, 5, 613–617. https://doi.org/10.1111/j.1553-2712.1998.tb02470.x

The President's National Infrastructure Advisory Council. (2018). *Surviving a catastrophic power outage*. https://www.cisa.gov/sites/default/files/publications/NIAC%20Catastrophic%20Power%20Outage%20Study_FINAL.pdf

Smart, R., & Schell, T. L. (2021). *Mass shootings in the United States*. https://www.rand.org/research/gun-policy/analysis/essays/mass-shootings.html

Toole, M. J., & Waldman, R. J. (0997). The public health aspects of complex emergencies and refugee situations. *Annual Reviews of Public Health*, 18, 283–312. https://doi.org/10.1146/annurev.publhealth.18.1.283

Wei-Haas, M. (2018). *Volcanoes, explained*. https://www.nationalgeographic.com/environment/article/volcanoes

Wikipedia. (2021). *2015 San Bernadino attack*. https://en.wikipedia.org/wiki/2015_San_Bernardino_attack

EPILOGUE

As of this writing, September 2021, the COVID-19 coronavirus pandemic, which began in January of 2020, continues in the United States and around the world. Rates of COVID-19 infection are surging in nearly every state, as the Delta variant of the virus attacks primarily persons who refused to be vaccinated against the disease. Again, similar to the past year, in some areas with high levels of community transmission, hospitals are reaching capacity, medical and support staff are suffering from prolonged stress, and staffing and material shortages are once again concerns.

In reflecting back to July 2020 after the Fourth of July holiday weekend, COVID-19 rates were skyrocketing. In that month alone, more than 1.9 million new infections were reported, nearly 42% of the total reported cases at the time and double the number observed in previous months. Yet, states were reopening businesses, and segments of the population staged protests and threatened violence to public officials who desired to continue such mitigation strategies as masking and physical distancing to minimize viral exposure.

The current trajectory of COVID-19 looks eerily similar, with rates trending upward after a steep decline in the spring, and the false sense of security garnered by the availability of vaccines and lifting of masking mandates for persons who were fully vaccinated. It was no surprise that people who had refused vaccines abandoned mask use as well, and in random public interactions there is no way to tell the difference between the vaccinated and not vaccinated. In southern states where vaccination rates are particularly low, the new COVID-19 variant rates are the highest, and in those states resistance to public health prevention measures has also been a common phenomenon. Eschewing mask wearing and rejecting vaccines have become symbols of rugged individualism and determination to resist any effort of government officials to influence behaviors—ironically, lifesaving ones.

How did we get to this point, and where do we go from here? How are public health measures designed to protect the nation connected to fears of losing rights and attacks on individual freedoms? In the 21st century, we have witnessed a resurgence of antiquated ideas including mistrust of science and expertise, a reliance on conspiracy theories rather than on facts, and fear and mistrust of governments, all of which are becoming orthodoxy in some communities, largely spread by social and other media outlets. It should be noted that some segments of the population will likely never be exposed to verifiable facts due to media market segmentation that provides crafted "news" programming to match political perspectives, and social media algorithms, which feed consumers content based on past consumption of ideas. These strategies are profit-driven and not designed to convey factual information but subliminally steer viewers toward purchasing products through exposure to and affirmation of deeply held biases.

At the close of this volume, we call for a national paradigm shift of Copernican proportions. We call for a reaffirmation of science and the application of science to public health emergency preparedness activities. We acknowledge that science and public health emergency preparedness are not static but rather are ever changing as new ideas and additional information are acquired. We also acknowledge that preparedness is much more than bureaucratic notions of structural capabilities. Public health emergency preparedness is the sum total of a nation's commitment for taking care of its people during normal times, paired with systems in place to maintain public safety and reduce morbidity and mortality during the stressful experiences of emergencies—especially for the most vulnerable in our communities. If a nation's "safety net" is marginally functioning in normal times, any stress to the system will make it falter and break. Resilience is based on existing strengths. Preparedness should be built by first strengthening the lives of the population by ensuring people have access to fulfilling basic human needs and healthcare in communities and layering on whole-community approaches for protecting lives during emergencies.

Tanya Telfair LeBlanc

Robert J. Kim-Farley

GLOSSARY

Access and Functional Needs—Physical or structural restrictions, limitations, or other barriers to self-protection experienced by human beings that will necessitate assistance before, during, and after an emergency.

Acute Radiation Syndrome (ARS)—"[S]ometimes known as radiation toxicity or radiation sickness), it is an acute illness caused by irradiation of the entire body (or most of the body) by a high dose of penetrating radiation in a very short period of time (usually a matter of minutes)." https://www.cdc.gov/nceh/radiation/emergencies/pdf/ars.pdf

Advanced Marginality—A multigenerational socioeconomic condition in which individuals or groups are systemically restricted from obtaining life sustainable work, are not able to enjoy the benefits of a society, are isolated from more advantaged people and groups, and are stigmatized because of their status; it is caused by structural inequalities in an economic or social system that serve as barriers to improvement of life chances and opportunities.

***Aedes aegypti* Mosquito**—A species of mosquito that can serve as a vector to transmit viruses that cause a number of diseases to humans including Dengue fever, chikungunya, Zika fever, Mayaro and yellow fever viruses, and other diseases.

Airways Hyperresponsiveness—Increased sensitivity and reactivity of the airways to numerous types of stimuli, which is characteristic of severe asthma.

Aldicarb Oxime—A hazardous insecticide, especially for infants and children. Its use was banned in 2010 but was reinstated for use on citrus fruit on January 13, 2021.

Anthropogenic Sources—Environmental changes and pollution caused by human activities, directly or indirectly.

Aqueous Ammonia—A solution of ammonia in water.

Association for Professionals in Infection Control (APIC)—The leading professional association for infection preventionists with more than 15,000 members whose mission is to advance the science and practice of infection prevention and control. https://apic.org/about-apic/about-apic-overview

Avian Influenza—Strains of influenza viruses that primarily infect birds but can also infect humans.

Backbone Organization—An organization, generally a state or local public health agency, in charge of convening and coordinating roles for an entire jurisdictional preparedness system, providing a wide variety of administrative functions for day-to-day activities, including managing financial and human resources and fiscal arrangements, community relationships, volunteer recruitment and trainings, logistics, strategic planning, and more.

Beta-Lactam Antibiotics—β-lactam antibiotics were some of the first antibiotics developed; they attack bacterial cell walls as they attempt to multiply in the body. They include penicillins, cephalosporins, monobactams, and carbapenems.

Borrelia burgdorferi—A corkscrew-shaped bacteria that causes Lyme disease.

Botulism—A rare but serious illness caused by a toxin that attacks the body's nerves and causes difficulty breathing, muscle paralysis, and even death. This toxin is made by *Clostridium botulinum* and sometimes *Clostridium butyricum* and *Clostridium baratii* bacteria.

Bubonic Plague—Plague is a potentially lethal infection caused by the *Yersinia pestis* bacteria, which is common in rodents and their fleas. Bubonic plague is the most common form of the disease and is so named because it causes painful swelling of the lymph nodes, called "buboes."

Built Environment—Man-made structures, features, and facilities viewed collectively as an environment in which people live and work.

California Code of Regulations (CCR)—"[I]s the official compilation and publication of the regulations adopted, amended or repealed by California state agencies pursuant to the Administrative Procedure Act. Properly adopted regulations that have been filed with the Secretary of State have the force of law." https://oal.ca.gov/publications/ccr

California Emergency Medical Services Authority (EMSA)—Charged with providing leadership in developing and implementing emergency medical services (EMS) systems throughout California and setting standards for the training and scope of practice of various levels of EMS personnel. https://emsa.ca.gov/about_emsa

***Campylobacter* Infection**—A common foodborne illness, contracted by ingesting undercooked or raw poultry, or by drinking contaminated water or raw milk.

Candida auris—Type of yeast that is naturally occurring in human skin and mucous membranes that can cause fungal illness in immunocompromised humans and under conditions of overgrowth. Some strains are multiresistant to available treatments.

Carbapenem-Resistant *Enterobacteriaceae* (CRE)—"Enterobacterales are a large order of different types of germs (bacteria) that commonly cause infections in healthcare settings. . . . When Enterobacterales develop resistance to the group of antibiotics called carbapenems, the germs are called carbapenem-resistant Enterobacterales (CRE). CRE are difficult to treat because they do not respond to commonly used antibiotics." https://www.cdc.gov/hai/organisms/cre/index.html

CARES Act—The Coronavirus Aid, Relief, and Economic Security (CARES) Act (2020) and the Coronavirus Response and Consolidated Appropriations Act (2021) were federal government economic stimulus packages that provided fast and direct economic assistance for American workers, families, small businesses, and industries. The CARES Act implemented a variety of programs to address issues related to the onset of the COVID-19 pandemic.

Catheters—Thin, flexible tubes that can put fluids into your body or take them out. A urinary catheter that goes into the bladder can rid the body of urine.

CDC Quarantine Station—"U.S. Quarantine Stations are part of a comprehensive Quarantine System that serves to limit the introduction of infectious diseases into the United States and to prevent their spread. U.S. Quarantine Stations are located at 20 ports of entry and land-border crossings where international travelers arrive. They are staffed with quarantine medical and public health officers from CDC." https://www.cdc.gov/quarantine/quarantinestations.html

CDC's Operational Readiness Review (ORR) Process—"[I]s a rigorous, evidence-based assessment that evaluates state, local, and territorial planning and operational functions. Currently, the ORR primarily focuses on evaluating a jurisdiction's ability to execute a large response requiring medical countermeasure (MCM) distribution and dispensing." https://www.cdc.gov/cpr/readiness/orr.html

CDC's Set of 15 Public Health Emergency Preparedness and Response Capabilities—Are "capabilities that serve as national standards for public health preparedness planning . . . these capability standards have served as a vital framework for state, local, tribal, and territorial preparedness programs as they plan, operationalize, and evaluate their ability to prepare for, respond to, and recover from public health emergencies." They include community preparedness, community recovery, emergency operations coordination, emergency public information and warning, fatality management, information sharing, mass care, medical countermeasures dispensing and administration, medical materiel management and distribution, medical surge, nonpharmaceutical interventions, public health laboratory testing, public health surveillance and epidemiological investigation, responder safety and health, and volunteer management. https://www.cdc.gov/cpr/readiness/capabilities.htm

Chief Complaint—The principal reason a person seeks medical care.

Chloramine—A compound containing chlorine and nitrogen; used as an antiseptic in wounds.

Chronic Disease—A human health condition that is persistent or long lasting. Disease that lasts a year or more and requires ongoing medical attention.

Chronic Obstructive Pulmonary Disease—A chronic inflammatory lung disease that causes obstructed airflow from the lungs. Symptoms include breathing difficulty, cough, mucus (sputum) production, and wheezing.

Clostridium difficile—Often referred to as *C. difficile* or *C. diff*, it is a bacterium that can cause symptoms ranging from diarrhea to life-threatening inflammation of the colon. This is a common hospital-borne infection.

Cluster Analysis—A set of statistical tools and algorithms used to group objects or participants that share characteristics on selected criteria.

C-MIST—A comprehensive framework for understanding and planning for access and functional needs during an emergence. The acronym stands for communication, medical, independence, supervision, and transportation needs.

Coalition—An alliance of stakeholders for a common purpose or action.

Coccidioidomycosis—Also called Valley fever, "it is an infection caused by the fungus Coccidioides. The fungus is known to live in the soil in the southwestern United States and parts of Mexico and Central and South America. The fungus was also recently found in south-central Washington." https://www.cdc.gov/fungal/diseases/coccidioidomycosis/index.html

Cognitive Behavioral Therapy—A type of psychotherapy in which negative patterns of thought about the self and the world are challenged in order to alter unwanted behavior patterns or treat mood disorders such as depression.

Cognitive Disabilities—Impairments in mental functioning, thinking, or memory processes that may limit communication, self-care, or social skills.

Cold War—The period following World War II, approximately 1947 to 1991, characterized by geopolitical tension between the United States and its allies and the Soviet Union and its allies.

Community Assessment for Public Health Emergency Response (CASPER)—"[I]s an epidemiologic technique designed to provide public health leaders and emergency managers with household-based information about a community. It is quick, reliable, relatively inexpensive, and flexible." https://www.cdc.gov/nceh/casper/default.htm

Community Health Assessment (CHA)—"[A]lso known as community health needs assessment (sometimes called a CHNA), refers to a state, tribal, local, or territorial health assessment that identifies key health needs and issues through systematic, comprehensive data collection and analysis." https://www.cdc.gov/publichealthgateway/cha/plan.html

Community Health Improvement Plan (CHIP)—"[I]s a long-term, systematic effort to address public health problems based on the results of community health assessment activities and the community health improvement process. A plan is typically updated every three to five years." https://www.cdc.gov/publichealthgateway/cha/plan.html

Community Health Resilience (CHR)—The ability of a community to use its assets to strengthen public health and healthcare systems and to improve the community's physical, behavioral, and social health to withstand, adapt to, and recover from adversity.

Community Resilience—The sustained ability of communities to withstand, adapt to, and recover from adversity.

Complex Coordinated Terrorist Attacks (CCTAs)—"[A]cts of terrorism that involve synchronized and independent team(s) at multiple locations, sequentially or in close succession, initiated with little or no warning, and employing one or more weapon systems: firearms, explosives, fire as a weapon, and other nontraditional attack methodologies that are intended to result in large numbers of casualties." https://www.fema.gov/sites/default/files/2020-07/planning-considerations-complex-coordinated-terrorist-attacks.pdf

Continuity of Government (COG) Plans—"A coordinated effort within the executive, legislative, or judicial branches to ensure that essential functions continue to be performed before, during, and after an emergency or threat. Continuity of government is intended to preserve the statutory and constitutional authority of elected officials at all levels of government across the United States." https://www.fema.gov/emergency-managers/national-preparedness/continuity/terms

Continuity of Operations (COOP) Plans—"[D]efined in the National Continuity Policy Implementation Plan (NCPIP) and the National Security Presidential Directive 51/Homeland Security Presidential Directive 20 (NSPD-51/HSPD-20), is an effort within individual executive departments and agencies to ensure that Primary Mission Essential Functions (PMEFs) continue to be performed during a wide range of emergencies." https://www.fema.gov/pdf/about/org/ncp/coop_brochure.pdf

Cooperative Agreement—A monetary award from a funding institution to a university, governmental agency, community-based organization, or other qualified organization that initiates a partnership between the funder and the awardee, with both entities working together toward specific programmatic goals for public good. The funder issues a "call for proposals" or a "request for applications" to select qualified recipients capable of performing functions required to accomplish the goals of the program and, upon selection, provides technical assistance to the awardee in the interest of achieving the outcomes.

COVID-19—An infectious disease caused by the novel SARS-CoV-2 virus emerging in late 2019 and causing a global pandemic in 2020.

Crisis Standards of Care (CSC)—"[P]rovides a framework for a systems approach to the development and implementation of CSC plans, and addresses the legal issues and the ethical, palliative care, and mental health issues that agencies and organizations at each level of a disaster response should address." https://pubmed.ncbi.nlm.nih.gov/24830057

Cryptosporidiosis—A tiny one-celled parasite that causes diarrhea in humans. The disease can be much more serious for persons with compromised immune systems. The parasite may be found in water sources, such as swimming pools, recreation water parks, lakes, streams, and ponds.

Cryptosporidium—A parasite that causes gastrointestinal and respiratory diseases.

***Culex* Species**—A species of mosquitoes that are vectors for diseases in humans, birds, and other animals.

Cumulative Health Vulnerability Index (CVHI)—Developed by Colleen Reid and colleagues, this index uses factor analysis on six demographic characteristics and two household air-conditioning variables, vegetation cover from satellite images, and diabetes prevalence from a national survey. They assigned values of increasing vulnerability for the four resulting factors to each of 39,794 census tracts and added the four factor scores to obtain a cumulative heat vulnerability index value.

Cyprofloxacin—A strong antibiotic used to treat bacterial infections.

Cytokines—Cell-signalling molecules that aid cell-to-cell communication in immune responses and stimulate the movement of cells toward sites of inflammation, infection, and trauma.

Defense Production Act (DPA)—"[I]s the primary source of presidential authorities to expedite and expand the supply of materials and services from the U.S. industrial base needed to promote the national defense. DPA authorities are available to support emergency preparedness activities conducted pursuant to Title VI of the Stafford Act; protection or restoration of critical infrastructure; and efforts to prevent, reduce vulnerability to, minimize damage from, and recover from acts of terrorism within the United States." https://www.fema.gov/disaster/defense-production-act

Department Operations Center (DOC)—"Per the National Incident Management System (NIMS), Department Operations Centers (DOC) are established and activated by individual departments to coordinate and control actions specific to that department during an emergency event." https://www.cidrap.umn.edu/practice/health-department-operations-center

Dialysis—(More formally, hemodialysis) Is a medical procedure that artificially replicates the action of the kidneys to filter and cleanse the blood of impurities and waste.

Disability—A physical or mental condition that may limit a person's movement, senses, or activities.

Disaster—"An occurrence of a natural catastrophe, technological accident, or human caused event that has resulted in severe property damage, deaths, and/or multiple injuries." https://www.fema.gov/pdf/plan/glo.pdf

Disaster Medical Assistance Teams (DMATs)—"[P]rovide high-quality rapid-response medical care when public health and medical emergencies overwhelm state, local, tribal, or territorial resources. In the aftermath of natural and technological disasters, acts of terrorism, and during disease outbreaks, DMAT members are on location protecting health and saving lives." https://www.phe.gov/Preparedness/responders/ndms/ndms-teams/Pages/dmat.aspx

Disaster Mortuary Operational Response Team (DMORT)—"[S]upport local mortuary services on location, working to quickly and accurately identify victims and reunite victims with their loved ones in a dignified, respectful manner. DMORTs are deployed to supplement federal, state, local, tribal and territorial resources at the request of local authorities." https://www.phe.gov/Preparedness/responders/ndms/ndms-teams/Pages/dmort.aspx

Disinformation—False information spread with the conscious intent to mislead an audience. Disinformation involves knowingly spreading false information.

Dispersant—A substance used to aid in spreading another substance.

Division of Occupational Safety and Health (Cal/OSHA)—"[P]rotects and improves the health and safety of working men and women in California and the safety of passengers riding on elevators, amusement rides, and tramways – through . . . setting and enforcing standards; providing outreach, education, and assistance; and issuing permits, licenses, certifications, registrations, and approvals." https://www.dir.ca.gov/dosh

Doctor's First Report (DFR) of Occupational Injury or Illness—"Every physician who treats an injured employee must file a complete . . . DFR with the employer's claims administrator within five days of the initial examination." https://www.dir.ca.gov/dwc/Electronic-Reporting-System-for-DFR/Index.htm

Doxycycline—A class of medications called tetracycline antibiotics. They work to treat infections by preventing the growth and spread of bacteria.

Ebola Virus Disease—A severe, often fatal illness affecting humans and other primates. The virus is transmitted to people from wild animals (such as fruit bats, porcupines, nonhuman primates) and then spreads in the human population through direct contact with the blood, secretions, organs, or other bodily fluids of infected people and with surfaces and materials (e.g., bedding, clothing) contaminated with these fluids. The average EVD case fatality rate is around 50%. Case fatality rates have varied from 25% to 90% in past outbreaks.

Electromagnetic Pulse (EMP)—"In a nuclear explosion an electromagnetic pulse, or EMP, is possible. An EMP is a side effect of a nuclear detonation that produces a surge of energy. This surge can damage electronic devices." https://www.cdc.gov/nceh/radiation/emergencies/waystostaytuned.htm

Emergency Alert System (EAS)—"[A] national public warning system commonly used by state and local authorities to deliver important emergency information, such as weather and AMBER alerts, to affected communities. EAS participants—radio and television broadcasters, cable systems, satellite radio and television providers, and wireline video providers—deliver local alerts on a voluntary basis, but they are required to provide the capability for the [p]resident to address the public during a national emergency." https://www.fcc.gov/emergency-alert-system

Emergency Operations Center (EOC)—"The physical location at which the coordination of information and resources to support incident management (on-scene operations) activities normally takes place. An EOC may be a temporary facility or may be located in a more central or permanently established facility, perhaps at a higher level of organization within a jurisdiction." https://training.fema.gov/programs/emischool/el361toolkit/glossary.htm

Emergency Operations Plans (EOPs)—"An ongoing plan for responding to a wide variety of potential hazards. An EOP describes how people and property will be protected; details who is responsible for carrying out specific actions; identifies the personnel, equipment, facilities, supplies, and other resources available; and outlines how all actions will be coordinated." https://training.fema.gov/programs/emischool/el361toolkit/glossary.htm

Emergency Preparedness Capabilities—A number of conceptual models defining the structural components of national safety and security and requirements for ensuring protection of citizens during emergencies, used by federal agencies to frame funded preparedness activities. https://training.fema.gov/programs/emischool/el361toolkit/glossary.htm

Emergency Support Functions (ESF)—"[P]rovide the structure for coordinating Federal interagency support for a Federal response to an incident. They are mechanisms for grouping functions most frequently used to provide Federal support to States and Federal-to-Federal support, both for declared disasters and emergencies under the Stafford Act and for non-Stafford Act incidents." https://training.fema.gov/programs/emischool/el361toolkit/glossary.htm

There are 15 societal components outlined in the National Response Framework to provide the structure for coordinating federal interagency support for a federal response to an incident.

ESF #1: Transportation
ESF #2: Communications

ESF #3: Public Works and Engineering
ESF #4: Firefighting
ESF #5: Information and Planning
ESF #6: Mass Care, Emergency Assistance, Temporary Housing, and Human Services
ESF #7: Logistics
ESF #8: Public Health and Medical Services
ESF #9: Search and Rescue
ESF #10: Oil and Hazardous Materials Response
ESF #11: Agriculture and Natural Resources Annex
ESF #12: Energy
ESF #13: Public Safety and Security
ESF #14: Cross-Sector Business and Infrastructure
ESF #15: External Affairs

Emergency Support Function #8 (ESF #8)—One of 15 Emergency Support Functions for national preparedness and security identified by the Federal Emergency Management Association (FEMA); it is assigned to the Department of Health and Human Services for administration. ESF #8 provides the mechanism for federal assistance to supplement local, state, tribal, and territorial resources in response to a disaster, emergency, or incident that may lead to a public health, medical, behavioral, or human service emergency.

Emergency System for Advance Registration of Volunteer Health Professionals (ESAR-VHP)—"[A] federal program created to support states and territories in establishing standardized volunteer registration programs for disasters and public health and medical emergencies. The program, administered on the state level, verifies health professionals' identification and credentials so that they can respond more quickly when disaster strikes." https://www.phe.gov/esarvhp/pages/about.aspx#:~:text=Main%20Content-,The%20Emergency%20System%20for%20Advance%20Registration%20of%20Volunteer%20Health%20Professionals,public%20health%20and%20medical%20emergencies

Endotrachael Tube—An endotracheal tube is a flexible plastic tube that is placed through the mouth into the trachea (windpipe) to help a patient breathe.

Enhanced Fujita Scale—The original F scale, developed by Dr. Tetsuya Theodore Fujita, estimates tornado wind speeds based on damage left behind by a tornado. Building on this work, the Enhanced Fujita (EF) Scale, developed by a forum of nationally renowned meteorologists and wind engineers, makes improvements to the original F scale by taking into account additional indicators for evidence of tornado destruction.

Environmental Hazards—A condition, process, state, or exposure that threatens the air, water, soil, or place that may cause widespread harm to human beings.

Enzyme-Linked Immunosorbent Assay (ELISA)—Enzyme-linked immunosorbent assay, a rapid immunochemical test that involves an enzyme used for measuring a wide variety of tests of body fluids.

ESSENCE—Electronic Surveillance System for the Early Notification of Community-Based Epidemics (ESSENCE) software is a system that inputs electronic emergency department (ED) data for the purpose of syndromic surveillance. ESSENCE groups chief complaints from electronic ED data into "syndrome" categories. This information is used to determine if the number of visits is greater than expected for that facility based on historical data and statistical analyses to conduct early event detection. Syndrome groups used include botulism-like exposure, fever, gastrointestinal issues, hemorrhagic illness, influenza-like illness, injury, neurological issues, rash, records of interest, respiratory issues, and shock/coma. ESSENCE can also be used for situational awareness during known health events by querying all ED visits for a particular syndrome or by keyword (such as carbon monoxide, animal bite, injury, etc.).

Essential Community Lifelines—"The integrated network of assets, services, and capabilities that provide lifeline services are used day-to-day to support the recurring needs of the community and enable all other aspects of society to function." The Federal Emergency Management Agency (FEMA) identifies seven community lifelines: "Safety and Security; Food, Water, and Sheltering; Health and Medical; Energy; Communications; Transportation; and Hazardous Materials." https://www.fema.gov/emergency-managers/practitioners/lifelines

Essential Public Health Services—Originally developed in 1994 by a federal working group, the 10 Essential Public Health Services were revised on September 9, 2020, as part of *The Futures Initiative: The 10 Essential Public Health Services*, the de Beaumont Foundation, Public Health National Center for Innovations, and a task force of public health experts. This revision "now centers equity and incorporates current and future public health practice." http://phnci.org/national-frameworks/10-ephs

Federal Emergency Management Agency (FEMA)—"[S]upports citizens and emergency personnel to build, sustain, and improve the nation's capability to prepare for, protect against, respond to, recover from, and mitigate all hazards." https://www.usa.gov/federal-agencies/federal-emergency-management-agency

Federal Radiological Monitoring and Assessment Center (FRMAC)—"[A] federal asset available on request by the Department of Homeland Security (DHS) to respond to nuclear and radiological incidents as described in the National Response Framework (NRF)." https://www.nnss.gov/pages/programs/FRMAC/FRMAC.html

FEMA's Comprehensive Preparedness Guide—"[P]rovides guidance for developing emergency operations plans. It promotes a common understanding of the fundamentals of risk-informed planning and decision making to help planners examine a hazard or threat and produce integrated, coordinated, and synchronized plans." https://www.fema.gov/sites/default/files/2020-05/CPG_101_V2_30NOV2010_FINAL_508.pdf

FEMA's Whole Community Approach—A means by which residents, emergency management practitioners, organizational and community leaders, and government officials can collectively understand and assess the needs of their respective communities and determine the best ways to organize and strengthen their assets, capacities, and interests. By doing so, a more effective path to societal security and resilience is built. In a sense, Whole Community is a philosophical approach on how to think about conducting emergency management. Benefits to a community include the following:

- shared understanding of community needs and capabilities
- greater empowerment and integration of resources from across the community

- stronger social infrastructure
- establishment of relationships that facilitate more effective prevention, protection, mitigation, response, and recovery activities
- increased individual and collective preparedness
- greater resiliency at both the community and national levels

Flaviviruses—A large group of heterogeneous viruses known for their ability to infect humans through various arthropod vectors. Arthropod vectors include mosquitoes, flies, biting midges, ticks, mites, fleas, bugs, lice, and other arthropods that carry and transmit disease-causing organisms, or pathogens, from one host to another.

Foundational Competencies—The 22 2021 MPH Foundational Competencies developed by the Council on Education for Public Health (CEPH), and used in the CEPH accreditation process for schools of public health and public health programs, serve as the basis for the competencies to provide the Essential Public Health Services in public health emergency settings in this book. These competencies are informed by the traditional public health core knowledge areas (biostatistics, epidemiology, social and behavioral sciences, health services administration and environmental health sciences), as well as cross-cutting and emerging public health areas.

Free Radicals—A free radical can be defined as any molecular species capable of independent existence that contains an unpaired electron in an atomic orbital. Many radicals are unstable and highly reactive. Free radicals attack important macromolecules leading to cell damage and homeostatic disruption.

Gig Worker—Independent contract workers who perform temporary, on-demand work, usually in the service sector.

Global Warming—The gradual increase in the overall temperature of the earth's atmosphere generally attributed to the greenhouse effect caused by increased levels of carbon dioxide, chlorofluorocarbons, and other pollutants.

Greenhouse Gas—Any gas that has the property of absorbing infrared radiation (net heat energy) emitted from Earth's surface and reradiating it back to the earth's surface, thus contributing to the greenhouse effect.

Guillain-Barré Syndrome—A rare neurological disorder in which the body's immune system mistakenly attacks part of its peripheral nervous system—the network of nerves located outside of the brain and spinal cord. The condition may be triggered by an acute bacterial or viral infection.

Hazard—"Something that is potentially dangerous or harmful, often the root cause of an unwanted outcome." https://training.fema.gov/programs/emischool/el361toolkit/glossary.htm

Hazard Risk Assessment Instrument (HRAI)—"[A] guide to enable state and local public health agencies to conduct a risk assessment of their community. The tool is designed for use as a standard approach to hazard risk assessment that is adapted to the public health impacts of hazards." https://fachc.memberclicks.net/assets/docs/Emergency-Management-Knowledgebase/hra_instrument_wbkucla.pdf

Hazard Vulnerability Assessment (HVA) Tool—"[P]rovides a systematic approach to analyzing hazards that may affect demand for hospital services, or a facility's ability to provide those services, helping to prioritize planning, mitigation, response, and recovery activities." https://asprtracie.hhs.gov/technical-resources/resource/250/kaiser-permanente-hazard-vulnerability-analysis-hva-tool

Health Equity—An aspirational goal to ensure that everyone in a society has an opportunity to pursue and achieve optimal health. Health equity is operationalized by combating social, economic, and societal structures that contribute to health disparities in some population segments.

Health Hazard Assessment and Prioritization Tool (hHAP)—An "instrument to provide a practical and innovative approach to hazard vulnerability assessment through use of a 6-step process to identify, assess and analyze the potential risk of 62 unique potential hazards facing a community." http://publichealth.lacounty.gov/eprp/hazardassessment.htm

Health Officer Orders—Legally appointed health officers at state and local levels have varying degrees of authority and power to issue orders (e.g., including quarantine and isolation) depending on the laws and ordinances of the jurisdiction. In California, "the sheriff of each county, or city and county, may enforce within the county, or the city and county, all orders of the local health officer issued for the purpose of preventing the spread of any contagious, infectious, or communicable disease." https://leginfo.legislature.ca.gov/faces/codes_displayText.xhtml?lawCode=HSC&division=101.&title=&part=3.&chapter=2.&article=1

Homeland Security Act of 2002—Created the Department of Homeland Security. https://www.dhs.gov/homeland-security-act-2002

Horizontal Alignment—"[E]nsures that individual facilities can interface successfully with the public health agency during emergencies for tasks such as information exchange, requests for assistance, sharing of equipment and personnel, and implementation of emergency orders and regulations." (See Chapter 5.)

Hospital Infection Prevention and Control (IPC)—An IPC "program, implemented within a healthcare facility, is critical not only to prevent healthcare-associated infections (HAIs) but also to prepare for and respond to communicable diseases crises." https://www.who.int/csr/resources/publications/AM_CoreCom_IPC.pdf

Immunocompromised—Having an impaired or weakened immune system, for example, persons with HIV/AIDS or cancer.

Incident Command System (ICS)—"A standardized on-scene emergency management construct specifically designed to provide an integrated organizational structure that reflects the complexity and demands of single or multiple incidents, without being hindered by jurisdictional boundaries. The Incident Command System is the combination of facilities, equipment, personnel, procedures, and communications operating within a common organizational structure, designed to aid in the management of resources during incidents." https://training.fema.gov/programs/emischool/el361toolkit/glossary.htm

Injury and Illness Prevention Program (IIPP)—A California law states that "every employer shall establish, implement and maintain an effective

Injury and Illness Prevention Program . . . in writing and, shall, at a minimum: (1) Identify the person or persons with authority and responsibility for implementing the Program; (2) Include a system for ensuring that employees comply with safe and healthy work practices. . . .; and (3) Include a system for communicating with employees in a form readily understandable by all affected employees on matters relating to occupational safety and health." https://www.dir.ca.gov/title8/3203.html

Interagency Modeling and Atmospheric Assessment Center (IMAAC)—"[C]oordinates and disseminates federal atmospheric dispersion modeling and hazard prediction products. . . . Through plume modeling analysis, the IMAAC provides emergency responders with predictions of hazards associated with atmospheric releases to aid in the decision making process to protect the public and the environment." https://www.fema.gov/emergency-managers/practitioners/hazardous-response-capabilities/imaac

In Vitro–In Vivo—*In vivo* refers to when research or work is done with or within an entire, living organism. *In vitro* is used to describe work that's performed outside of a living organism.

Isolation—"[S]eparates sick people with a contagious disease from people who are not sick." https://www.cdc.gov/quarantine/index.html

Ixodes scapularis—The scientific name for a deer tick. The deer tick is a vector for human pathogens, including Lyme disease.

Joint Information Center (JIC)—"A facility established to coordinate critical emergency information, crisis communications, and public affairs functions. The Joint Information Center is the central point of contact for all news media. The Public Information Officer may activate the JIC to better manage external communication." https://training.fema.gov/programs/emischool/el361toolkit/glossary.htm

Kawasaki Disease—An illness that causes inflammation (swelling and redness) in blood vessels throughout the body; more common in infants and children.

Listeria—Bacteria found in soil, water, and some animals, including cattle and poultry, that cause food poisoning.

Low-Pressure Center—An area that has lower atmospheric pressure than its surrounding area. Atmospheric pressure is measured with a barometer.

Machine Learning—The use and development of computer systems that are able to learn and adapt without following explicit instructions, by using algorithms and statistical models to analyze and draw inferences from patterns in data.

Medical Countermeasures—FDA-regulated drugs, devices, biologics, or other medical supplies used in response to mass medical emergencies. **Biologic products** are vaccines, blood products, and antibodies. **Drugs** are antimicrobials or antivirals, for example. **Devices** include diagnostic tests to identify threat agents, and personal protective equipment (PPE), such as gloves, respirators (certain face masks), and ventilators.

Medical Reserve Corps—"A national network of local groups of volunteers engaging local communities to strengthen public health, reduce vulnerability, build resilience, and improve preparedness, response and recovery capabilities." https://mrc.hhs.gov/pageviewfldr/About

Medically Sensitive Populations—Persons with chronic medical conditions, such as diabetes, hypertension, heart disease, cancer, or other conditions that may include adverse reactions to medicines or chemical exposures; this category would also include pregnant women and those with disabilities, requiring special considerations for provision of medical care during emergencies.

Memorandum of Understanding—An agreement between two or more parties, clearly outlining responsibilities and expectations for each party in a written document.

MERS—Middle East Respiratory Syndrome (MERS) is a viral respiratory illness that is relatively new to humans. It was first reported in Saudi Arabia in 2012 and has since spread to at least 27 other countries, including the United States, leading to 858 known deaths. Most people infected with MERS-CoV developed severe respiratory illness, including fever, cough, and shortness of breath. The dromedary camel is suspected as a transmitter of the virus.

Methyl Isocyanate—A colorless, highly flammable toxic liquid that evaporates quickly when exposed to the air. It has a sharp, strong odor. Methyl isocyanate is used in the production of pesticides, polyurethane foam, and plastics.

Metropolitan Statistical Area—Areas delineated by the U.S. Office of Management and Budget as having at least one urbanized **area** with a minimum population of 50,000. **Metropolitan statistical area** (MSA) is the formal **definition** of a **region** that consists of a city and surrounding communities linked by social and economic factors. https://www.census.gov/programs-surveys/metro-micro/about/omb-bulletins.html

Microcephaly—A condition in which a baby's head is much smaller than expected, often due to abnormal brain development. Causes of microcephaly include infections, malnutrition, or exposure to toxins.

Symptoms vary and include intellectual disability and speech delay. In severe cases, there may be seizures and abnormal muscle functionality.

Micro-Orifice Uniform Deposit Impactor (MOUDI)—Used for precision, high-accuracy aerosol sampling, and collecting size fractionated particle samples for gravimetric and/or chemical analysis.

Millibar—The standard unit of measure for atmospheric pressure.

Misinformation—False information that is spread, with or without the intent to mislead. Misinformation may take the form of misinterpreting statistics or not understanding information clearly and restating it to change the original intent. Disinformation is defined as false information spread, with deliberate intent to mislead.

Mitigation—Reducing the risks or potential harms of an adverse event. In public health emergency preparedness, it refers to efforts for reducing the loss of life and property and prevention of physical harm to living beings by lessening the impact of a disaster.

Mitigation and Preparedness—Aim to put structure, process, policy, and laws in place to facilitate response to an adverse event and create agency and community resilience.

Model State Emergency Health Powers Act (MSEHPA) of 2001—The Center for Law and the Public's Health (CLPH) at Georgetown and Johns Hopkins

Universities drafted the Model State Emergency Health Powers Act ("MSEHPA" or the "Model Act") at the request of the "Centers for Disease Control and Prevention (CDC) and in collaboration with members of national organizations representing governors, legislators, attorneys general, and health commissioners. . . . It provides responsible state actors with the powers they need to detect and contain a potentially catastrophic disease outbreak and, at the same time, protects individual rights and freedoms." https://scholarlycommons.law.case.edu/cgi/viewcontent.cgi?article=1387&context=healthmatrix

Moratoria—Plural of *moratorium* and refers to temporary prohibition of an activity or activities.

Moulage—In the context of training for emergencies, *moulage* means applying makeup, bandages, or other special effects to a person acting as an injury victim for the purpose of the training exercise.

Multidrug-Resistant Organism (MDRO)—"[M]icroorganisms, mainly bacteria, that are resistant to one or more classes of antimicrobial agents. . . . MDROs' resistances limit treatment options for patients, making infection critical to preventing further harms." https://www.ncbi.nlm.nih.gov/books/NBK555533

Multisystem Inflammatory Syndrome—Multisystem inflammatory syndrome in children (MIS-C) is a condition in which different body parts can become inflamed, including the heart, lungs, kidneys, brain, skin, eyes, or gastrointestinal organs.

Mustard Gas—A chemical warfare agent that can cause blisters on exposed skin and in the lungs.

Mycoplasma Pneumonia—*Mycoplasma pneumoniae* bacteria commonly cause mild infections of the respiratory system (the parts of the body involved in breathing). The most common illness caused by these bacteria, especially in children, is tracheobronchitis (chest cold). Lung infections caused by *M. pneumoniae* are sometimes referred to as "walking pneumonia" since symptoms are generally mild. Sometimes *M. pneumoniae* can cause more serious lung infections that require care in a hospital.

Myocardial Infarction—The scientific name for a heart attack. A heart attack usually occurs when a blood clot blocks blood flow to the heart.

Nasogastric Tube—A nasogastric (NG) tube is a flexible tube of rubber or plastic that is passed through the nose, down through the esophagus, and into the stomach. It can be used to either remove substances from or add them to the stomach.

National Disaster Medical System (NDMS)—"At a state's request, NDMS provides personnel, equipment, supplies, and a system of partner hospitals to work together with state and local personnel to provide care when Americans need it most." https://www.phe.gov/Preparedness/responders/ndms/Pages/default.aspx

National Emergencies Act (NEA)—"[A]uthorizes the president to declare a national emergency, which declaration activates emergency powers contained in other federal statutes." https://www.astho.org/Programs/Preparedness/Public-Health-Emergency-Law/Emergency-Authority-and-Immunity-Toolkit/National-Emergencies-Act,-Sections-201-and-301-Fact-Sheet

National Health Security Preparedness Index (NHSPI)—"[A]ims to provide an accurate portrayal of the nation's health security using relevant, actionable information to help guide efforts to achieve a higher level of health security and preparedness." https://nhspi.org/about

National Incident Management System (NIMS)—"A set of principles that provides a systematic, proactive approach guiding government agencies at all levels, nongovernmental organizations, and the private sector to work seamlessly to prevent, protect against, respond to, recover from, and mitigate the effects of incidents, regardless of cause, size, location, or complexity, in order to reduce the loss of life or property and harm to the environment." https://training.fema.gov/programs/emischool/el361toolkit/glossary.htm

National Multi-Agency Coordinating Group—A national, regional, or local management group for interagency planning, coordination, and operations leadership for incidents. Provides an essential management mechanism for strategic coordination to ensure incident resources are efficiently and appropriately managed in a cost-effective manner.

National Preparedness Goal—"A secure and resilient Nation with the capabilities required across the whole community to prevent, protect against, mitigate, respond to, and recover from the threats and hazards that pose the greatest risk." https://www.fema.gov/sites/default/files/2020-06/national_preparedness_goal_2nd_edition.pdf

National Preparedness System—"[A]n organized process for everyone in the whole community to move forward with their preparedness activities and achieve the National Preparedness Goal. . . . It has six parts: identifying and assessing risk, estimating capability requirements, building and strengthening capabilities, planning to deliver capabilities, validating capabilities, and reviewing and updating." https://www.fema.gov/emergency-managers/national-preparedness/system

National Response Framework (formerly the National Response Plan)—Developed by the Federal Emergency Management Agency (FEMA), it is a guide to how the nation responds to various types of disasters. It specifies 15 Emergency Support Functions covering a broad range of societal components and is designed to help jurisdictions develop whole community plans, integrate continuity plans, build capabilities to respond to cascading failures among businesses, supply chains, and infrastructure sectors, and collaborate to stabilize community lifelines and restore services. https://www.fema.gov/emergency-managers/national-preparedness/frameworks/response#esf

Nongovernmental Organizations (NGOs)—Organizations that are independent of government involvement. Many community-based organizations are NGOs.

Nonpharmaceutical control measures—Strategies to prevent or control the spread of diseases that do not require medicines. In the case of a pandemic, wearing masks is a nonpharmaceutical control measure.

Novel Coronavirus—Coronaviruses are a family of viruses named for the crown-like spikes on their surface. The word "corona" itself means "crown." Although most coronaviruses are found in animals, the first human coronaviruses were identified in the mid-1960s, and seven, including SARS-CoV-2, are known to affect humans today. When animal coronaviruses evolve and are able to infect humans, these viruses are considered to be novel.

Office of Emergency Services (OES)—"[C]oordination of overall state agency response to disasters. Assuring the state's readiness to respond to, recover from all hazards and assisting local governments in their emergency preparedness, response, recovery and mitigation." Such offices may also exist at local levels of government. https://www.caloes.ca.gov/cal-oes-divisions

Oocyst—A cyst containing a parasitic protozoan zygote.

Oxidized Low-Density Lipoprotein (OxLDL)—A potentially harmful type of cholesterol that is produced in the body when normal LDL cholesterol is damaged by chemical interactions with free radicals. Together with inflammatory responses, free radicals can result in hardening of the arteries.

Pandemic and All-Hazards Preparedness Act (PAHPA) of 2006—Its purpose is "to improve the Nation's public health and medical preparedness and response capabilities for emergencies, whether deliberate, accidental, or natural." "[T]he Act amended the Public Health Service Act to establish within the Department a new Assistant Secretary for Preparedness and Response (ASPR); provided new authorities for a number of programs, including the advanced development and acquisitions of medical countermeasures; and called for the establishment of a quadrennial National Health Security Strategy." https://www.phe.gov/Preparedness/legal/pahpa/Pages/default.aspx

***Parens patriae* power**—"A doctrine that grants the inherent power and authority of the state to protect persons who are legally unable to act on their own behalf." https://law.jrank.org/pages/9014/Parens-Patriae.html

Paris Climate Agreement—A 2015 international agreement among 195 countries to reduce emissions of gasses that contribute to global warming.

Pathogen—A virus, bacterium, or other microorganism that causes diseases.

Patient Unified Lookup System for Emergencies (PULSE)—"[A]n effort to create national resilience through access to health information during disasters, including public health emergencies. PULSE provides a process for states and localities to grant response personnel (e.g., epidemiologists, emergency medical services, and health care volunteers) secure access to vital health information during disasters, ensuring patients can continue to receive care when and where they need it." https://www.healthit.gov/topic/health-it-health-care-settings/public-health/patient-unified-lookup-system-for-emergencies-pulse

Pennsylvania Public Health Risk Assessment Tool (PHRAT)—"[D]eveloped to help public health planners prioritize their planning efforts for emergencies that impact the health of the public. In order to inform these decisions, the PHRAT guides planners through an analysis of the health-related impacts of various hazards that can occur in their jurisdictions. It assesses the planning that is necessary to ensure access to emergency response and preparedness resources, taking into account the services provided by public health agencies and the healthcare system." https://www.health.pa.gov/topics/Documents/Health%20Planning/PHRAT%20Guide.pdf

Permafrost—A thick subsurface layer of soil that remains frozen throughout the year, occurring chiefly in polar regions.

Personal Protective Equipment (PPE)—"[E]quipment worn to minimize exposure to hazards that cause serious workplace injuries and illnesses. These injuries and illnesses may result from contact with chemical, radiological, physical, electrical, mechanical, or other workplace hazards. Personal protective equipment may include items such as gloves, safety glasses and shoes, earplugs or muffs, hard hats, respirators, or coveralls, vests and full body suits." https://www.osha.gov/personal-protective-equipment

Persons Under Investigation (PUI)—"[A] patient who presents with both clinical and epidemiological risk factors for a specific infectious disease." https://www.ncbi.nlm.nih.gov/pmc/articles/PMC7123748

Plasmodium species—Parasites that cause malaria.

Plume Mappers Group—A group of subject matter experts in plume modeling and mapping brought together in Ventura County, California, that is prepared to assist in developing backup plume maps for radioactive fallout in a radiological emergency.

Police Power—In the United States, state police power comes from the Tenth Amendment to the Constitution, which gives states the rights and powers "not delegated to the United States." States are thus granted the power to establish and enforce laws protecting the welfare, safety, and health of the public." https://www.law.cornell.edu/wex/police_powers

Posttraumatic Stress Disorder—A condition of persistent mental and emotional stress occurring as a result of injury or severe psychological shock, typically involving disturbance of sleep and constant vivid recall of the experience, with dulled responses to others and to the outside world.

Prediction Science—The ability to predict a future event based on scientific evidence. In the context of earthquakes, the U.S. Geological Survey "scientists can only calculate the probability that a significant earthquake will occur in a specific area within a certain number of years." https://www.usgs.gov/faqs/can-you-predict-earthquakes?qt-news_science_products=0#qt-news_science_products

Preemption—"[R]efers to laws at one level of government taking precedence over laws of a lower level. As such, no entity at the lower level can pass a law that allows action that would violate the higher-level law." https://www.cdpr.ca.gov/docs/pressrls/dprguide/preemption.pdf

Principal Federal Official (PFO)—A PFO is appointed "for catastrophic or unusually complex incidents that require extraordinary coordination. When appointed, the PFO interfaces with Federal, State, tribal, and local jurisdictional officials regarding the overall Federal incident management strategy and acts as the primary Federal spokesperson for coordinated media and public communications. The PFO serves as a member of the Unified Coordination Group and provides a primary point of contact and situational awareness locally for the Secretary of Homeland Security." https://www.fema.gov/pdf/emergency/nrf/nrf-core.pdf

Prognosis—A medical term meaning the likely course or forecast of a disease or condition, which would include whether the symptoms will improve.

Prophylactic Potassium Iodide (KI)—"KI (potassium iodide) is a salt of stable (not radioactive) iodine that can help block radioactive iodine from being absorbed by the thyroid gland, thus protecting this gland from radiation injury. The thyroid gland is the part of the body that is most sensitive to radioactive iodine." https://www.cdc.gov/nceh/radiation/emergencies/ki.htm

Prophylaxis—An action taken to prevent disease.

Protozoan—A single-cell, microscopic animal that may be parasitic.

Public Health Accreditation Board (PHAB)—"PHAB's national accreditation program fosters health departments' commitment to quality improvement, performance management, accountability, transparency, and the capacity to deliver the Ten Essential Public Health Services." https://phaboard.org/?gclid=Cj0KCQjwiqWHBhD2ARIsAPCDzakHjUv6VYc5e8S2_p8DrYiBDpLhwAw7NE_q46Sap-Jf36q-ki3cxVMaAt-REALw_wcB

Public Health Emergency of International Concern (PHEIC)—"[A]n extraordinary event which is determined," as provided in the WHO International Health Regulations, "to constitute a public health risk to other States through the international spread of disease and to potentially require a coordinated international response." https://www.who.int/publications/i/item/9789241580496

Public Health Emergency Preparedness—A set of ever-changing strategies and structures, processes, and plans utilized by the public health and health-care sectors, governments, communities, and individuals, in collaboration, to prevent, protect against, quickly respond to, and recover from a vast and unknowable range of large-scale health emergencies, particularly those whose scale, timing, or unpredictability threatens to overwhelm routine daily life functions.

Public Health Emergency Preparedness (PHEP) Program—A cooperative agreement program of the Centers for Disease Control and Prevention that "is a critical source of funding for state, local, and territorial public health departments. . . . This helps health departments build and strengthen their abilities to effectively respond to a range of public health threats, including infectious diseases, natural disasters, and biological, chemical, nuclear, and radiological events. Preparedness activities funded by the PHEP cooperative agreement specifically targeted the development of emergency-ready public health departments that are flexible and adaptable." https://www.cdc.gov/cpr/readiness/phep.htm

Public Health Law—The field of law "that focuses legal practice, scholarship and advocacy on issues involving the government's legal authorities and duties 'to ensure the conditions for people to be healthy,' and how to balance these authorities and duties with 'individual rights to autonomy, privacy, liberty, property and other legally protected interests.' The scope of public health law is broad. Public health law issues range from narrow questions of legal interpretation to complex matters involving public health policy, social justice and ethics." https://www.apha.org/-/media/Files/PDF/factsheets/What_is_Public_Health_Law_factsheet.ashx#:~:text=Public%20health%20law%20is%20a,%2C%20privacy%2C%20liberty%2C%20property%20and

Public Health Nurses (PHNs)—"[R]epresent the single largest group of public health practitioners working in U.S. state health departments (SHDs) and local health departments (LHDs). . . . PHNs are vital to the delivery of essential public health services for populations, and often possess diverse skills to carry out job tasks related to clinical diagnostics and treatment, epidemiology, statistics, health promotion, disease surveillance, community health assessment, and policy development." https://www.ncbi.nlm.nih.gov/pmc/articles/PMC4716482

Public Health Service Act (PHSA)—"[P]rovides the legal authority for the Department of Health and Human Services (HHS), among other things, to respond to public health emergencies. The act authorizes the HHS secretary to lead federal public health and medical response to public health emergencies, determine that a public health emergency exists, and assist states in their response activities." https://www.astho.org/Programs/Preparedness/Public-Health-Emergency-Law/Emergency-Authority-and-Immunity-Toolkit/Public-Health-Service-Act,-Section-319-Fact-Sheet

Public Readiness and Emergency Preparedness (PREP) Act—"[A]uthorizes the Secretary of the Department of Health and Human Services to issue a PREP Act declaration. The declaration provides immunity from liability (except for willful misconduct) for claims" . . . and "is specifically for the purpose of providing immunity from liability, and is different from, and not dependent on, other emergency declarations." https://www.phe.gov/Preparedness/legal/prepact/Pages/default.aspx

Quarantine—"[S]eparates and restricts the movement of people who were exposed to a contagious disease to see if they become sick." https://www.cdc.gov/quarantine/index.html

Radiological Assistance Program (RAP)—"[T]he Nation's premier first responder organization for assessing radiological incidents. RAP advises federal, state, local, and tribal public safety officials, first responders, and law enforcement personnel on steps to protect public health and safety or the environment during incidents involving radioactive materials." https://www.energy.gov/nnsa/nuclear-emergency-support-team-nest

Reportable Diseases and Conditions List—"[I]s compiled through collaborative efforts among state health departments and the Centers for Disease Control and Prevention (CDC). Reporting of diseases is mandated by state legislation and regulations, therefore diseases that are considered notifiable vary from state to state. Internationally notifiable diseases (i.e., cholera, plague, and yellow fever) are also reportable in compliance with the World Health Organization's International Health Regulations." https://www.cdc.gov/healthywater/statistics/surveillance/notifiable.html

Risk—"[I]s most commonly defined as the result of the interaction of a hazard (e.g., flood, hurricane, earthquake, etc.) and the vulnerability of the system or element exposed, including the probability of the occurrence of the hazard phenomena. . . . Risk is estimated by combining the probability of a hazard occurrence, such as the likelihood of a flood (with a specific magnitude or intensity) and the potential scale of consequences (e.g., injury, damage, and loss) that would arise if the event strikes society or exposed elements. https://link.springer.com/referenceworkentry/10.1007%2F978-1-4020-4399-4_296

Rugged Individualism—Belief that all or most individuals are able-bodied and can succeed in life on their own, without assistance. Also, the practice or advocacy of individualism in social and economic relations emphasizing personal liberty and independence, self-reliance, resourcefulness, self-direction of the individual, and free competition in enterprise.

Salmonella—*Salmonella* infection (salmonellosis) is a common bacterial disease that affects the intestinal tract. *Salmonella* bacteria typically live in animal and human intestines and are shed through feces. Humans become infected most frequently through contaminated water or food.

Sarin Gas—A highly toxic organophosphorus nerve agent that was developed for chemical warfare during World War II and can cause death in minutes after inhaling a lethal dose.

SARS—Severe acute respiratory syndrome (SARS) is a viral respiratory disease caused by a SARS-associated coronavirus. It was first identified at the end of February 2003 during an outbreak that emerged in China and spread to four other countries.

Serological Studies—Test on blood samples to identify diseases or deficiencies.

Social Capital—Benefits, assets, and resources acquired in community social and business networks, shared among people with established and trusted relationships. An example of social capital is the local owner of a business sponsoring Little League Baseball team uniforms for his son's school team. The school team gets to wear the uniforms. The business gets to advertise on the jerseys.

Social Determinants of Health (SDoH)—The conditions in which people are born, grow, live, play, work, worship, and age and influence many health outcomes. Social determinants of health include income, education, housing conditions, access to healthcare, access to food and clean water, and so on.

Social Vulnerabilities—Refer to threats to community resilience due to multiple life stressors to which members of the community are exposed. Social vulnerabilities include poverty, a lack of education and marketable skills, a lack of access to medical care, a lack of access to transportation, language barriers, and many others. Social vulnerabilities may impede preparedness, response, and recovery to medical emergencies.

Society for Healthcare Epidemiology of America (SHEA)—"[A] professional society that improves public health by establishing infection prevention measures and supporting antibiotic stewardship among healthcare providers." Its "mission is to promote the prevention of healthcare-associated infections and antibiotic resistance and to advance the fields of healthcare epidemiology and antibiotic stewardship." https://www.shea-online.org/index.php/about/mission-history

Sodium Hydroxide—The scientific name for lye, a caustic substance that degrades proteins and causes chemical burns if exposed to skin,

Spin Trap—A chemical that holds free radicals in a temporary stable form so they can be measured using electron paramagnetic resonance (EPR). Spin trapping is an analytical technique employed in chemistry and biology for the detection and identification of short-lived free radicals through the use of electron paramagnetic resonance (EPR) spectroscopy.

Stafford Act (Robert T. Stafford Disaster Relief and Emergency Assistance Act)—Signed into law November 23, 1988, and amended the Disaster Relief Act of 1974; it provides the statutory authority for most federal disaster response activities and authorizes the delivery of federal technical, financial, logistical, and other assistance to states and localities during declared major disasters or emergencies.

Stochastic Effects—"Effects that occur by chance, generally occurring without a threshold level of dose, whose probability is proportional to the dose and whose severity is independent of the dose. In the context of radiation protection, the main stochastic effects are cancer and genetic effects." https://www.nrc.gov/reading-rm/basic-ref/glossary/stochastic-effects.html

Strategic National Stockpile—(formerly the National Pharmaceutical Stockpile) The national repository of antibiotics, vaccines, chemical antidotes, antitoxins, and other critical medical supplies for use during mass medical emergencies.

Syndromic Surveillance—Using information collected during routine patient care, for example, clinical signs, symptoms and preliminary diagnoses as proxy measures, syndromic surveillance allows for a real-time (or near-real-time) collection, analysis, interpretation, and dissemination of health-related data to enable the early identification of a disease outbreak or health impact.

Telehealth—The use of electronic information and telecommunications technologies to support long-distance clinical healthcare, patient and professional health-related education, public health and health administration.

The President's National Infrastructure Advisory Council (NIAC)—Includes executive leaders from private industry and state/local government who advise the White House on how to reduce physical and cyber risks and improve the security and resilience of the nation's critical infrastructure sectors. https://www.cisa.gov/niac

Threat—"Natural, technological, or human-caused occurrence, individual, entity, or action that has or indicates the potential to harm life, information, operations, the environment, and/or property." https://training.fema.gov/programs/emischool/el361toolkit/glossary.htm

Threat and Hazard Identification and Risk Assessment (THIRA)—"[A] three-step risk assessment process that helps communities understand their risks and what they need to do to address those risks by answering the following questions: What threats and hazards can affect our community? If they occurred, what impacts would those threats and hazards have on our community? Based on those impacts, what capabilities should our community have?" https://www.fema.gov/emergency-managers/risk-management/risk-capability-assessment

Toxic Shock Syndrome—A sudden, potentially fatal condition caused by the release of toxins from an overgrowth of bacteria called *Staphylococcus aureus*, or staph, found in many women's bodies. Toxic shock syndrome affects menstruating women, especially those who use super-absorbent tampons.

Underrepresented and Marginalized Communities—Community subsets, generally based on gender, race, ethnicity, income, or some other characteristic, within a larger population who are not sufficiently included in leadership or decision-making activities that affect their lives or have restricted access to full participation and benefits in a society.

Vertical Alignment—"[I]ncludes protocols for requesting public health assistance from higher levels of government, as well as protocols for delivering requested assistance to lower levels of government." (See Chapter 5.)

Vulnerability—"The characteristics and circumstances of a community, system or asset that make it susceptible to the damaging effects of a hazard." https://www.unisdr.org/files/7817_UNISDRTerminologyEnglish.pdf

Watershed—An area or ridge of land that separates waters flowing to different rivers, basins, or seas.; an area or region drained by a river, river system, or other body of water

Whole Community Approach to Public Health Emergency Preparedness—Drawing from FEMA's Whole Community Approach Model of General Preparedness, the approach is applied in the public health sphere to activate interest and build coalitions among entire communities, healthcare organizations, governmental agencies, nonprofit organizations, faith-based groups, hospitals, health departments, laboratories, community health workers, doctors, nurses, academia, businesses, and others in working toward preparing for mass medical emergencies to reduce morbidity and mortality associated with any catastrophic event.

Whole Genome Sequencing—A laboratory process that determines the entire or nearly entire sequence of an organism's DNA sequence or pattern.

World Health Organization—An agency within the United Nations responsible for international public health. https://www.who.int/about/what-we-do

YouTube Channels—YouTube is an online video-sharing platform owned by Google to which users can upload and share original video content with millions of others.

THE 10 ESSENTIAL PUBLIC HEALTH SERVICES

Essential Services of Public Health 2020 Update
1. Assess and monitor population health status, factors that influence health, and community needs and assets (Assessment)
2. Investigate, diagnose, and address health problems and hazards affecting the population (Assessment)
3. Communicate effectively to inform and educate people about health, factors that influence it, and how to improve it (Policy Development)
4. Strengthen, support, and mobilize communities and partnerships to improve health (Policy Development)
5. Create, champion, and implement policies, plans, and laws that impact health (Policy Development)
6. Utilize legal and regulatory actions designed to improve and protect the public's health (Policy Development)
7. Assure an effective system that enables equitable access to the individual services and care needed to be healthy (Assurance)
8. Build and support a diverse and skilled public health workforce (Assurance)
9. Improve and innovate public health functions through ongoing evaluation, research, and continuous quality improvement (Assurance)
10. Build and maintain a strong organizational infrastructure for public health (Assurance)

CEPH FOUNDATIONAL COMPETENCIES

Evidence-Based Approaches to Public Health
1. Apply epidemiological methods to settings and situations in public health practice.
2. Select quantitative and qualitative data collection methods appropriate for a given public health context.
3. Analyze quantitative and qualitative data using biostatistics, informatics, computer-based programming, and software, as appropriate.
4. Interpret results of data analysis for public health research, policy, or practice.
Public Health and Healthcare Systems
5. Compare the organization, structure, and function of healthcare, public health, and regulatory systems across national and international settings.
6. Discuss the means by which structural bias, social inequities, and racism undermine health and create challenges to achieving health equity at organizational, community, and systemic levels.
Planning and Management to Promote Health
7. Assess population needs, assets, and capacities that affect communities' health.
8. Apply awareness of cultural values and practices to the design, implementation, or critique of public health policies or programs.
9. Design a population-based policy, program, project, or intervention.
10. Explain basic principles and tools of budget and resource management.
11. Select methods to evaluate public health programs.
Policy in Public Health
12. Discuss the policy-making process, including the roles of ethics and evidence.
13. Propose strategies to identify stakeholders and build coalitions and partnerships for influencing public health outcomes.
14. Advocate for political, social, or economic policies and programs that will improve health in diverse populations.
15. Evaluate policies for their impact on public health and health equity.

Leadership
16. Apply leadership and/or management principles to address a relevant health issue.
17. Apply negotiation and mediation skills to address organizational or community challenges.
Communication
18. Select communication strategies for different audiences and sectors.
19. Communicate audience-appropriate (i.e., non-academic, non-peer audience) public health content, both in writing and through oral presentation.
20. Describe the importance of cultural competence in communicating public health content.
Interprofessional and/or Intersectoral Practice
21. Integrate perspectives from other sectors and/or professions to promote and advance population health.
Systems Thinking
22. Apply a systems thinking tool to visually represent a public health issue in a format other than standard narrative.

INDEX